D0849737

Acquired Immune Hemolytic Anemias

Acquired Immune Hemolytic Anemias

LAWRENCE D. PETZ, M.D.
Chairman, Division of Medicine
City of Hope National Medical Center
Duarte, California

GEORGE GARRATTY, F.I.M.L.S., M.R.C. Path.
Scientific Director
Los Angeles–Orange Counties
Red Cross Blood Services
Los Angeles, California

Churchill Livingstone   1980
New York, Edinburgh, and London

© Churchill Livingstone Inc.   1980

Distributed in the United Kingdom by Churchill Livingstone, Robert Stevenson House, 1–3 Baxter's Place, Leith Walk, Edinburgh EH1 3AF and by associated companies, branches and representatives throughout the world.

First published 1980

Printed in USA

ISBN 0 443 08051 8

7   6   5   4   3   2

Library of Congress Cataloging in Publication Data

Petz, Lawrence D
    Acquired immune hemolytic anemias.

    Bibliography: p.
    Includes index.
    1. Hemolytic anemia, Autoimmune.   I.   Garratty, George, joint author.   II.   Title.
RC641.7.H4P47   616.1'52   79-19235
ISBN 0-443-08051-8

Preface

This book is intended to be a useful source of information for those who care for patients who have immune hemolytic anemias, i.e., clinicians with primary responsibility for patient management, physicians concerned with laboratory medicine, including blood bank directors, and the technical staff of such laboratories. It is not intended as an encyclopedic review nor as a "tour de force" exposition of facts that are of interest primarily to those with extensive background and a highly specialized interest in the field.

Patients with immune hemolytic anemias are sufficiently common as to constitute an important problem but, on the other hand, are sufficiently unusual that it is difficult for many individuals outside of referral centers to acquire adequate experience to feel at ease in managing the multitude of problems such patients may present. We have had a special interest in these disorders and we earnestly hope that sharing our experiences through the medium of this book will be of value to others who confront such problems less commonly. We include previously unpublished data concerning our experiences with various phases of the diagnosis and management of more than 300 patients, as well as a review of relevant information available in the medical literature.

Although the primary purpose of this book is, therefore, to be a source of information that will be of value in management of patients, this purpose cannot be adequately served merely by a superficial exposition of "practical" facts, and we do not intend this book to be a manual of patient care. We trust that the interested reader would demand an adequately detailed scientific background to make meaningful the recommended laboratory procedures and their clinical interpretation. For example, the knowledge that the direct antiglobulin (Coombs') test performed on red cells from patients with cold agglutinin syndrome is invariably positive using anti-C3d antiglobulin serum and invariably negative using anti-IgG antiglobulin serum is of some clinical value (Ch. 6). When such information is augmented by an understanding of pertinent aspects of the serum complement system (Ch. 3) and the mechanisms of immune hemolysis (Ch. 4), one then has a basis for understanding such facts and their clinical significance.

Writing this book presents a unique problem. That is, one of the important aspects of diagnosis and management of patients with immune hemolytic anemias is that the care of such patients depends upon a knowledge of some aspects of both clinical and laboratory medicine. Although this is true throughout medicine, a problem of unusual magnitude is created by the fact that most clinicians have very little exposure to immunohematology. Results of direct antiglobulin tests with monospecific antiglobulin sera and the characterization of serum antibody specificity and thermal range is information that is difficult or impossible for most practicing physicians to utilize. This problem is augmented by the fact that laboratory personnel are faced with difficult technical tasks, and, in the very best of hands, uncertainties may remain. For example, in regard to blood transfusion (Ch. 10), what is the probability of not detecting a red cell alloantibody in the serum of a patient with autoimmune hemolytic anemia when the serum reacts with all donor cells tested, and what is the risk of transfusion of blood that is incompatible because of the presence of an autoantibody? One of the prime purposes of this book, and one of the more difficult tasks we faced in writing it, is to present both the laboratory and clinical aspects of immune hemolytic anemias in a single volume in a manner that is understandable by those in both fields. Neither laboratory personnel (including physicians) nor clinicians can optimally contribute to the care of patients with immune hemolytic anemias without an understanding of both aspects of the subject. Therefore, it is our firm opinion that, with few exceptions (e.g., some sections concerning technical details which may justifiably be ignored by clinicians, and some aspects of therapy which may not be essential knowledge for technologists), the information herein is important to those in both clinical and laboratory medicine for proper management of patients with immune hemolytic anemias.

Lawrence D. Petz
George Garratty

Acknowledgements

We are both indebted to Professor Sir John Dacie for the privilege of working in his laboratory at the Royal Postgraduate Medical School and Hammersmith Hospital in London. His teachings served as a foundation for our work and, moreover, we have attempted to emulate his dedication and precision in scientific investigation.

Grateful acknowledgement is also due to the numerous physicians and technologists who were kind enough to refer interesting and challenging immunohematology problems to our laboratory. Without this continued support, it would have been impossible to acquire the experience and data necessary to compile this volume. In addition to those individuals cited in the text in regard to an individual patient, particular thanks are due to Drs. Neil Culp, Hunter Cutting, Patrick Flannery, Paul Ness, Herbert Perkins, Ernest Rosenbaum, Curt Ries, Ralph Wallerstein, and Lee Wilkinson.

Among the numerous technologists who shared their problems with us were Edith Bossom, Betsy Haffleigh, Mary Meyers, Phyllis Morel, Mildred Sattler, and Eleanor Willbanks.

Drs. Peter Spath, Jörg Fischer, and Lee Wilkinson developed significant data while working in our laboratory. Although their pertinent published studies are cited, their initiative and enthusiasm were additional contributions which permeated other aspects of our work.

Technologists whose proficiency we justifiably relied upon include Eleanor Lloyd, Alice Steers, Priscilla Yam, Nita Hoops, and Mary Webb. Their contribution consisted of more than the mere performance of assigned tasks; their development of new techniques and critical review of data were essential aspects of our laboratory.

We are also indebted to Drs. Neil Cooper, Herbert Perkins, Hugh Chaplin, and Scott N. Swisher for making helpful suggestions after kindly agreeing to review portions of the text.

The art work was done by Jim Brodale and photography by Helen Sullivan and Dr. Thomas Jackson.

The innumerable typings and revisions done within a rather tight schedule were handled at a sometimes frantic pace by our imperturbable secretary, Kathy De Brabant, who, after a period of absence, agreed to return to our laboratory to assist with this text. For reasons which perhaps should be evident to us, she changed occupations after completion of the book.

Finally, since a seemingly endless number of evenings and weekends were spent struggling with data, books, reprints, manuscript drafts, and galley proofs we would particularly like to acknowledge our gratitude to our wives whose patience and understanding were essential to the completion of this book.

Acknowledgement

The authors wish to thank Ortho Diagnostics, Inc., for a generous grant which made it possible for them to devote the time necessary to the writing of this book. The grant was strictly supportive and was in no way used to influence the content or format of the book. The authors commend the valuable contributions Ortho Diagnostics, Inc. has made and continues to make to further education in the fields of Immunohematology and Blood Transfusion.

Contents

Table of Contents of Methods   xvii

1. THE DIAGNOSIS OF HEMOLYTIC ANEMIA   1

Definitions   1
Determination of the Hemolytic Nature of the Anemia   4
    The Blood Count   5
    Bilirubin   7
    Serum Haptoglobin   8
    Serum Lactic Dehydrogenase   8
    Other Tests   9
Establishing a Tentative Diagnosis of the Cause of the Hemolytic
    Anemia   9
    History and Physical Examination   13
    The Peripheral Blood Film   15
    Features of Intravascular Hemolysis   20
    The Direct Antiglobulin Test   22
Specific Confirmatory Tests   23

2. CLASSIFICATION AND CLINICAL CHARACTERISTICS OF AUTOIMMUNE HEMOLYTIC ANEMIAS   26

Classification   26
Clinical Characteristics of Autoimmune Hemolytic Anemias   28
    Warm Antibody AIHA   29
    Cold Agglutinin Syndrome   37
    Paroxysmal Cold Hemoglobinuria   50

3. COMPLEMENT: A REVIEW FOR THE IMMUNO-HEMATOLOGIST   64

The Classical Pathway of Complement Activation   65
    Physicochemical Properties of Proteins Participating in the
    Classical Pathway   65
    Reaction Mechanisms of the Classical Pathway   67
The Alternative Pathway of Complement Activation   73
    Proteins Participating in the Alternative Pathway of Comple-
    ment Activation   74
    Reaction Mechanisms of the Alternative Complement Pathway   75

Biological Activities of Complement   79
Complement in Human Disease   83
  Inborn Abnormalities   83
  Acquired Abnormalities   84
Measurement of Complement Activity   84
The Role of Complement in Immunohematology   87
  Complement Activated by Antibodies   87
  Complement Activation by Immune Complexes   89
  Non-Immune Sensitization of Red Cells with Complement   89
  The Role of Complement in the Antiglobulin Test   91
Complement Receptors and Cell Associated Complement Com-
  ponents   99
The Stability of Complement in Stored Human Serum   101
The Effect of Heparin on Complement   102

4. MECHANISMS OF IMMUNE HEMOLYSIS   **110**

Intravascular Immune Red Cell Destruction   110
Extravascular Immune Red Cell Destruction   111
  Macrophage Receptors   112
  Effect of Type of Protein Causing Red Cell Sensitization 116
  Variation in Macrophage Activity   128
Other Possible Mechanisms of Immune Red Cell Destruction   130
  Possible Role of Lymphocytes in Immune Red Cell Destruction 130
  Macrophage/Monocyte Cytotoxicity   131
  In Vivo Agglutination of Red Cells   132

**5. THE SEROLOGIC INVESTIGATION OF AUTOIMMUNE
HEMOLYTIC ANEMIA**   **139**

The Structure and Function of Immunoglobulins   139
Role of Albumin and Enzymes in Antibody Detection   144
The Antiglobulin Test   148
  Principles of the Antiglobulin Test   148
  Monospecific Antiglobulin Reagents   150
  The Significance of Positive Direct Antiglobulin Tests 151
Causes of Positive Direct Antiglobulin Tests   151
Causes of False Negative Directs Antiglobulin Tests   152
Methods for Standardization and Evaluation of Antiglobulin
  Sera   153
  Anti-IgG Activity   153
  Anti-IgA and Anti-IgM Activity   155
  Anti-Complement Activity   156
  Daily Quality Control of Antiglobulin Serum   158

General Serologic Investigations in Autoimmune Hemolytic
  Anemia   158
Collection of Blood   159
ABO and Rh Grouping   159
Typing Red Cells for Antigens When Only Antiglobulin Reac-
  tive Antisera Are Available   160
The Direct Antiglobulin Test   162
Method   162
Determination of Type and Amount of Protein on Patient's
  Red Cells   163
Characterization of Antibodies in Serum and Eluate in Au-
  toimmune Hemolytic Anemia   164
Serum Screen to Determine Serum Antibody Characteristics   165
Cold Agglutinin Titer/Thermal Range/Ii Specificity   168
Titration of Hemolysins   169
Determining Specificity of Autoantibodies   170
Warm Type Autoimmune Hemolytic Anemia   172
Cold Agglutinin Syndrome   174
Paroxysmal Cold Hemoglobinuria   175
The Use of the Autoanalyzer for Studying Autoimmune
  Hemolytic Anemia   178

**6. DIFFERENTIAL DIAGNOSIS OF IMMUNE HEMOLYTIC
ANEMIAS**   **185**

Distinctive Clinical and Routine Laboratory Features   185
Laboratory Diagnosis of Immune Hemolytic Anemias   188
The Significance of the Direct Antiglobulin Test in the Differ-
  ential Diagnosis of Immune Hemolytic Anemias   188
Results Using Polyspecific and Monospecific Antiglobulin
  Reagents   189
Antiglobulin Test Titrations and Scores   194
An Approach to the Characterization of Antibodies in Serum
  and Red Cell Eluate in Immune Hemolytic Anemias   206
Characterization of Antibodies in Serum and Red Cell Eluate
  in Warm Antibody AIHA   208
Essential Diagnostic Tests   208
Additional Important Aspects of Serologic Tests   211
Characterization of Antibodies in the Cold Agglutinin Syn-
  drome   213
Development of Criteria to Distinguish Benign Cold Ag-
  glutinins from Those Associated with In Vivo Hemolysis   214
Additional Comments Regarding Serologic Tests   222
Laboratory Diagnosis of Paroxysmal Cold Hemoglobinuria   223
Essential Diagnostic Tests   223

Comparison of Paroxysmal Cold Hemoglobinuria and the
Cold Agglutinin Syndrome   227

7. SPECIFICITY OF AUTOANTIBODIES   232

Specificity of Autoantibodies Associated With Warm-Antibody
Type Autoimmune Hemolytic Anemia   232
Early Observations   232
Observations During the Last Decade   234
Autoantibody Specificity Not Associated with Rh   237
Autoantibodies Mimicking Alloantibodies   246
Changes in Specificity of Autoantibodies   250
Specificity of Autoantibodies Associated With Cold Agglutinin
Syndrome   250
Ii Blood Group "System"   250
Chemistry of Ii Antigens   254
Other Autoantibody Specificities Associated With Cold Ag-
glutinin Syndrome   256
Chemistry of Pr Blood Groups   258
Isolated Examples of Antibodies Other Than Anti-I, -i, or -Pr
Associated With Cold Agglutinin Syndrome   259
Autoantibody Specificity Associated With Paroxysmal Cold
Hemoglobinuria   260

8. DRUG-INDUCED IMMUNE HEMOLYTIC ANEMIA   267

Immunologic Mechanisms   267
General Concepts Regarding Drug-Induced Immune
Cytopenias   267
Mechanisms of Drug-Induced Positive Direct Antiglobulin Tests
and Immune Hemolysis   272
Immune Complex Mechanism   272
Drug Absorption Mechanism   273
Nonimmunologic Protein Absorption   283
Autoimmune Hemolytic Anemia Caused by Drugs   285
Methods of Diagnosis   289
History   289
Laboratory Tests   290
Methyldopa, L-Dopa, and Mefenamic Acid   290
Penicillins   291
Cephalosporins   293
Other Drugs   293
Compatibility Testing in Patients With Drug-Induced Immuno-
hematologic Abnormalities   294
Management and Prognosis   295

9. UNUSUAL PROBLEMS REGARDING AUTOIMMUNE HEMOLYTIC ANEMIAS — 305

Autoimmune Hemolytic Anemia Associated With a Negative Direct Antiglobulin Test — 305
Autoimmune Hemolytic Anemia During Pregnancy — 321
The Differentiation Between a Delayed Hemolytic Transfusion Reaction and Autoimmune Hemolytic Anemia — 327
The Development of Autoimmune Hemolytic Anemia Following Blood Transfusion — 331
Serum Complement in Autoimmune Hemolytic Anemia — 337
Chronic Idiopathic Paroxysmal Cold Hemoglobinuria — 341
Warm Antibody Autoimmune Hemolytic Anemia Associated with Abnormal Cold Agglutinins — 344
Warm Antibody Autoimmune Hemolytic Anemia in Patients Whose Direct Antiglobulin Test Is Positive Only With Anti-IgA Antiserum — 348
Autoimmune Hemolytic Anemia in Infancy and Childhood — 349

10. BLOOD TRANSFUSION IN AUTOIMMUNE HEMOLYTIC ANEMIAS — 358

General Principles Concerning Indications for Transfusions — 359
Assessing the Need for Transfusion in Patients With Autoimmune Hemolytic Anemia — 362
Assessing the Acuteness of Onset and Rapidity of Progression of Anemia in Patients with AIHA — 362
The Risks of Transfusion in Patients With Autoimmune Hemolytic Anemia — 364
The Selection of Donor Blood for Transfusion in Specific Kinds of Autoimmune Hemolytic Anemia — 365
Warm Antibody Autoimmune Hemolytic Anemia — 365
ABO and Rh Cell Typing — 365
Detection of Alloantibodies — 366
Significance of Autoantibody Specificity — 372
Cold Agglutinin Syndrome — 376
Paroxysmal Cold Hemoglobinuria — 382
In Vivo Compatibility Testing — 382
Optimal Volume of Blood to Be Transfused — 384
The Use of Warm Blood for Patients With Cold Agglutinin Syndrome and Paroxysmal Cold Hemoglobinuria — 387
Use of Washed Red Blood Cells — 388

11. MANAGEMENT OF AUTOIMMUNE HEMOLYTIC ANEMIAS 392

Warm Antibody Autoimmune Hemolytic Anemia 392
  Corticosteroid Therapy 392
    Initial Management 392
    Remission Maintenance 393
    Mechanisms of Corticosteroid Response 394
  Splenectomy 397
    Clinical Response 397
    Mechanisms of Response to Splenectomy 398
    The Value of Radiolabelled Red Cell Studies in the Selection
      of Patients for Splenectomy 399
    Adverse Effects of Splenectomy 400
  Immunosuppressive Drugs 403
    Effectiveness 403
    Indications and Therapeutic Regimens 404
    Adverse Effects 405
  Other Therapies 408
    Heparin Therapy 408
    Thymectomy 414
    Antilymphocyte Globulin 416
    Splenic Irradiation 416
    Vinblastine-Laden Platelets 416
    Plasma Exchange 418
Cold Agglutinin Syndrome 420
  Avoidance of Cold 420
  Corticosteroid Therapy 420
  Immunosuppressive Drugs 422
  Plasma Exchange 424
  Penicillamine 425
  Splenectomy 426
Paroxysmal Cold Hemoglobinuria 427
Secondary Autoimmune Hemolytic Anemias 429
  Mycoplasma Pneumoniae Infections and Infectious Mono-
    nucleosis 429
  Ovarian Tumors 430
  Ulcerative Colitis 430
  Systemic Lupus Erythematosus 431
  Lymphoreticular Malignant Disease 431
  A Summary of Therapeutic Principles in the Management of
    Patients with Autoimmune Hemolytic Anemia 431

INDEX 441

Table of Contents of Methods

NOTE: Although this book is not intended primarily as a laboratory manual, pertinent methods are described in detail.

In keeping with our philosophy of integrating clinical and laboratory aspects of medicine, we have included the description of these methods in the most relevant chapters rather than developing a separate "technical appendix." In order to assist the reader in location of these methods, we offer this table of contents of methods.

CHAPTER 5: THE SEROLOGIC INVESTIGATION OF AUTOIMMUNE HEMOLYTIC ANEMIA

Standardization and Evaluation of Antiglobulin Sera
Anti-IgG Activity 153
Anti-IgA and Anti-IgM Activity 155
Anti-Complement Activity 156
Daily Quality Control of Antiglobulin Serum 158
General Serologic Investigations in Autoimmune Hemolytic Anemia
Collection of Blood 159
ABO and Rh Grouping 159
Typing Red Cells for Antigens When Only Antiglobulin Reactive Antisera Are Available 160
The Direct Antiglobulin Test 162
Semiquantitative Direct Antiglobulin Test (Antiglobulin Test Titration Scores) 163
Screening Tests for Determining Serum Antibody Characteristics 165
Cold Agglutinin Titers, Thermal Range and Ii Specificity 168
Titration of Hemolysins 169
Preparation of Red Cell Eluates 170
Determining the Specificity of Autoantibodies
Warm Type Autoimmune Hemolytic Anemia 172
Cold Agglutinin Syndrome 174
Paroxysmal Cold Hemoglobulinuria 175
Donath-Landsteiner Test 175

CHAPTER 8: DRUG-INDUCED IMMUNE HEMOLYTIC ANEMIA

Autoimmune Hemolytic Anemias Caused by Drugs 290
Penicillin-Induced Immune Hemolytic Anemia 291
Cephalosporin-Induced Immune Hemolytic Anemia 293
Other Drugs 293

CHAPTER 10: BLOOD TRANSFUSION IN AUTOIMMUNE HEMOLYTIC ANEMIAS

Selection of Donor Blood for Transfusion in Autoimmune Hemolytic Anemia
Warm Antibody Autoimmune Hemolytic Anemia ... 365
  ABO and Rh Cell Typing ... 365
  Detection of Alloantibodies ... 366
    Comparison of Direct and Indirect Antiglobulin Tests ... 366
    Testing of Patient's Serum Against a Red Cell Panel ... 366
    Warm Autoabsorption Technique ... 366
    Dilution Technique ... 370
    Differential Absorption Technique ... 371
  Significance of Autoantibody Specificity ... 372
Cold Agglutinin Syndrome ... 376
  Performing Compatibility Test at 37°C in Saline ... 376
  Cold Autoabsorption Method ... 377
  Other Methods ... 379
Paroxysmal Cold Hemoglobulinuria ... 382

Acquired Immune Hemolytic Anemias

1

The Diagnosis of Hemolytic Anemia

This chapter offers an approach to the diagnosis of hemolytic anemia that enables the physician to make an accurate diagnosis without superfluous steps. In addition to findings elicited in the history and physical examination, there are a large number of laboratory tests available that are relevant to the diagnosis of hemolytic anemia. These tests include the examination of the blood and bone marrow, serum haptoglobin, serum bilirubin, urinary urobilinogen, fecal stercobilinogen, plasma hemoglobin, urinary hemoglobin and hemosiderin, methemalbumin, measurement of survival of radiolabelled red cells, measurement of endogenous production of carbon monoxide, autohemolysis for 48 hours with and without added glucose, osmotic fragility before and after incubation for 24 hours at 37°C, direct and indirect antiglobulin (Coombs') tests, cold agglutinin titer, determination of the thermal amplitude and specificity of antibodies in the patient's serum and eluate, Ham's acid-serum test, the sucrose hemolytic test, Donath-Landsteiner test, hemoglobin electrophoresis, measurement of red cell enzymes, studies of membrane lipids, genetic studies, etc. The availability of such a bewildering array of laboratory tests makes their optimal utilization a difficult task for the physician who encounters such a patient only occasionally.

To put some order into what is often a rather disorganized approach, it is useful to think in terms of three separate steps: (1) determine whether or not the patient's anemia is due to hemolysis; (2) utilize a limited number of clinical and laboratory findings to develop a tentative diagnosis concerning the cause of the hemolysis; and (3) perform confirmatory tests to establish the specific etiology.

However, before proceeding to a consideration of each of these three aspects of diagnosis, a review of some definitions is appropriate.

DEFINITIONS

Hemolysis. Hemolysis is defined as a reduction of the average red cell life span to less than the normal range of 100 to 120 days.

1

Compensated Hemolytic Disease. A shortened red cell life span does not necessarily result in anemia since compensatory increase in erythropoiesis by the bone marrow may be adequate to prevent the development of anemia.

Anemia with a Hemolytic Component. Studies of red cell survival have shown that red cell life span is often shortened in a number of chronic anemias. They include the anemias associated with disseminated malignant disease, leukemias, lymphomas, renal insufficiency, liver disease, rheumatoid arthritis, and the megaloblastic anemias. Thus the mechanism of the anemia in many patients includes a mild decrease in red cell survival, but is primarily due to inadequate marrow production (relative marrow failure). It is customary not to classify such patients as having hemolytic anemia.

Hemolytic Anemia. The diagnosis of hemolytic anemia is justified if a major mechanism in causation of a patient's anemia is a shortened red cell life span.

Acquired Hemolytic Anemias. All hemolytic anemias except those caused by a hereditary defect are referred to as acquired. Acquired hemolytic anemias do not necessarily have an immune pathogenesis, and it is inappropriate to use this term as a synonym for autoimmune hemolytic anemia.

Hereditary Hemolytic Anemias. These hemolytic anemias are caused by a hereditary abnormality, usually affecting the red cell intracellular contents or membrane structure.

Congenital Hemolytic Anemias. Although the words congenital and hereditary are often used synonymously, congenital is defined as existing at birth regardless of the causation. Hemolytic disease of the newborn is thus a congenital but not hereditary hemolytic anemia.

Intravascular Hemolysis. In some diseases, such as mechanical hemolytic anemia, paroxysmal nocturnal hemoglobinuria, and paroxysmal cold hemoglobinuria, the destruction of red cells appears to take place primarily in the intravascular space with a release of free hemoglobin into the blood. Signs of intravascular hemolysis include increased plasma hemoglobin, hemoglobinuria, and hemosiderinuria; even with only minimal hemolysis the serum haptoglobin will be low or absent (Fig. 1-1).[3, 9]

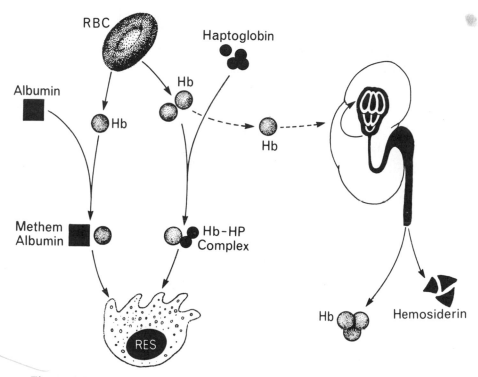

Figure 1-1. *The destruction of red cells intravascularly results in the liberation of hemoglobin from the red cell. The hemoglobin combines with haptoglobin, and the haptoglobin-hemoglobin complexes are rapidly catabolized in the reticuloendothelial system (RES), resulting in low levels of serum haptoglobin. Also, when hemoglobin is liberated into the plasma in large quantities, some of the heme combines with plasma albumin, resulting in the formation of methemalbumin. When haptoglobin has been saturated and the level of plasma hemoglobin exceeds the renal threshold, hemoglobin appears in the urine. Hemoglobinuria persisting for at least several days results in the deposition in the renal tubules of hemosiderin derived from the breakdown of hemoglobin. This hemosiderin may be excreted in the urine, probably as a result of the desquamation of renal tubular cells.* (Hb = hemoglobin; HP = haptoglobin.)

Extravascular Hemolysis. In most hemolytic anemias, erythrocyte destruction takes place predominantly in the cells of the reticuloendothelial system. In such cases hemoglobinemia and hemoglobinuria are not found, but there is an increase in serum bilirubin and in bilirubin degradation products in the urine and stool (Fig. 1-2). However, with brisk hemolysis of any etiology, some manifestations of intravascular hemolysis may be present, especially low serum haptoglobin.

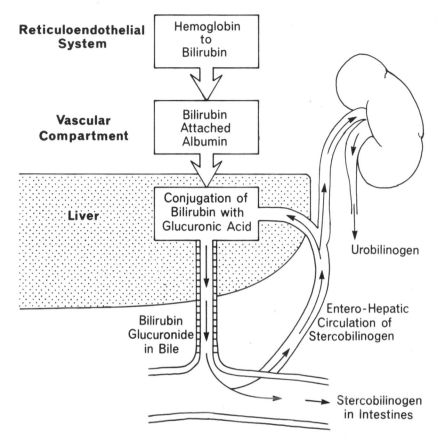

Figure 1-2. *The destruction of red cells extravascularly within the cells of the reticuloendothelial system results in the degradation of hemoglobin and the production of bilirubin. The bilirubin passes into the plasma, forms a loose complex with albumin, and is taken up by the liver, where it is conjugated with glucuronic acid. Conjugated bilirubin gives a positive direct van den Bergh test, whereas unconjugated bilirubin gives a positive indirect reaction. Only conjugated bilirubin is readily excreted into the urine. Conjugated bilirubin largely passes via the hepatic ducts to the intestine, where it is reduced to stercobilinogen and is excreted. Part of the stercobilinogen is absorbed from the bowel and is re-excreted by the liver (enterohepatic circulation). Some absorbed stercobilinogen is excreted by the kidneys as urobilinogen.*

In hemolytic anemia, the increased catabolism of bilirubin characteristically results in increased concentrations of unconjugated bilirubin in the plasma and increased concentrations of bilirubin degradation products in feces and urine.

DETERMINATION OF THE HEMOLYTIC NATURE OF THE ANEMIA

The patient's history and physical examination may suggest the possibility of a hemolytic anemia (symptoms of anemia, acholuric jaundice, splenomegaly), but usually the manifestations are non-specific and the initial work-up involves a laboratory evaluation of anemia. Although the presence of hemolysis can be determined by direct measurement of red cell life span, red cell survival studies are rarely necessary.[37] Instead, indirect indications of hemolysis are sought by tests that yield evidence of increased hemoglobin breakdown and of bone marrow regeneration. These features are common to all hemolytic anemias, regardless of their etiology.

In this era of extraordinarily sophisticated laboratory technology, it seems incongruous that a few easily performed studies usually suffice in the decision of whether the patient's anemia is hemolytic in nature. The most helpful of the readily available laboratory tests are: (1) a complete blood count (or serial blood counts) with emphasis on the reticulocyte count and on the red cell morphology in the peripheral blood film; (2) serum bilirubin; (3) serum haptoglobin; and (4) serum lactic dehydrogenase.

The Blood Count

Reticulocyte Count. An elevated reticulocyte count is a reflection of the compensatory increase in erythropoiesis by the bone marrow, and it is therefore an indirect indication of shortened erythrocyte life span. In the normal person the reticulocyte count is approximately 0.5 to 1.5 percent. Using the value of 5,000,000 per μl as a normal red blood cell count, a reticulocyte percentage of 0.5 to 1.5 represents 25,000 to 75,000 reticulocytes per μl or a mean value of 50,000 per μl. In hemolytic anemia, the percentage is frequently 10 to 20 percent and may even reach levels of 80 percent or more.

The ratio of the number of reticulocytes per μl to the normal mean number of 50,000 per μl may be used as an estimate of the rate of red cell production, and is one means of calculating the "corrected reticulocyte count." Thus, production is increased threefold in a patient with a reticulocyte count of 5 percent and a red blood cell count of 3,000,000 per μl (3,000,000 x .05 = 150,000; 150,000 ÷ 50,000 = 3). Since red blood cell counts had a high percentage of error prior to the development of automated cell counters, the corrected reticulocyte count has more traditionally been obtained by multiplying the reticulocyte count by the ratio of the patient's hematocrit to the mean normal hematocrit value—corrected reticulocyte count = percent reticulocytes $\times \dfrac{\text{patient's hematocrit}}{45}$.

Estimating red cell production by the use of the corrected reticulocyte count may result in misleadingly high values in patients in whom there is premature release of reticulocytes from the marrow, as occurs in severe anemia. In this case, Hillman and Finch [18] suggest that a better estimate of red cell production is obtained by dividing the corrected reticulocyte count by an additional correction factor that varies depending on the severity of the anemia. Thus one may divide the corrected reticulocyte count by 1.5 if the hematocrit is 25 to 35 percent, by 2.0 if the hematocrit is 15 to 25 percent, and by 2.5 if the hematocrit is less than 15 percent. The value thus obtained is called the reticulocyte production index, and hemolytic anemia is the most likely diagnosis if the reticulocyte production index is greater than 3.[18]

These arithmetic manipulations may impart a false sense of scientific precision. In reality, hemolytic anemia may well be present even though the reticulocyte production index is less than 3. For example, a patient with a hematocrit of 15 and a reticulocyte count of 18 percent very likely has hemolytic anemia, but the reticulocyte production index is only 2.4 ($18 \times \frac{15}{45} \div 2.5$ = 2.4). Similarly, in order for the reticulocyte production index to be greater than 3 in a patient with a hematocrit of 20, the reticulocyte count must be at least 13.6 percent. As a simpler, but perhaps as accurate a guideline, one should suspect hemolytic anemia wherever the reticulocyte count is greater than 5 percent. The probability of hemolytic anemia rapidly increases with greater degrees of reticulocytosis and, if the reticulocyte count is greater than 10 percent, the diagnosis is very likely.

Although observation of the initial reticulocyte count accurately indicates the presence or absence of hemolytic anemia in a surprisingly high percentage of patients, exceptions do, of course, occur. A reticulocytosis can occur for other reasons, e.g., as a result of blood loss or recent treatment of megaloblastic anemia. However, blood loss causes a problem in differential diagnosis rather infrequently because sustained bleeding of sufficient volume and duration to result in a reticulocyte count high enough to cause a strong suspicion of hemolysis can result only from clinically evident blood loss. Similarly, the confusion of treated megaloblastic anemia with hemolytic anemia is an infrequent clinical problem. In cases in which there is doubt, repeat blood counts will be of value since an elevated reticulocyte count without an increase in hemoglobin and in the absence of blood loss is diagnostic of hemolysis.

Reticulocytopenia in the presence of hemolytic anemia presents a more difficult problem. If the hemolysis is of abrupt onset, at least several days must elapse before the development of a reticulocytosis. Patients with hemolytic anemia less acute in onset may also have reticulocytopenia because of bone marrow suppression for various reasons, included among which may be autoantibody reactivity against erythroid precursors (see Chapter 2). Although the initial reticulocyte count may misleadingly suggest that hemolytic anemia is not present, the diagnosis of hemolysis can nevertheless be made just from the blood count if serial determinations are made over a period of several days or more. This is true because the combination of hemolysis and reticulocytopenia results in a rapidly falling hemoglobin and hematocrit level, which can result only from hemolysis, providing significant blood loss is excluded.

Thus, hemolytic anemia can usually be diagnosed or excluded from consideration on the basis of routine blood counts, and, indeed, this remains the single most important means of doing so.

Red Blood Cell Morphology. The erythrocyte morphology in the peripheral blood film not only frequently substantiates the impression of hemolysis, but often suggests a specific diagnosis or a limited number of diagnostic possibilities. Morphologic findings are discussed in more detail below.

Bilirubin

Bilirubin is formed mainly in the reticuloendothelial system by enzymatic degradation of hemoglobin from senescent erythrocytes. About 15 percent, the so-called early labeled pigment or shunt bilirubin, is produced in the liver from non-hemoglobin heme, such as the cytochromes, or in the bone marrow from erythrocyte precursors, as in intramedullary hemolysis or ineffective erythropoiesis. Unconjugated bilirubin in the serum is bound to albumin and is transported to the liver, where it is taken up by hepatic acceptor protein. The hepatic microsomal enzyme, glucuronyl transferase, transforms unconjugated bilirubin to water soluble conjugated bilirubin, primarily bilirubin diglucuronide, which is then excreted in the bile.[27] In general the conjugated bilirubin is measured by the direct reacting fraction and the unconjugated bilirubin by the indirect reacting fraction.

Hyperbilirubinemia is usual in hemolytic anemia, but it is not a constant finding so that its absence does not exclude the diagnosis. The greatest importance of the serum bilirubin level in regard to the diagnosis of hemolytic anemia lies in the fact that if a patient has a significantly elevated serum bilirubin level (characteristically, but not invariably, between 1 and 5 mg per dl), which is almost exclusively of the unconjugated or indirect reacting type, the presence of hemolysis is almost assured. Perhaps the only exception to this rule is constitutional hepatic dysfunction (Gilbert's disease); in other syndromes with unconjugated hyperbilirubinemia such as primary shunt hyperbilirubinemia,[22] some cases of sideroblastic anemia,[19] thalassemia,[39] and dyserythropoietic jaundice,[8] the hyperbilirubinemia is due at least in part to hemolysis including destruction of erythroid precursors in the bone marrow.

Tisdale et al.[36] performed 77 bilirubin determinations in 46 patients with hemolytic anemia and found that the direct-reacting fraction constituted less than 15 percent of the total in most patients, especially if the total bilirubin was 4.0 mg/dl or greater. The direct-reacting fraction exceeded 1.2 mg/dl in only five instances unless there was definite evidence of concomitant hepatic disease.

Allgood and Chaplin[1] found that the indirect-reacting bilirubin was less than 1.0 mg per dl in only 13 percent of 47 patients with autoimmune hemolytic anemia. It varied from less than 0.8 to 8.6 mg per dl, and in 9 of the 47 patients it was greater than 4 mg per dl. The direct-reacting fraction was significantly elevated in only five patients, and the highest value was 3.6 mg per dl. In two of these patients there was definite evidence of underlying liver disease and, in the other three, it was suspected.

Although indirect-reacting hyperbilirubinemia is characteristic of hemolytic anemia, an increase in conjugated (direct-reacting) bilirubin does occur in a minority of patients, even in the absence of liver dysfunction.[27, 31, 32, 36] Even less well recognized is the fact that bilirubinuria is seen occasionally in patients with uncomplicated hemolytic jaundice.[32, 36]

Other aspects of bilirubin metabolism that may be studied in considering the diagnosis of hemolytic anemia are fecal stercobilinogen and urinary urobilinogen. Fecal stercobilinogen is affected by constipation, diarrhea, the administration of antibiotics, and the difficulties of stool collection, and urinary urobilinogen excretion depends more on liver function than on the rate of red cell destruction.[12] Although raised values are considered valid indications of hemolysis, the tests are difficult to perform accurately and are usually not necessary.

Serum Haptoglobin

Serum haptoglobins are alpha$_2$-glycoproteins that have the property of combining with hemoglobin.[9, 24, 33] The normal range of serum haptoglobin is about 50 to 150 mg/dl. Haptoglobin-hemoglobin complexes are rapidly catabolized at a rate of approximately 15 mg hemoglobin per 100 ml plasma per hour [16, 17] and, if hemoglobin is liberated into plasma at a sufficiently fast rate, the rate of production of haptoglobin (probably in the liver) [2, 30] is unable to keep pace with the rate of destruction, and this results in a low level of serum haptoglobin. When hemoglobin destruction exceeds two or three times the normal rate, the serum haptoglobin level will usually be low [12] and even less hemolysis is necessary to result in low serum haptoglobin if the hemolysis is intravascular. Thus the level of serum haptoglobin can be considered a reasonably sensitive indicator of hemolysis, although it must be kept in mind that even greater rates of hemoglobin breakdown may be necessary to depress the level of serum haptoglobin in situations in which there is apparently an increased rate of synthesis, such as in acute or chronic inflammatory disease, neoplasia including lymphomas, or steroid administration. Also, in severe hepatocellular disease, the serum haptoglobin level may be low, probably as a result of decreased production.

Serum Lactic Dehydrogenase

Serum lactic dehydrogenase has also beeen utilized in the diagnosis of hemolytic anemia. Stein [34] studied serum lactic dehydrogenase activity in patients with hemolytic anemia, including patients with primarily intravascular hemolysis (e.g., prosthetic heart valves, paroxysmal nocturnal hemoglobinuria) or primarily extravascular hemolysis (e.g., hereditary spherocytosis) (Table 1-1). The level of lactic dehydrogenase elevation in hereditary spherocytosis was modest even with severe hemolysis, although intravascular hemolysis always produced a marked elevation.

Table 1-1. SERUM LACTIC DEHYDROGENASE IN HEMOLYTIC ANEMIA

Patient	Diagnosis	PCV (%)	Reticulocyte Count (%)	Serum LDH N = 250–800 U/ml
1	3 artificial heart valves	27	7.4	5,040
2	2 artificial heart valves	27	10.4	4,200
3	1 artificial heart valve	25	10.0	8,250
4	Paroxysmal nocturnal hemoglobinuria	24	9.0	9,720
5	Paroxysmal nocturnal hemoglobinuria	12	22.4	22,800
6	Paroxysmal nocturnal hemoglobinuria	27	8.2	8,520
7	Acid ingestion	40	2.1	4,960
8	Chemical abortion	19	3.7	4,400
9	Burns	31	3.0	9,390
10	Vasculitis	27	7.4	7,020
11	Hereditary spherocytosis	28	6.8	700
12	Hereditary spherocytosis	29	10.0	450
13	Hereditary spherocytosis	21	28.4	1,340
14	Beta-thalassemia	22	10.5	1,500
15	Sickle cell anemia	18	10.7	2,550

Other Tests

Fehr and Knob [16a] have recently evaluated the use of red cell creatine as an indicator of the severity of hemolytic disease. In patients with steady-state hemolysis, there was a better correlation between red cell survival and red cell creatine than there was between red cell survival and the reticulocyte count. The authors suggest that this simple chemical assay may be used to obtain a useful estimation of red cell survival.

For further evidence of hemolysis one might look for erythroid hyperplasia of the bone marrow or perform red cell survival studies with ^{51}Cr or ^{32}P-diisopropyl fluorophosphate (DFP).[28] Also, measurement of the rate of endogenous production of carbon monoxide may be used to calculate the red cell life span.[10, 15, 23, 26] However, these tests are usually not necessary to establish the presence or absence of hemolysis.[37]

ESTABLISHING A TENTATIVE DIAGNOSIS OF THE CAUSE OF THE HEMOLYTIC ANEMIA

When it has been established that the patient has a hemolytic anemia, the cause of the hemolysis should be sought next. One should consider the differential diagnosis of hemolytic anemias and develop a preliminary diagnosis.

Table 1-2. CLASSIFICATION OF HEMOLYTIC ANEMIAS

Intracellular Abnormalities	Membrane Abnormalities	Extracellular Abnormalities
	Hereditary	
Enzyme defects	Hereditary spherocytosis	Lipid Abnormalities
Glucose-6-phosphate dehydrogenase,	Hereditary stomatocytosis	Abetalipoproteinemia (acanthocytosis)
pyruvate kinase deficiency, triosephos-	Rh_{null} syndrome	Lecithin: cholesterol acyl transferase (LCAT)
phate isomerase deficiency, glucose	Hereditary elliptocytosis	deficiency
phosphate isomerase deficiency, 2,3-	Abnormal cation permeability	
diphosphoglycerate mutase deficiency,	Hydrocytosis and dessiccytosis	
etc.	High phosphatidyl choline hemolytic	
Globin disorders	anemia	
Defects in globin structure (sickle cell	Calcium leak with extreme microcytosis	
anemia, hemoglobin S-C disease,	Muscular dystrophies	
hemoglobin S-D disease, hemoglobin C	Congenital dyserythropoietic anemias	
disease, etc.; unstable hemoglobins		
such as hemoglobin Köln, Ham-		
mersmith, Philly, and Zürich)		
Defects in globin synthesis (thalassemias)		
Heme disorders (porphyrias)		
Erythropoietic protoporphyria		
Congenital erythropoietic porphyria		
(erythropoietic uroporphyria)		
	Acquired	
Environmental factors influencing	Paroxysmal nocturnal hemoglobinuria	Immune hemolytic
metabolism	Membrane lipid abnormalities	anemias
Hypophosphatemia	Liver disease	Autoimmune
Wilson's disease (high serum copper)		Alloimmune
		Drug-induced

Lead poisoning
Uremia
Severe iron deficiency anemia

Clostridial infection
Anorexia nervosa
Vitamin E deficiency

Drugs (non-immune),
Chemicals, venoms

Mechanical hemolytic
anemia
Prosthetic cardiovascular materials
March hemoglobinuria
Microangiopathic hemolytic anemia
Thrombotic throm-
bocytopenic purpura
Hemolytic uremic syndrome
Malignant hypertension
Carcinomatosis
Hemangioma

Heat (severe burns)

Infectious agents
Malaria
Leishmaniasis
Toxoplasmosis

Hypersplenism

Hereditary and Acquired

Hereditary Factor		Acquired Factor
Metabolic defects (Enzymopathies especially glucose 6-phosphate dehydrogenase deficiency)	in conjunction with	Oxidant drugs, favism, infections (e.g., viral hepatitis), diabetic ketoacidosis
Unstable hemoglobins (Zürich, H, Torino, Köln, Shepherds Bush, etc.)	in conjunction with	Drugs, infections

[11]

Hemolytic anemias have been classified in a number of ways. Traditionally they are divided into intracorpuscular and extracorpuscular defects or into hereditary and acquired disorders. More recently, efforts have been made to extend these classifications by incorporating present day knowledge of the site of the basic defect in reference to the red cell membrane.[5] Thus, hemolytic disorders may be caused by intracellular abnormalities, defects of the red cell membrane, or extracellular abnormalities. Taking into account all the information stated above, we have developed the classification in Table 1-2, which considers not only the site of the basic defect, but also the hereditary or acquired nature of many of the recognized causes of hemolytic anemia.

Although such a classification is comprehensive, it is rather cumbersome, and many of the disorders listed are extremely rare. Thus, when determining the cause of a patient's hemolytic anemia, it is more practical to emphasize consideration of a more limited number of relatively common disorders, and we find the comparatively simple classification listed in Table 1-3 useful for this purpose.

Table 1-3. A SIMPLIFIED CLASSIFICATION OF HEMOLYTIC ANEMIAS

Hereditary hemolytic anemias
    Hereditary spherocytosis
    Hereditary elliptocytosis
    Thalassemias
    Hemoglobinopathies
    Enzyme deficiency hemolytic anemias
Acquired hemolytic anemias
    Immune hemolytic anemias
        Autoimmune hemolytic anemias (AIHA)
            Warm antibody AIHA
            Cold agglutinin syndrome
            Paroxysmal cold hemoglobinuria
        Alloimmune hemolytic anemias
            Hemolytic disease of the newborn
            Hemolytic transfusion reactions
        Drug-induced immune hemolytic anemia
    Drug-induced hemolytic anemias (non-immunologic mechanisms)
        Direct toxic effect
        Idiosyncrasy mechanism
    Hemolytic anemias associated with numerous irregularly contracted erythrocytes in the
        blood film
        Mechanical hemolytic anemia
        Microangiopathic hemolytic anemias
    Paroxysmal nocturnal hemoglobinuria
    Miscellaneous
        Infectious agents (uncommon)
            Protozoal parasites: malaria
            Bacteria: Clostridium perfringens (welchii)

Since the number of causes of hemolytic anemia is large, even when considering the simplified classification, it is evident that it is necessary to have a more restricted list of possibilities in mind before performing specific diagnostic tests. A tentative or working diagnosis should be formulated after careful consideration of four important points: (1) a review of the history and physical examination, (2) a review of the peripheral blood film, (3) findings of intravascular hemolysis, and (4) the direct antiglobulin test.

History and Physical Examination

Since hemolytic anemia is often not suspected on the basis of the initial history and physical examination, it is important to review them with emphasis on specific points after a diagnosis of hemolysis has been made.

A history of anemia or of splenectomy in members of the family suggests a hereditary hemolytic anemia. If present in successive generations, an autosomal disorder (such as hereditary spherocytosis) or a condition that is manifested in the heterozygous state (such as the unstable hemoglobins) [20] should be considered. The most common hereditary red cell enzyme defects, glucose-6-phosphate dehydrogenase deficiency and pyruvate kinase deficiency, are clinically manifested in the sex-linked hemizygous (or rare homozygous) and homozygous state, respectively, In these instances, the examination of other family members is of obvious importance. A history of jaundice at birth and longstanding or recurring anemia and/or jaundice may also be obtained in hereditary hemolytic states.

In contrast, the presence of acquired hemolysis may be indicated by the knowledge of a previously normal blood count or by the history of the acute onset of constitutional symptoms such as fever, malaise, or pain in the back, legs, or abdomen. A history of dark urine suggests the presence of hemoglobinuria, dipyrroluria [38] or, rarely, porphyrinuria. The relationship, if any, of hemoglobinuria to sleep (paroxysmal nocturnal hemoglobinuria), cold (cold agglutinin syndrome or paroxysmal cold hemoglobinuria), and exertion (march hemoglobinuria) should also be noted.

Details of the taking of drugs or exposure to chemicals must be obtained, as hemolysis can result from a direct toxic effect on red cells, oxidative injury (especially when an enzyme defect or unstable hemoglobin is present), or immunologic damage. However, a history of ingestion of drugs such as analgesics may not always be easy to obtain.[4] Several types of hemolytic anemia have been described in alcoholism, particularly when there is associated liver disease.[14, 35]

Symptoms and signs suggestive of systemic lupus erythematosus, lymphomas, chronic lymphocytic leukemia, or infectious mononucleosis are important because of the association of autoimmune hemolytic anemias with these diseases. Raynaud's phenomenon and, less frequently, cold urticaria may be present in autoimmune hemolytic anemias caused by cold antibodies. Occasionally, infections are associated with a hemolytic state,[6, 29] or they may provoke acute hemolysis in subjects with an intrinsic red cell defect.

Microangiopathic hemolytic anemia is suggested by the presence of certain underlying disorders as indicated in Table 1-4.

The classical physical findings of hemolytic anemia are pallor, jaundice, and splenomegaly. However, in milder degrees of hemolysis these findings are often absent. Leg ulcers or their residual pigmentation, typically over the malleoli, may be present in chronic hemolytic anemias. Thickening of the skull as a result of bone marrow expansion may occur in severe hereditary hemolytic states, and a radiologic examination will show thinning of cortical bone with expansion and trabeculation of the medulla, sometimes with the typical hair-on-end appearance.

Although splenomegaly occurs in many hemolytic anemias, massive splenomegaly suggests thalassemia major, lymphoma, myelofibrosis, or chronic leukemias. Dusky cyanosis is associated with the M hemoglobins [21] or unstable hemoglobins with low oxygen affinity. Purpura may be seen in hemolytic anemias associated with systemic lupus erythematosus, thrombotic thrombocytopenic purpura, or Evans' syndrome.

Table 1-4. DIFFERENTIAL DIAGNOSIS IN HEMOLYTIC ANEMIAS ASSOCIATED WITH SPHEROCYTOSIS OR NUMEROUS IRREGULARLY CONTRACTED ERYTHROCYTES

Spherocytes
   Hereditary spherocytosis
   Immune hemolytic anemias
      Alloimmune hemolytic anemia, especially ABO hemolytic disease of the newborn
         and hemolytic transfusion reactions
      Autoimmune hemolytic anemia, especially warm antibody AIHA
      Drug-induced hemolysis (some cases)
   Severe burns
   Clostridium perfringens (welchii) septicemia
   Hypophosphatemia
Fragmented erythrocytes (schistocytes, helmet cells, burr cells)
   Chemical or drug-induced hemolytic anemia (some cases)
   Mechanical hemolytic anemia (prosthetic cardiovascular materials)
   Microangiopathic hemolytic anemia
      Hemolytic uremic syndrome
      Thrombotic thrombocytopenic purpura
      Disseminated intravascular coagulation
      Malignant hypertension
      Disseminated carcinomatosis
      Eclampsia
      Polyarteritis
      Systemic lupus erythematosus
Less characteristic irregularly contracted erythrocytes
   Severe megaloblastic anemia
   Severe iron deficiency
   Thalassemia major

The Peripheral Blood Film

The peripheral blood film is often very helpful in suggesting a specific diagnosis or a limited number of diagnostic possibilities. Spherocytes may be a prominent feature in several hemolytic anemias, as indicated in Table 1-4 and in Figures 1-3 and 1-4. Basophilic stippling, due to clumping of ribosomes, is encountered in many anemias but is prominent in β-thalassemias, and coarse stippling is seen in lead poisoning. Hypochromic red cells associated with a hemolytic state suggest thalassemic disorders, hemoglobinopathies, lead poisoning, and chronic intravascular hemolysis with urinary loss of iron. Target cells (Fig. 1-5) are present in patients with thalassemia or some of the hemoglobinopathies, especially hemoglobins C and E. They may also be found in patients with obstructive jaundice or hepatitis. Target cell formation is more pronounced after splenectomy. Sickle cells (Fig. 1-6) may be seen in patients with sickle cell anemia.

Fragmented erythrocytes (Fig. 1-7) are typically seen in microangiopathic, mechanical, and some drug-induced hemolytic anemias; irregularly contracted red cells of less characteristic appearance are also present in other hemolytic anemias (Table 1-4). In hereditary elliptocytosis (or ovalocytosis) (Fig. 1-8), 50 to 90 percent of the red cells are oval. In normal subjects, less than 15 percent of red cells are oval, and such cells are also present in a wide variety of anemias, which include iron deficiency, thalassemia, megaloblastic anemia, and myelofibrosis. However, the degree of elliptocytosis is most marked in the hereditary form.

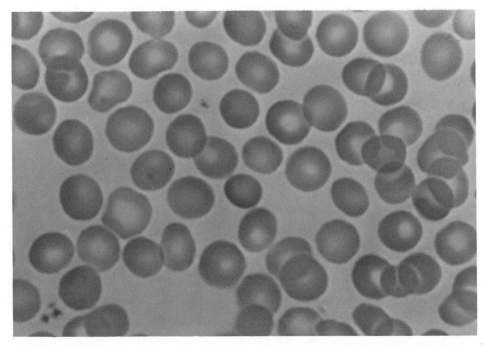

Figure 1-3. Hereditary spherocytosis. Numerously densely staining microspherocytes are present.

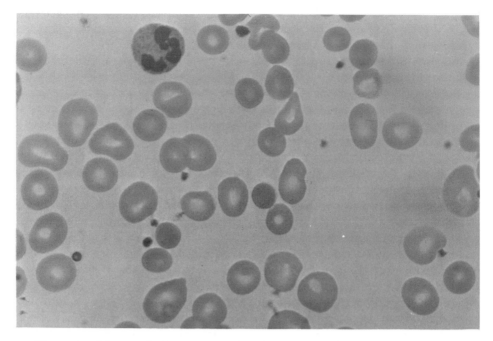

Figure 1-4. Warm antibody autoimmune hemolytic anemia. Spherocytes are evident, and the degree of poikilocytosis is generally more marked than in hereditary spherocytosis as a result of the interaction of antibody and/or complement sensitized red cells with macrophages (see Chapter 4).

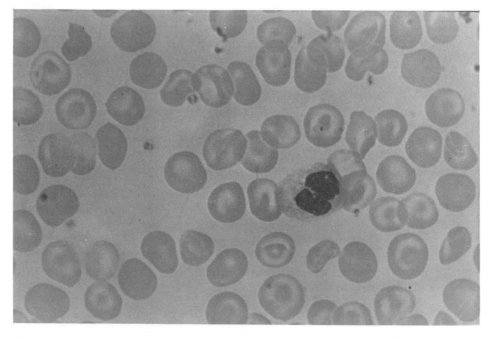

Figure 1-5. Hemoglobin C. Numerous target cells are present. Hemoglobin electrophoresis indicated that the patient was heterozygous for hemoglobin C.

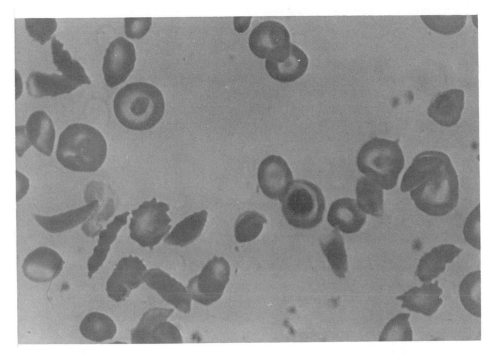

Figure 1-6. Hemoglobin S. Anisocytosis, poikilocytosis, and several sickle cells are illustrated.

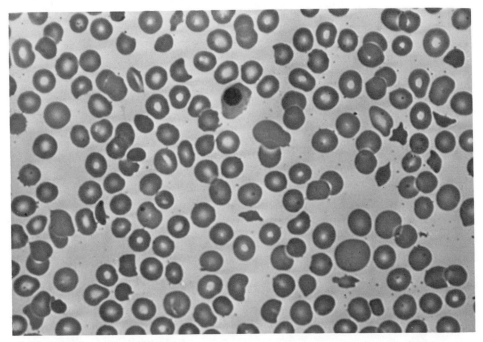

Figure 1-7. Thrombotic thrombocytopenic purpura. Numerous fragmented erythrocytes and a marked decrease in the number of platelets are characteristic features of the disorder. A nucleated red blood cell is also present.

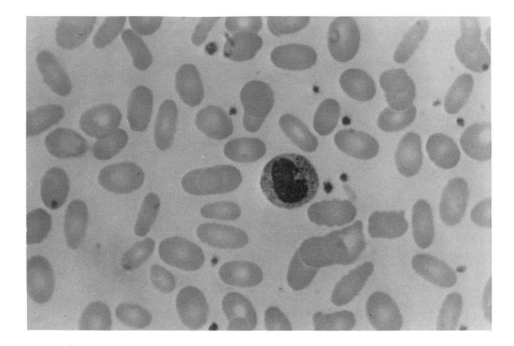

Figure 1-8. *Hereditary elliptocytosis. Occasional elliptocytes may be seen in a variety of anemias, but hereditary elliptocytosis is characterized by the marked degree of elliptocytosis illustrated here. About 15 percent of patients with hereditary elliptocytosis have hemolytic anemia.*

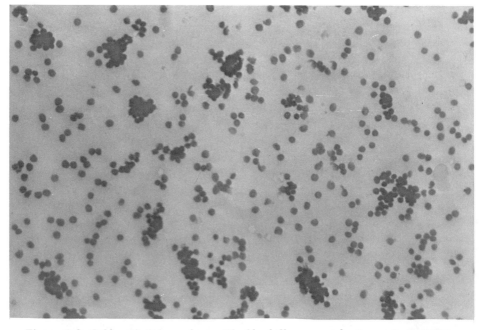

Figure 1-9. *Cold agglutinin syndrome. The blood film was made at room temperature and gross autoagglutination is evident.*

Stomatocytes are present in small numbers in many blood smears, but they occur in larger numbers in a rare hemolytic anemia associated with increased red cell sodium permeability [40] and in alcoholic liver disease. [13] Acanthocytes are characteristically seen in hereditary a-β-lipoproteinemia, but they also occur in malabsorption with hypo-β-lipoproteinemia and chronic liver diseases. [25] Cold agglutinin syndrome is suggested by finding gross agglutination in blood films made at room temperature, especially if agglutination is not present when the same sample of blood is warmed to 37°C prior to making the blood film (Figs. 1-9 and 1-10).

It is also true that findings other than red blood cell morphology may suggest the cause of a patient's hemolytic anemia. For example, findings may indicate the presence of chronic lymphatic leukemia or infectious mononucleosis. Also, a marked decrease in platelets in a patient with hemolytic anemia who has numerous fragmented red cells in the peripheral blood film suggests a diagnosis of thrombotic thrombocytopenic purpura or the hemolytic uremic syndrome, and thrombocytopenia in the presence of spherocytes suggests Evans' syndrome.

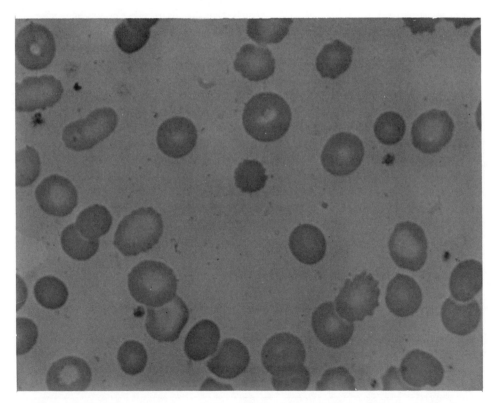

Figure 1-10. Cold agglutinin syndrome. Same patient as in Figure 1-9, but the blood film was made strictly at 37°C. Autoagglutination is not present. There is an occasional microspherocyte, moderate poikilocytosis, and anisocytosis with some macrocytes that are probably reticulocytes.

Features of Intravascular Hemolysis

Laboratory findings that indicate that the hemolysis is primarily intravascular in nature are helpful in that they suggest that the specific diagnosis is likely to be one of a limited number of disorders, particularly those listed in Table 1-5.

Constitutional symptoms (fever, backache, etc.) often accompany severe intravascular hemolysis, but they are much less common and marked in chronic hemoglobinuria and, indeed, they may be completely absent. The symptoms may occur shortly after the hemolysis begins and may be present before the appearance of hemoglobinuria.

Hemoglobinuria is always associated with hemoglobinemia. In normal subjects hemoglobin breakdown occurs mainly in the cells of the reticuloendothelial system, and therefore the level of free hemoglobin in the plasma is low, ranging from 2 to 5 mg/dl. When hemolysis occurs in the blood, the hemoglobin from the broken down red cells is liberated into the plasma, causing a rise of plasma hemoglobin with values rising to 100 to 200 mg/dl or even more. When the plasma hemoglobin level is markedly raised, the plasma has a pink or red color, depending on the concentration of the hemoglobin. When the rise is moderate, e.g., from 10 to 40 mg/dl, this color may be lacking, not only because of the relatively low concentration but also because other pigments such as bilirubin, which gives a yellow color, and methemalbumin, which gives

Table 1-5. CAUSES OF HEMOGLOBINURIA

Acute Hemoglobinuria
  Incompatible blood transfusion
  Transfusion of damaged blood (overheating or freezing, bacterial contamination, pump-oxygenation)
  Drugs and chemical agents (immune or non-immune mechanisms)
  Paroxysmal cold hemoglobinuria *
  Acute severe warm antibody AIHA
  Clostridium perfringens (welchii) infection
  Malaria (blackwater fever)
  Snake and spider bites
  Cold agglutinin syndrome †
  March hemoglobinuria
  Microangiopathic hemolytic anemia
  Hypotonic bladder irrigations during prostatic surgery
  Mistaken intravenous administration of water
Chronic Hemoglobinuria
  Paroxysmal nocturnal hemoglobinuria ‡
  Prosthetic cardiovascular materials

* In very rare instances may occur as a chronic disorder exacerbated by exposure to cold.
† Chronic low grade intravascular hemolysis is common with acute hemoglobinuria resulting from exposure to cold.
‡ Characteristically associated with intermittent episodes of grossly evident hemoglobinuria.

a brownish color, may mask the pink tint. When the level of plasma hemoglobin exceeds the renal threshold, hemoglobin appears in the urine—hemoglobinuria.

The urine may be pink, red, brown or almost black.[7] It contains two pigments, oxyhemoglobin and methemoglobin, which are produced by auto-oxidation of the hemoglobin in the urinary tract when the urine is acid. Oxyhemoglobin is bright red and methemoglobin dark brown; the color of the urine therefore depends on the concentration (which is related to the degree of hemolysis) and the relative proportions of the two pigments. Oxyhemoglobin predominates in alkaline urine and methemoglobin in acid urine. The term "blackwater" has been used clinically to describe the dark color of the urine that occurs in some patients with marked hemoglobinuria. The term has most commonly been applied in malaria, where hemolysis in association with an acute febrile episode has been called "blackwater fever." Hemoglobin in the urine can be identified by spectroscopic examination and by the positive reaction with benzidine and quaiac. Hemoglobinuria is accompanied by albuminuria, which disappears when hemoglobinuria ceases.[12]

Hemoglobinuria may be confused with hematuria, especially when the urine is bright red. The urine in hemoglobinuria is clear, but in hematuria it is smoky. The microscopic examination of a freshly voided centrifuged specimen will distinguish hematuria, as the sediment is seen to contain numerous red cells and the supernatant fluid is clear. Occasionally, however, the specific gravity of the urine is so low (less than 1.007) that the red cells rupture in the urine and cause the supernatant to be red. In such cases the inspection of a carefully collected centrifuged specimen of blood, taken with precautions to prevent hemolysis, will distinguish the two conditions. In hematuria the plasma is of normal color, while in hemoglobinuria the plasma is pink or red due to the hemoglobinemia.

In some patients with acute intravascular hemolysis the kidneys are damaged, which gives rise to acute renal failure due to acute tubular necrosis. This condition is characterized clinically by oliguria, which may progress to anuria, uremia, and sometimes death. Acute tubular necrosis is classically seen following intravascular hemolysis resulting from incompatible transfusion, which is by far the commonest cause of this syndrome; however, it occasionally occurs in other disorders causing acute intravascular hemolysis, especially when hemolysis is massive. Urinary output should be monitored in all cases of acute hemoglobinuria in order to detect early the onset of oliguria.

When hemoglobin is liberated into the plasma in large quantities, some of the heme combines with the plasma albumin to form a hematin-albumin complex known as methemalbumin. Methemalbumin does not occur in the plasma of normal persons, and its presence is diagnostic of intravascular hemolysis. Methemalbumin gives the plasma a golden to brown color, depending on its concentration. More definitive identification may be accomplished by biochemical tests.

Hemoglobinuria results in the deposition in the renal tubules, of hemosiderin derived from the breakdown of hemoglobin. This hemosiderin may be excreted in the urine, probably as a result of the desquamation of tubular cells. Hemosiderin granules can be demonstrated by staining a centrifuged urine sediment for iron. Hemosiderinuria is seen particularly in chronic hemoglobinemias, and is especially typical of paroxysmal nocturnal hemoglobinuria, in which hemosiderinuria persists even when hemoglobinuria is absent. Transient hemosiderinuria also occurs in acute hemoglobinuria, but it may not occur until several days after the onset of the hemoglobinuria.

The Direct Antiglobulin Test

The direct antiglobulin test should be performed in every patient in whom the presence of hemolysis has been established. Although some exceptions to this rule might be considered, as when the diagnosis of a congenital hemolytic anemia is evident, the antiglobulin test is a simple, quick, inexpensive test that yields useful information.

The presence of a positive direct antiglobulin test in a patient with hemolytic anemia does, of course indicate that the most likely diagnosis is one of the immune hemolytic anemias. It should be emphasized that the determination of the presence of hemolysis as described earlier in this chapter should logically precede the performance of the direct antiglobulin test, and that the purpose of the latter test is to indicate the presence or absence of an immune etiology in patients known to have hemolytic anemia.

Although the result of the direct antiglobulin test in a patient with hemolytic anemia generally indicates whether or not the hemolytic anemia is immunologically mediated, a positive antiglobulin test may occur as a coincidental finding in patients with hemolytic anemia caused by non-immune mechanisms, and some patients with immune hemolytic anemias have a negative direct antiglobulin test.

Moreover, although a positive direct antiglobulin test is very unusual in perfectly healthy persons, positive reactions are obtained in a significant number of hospitalized patients who do not have hemolytic anemia. Indeed, Dacie and Worlledge [11] reported that weakly positive reactions were obtained in 40 of 489 (8 percent) blood samples submitted for routine hematologic tests. We have recently performed a similar study using blood samples obtained in EDTA anticoagulant. We found that 8 of 100 hospitalized patients without evidence of hematologic disease had a weakly positive direct antiglobulin test using anti-C3 antiglobulin serum. In two of the eight patients, the reaction was 1+ and in the other six patients, it was weaker than 1+. Negative results were uniformly obtained using anti-IgG antiglobulin serum. In 100 normal persons, we obtained only one weakly positive reaction using anti-C3 (½+) and, using anti-IgG antiglobulin serum, one person had a 1+ result.

These findings emphasize that careful evaluation is required before a precise diagnosis can be made in patients who have a hemolytic anemia and a positive direct antiglobulin test. The details of such an evaluation are discussed in Chapters 5 and 6.

SPECIFIC CONFIRMATORY TESTS

On the basis of the evaluation indicated thus far, a provisional diagnosis or a limited number of diagnostic possibilities can usually be established with reasonable certainty. It is beyond the scope of this text to describe the details of the use of specific confirmatory tests for a wide variety of hemolytic anemias. However, a few examples may be cited to illustrate the use of the principles advocated in this chapter.

If, in a patient with hemolytic anemia, the history suggests a hereditary hemolytic anemia, the physical examination reveals splenomegaly, the peripheral blood film reveals spherocytes, features of intravascular hemolysis are absent, and the direct antiglobulin test is negative, a tentative diagnosis of hereditary spherocytosis is warranted. The best confirmatory evidence is the documentation of similar findings in family members. Also, osmotic fragility and autohemolysis tests will yield characteristic abnormalities, although similar results may be obtained in patients who have spherocytosis as a result of acquired disease.

If an adult patient with hemolytic anemia manifesting for the first time has a history of repeated episodes of dark urine and abdominal pain, a blood film that reveals no characteristic abnormalities, laboratory tests indicating features of intravascular hemolysis, and a negative direct antiglobulin test, the tentative diagnosis of paroxysmal nocturnal hemoglobinuria may be made. The diagnosis may be confirmed by the performance of the sucrose-hemolysis test and/or Ham's acid serum test. Further relevant tests are the documentation of hemoglobinuria and hemosiderinuria.

Another example is that of a patient who has an acquired hemolytic anemia; does not have a history of recent blood transfusion or drug ingestion, has an acute onset of systemic symptoms such as fever, malaise, and aching in the back and legs; a physical examination that reveals splenomegaly; a blood film revealing spherocytosis; no evidence of hemoglobinuria; and a strongly positive direct antiglobulin test. An autoimmune hemolytic anemia is the most likely diagnosis, and details of further diagnostic tests that should be performed are described in later chapters.

REFERENCES

1. Allgood, J. W., and Chaplin, H.: Idiopathic acquired autoimmune hemolytic anemia. Am. J. Med., *43*:254, 1967.
2. Alper, C. A., Peters, J. H., Birtch, A. G., and Gardner, F. H.: Haptoglobin synthesis. I. In vivo studies of the production of haptoglobin, fibrinogen, and γ-globulin by the canine liver. J. Clin. Invest., *44*:574, 1965.
3. Andersen, M. N., Gabrieli, E., and Zizzi, J. A.: Chronic hemolysis in patients with ball-valve prostheses. J. Thorac. Cardiov. Surg., *50*:501, 1965.
4. Azen, E. A., Bryan, G. T., Shahidi, N. T., Rossi, E. C., and Clatanoff, D. V.: Obscure hemolytic anemia due to analgesic abuse. Am. J. Med., *48*:724, 1970.
5. Ballas, S. K.: Disorders of the red cell membrane: A reclassification of hemolytic anemias. Am. J. Med. Sci., *276*:4, 1978.
6. Barrett-Connor, E.: Anemia and infection. Am. J. Med., *52*:242, 1972.

7. Berman, L. B.: When the urine is red. J.A.M.A., *237:*2753, 1977.
8. Berendsohn, S., Lowman, J., Sundberg, D., and Watson, C. J.: Idiopathic dysery-thropoietic jaundice. Blood, *24:*1, 1964.
9. Brus, I., and Lewis, S. M.: The haptoglobin content of serum in haemolytic anaemia. Br. J. Haematol, *5:*348, 1959.
10. Coburn, R. F., Williams, W. J., and Kahn, S. B.: Endogenous carbon monoxide production in patients with hemolytic anemia. J. Clin. Invest., *45:*460, 1966.
11. Dacie, J. V., and Worlledge, S. M.: Auto-immune hemolytic anemias. Progr. Hematol., *6:*82, 1969.
12. de Gruchy, G. C.: Clinical Haematology in Medical Practice. 3rd Ed. Oxford, Blackwell Scientific Publications, 1970.
13. Douglass, C. C., and Twomey, J. J.: Transient stomatocytosis with hemolysis: A previously unrecognized complication of alcoholism. Ann. Intern. Med., *72:*159, 1970.
14. Eichner, E. R.: The hematologic disorders of alcoholism. Am. J. Med., *54:*621, 1973.
15. Engel, R. R., Rodkey, F. L., and Krill, C. E.: Carboxyhemoglobin levels as an index of hemolysis. Pediatr., *47:*723, 1971.
16. Faulstick, D. A., Lowenstein, J., and Yiengst, M. J.: Clearance kinetics of haptoglobin-hemoglobin complex in the human. Blood, *20:*65, 1962.
16a. Fehr, J., and Knob, M.: Comparison of red cell creatine level and reticulocyte count in appraising the severity of hemolytic processes. Blood, *53:*966, 1979.
17. Gabrieli, E. R., and Pyzikiewicz, T.: Plasma hemoglobin clearance: A clinical study. J. Reticuloendothel. Soc., *3:*163, 1966.
18. Hillman, R. S., and Finch, C. A.: Erythropoiesis: Normal and abnormal. Seminars Hematol., *4:*327, 1967.
19. Horne, M. K., Rosse, W. F., Flickinger, E. G., and Saltzman, H. A.: "Early-peak" carbon monoxide production in certain erythropoietic disorders. Blood, *45:*365, 1975.
20. Huehns, E. R.: Diseases due to abnormalities of hemoglobin structure. Annual Rev. Med., *21:*157, 1970.
21. Huehns, E. R., and Shooter, E. M.: Human haemoglobins. J. Med. Genet., *2:*48, 1965.
22. Klaus, D., and Feine, U.: Primary shunt hyperbilirubinaemia. German Med. Monthly, *10:*89, 1965.
23. Landaw, S. A., and Winchell, H. S.: Endogenous production of ^{14}CO: A method for calculation of RBC lifespan in vivo. Blood, *36:*642, 1970.
24. Laurell, C. B., and Nyman, M.: Studies on the serum haptoglobin level in hemo-globinemia and its influence on renal excretion of hemoglobin. Blood, *12:*493, 1957.
25. Lessin, L. S., and Bessis, M.: Morphology of the erythron. *In* Hematology. Williams, W. J., Beutler, E., Erslev, A. J., and Rundles, W., Eds. New York, McGraw-Hill, 1972, Chapter 8.
26. Logue, G. L., Rosse, W. F., and Gockerman, J. P.: Measurement of the third component of complement bound to red blood cells in patients with the cold agglutinin syndrome. J. Clin. Invest., *52:*493, 1973.
27. Maldonado, J. E., Kyle, R. A., and Schoenfield, L. J.: Increased serum conjugated bilirubin in hemolytic anemia. Postgrad. Med., *55:*183, 1974.
28. McIntyre, P. A.: New developments in nuclear medicine applicable in hematology. Prog. Hematol., *10:*361, 1977.
29. Murdoch, J. McC., and Smith, C. C.: Infection. Clinics Hematol., *1:* 619, 1972.
30. Peters, J. H., and Alper, C. A.: Haptoglobin synthesis. II. Cellular localization studies. J. Clin. Invest., *45:*314, 1966.
31. Pirofsky, B.: Autoimmunization and the Autoimmune Hemolytic Anemias. Baltimore, Williams & Wilkins Company, 1969.

32. Schalm, L., and Weber, A. P.: Jaundice with conjugated bilirubin in hyperhaemolysis. Acta Med. Scand., *176:*549, 1964.
33. Shinton, N. K., Richardson, R. W., and Williams, J. D. F.: Diagnostic value of serum haptoglobin. J. Clin. Path., *18:*114, 1965.
34. Stein, I. D.: Serum lactate dehydrogenase isoenzymes: Stability, clearance, and diagnostic application in hemolytic anemia. J. Lab. Clin. Med., *76:*76, 1970.
35. Straus, D. J.: Hematologic aspects of alcoholism. Seminars in Hematol., *10:*183, 1973.
36. Tisdale, W. A., Klatskin, G., and Kinsella, E. D.: The significance of the direct-reacting fraction of serum bilirubin in hemolytic jaundice. Am. J. Med., *26:*214, 1959.
37. Todd, D.: Diagnosis of haemolytic states. Clinics Haematol., *4:*63, 1975.
38. White, J. M., and Dacie, J. V.: The unstable hemoglobins—molecular and clinical features. Progr. Hematol. *9:*69, 1971.
39. White, P., Coburn, R. F., Williams, W. J., Goldwein, M. I., Rother, M. L., and Shafer, B. C.: Carbon monoxide production associated with ineffective erythropoiesis. J. Clin. Invest., *46:*1986, 1967.
40. Zarkowsky, H. S., Oski, F. A., Sha'afi, R., Shohet, S. B., and Nathan, D. G.: Congenital hemolytic anemia with high sodium, low potassium red cells. I. Studies of membrane permeability. New Engl. J. Med., *278:*573, 1968.

2

Classification and Clinical Characteristics of Autoimmune Hemolytic Anemias

CLASSIFICATION

In this chapter we present a clinically useful classification of immune hemolytic anemias, and we review the clinical manifestations of each type of autoimmune hemolytic anemia (AIHA).

Numerous classifications of immune hemolytic anemias have been proposed. The purpose of a classification of any group of diseases should be to divide that group into clinically distinctive categories. The rather simple classification listed in Table 2-1 serves this purpose well since clinical manifestations, prognosis, and therapy are different among the diagnostic groups listed. Table 2-2 outlines some of these distinctions.

Some comments about the classification listed in Table 2-1 follow. We refer to AIHA as idiopathic if it is unassociated with any demonstrable underlying disease. If the AIHA is associated with an additional disorder and there is reason to suspect that the association is not merely fortuitous, we refer to the AIHA as secondary.

Among the patients with secondary cold agglutinin syndrome, those associated with infectious disorders consist of patients in whom the hemolytic anemia is predictably transient and remits after resolution of the associated infectious disease. The underlying diseases in patients with lymphoreticular malignancies are more chronic, and the course of the AIHA is less predictable. Another reason supporting a distinction between these two groups is that the IgM cold agglutinin in patients in the first group is almost always a polyclonal protein, in contrast to the monoclonal antibody that is characteristically found in patients in the second group, as well as in almost all idiopathic cases (also see page 47).

Paroxysmal cold hemoglobinuria is historically related to syphilis, but all reported cases in the recent medical literature are idiopathic or associated with a viral syndrome.

The ingestion of some drugs (e.g., methyldopa) causes hemolytic anemia that is clinically and serologically indistinguishable from other cases of warm

26

Table 2-1. CLASSIFICATION OF IMMUNE HEMOLYTIC ANEMIAS

Autoimmune hemolytic anemias (AIHA)
  Warm antibody AIHA
    Idiopathic
      Secondary (Chronic lymphocytic leukemia, lymphomas, systemic lupus erythe-
        matosus, etc.)
  Cold agglutinin syndrome
    Idiopathic
    Secondary
      Mycoplasma pneumoniae infection, infectious mononucleosis, virus infections
      Lymphoreticular malignant processes
  Paroxysmal cold hemoglobinuria
    Idiopathic
    Secondary
      Viral syndromes
      Syphilis
  Atypical AIHA
    Antiglobulin test negative AIHA
    Miscellaneous and unclassifiable
Drug-induced immune hemolytic anemia
Alloantibody-induced immune hemolytic anemia
  Hemolytic transfusion reactions
  Hemolytic disease of the newborn

antibody AIHA. In particular, the antibody in the patient's serum and in an eluate from the patient's red cells reacts with normal red cells similarly to warm autoantibodies, and no relationship between the drug and the antibody can be demonstrated *in vitro*. Therefore, these patients could justifiably be categorized as having secondary warm antibody AIHA or immune drug-induced hemolytic anemia. We prefer the latter in order to be consistent with the purpose of the classification; in particular, prognosis and therapy are those of drug-induced immune hemolytic anemias, and they are quite distinct from secondary warm antibody AIHA associated with underlying illnesses such as chronic lymphocytic leukemia or systemic lupus erythematosus.

Other drugs (e.g., penicillin) cause the development of an antibody that has specificity for the drug and does not react with intrinsic red cell antigens. These patients are clearly not afflicted with autoimmune hemolytic anemias since the antibody does not have specificity for self-antigens. (The mechanisms by which drug-related antibodies cause red cell destruction are discussed in Chapter 8.)

Alloantibody-induced hemolytic anemias are included in the classification in Table 2-1 for completeness, but they are beyond the scope of this text, except for a discussion of the differentiation of hemolytic transfusion reactions and AIHA (Chapter 9, page 327).

Table 2-2. SOME CHARACTERISTIC FEATURES OF AUTOIMMUNE AND DRUG-INDUCED IMMUNE HEMOLYTIC ANEMIAS

Warm antibody AIHA

> Clinical manifestations: Variable, usually symptoms of anemia, occasionally acute hemolytic syndrome
> Prognosis: Fair, with significant mortality
> Therapy: Steroids, splenectomy, immunosuppressive drugs

Cold agglutinin syndrome

> Clinical manifestations: Moderate chronic hemolytic anemia in middle-aged or elderly person, often with signs and symptoms exacerbated by cold
> Prognosis: Good, usually a chronic and quite stable anemia
> Therapy: Avoid cold exposure; chlorambucil

Paroxysmal cold hemoglobinuria

> Clinical manifestations: Acute hemolytic anemia, often with hemoglobinuria, particularly in a child with history of recent viral or viral-like illness
> Prognosis: Excellent after initial stormy course
> Therapy: Not well defined; steroids empirically and transfusions if required

Drug-induced immune hemolytic anemia

> Clinical manifestations: Variable, most commonly subacute in onset, but occasionally acute hemolytic syndrome
> Prognosis: Excellent
> Therapy: Stop drug; occasionally a short course of steroids empirically

Some authors have suggested much more detailed and complicated classifications of AIHA, often based not only on the results of direct antiglobulin tests with a battery of monospecific antiglobulin sera, but also on the immunochemical nature of the autoantibody and its serologic behavior. However, we agree with those who feel that the value of serologic classification by antiglobulin reaction has been overemphasized [36, 93] and that an over sophisticated classification is of no clinical relevance.[90]

CLINICAL CHARACTERISTICS OF AUTOIMMUNE HEMOLYTIC ANEMIAS

A review of the clinical manifestations of the various categories of autoimmune hemolytic anemia seems pertinent as a preliminary to the discussion of the means of diagnosis of these disorders (Chapters 5 and 6). A large majority of autoimmune hemolytic anemias may be readily classified as warm antibody AIHA, cold agglutinin syndrome, or paroxysmal cold hemoglobinuria, and these are discussed below.

Warm Antibody AIHA

Incidence. Autoimmune hemolytic anemias are relatively uncommon but certainly not rare disorders. Their significance in clinical medicine is far greater than a statistical evaluation of their incidence might imply because of the myriad of diagnostic and therapeutic problems that they present. Nevertheless, we offer the following information for the statistically minded reader.

In Portland, Oregon, Pirofsky [98] reported the findings in patients that were referred from a population of 2.3 million in the Pacific Northwest of the United States over an eight year period. He concluded that the minimum annual incidence of warm antibody AIHA is 1 per 80,000 population. Similarly, data obtained from a hospital in Odense, Denmark that received all medical cases from a population of 230,000 indicate an annual incidence of about 1 per 75,000 population. [98] A similar study during a 5-year period in one of Sweden's health care regions indicated an incidence of 2.6 patients per 100,000 persons per year. [13]

Warm antibody AIHA is by far the most common type of acquired immune hemolytic anemia; it comprises 70.3 percent of our 347 patients (Table 2-3). Dacie and Worlledge [36] reported 284 patients with AIHA (excluding drug-induced immune hemolytic anemias), and the incidence of warm antibody AIHA was 70 percent.

Table 2-3. INCIDENCE OF VARIOUS KINDS OF ACQUIRED IMMUNE HEMOLYTIC ANEMIAS IN OUR SERIES OF 347 PATIENTS

	Number of Patients	Percent of Total
Warm AIHA	244	70.3
Cold Agglutinin Syndrome	54	15.6
Paroxysmal Cold Hemoglobinuria	6	1.7
Drug-Induced IHA	43	12.4

DRUG-INDUCED IMMUNE HEMOLYTIC ANEMIA (43 PATIENTS)

	Number of Patients	Percent of Total
Methyldopa	29	67.4
Penicillin	10	23.3
L-Dopa	1	2.3
Quinine	1	2.3
Hydrochlorothiazide	1	2.3
Rifampin	1	2.3

Age Distribution. Subjects of all ages are affected, from infants in the first few months of life until old age. In Dacie's series [35] the youngest patient was aged 5 months and the oldest 78 years when their illness was first diagnosed. Pirofsky reported ages of onset of 1 month to 87 years.[99] Of these patients 73 percent were over 40 years of age, and the peak incidence appeared between the ages of 60 and 70.

As might be anticipated, the underlying disease process has a marked effect on the age distribution. In Allgood and Chaplin's report of idiopathic cases, the peak incidence was in the fourth to seventh decades, with the mean age of onset of 48.6 years.[1] However, patients with secondary warm antibody AIHA associated with chronic lymphatic leukemia or systemic lupus erythematosus will have the age distribution of the underlying disease. This finding emphasizes that clinical features of AIHA occurring in association with other diseases are frequently dominated by underlying pathologic states.

Autoimmune hemolytic anemia in the young is not a rarity, and a large literature is available that describes such patients.[66, 98] Although clinical and laboratory findings in children are quite similar to those in adults, there are some distinctive features that will be emphasized later (Chapter 9, page 349).

Race and Sex. There is no evidence that warm antibody AIHA is confined to any particular race. Most published case reports have dealt so far with Caucasians, but Blacks do develop the disease.[98] Lie-Injo and Pillay reported on autoimmune hemolytic anemia in Malaya and concluded that the disorder is not rare.[87]

Most observers have reported a somewhat higher incidence in females than in males. In idiopathic cases, Allgood and Chaplin [1] reported that 60 percent of 47 patients were female; Dausset and Colombani [39] reported that 61 percent of 93 patients were female (said to be significant at the 95 percent probability level); Pirofsky [98] indicates that 64 percent were female; and Dacie reports 58 percent of 108 patients were female.[35] In secondary warm antibody AIHA, the percentages are more variable, perhaps depending on the incidence of underlying diseases seen in referral centers. For example, Pirofsky reported that 80 percent of cases associated with systemic lupus erythematosus were in females, whereas a male predominance was found when patients with reticuloendothelial neoplasia were analyzed.[98]

Incidence of Idiopathic and Secondary Types of Warm Antibody AIHA. Many reports of the relative incidence of idiopathic and secondary forms of autoimmune hemolytic anemia are available. The reported incidence varies significantly, possibly depending on the nature of the center to which cases were referred and also in regard to an interpretation of what constitutes a related underlying disorder. Reports suggesting that idiopathic cases are more frequent include those of Dacie and Worlledge [36] and Dausset and Colombani.[39] Approximately an equal incidence is suggested by the reviews of Dameshek and Komninos,[38] Evans and Weiser,[52] and Bell et al. (excluding drug-induced).[9] Reports suggesting that secondary cases are more common are those of Chaplin and Avioli [23] and Pirofsky. [98, 99] Pirofsky's data are heavily influenced by the fact that his patient population was characterized by many patients with leukemia and lymphoma who were undergoing constant medical follow-up. Table 2-4 summarizes the data available in the previously cited series.

Table 2-4. COMPARATIVE INCIDENCE OF IDIOPATHIC AND SECONDARY WARM ANTIBODY AIHA

Reference	Number of Cases	Idiopathic		Secondary	
		Number	Percent	Number	Percent
Dameshek and Komninos [38]	43	21	50	22	50
Dacie and Worlledge [36]	199	111	56	88	44
Dausset and Colombani [39]	106	83	78	23	22
Evans and Weiser (13) [52]	37	15	41	22	59
Bell et al [9]	37	18	49	19	51
Pirofsky [98]	234	44	19	190	81
Totals	656	292	45	364	55

Associated Diseases. Autoimmune hemolytic anemias are classified as secondary for any of several reasons. One reason is the association of AIHA with an underlying disease with a frequency greater than can be explained by chance alone. For example, all authors agree that the incidence of warm antibody AIHA is higher in patients with reticuloendothelial neoplasms and systemic lupus erythematosus than in the general population.

Another criterion for categorizing a given case of AIHA as secondary is the reversal of the hemolytic anemia simultaneously with the correction of the associated disease. Ovarian tumors are a good example; well documented cases of cure of the AIHA after surgical removal of the tumor have been reported. [4, 16, 40] (See Chapter 11, page 430.)

Still another reason for suspecting a relationship between the occurrence of AIHA and an associated disease consists of evidence of immunologic aberration as part of the underlying disorder, especially if the associated disease is thought to have an autoimmune pathogenesis. However, when the coexistence of two immunologic disorders in a single patient is infrequent, the pathogenetic significance is conjectural and interpretations vary. Allgood and Chaplin [1] noted the presence of ulcerative colitis and rheumatoid arthritis in some of their patients but still considered the AIHA idiopathic, whereas Pirofsky [98] included these and numerous other disorders among patients classified as having secondary AIHA. Indeed, rheumatoid arthritis is an extremely common disorder and there are only occasional reports of an associated AIHA, so the combination may well be coincidental. In ulcerative colitis, four reports of resolution of the hemolytic anemia after colectomy, [114] the frequent further association with other immunologically mediated abnormalities, and the frequent sequential development of immunologic abnormalities in a single patient lend weight to speculations that ulcerative colitis and AIHA should be considered as only two parts of a complex, immunologically mediated multi-system disease state.[98] In general, the evidence for a relationship between immunologic disorders, including immune deficiency states, and AIHA is strong [12, 37, 59–61, 83, 98, 103] although the pathogenetic basis for such a relationship has not been clarified.

The significance of the relationship between other associated diseases and AIHA is far less clear in many reported cases of "secondary" AIHA. Occasionally reported associated diseases that are not clearly of significance include leukemias other than chronic lymphocytic leukemia, thyroid disease, myeloproliferative disorders, pernicious anemia, cirrhosis of the liver, carcinomas, and bacterial infections.[37]

On the basis of the preceding information, we believe that warm antibody AIHA may reasonably be classified as secondary when associated with the diseases listed in Table 2-5.

Table 2-5. DISORDERS FREQUENTLY ASSOCIATED WITH WARM ANTIBODY AIHA *

Reticuloendothelial neoplasms

    Chronic lymphocytic leukemia
    Hodgkin's disease
    Non-Hodgkin's lymphomas
    Thymomas
    Multiple myeloma
    Waldenström's macroglobulinemia

Collagen diseases

    Systemic lupus erythematosus
    Scleroderma
    Rheumatoid arthritis

Infectious diseases, especially childhood viral syndromes

Immunologic diseases

    Hypogammaglobulinemia
    Dysglobulinemias
    Other immune deficiency syndromes

Gastrointestinal disease
    Ulcerative colitis

Benign tumors
    Ovarian dermoid cyst

---

* Although some drugs cause hemolytic anemia with laboratory findings similar to warm antibody AIHA, we prefer to consider them under the heading of drug-induced immune hemolytic anemias (see page 26).

Presenting Symptoms. Warm antibody AIHA is an extremely variable disorder, and almost every grade of severity may be encountered. In some patients the onset is slow and insidious over a period of months, with the ultimate emergence of symptomatic anemia. In other patients the onset is sudden, with fever, abdominal or back pain, malaise, and manifestations of rapidly increasing anemia. In severe anemia, neurologic manifestations may occur that progress from obtundation to coma and death. In children, the disease not infrequently appears as an acute and sometimes fulminating disorder. Although such acute manifestations are serious and present difficult problems in management, they may be of short duration, with complete recovery within a few weeks.[35, 66]

In patients with secondary AIHA, the associated pathologic state may cause the most prominent of the patient's symptoms and obscure the symptoms of the hemolytic anemia. Considering the diversity of underlying diseases associated with AIHA, a complete list of presenting symptoms would be encyclopedic and of little or no value. But considering only those symptoms that may relate specifically to the hemolytic state, weakness is the most common complaint; it occurs in 87 percent of Pirofsky's series.[98] Other common symptoms are fever and jaundice, although neither of these symptoms occurs in a majority of patients.

Symptoms relating directly to the presence of anemia and that resolve upon improvement in the level of hemoglobin include dizziness, palpitations, and dyspnea on exertion. Angina, edema, and frank congestive heart failure occur in a small percentage of patients.

A history of dark urine may be elicited; this condition may result from the presence of bile pigments or hemoglobinuria (also see Chapter 1). Hemolytic jaundice is classically regarded as acholuric but, in seriously ill patients, significant amounts of conjugated bilirubin may circulate in the plasma, and bile pigment may appear in the urine.[35, 41] Furthermore, urobilinogen frequently darkens the color of the urine, especially on standing.[41] Hemoglobinuria may cause the urine to be pink, red, brown, or almost black, depending on the concentration and relative proportions of oxyhemoglobin, which is bright red, and methemoglobin, which is dark brown. The final color of the urine is determined by the concentration of hemoglobin, the pH of the urine, and duration of contact between hemoglobin and urine.[10] Hemoglobinuria is quite unusual in adults, but it is a prominent finding in the most seriously ill patients. It is much more common in children.

Physical Signs. The diagnosis of anemia on the basis of physical signs is remarkably difficult, and the classic observation of pallor is quite unreliable. Jaundice is more commonly observed; it occurred as a presenting sign in 39 percent of the patients in Pirofsky's series.[98] Splenomegaly is present in a slight majority of patients, reported by Allgood and Chaplin[1] in 57 percent of patients with idiopathic warm antibody AIHA, and by Pirofsky[98] in just over 50 percent of the patients with either idiopathic or secondary AIHA. The organ is generally firm, non-tender, and only slightly to moderately enlarged. It is unusual for an enlarged spleen to reach the umbilicus and, on the whole, the degree of splenomegaly is less than that found in hereditary spherocytosis.

Hepatomegaly occurs in about one third of the patients with idiopathic AIHA, and the organ is usually firm and non-tender. Liver enlargement is generally moderate, and massive hepatomegaly is rare.[99] The incidence of lymphadenopathy varies in reported series depending, at least in part, on the relative proportion of idiopathic and secondary cases. In Dacie's series of predominantly idiopathic warm antibody AIHA, the enlargement of lymph nodes was distinctly unusual.[35] In contrast, Pirofsky[98] reported lymphadenopathy in 37 percent of the patients with secondary AIHA, a majority of whom had reticuloendothelial neoplasia. However, Pirofsky also found that 23 percent of the patients with idiopathic warm antibody AIHA had lymphadenopathy, and that, overall, enlargement of the various reticuloendothelial structures was the most consistent abnormality on physical examination. Only 26 percent of all patients manifested no enlargement of spleen, liver, or lymph nodes.

The Blood Picture. The degree of anemia is variable, but it is not infrequently severe. Allgood and Chaplin [1] reported that the initial hemoglobin concentration in 21 of 47 patients was less than 7 gm/dl. Although only a moderate anemia may be present on admission, a meticulous follow-up is required, particularly when the patient is first observed. Progression of the severity of the anemia frequently occurs before therapy becomes effective, and the fall in hemoglobin and hematocrit may be rapid, justifying the terms "acute hemolytic anemia" or "hemolytic crisis." Indeed, Pirofsky [99] emphasizes that among 213 patients, the lowest hematocrit ranged from 7.5 percent to 41.5 percent, but with a median value of only 19 percent. A hematocrit of 15 percent or less was observed in 49 patients! Similarly, Crosby and Rappaport [32] reported hemoglobin values of 5 gm/dl or less in 15 of 34 patients.

Autoagglutination *in vitro* is a phenomenon occasionally observed, particularly in more severely affected patients. The agglutination typically consists of rather fine clumps of red cells that may be visible to the naked eye on close observation and, in contrast to those caused by cold agglutinins, they do not change after incubation at 37°C (also see Chapter 6, page 186).

The white blood count is normal in more than half of the patients with idiopathic AIHA [1, 98] but, of course, it varies greatly among patients with secondary AIHA, depending on the underlying disease. Even in patients with idiopathic disease, a range of values extending from 1,400 to 37,000 per μl was obtained in Pirofsky's series.[98] Leukocyte counts of less than 2,000 per μl were observed in 6 of 38 patients. These results occurred in a pattern of peripheral pancytopenia with hypoplastic or normal bone marrows and may be a manifestation of an immune pancytopenia.

In acute hemolytic episodes, however, leukocytosis is frequent, with counts usually ranging from 15,000 to 25,000 per μl. This finding is chiefly the result of an increase in neutrophils with occasional metamyelocytes and myelocytes as part of a leukemoid reaction.

Counts considerably in excess of the preceding figures have been reported, especially in children.[35] The highest white cell count in Pirofsky's series[98] was a 2½ year old infant in whom the count was 37,000 per μl, chiefly lymphocytes. Twenty-two of 46 patients reported by Habibi et al.[66] had leukocytosis with total white cell counts as high as 40,000 per μl and with promyelocytes and myelocytes accounting for up to 20 percent of the total.

Platelet counts are usually normal in idiopathic warm antibody AIHA. A minority of patients have thrombocytosis which, on occasion, reaches impressive heights. Allgood and Chaplin[1] reported that 24 percent of their patients had thrombocytosis at the time of presentation, with the highest value recorded being 1,900,000 per μl. Pirofsky[99] reports that 17 percent of his patients with AIHA in the absence of malignant lymphoid disease had thrombocytosis, with the highest value being greater than 1,000,000 per μl.

Thrombocytopenia occurs in some patients in all large series of warm antibody AIHA. In 1949, Evans and Duane[51] called attention to this association, and the simultaneous occurrence of thrombocytopenia and AIHA is now well recognized and is frequently referred to as "Evans' syndrome." Dausset and Colombani,[39] in a review of 83 patients with idiopathic warm antibody anemia, encountered thrombocytopenic purpura in 11 (13.2 percent). Allgood and Chaplin[1] reported thrombocytopenia in 3 of 47 patients at the time of diagnosis of the hemolytic anemia; 3 others either had a history of thrombocytopenia, or thrombocytopenia developed at some time after the diagnosis of AIHA was made.

In addition to these clinical observations, Zucker-Franklin and Karpatkin[136] presented data indicating that autoimmune mechanisms may be directed against erythrocytes as well as platelets in most patients with severe idiopathic autoimmune thrombocytopenia. They noted that routine blood smears of patients with chronic autoimmune thrombocytopenic purpura (idiopathic thrombocytopenic purpura) commonly showed platelets larger than normal with many giant forms, but Coulter-counter volume measurements of platelets also revealed a distinct peak in the area in which particles with volumes much below those of normal platelets would be located. By electron microscopy, erythrocyte as well as platelet fragments were found in the 27,000 × g plasma sediment of 15 patients with severe disease. These fragments were not observed in the plasma sediment of 12 normal subjects, 2 healthy asplenic subjects, 3 patients with thrombocytopenia of nonimmunologic origin, and 2 with autoimmune thrombocytopenic purpura in remission.

Both Dacie[35] and Pirofsky[98] emphasize that anemia and thrombocytopenia do not necessarily appear at the same time; several years may elapse between these two manifestations. Several cases have been reported in which AIHA supervened in patients who had undergone splenectomy several years earlier for thrombocytopenic purpura.[35] Allgood and Chaplin mentioned one patient who developed AIHA 25 years after splenectomy for thrombocytopenic purpura, and they emphasized that the two disorders may be entirely unrelated in respect to time of onset and response to steroid therapy and/or splenectomy.[1]

Crosby [31] and Crosby and Rappaport [32] have pointed out that the prognosis appears worse when thrombocytopenia is present in AIHA. Of the patients they reviewed, 12 of 17 patients with thrombocytopenia died, compared with 5 of 16 patients who did not have thrombocytopenia. Chertkow and Dacie [24] derived a similar conclusion from their data, but Allgood and Chaplin [1] found no relationship between initial platelet count and mortality.

Reticulocytes. As in other types of hemolytic anemias, a persistently raised reticulocyte count is a typical and characteristic finding in patients with warm antibody AIHA. On occasion the count may exceed 50 percent. However, reticulocytopenia is recognized as an important although uncommon manifestation of AIHA. Diagnosis is difficult since AIHA does not seem to be a logical consideration in the presence of reticulocytopenia, especially if it is associated with pancytopenia and a hypoplastic bone marrow. However, serologic findings typical of warm antibody AIHA, followed by an excellent therapeutic response to corticosteroids have been reported in just such cases. [98]

Both acute aplastic crises [15, 113] and more prolonged crises with severe reticulocytopenia [18, 48, 86] have been observed. Burston et al. [18] reported two patients in whom AIHA was accompanied by reticulocytopenia, leukopenia, thrombocytopenia (in one patient), and marrow aplasia. The first patient gradually recovered following steroid therapy; the second, who had reticulocytopenia and leukopenia only, died of tuberculosis that may have been reactivated by corticosteroid therapy. In other patients, AIHA and reticulocytopenia associated with pure red cell aplasia in the bone marrow have been reported. [48, 89, 98]

Not all patients with hemolysis and reticulocytopenia have hypoplastic bone marrows. Hegde et al. [69] reported three patients with acquired hemolytic anemia who had low reticulocyte counts at a time when their bone marrows showed normal or even increased numbers of erythroid precursors.

The cause of reticulocytopenia in AIHA has been investigated, and experimental studies suggest that antigenic determinants on erythrocyte precursors can react with erythrocyte autoantibodies. Pisciotta and Hinz [100] and Yunis and Yunis [135] have demonstrated that erythrocyte autoantibodies can interact with nucleated erythrocytes. More recently, Meyer et al. [89] described a patient with systemic lupus erythematosus and autoimmune hemolytic anemia complicated by periodic episodes of red cell hypoplasia. These investigators demonstrated that erythroid colony formation by normal human bone marrow cells *in vitro* was inhibited by both the patient's serum and an eluate from his red cells. Autoantibodies from other patients with AIHA but without pure red cell aplasia did not cause such inhibition.

Pancytopenia and bone marrow aplasia may also be due to immune mechanisms. Leukocyte antibodies and thrombocyte antibodies have been documented in patients with autoimmune hemolytic anemia. [54] It is therefore possible for antibody formation, either multiple or single, to result in leukopenia, thrombocytopenia, or pancytopenia with hypoplastic bone marrow.[2] This immunologic explanation is an expansion of earlier views of Fisher [57] and Evans and Duane.[51]

Crosby and Rappaport [32] have reported that reticulocytopenia at the time of intense hemolysis carries a high mortality rate, even in the face of bone marrow erythrocytic hyperplasia. Dausset and Colombani [39] made a similar observation, whereas Allgood and Chaplin [1] found no relationship between mortality and the initial reticulocytic count.

Prognosis and Survival. The natural history of warm antibody AIHA is unpredictable, with no firm conclusions possible regarding clinical, hematologic, or serologic features that would enable one to predict the ultimate course in a patient once the diagnosis has been made. Some early suggestions that mortality is increased in patients who have a positive indirect antiglobulin test [39] or who have reticulocytopenia [32] have not been confirmed in more recent series.[1, 115]

The mortality rate in most series is quite high, but it is perhaps gradually improving in recent years. Early reviews on prognosis were discouraging, with reports by Crosby and Rappaport in 1957 [32] of a 32 percent mortality in 50 patients, a 31 percent mortality in 83 cases reported by Dausset and Colombani in 1959,[39] and a 46 percent mortality rate in 50 cases reported by Dacie in 1962.[35] However, some of these patients did not receive corticosteroids, or they received inadequate trials of therapy.

However, prognosis even in more recent series has not been good. Pirofsky, in reviewing patients studied between 1958 and 1966, reported a mortality rate of 38 percent in patients with idiopathic AIHA, and a mortality twice as great in secondary AIHA (primarily associated with reticuloendothelial neoplasia).[98] The mortality reported by Allgood and Chaplin was 38 percent in their 47 patients with idiopathic AIHA observed between 1955 and 1965.[1]

Some more encouraging reports have appeared. In 1974, Worlledge [133] suggested that prognosis may have improved with modern therapy since the mortality was only 14 percent in 85 patients followed for periods of 3 months to 7 years. This finding compares favorably with the earlier report from the same institution of a 46 percent mortality.[35] Silverstein et al.[115] analyzed the records of 117 patients observed between 1955 and 1965. Using actuarial survival curves, they concluded that the lethality of acquired hemolytic anemia is much less than previously reported. The survival rate was 91 percent at 1 year, 76 percent at 5 years, and 73 percent at 10 years.

Cold Agglutinin Syndrome

History. Cold agglutinins were initially demonstrated by Landsteiner in 1903 [84] but their significance in human disease was not accurately appreciated until several decades later. A recognition of the relationship between cold agglutinins, hemolytic anemia, Raynaud's phenomenon, and hemoglobinuria began to emerge with the case reports of Iwai and Mei-Sai in 1925 and 1926.[75, 76] Their first patient was a 36-year-old Chinese man giving a 6-year history of Raynaud's disease. His serum contained a cold agglutinin that reacted to a titer of 1,000 at 0°C and reacted up to 30°C against normal red cells as well as those of the patient. They demonstrated that the circulation of the patient's blood through fine tubes was impeded when the blood was cooled to 5°C and suggested that the Raynaud's phenomenon might be related to mechanical obstruction by autoagglutinated red cells. In their second patient, a woman aged 78, they showed that cooling of the fingers was associated with breaking of the column of blood in the capillaries of the nail bed. However, in neither case did the authors describe hemoglobinuria or anemia.

Roth, in 1935, reported a 59-year-old man who suffered from Raynaud's phenomenon affecting his hands, feet, and nose when exposed to mild degrees of cold.[110] More severe chilling produced hemoglobinuria. The author noted that the patient's blood underwent rapid autoagglutination after withdrawal, which was reversed by warming.

In the same year Ernstene and Gardner [50] reported a 38-year-old man who had attacks of hemoglobinuria and Raynaud's phenomenon on exposure to cold. Autoagglutination of his blood was noted at room temperature, red blood cell counts were difficult to perform, the cold agglutinin titer was 1280, and he was anemic with a hemoglobin of 10.5 gm/dl.

In spite of these early reports, the syndrome did not receive wide recognition and the pathogenetic role of cold agglutinins was not well accepted. Indeed, as late as 1943, Stats and Wasserman [116] published a review of cold hemagglutination in which they expressed the then prevalent viewpoint that cold agglutinins were not the cause of hemolytic disease but only a secondary phenomenon. An accurate description of the syndrome and features that distinguished it from other forms of AIHA appeared during the 1950's. The hemolytic activity of serum of patients with cold agglutinin disease had not been well recognized because the pH of blood rapidly rises to pH 8 and higher *in vitro* following the loss of CO_2, and the antibodies do not cause optimal lysis at alkaline pH. Dacie demonstrated the presence of cold hemolysis in sera containing cold agglutinins by adding a trace of hydrochloric acid to produce a slightly acid pH value.[33] However, he still used the two-step temperature arrangement in the classic Donath-Landsteiner test. In 1952 Schubothe pointed out that hemolysis caused by the cold agglutinins does not have a bithermic mode of action but takes place monothermically.[112] He introduced the term "cold hemagglutinin disease" to separate the disorder from other acquired hemolytic anemias.

More recently, numerous case reports and detailed reviews of clinical findings, laboratory features, serologic and immunochemical characterization of the antibodies, and the pathogenesis of the disorder have been published.[28, 29, 35, 58, 67, 77, 88, 101, 106, 130]

Age, Sex, and Incidence. Patients with cold agglutinin disease are typically middle-aged or elderly. Schubothe [112] noted a peak incidence of onset from ages 51 to 60. However, 26 percent of the patients were less than 41 years of age, a finding possibly resulting from the inclusion of patients with the acute transient variant of the disease who are more frequently younger. In Dacie's series,[35] only 3 of 21 patients with idiopathic cold agglutinin syndrome were younger than 50, whereas 9 of 12 post-pneumonia cases occurred in patients between the ages of 20 and 45.

Both sexes are affected, and there is no clear predominance in males or females.

The cold agglutinin syndrome is relatively uncommon compared with warm antibody AIHA, but it occurs much more frequently than paroxysmal cold hemoglobinuria. In our series of 347 patients with acquired immune hemolytic anemias (including drug-induced immune hemolytic anemia), 54 patients (15.6 percent) had cold agglutinin syndrome (Table 2-3). Dacie and Worlledge [36] reported that 25 percent of their patients with AIHA had cold agglutinin syndrome, whereas van Loghem et al.[123] and Dausset and Colombani [39] reported an incidence of only 7.7 percent.

Symptoms and Signs. Symptoms are frequently just those of a chronic anemia. In idiopathic cases, the disorder usually remains quite static and at worst only progresses slowly in intensity.

Patients may experience hemoglobinuria, particularly in cold weather, and this finding is prominent among manifestations listed in reviews of the disorder. However, its incidence is difficult to determine, and in many patients hemoglobinuria is never observed. This finding is true even in some patients with severe Raynaud's phenomenon. When an episode of intravascular hemolysis does occur after cold exposure, it is not associated with fever, chills, or acute renal insufficiency.[98, 112] This phenomenon contrasts with the marked constitutional symptoms associated with hemoglobinuria in paroxysmal cold hemoglobinuria or in those few patients with warm antibody AIHA who have hemoglobinuria.

Many affected patients complain of acrocyanosis of the ears, the nose tip, fingers, and toes in cold temperatures, a condition that vanishes quickly on warming. These symptoms are caused by autoagglutination of the patient's erythrocytes in the skin capillaries causing local blood stasis. As blood flows through the capillaries of the skin and subcutaneous tissue, the temperature of the blood falls to as low as 28°C if the ambient temperature is low.[3] Since the cold antibody is active at this temperature in patients with *in vivo* hemolysis (see Chapter 6, page 213), it agglutinates cells and fixes complement. *In vivo* agglutination can be directly demonstrated by microscopy of conjunctival vessels after local administration of ice-cold saline or by finger plethysmography after local exposure to cold.[67]

The acrocyanosis associated with cold agglutinins may be distinguished from the much more common Raynaud's phenomenon that may be idiopathic or associated with diseases such as collagen vascular disorders. In the former, the exposed distal fingers or toes turn a dusky blue that either quickly reverts to normal on warming or may progress to blanching after more prolonged or more severe cold exposure. In the latter event, the digits characteristically turn white and then, as ischemica is resolving, turn blue; this change may be followed by a hyperemic phase in which the exposed parts become reddened. Further, exposure to moderate degrees of cold in patients with cold agglutinins will cause all digits to be equally affected, whereas Raynaud's phenomenon not associated with cold agglutinins may cause marked blanching of one or two fingers with the others remaining normal.

Occasionally actual gangrene, particularly of a digit or digits, has been observed.[35] Although the occurrence of gangrene after prolonged exposure to cold would appear to be a logical consequence of vascular insufficiency caused by autohemagglutination, there is some question as to whether the presence of cryoglobulins may not be critical instead. In a minority of patients with cold agglutinin syndrome, the cold antibody is a cold precipitable protein.[101] Ferriman et al.,[55] Rørvik,[107] and Gaddy and Powell[62] all reported cases of cold agglutinin syndrome associated with tissue gangrene in which cryoglobulins were present.

Physical findings are infrequent. Pallor and jaundice may, of course, be present, but hepatosplenomegaly and lymphadenopathy are not prominent findings. Dacie[35] reports that the spleen is palpably enlarged only in a minority of patients, whereas Schubothe[112] states that usually the spleen and sometimes the liver are slightly enlarged. Dausset and Colombani[39] noted splenomegaly in 6 of 10 patients.

Laboratory Findings. Autoagglutination of blood samples that occurs quickly as blood cools to room temperature is characteristic and is frequently the first observation made to suggest the diagnosis. The agglutination creates problems in making satisfactory blood films and performing blood counts. However, it should be stressed that the mere observance of cold autoagglutination is not diagnostic of the disorder, and that the cold antibodies must be further characterized as described in Chapter 6, page 213.

In classic cases the degree of anemia varies with the degree of cold exposure, and seasonal anemia has been described.[35] More commonly, the patient has a chronic, fairly stable anemia that is mild or moderate in severity. For example, in only 2 of the 12 patients reviewed by Ferriman et al.[55] did the hemoglobin fall below 7.4 gm/dl. Similarly, Schubothe[112] reported 16 patients followed for "several years," and every patient had a hemoglobin of 9 mg/dl or greater at some time during the period, and in only 2 patients did the hemoglobin fall below 6.5 gm/dl at any time. This finding contrasts strikingly with hemoglobin values in warm AIHA or paroxysmal cold hemoglobinuria (see pages 34 and 56, respectively).

Erythrocyte morphology is less abnormal than in patients with warm antibody AIHA, with lesser degrees of anisocytosis and poikilocytosis. Similarly, spherocytosis is less intense but has been noted by Leddy and Swisher,[85] Schreiber et al.,[111] and Rosse.[109] Reticulocytosis usually is in proportion to the severity of hemolysis, and reticulocytopenia is rare. Leukocyte and platelet counts are usually normal. Bilirubinemia of mild degree is common.

Hemosiderinuria may occur even in patients without gross hemoglobinuria and is a reflection of less intense intravascular hemolysis.

Bone marrow morphology is discussed later in this chapter (page 48).

Prognosis. The prognosis in patients with idiopathic cold agglutinin syndrome is significantly better than it is in patients with warm antibody AIHA. Schubothe [112] describes the course of the disease as "monotonous," and patients may survive many years, suffering minimal disability. Most patients tolerate their mild or moderate anemia quite well. In more severe cases, however, death may ensue from complications of slowly progressive anemia, or from complications of blood transfusion. Therapy, as reviewed in detail in Chapter 11, usually has little effect on the outcome of the disease.

Associated Diseases. *Reticuloendothelial Neoplasia.* The association of hemolytic anemia, high titer cold agglutinins and reticuloendothelial neoplasia is uncommon. Nevertheless, occasional cases have been described in association with chronic lymphatic leukemia, "lymphosarcoma," "reticulum cell sarcoma," Hodgkin's disease, and multiple myeloma.[98] In these disorders the course is primarily determined by the activity of the underlying malignant disease. The relationship of cold agglutinin syndrome and Waldenström's macroglobulinemia is discussed separately (see page 48).

The cold agglutinin syndrome may also occur as a transient disorder in association with a number of underlying infectious diseases, particularly *Mycoplasma pneumoniae* infections and infectious mononucleosis.

Mycoplasma Pneumoniae Infections. Approximately half the patients with *M. pneumoniae* pneumonia have elevated titers of cold hemagglutinins (titers greater than 64) or a fourfold or greater increase in titer. An acute cold agglutinin response is sometimes seen in viral infections such as influenza A and infectious mononucleosis, but very high titers are seen almost exclusively in mycoplasmal pneumonia. Subclinical hemolysis may be common, but only 51 cases of overt immune hemolytic anemia have been reported in the world literature.[118]

When cold agglutinin syndrome occurs in association with *Mycoplasma pneumoniae* infection, it does so usually in the second or third week of the patient's illness. A rapid onset of hemolysis is frequently observed, and abnormal IgM cold agglutinins (which characteristically have anti-I specificity) are present. The patient may already be recovered from his respiratory infection, but he becomes ill once more with increasing pallor and jaundice. Splenomegaly is generally present; acrocyanosis and hemoglobinuria are unusual,[98] and gangrene on exposure to cold is very rare. Hemolysis is self-limiting and usually resolves in two to three weeks. However, the hemolytic anemia may proceed at an alarming rate and, indeed, several fatalities have been reported.[35, 118] The disorder may be more pronounced in patients with glucose-6-phosphate dehydrogenase deficiency and sickle-cell disease.[118]

The mechanism by which cold agglutinins are elicited by *M. pneumoniae* has been studied by several groups of investigators. The cold agglutinin produced in response to human infection with the organism, as well as the antibody found in idiopathic cold agglutinin syndrome, usually have specificity for the blood group I antigen contained in red cell glycoproteins. Janney et al.[78] reported results of experiments consistent with the hypothesis that the cold agglutinin that arises during *M. pneumoniae* infection and that is inhibited by erythrocyte glycoprotein is a cross-reactive response to mycoplasmal antigens, as had previously been proposed by others.

Management consists primarily of keeping the patient warm. If blood transfusion seems necessary, the principles and techniques reviewed for cold agglutinin syndrome in Chapter 10 should be followed. Steroids have been used, but most investigators consider them to be ineffective. Tetracycline and erythromycin are effective against *M. pneumoniae,* but at the time hemolysis begins the pneumonia may be resolved. Nevertheless, in some patients who delay seeking medical attention for their respiratory symptoms, antibiotic therapy has seemed to promptly resolve both the pneumonia and the hemolytic anemia. Further details of therapy are described in Chapter 11.

Infectious Mononucleosis. Clinical Findings: Acute hemolytic anemia complicating infectious mononucleosis is an infrequent but well described occurrence. Worlledge and Dacie[134] estimated the incidence of major hemolysis as less than 1 in 1,000 cases. Hoagland[70] stated that approximately 3 percent of the patients in his series of 500 patients with infectious mononucleosis had hemolytic anemia, and that minor degrees of hemolysis possibly occur more frequently than this.[22] Some of the clinical features of hemolytic anemia occurring in association with infectious mononucleosis[134] are listed in Table 2-6. Signs of hemolysis usually develop one to two weeks after the onset of symptoms of infectious mononucleosis; less frequently, both develop simul-

TABLE 2-6. CLINICAL FINDINGS IN HEMOLYTIC ANEMIA ASSOCIATED WITH INFECTIOUS MONONUCLEOSIS

Onset of hemolysis in	1 week	28%
relation to the onset	7–13 days	44%
of infectious mononucleosis	14–21 days	15%
	21 days	13%
Duration of hemolysis	under 1 month	71%
	1–2 months	25%
	more than 2 months	4%
Enlargement of spleen	palpable	74%
	not palpable	26%
Enlargement of liver	palpable	74%
	not palpable	26%

taneously. Occasionally hemolytic anemia becomes obvious as late as two months after the initial symptoms. The usual history is that of an acute illness, with high fever, followed by weakness, anemia, and jaundice. Sore throat, lymphadenopathy and hepatosplenomegaly are common. Some patients have had hemoglobinuria.[82]

Laboratory Findings: The degree of anemia may be mild to severe, with a corresponding rise in reticulocyte count after the initial stages. Spherocytosis and an accompanying increased fragility of red cells have often been reported.

Serologic findings are varied, and the knowledge of the characteristics of the autoantibodies in this disorder has undergone a particularly interesting evolution. Jenkins et al.[79] in 1965 first reported a case of hemolytic anemia in infectious mononucleosis that was apparently mediated by the temporary production of a high thermal amplitude cold agglutinin of anti-i specificity. In the same year Calvo et al.[19] reported a second case of hemolytic anemia complicating infectious mononucleosis in which an anti-i cold agglutinin was implicated. The latter group described the presence of anti-i cold agglutinins in 23 of 38 uncomplicated cases of infectious mononucleosis. Other reports [108, 132] confirmed and extended these findings. Troxel et al.[121] were the third group to report anti-i antibodies in a case of hemolytic anemia in infectious mononucleosis. They found an IgM autoagglutinin of anti-i specificity in their patient's serum to a titer of 128 at 37°C. These authors also suggested the possibility that previously reported cases of hemolytic anemia in infectious mononucleosis with negative direct antiglobulin tests might represent the absence of anticomplement activity in the antiglobulin sera used.

The preceding reports led to the general acceptance of the concept that anti-i played a major role in the hemolytic anemia that is occasionally a part of infectious mononucleosis.[134] This conclusion was facilitated by the ready analogy apparent in the hemolytic anemia that may complicate pneumonia due to *Mycoplasma pneumoniae* which is mediated by anti-I cold agglutinins. That is, it was suggested that a large percentage of patients with infectious mononucleosis develop anti-i (analogous to the development of anti-I in the case of *Mycoplasma pneumoniae* infections), but only occasionally is the antibody of sufficient titer and thermal amplitude to mediate *in vivo* hemolysis.

In contrast to these reports regarding IgM antibodies, Goldberg and Barnett [64] and Capra et al.[20] have presented data implicating an IgG anti-i in the hemolytic anemia of infectious mononucleosis. The recognition of a patient with hemolytic anemia complicating infectious mononucleosis who had an incomplete IgG cold agglutinin of anti-i specificity prompted the latter investigators to investigate the prevalence of IgG anti-i in infectious mononucleosis. They demonstrated such antibodies reactive at 4°C in the sera of 45 of 50 patients with infectious mononucleosis. In addition, they reported the presence of a "19S" anti-IgG in 72 percent of these patients, and postulated an interaction of the IgG anti-i and the IgM anti-IgG in most instances of infectious mononucleosis. However, these authors do not present any data indicating that these antibodies were reactive at physiologic temperatures. Indeed, thermal amplitude studies revealed only "slight activity" of anti-i at 25°C in just 2 of the 4 eluates tested. Goldberg and Barnett [64] point out that at room temperature they could detect "very slight" IgG anti-i activity, and the IgM anti-globulin reactivity occurred exclusively at 4°C. Such antibodies would therefore appear to be of little clinical significance.

More recently, Wilkinson, Petz and Garratty [128] reported a detailed serologic evaluation of three patients during moderate to severe hemolytic anemia in infectious mononucleosis. These studies revealed high thermal amplitude anti-i in only one. This patient's direct antiglobulin test (Patient, T.W., Table 2-7) was negative using anti-IgG but was 3+ using anti-C3 and anti-C4. The serum antibody titer against i adult or i cord red cells was 256–512 at 4°C and 4 at 31°C (Table 2-8). The anti-i was inhibited by mercaptoethanol, and anti-IgG was not found in the patient's serum. Patient H.P. had a negative direct antiglobulin test, and patient W.R. had a 2+ direct antiglobulin test using anti-C3 and anti-C4. Anti-i was present only in low titer at 4°C and was unreactive at 20°C in these patients's sera. It was inhibited by mercaptoethanol. The sera of patients H.P. and W.R. contained anti-IgG antibodies. In none of our patients were warm autoantibodies detected. These data demonstrate that hemolytic anemia in infectious mononucleosis is not necessarily associated with high thermal amplitude anti-i. Further, since the anti-i antibodies in patients H.P. and W.R. were of low titer, were inhibited by mercaptoethanol, and did not react at physiologic temperatures, the mechanism of hemolysis in these patients did not seem related to the interaction of IgM anti-IgG antibodies and IgG anti-i antibodies.

Thus, although high thermal amplitude anti-i antibodies are associated with some cases of hemolytic anemia in infectious mononucleosis, our data indicated instances in which hemolysis cannot be attributed either to temporary production of high thermal amplitude cold agglutinins of anti-i specific-

Table 2-7. DIRECT ANTIGLOBULIN TESTS IN THREE PATIENTS WITH INFECTIOUS MONONUCLEOSIS AND HEMOLYTIC ANEMIA

Antisera	Patient	Dilutions of Antiglobulin sera						Score
		4	8	16	32	64	128	
Anti-IgG	T.W.	0	0	0	0	0	0	0
	H.P.	0	0	0	0	0	0	0
	W.R.	0	0	0	0	0	0	0
Anti-C3	T.W.	3+	3+	2½+	2+	1+	0	33
	H.P.	0	0	0	0	0	0	0
	W.R.	2+	1½+	1+	1+	½+	0	21
Anti-C4	T.W.	3+	2+	1+	0	0	0	18
	H.P.	0	0	0	0	0	0	0
	W.R.	2+	1½+	1+	1+	0	0	19

Agglutination reactions are graded as ½+ to 4+.
(Wilkinson, L. S., Petz, L. D., and Garratty, G.: Reappraisal of the role of anti-i in haemolytic anaemia in infectious mononucleosis. Brit. J. Haematol., 25:715, 1973.)

Table 2-8. COLD AGGULUTININ CHARACTERISTICS IN 3
PATIENTS WITH INFECTIOUS MONONUCLEOSIS AND
HEMOLYTIC ANEMIA

| Cells | Temperature (°C) | Agglutination Titer | | |
| | | Patient | | |
		T.W.	H.P.	W.R.
I Adult	4	64	0	0
	22	2	0	0
	31	0	0	0
	37	0	0	0
i Cord	4	512	1	4
	22	64	0	0
	31	4	0	0
	37	0	0	0
i Adult	4	256	1	4
	22	64	0	0
	31	4	0	0
	37	0	0	0

(Wilkinson, L. S., Petz, L. D., and Garratty, G.: Reappraisal of the role of
anti-i in haemolytic anaemia in infectious mononucleosis. Brit. J. Haematol.,
25:715, 1973.)

ity or to the interaction of anti-IgG with IgG anti-i antibodies at physiologic
temperatures. It seems unlikely that a single mechanism is operative in all
cases of hemolytic anemia in infectious mononucleosis. This idea is further
evidenced by reports of infectious mononucleosis complicated by acute
hemolytic anemia with a positive Donath-Landsteiner reaction [49, 131] and by a
case associated with an auto anti-N antibody. [14]

Further studies of the cold agglutinins in infectious mononucleosis and
heterophil-antibody-negative mononucleosis-like syndromes were carried out
by Horwitz et al. [72] These investigators studied the sera of 150 patients with
heterophil-antibody-positive infectious mononucleosis; 7 patients with
heterophil-negative, Epstein-Barr virus-induced infectious mononucleosis; 31
patients with heterophil-antibody-negative mononucleosis-like syndrome due
to cytomegalovirus or unspecified agents; and 1,250 controls. They found
that anti-i was reasonably specific for Epstein-Barr virus-induced infectious
mononucleosis and that it occurred in 31.8 percent of heterophil-positive and
heterophil-negative patients, but in only 0.8 percent of controls. Anti-i was not
found in patients with cytomegalovirus-induced disease. In agreement with
the findings of Wilkinson et al., [128] they were unable to demonstrate IgG anti-i
antibodies, but their serum specimens were obtained mainly from patients
without obvious hemolysis.

Some authors emphasize that evidence for an immune mechanism is
scanty in many cases. Indeed, the direct antiglobulin test was negative in 39
percent of the patients reviewed by Worlledge and Dacie. [134] Some of these

negative reactions may be related to the fact that, in earlier years, it was not realized that the detection of complement components on the red cell surface may indicate a previous antigen-antibody reaction. However, even more recent reports [134] (including our own previously cited study [128]) document that some patients with hemolytic anemia have a negative direct antiglobulin test even when it is performed with polyspecific and monospecific antiglobulin sera used in serial dilutions.

One further interesting facet of the hemolytic anemia associated with infectious mononucleosis is related to the findings of Giblett and Crookston [63] who found that patients suffering from various blood diseases, including thalassemia and hereditary spherocytosis, often show increased agglutinability by anti-i. This increased agglutinability by anti-i probably accounts for the fact that occurrences of hemolytic anemia in infectious mononucleosis have been reported in patients who also have hereditary spherocytosis [6, 42] and thalassemia. [19, 119] However, anti-i was not present in three patients with infectious mononucleosis and hemolytic anemia associated with hereditary spherocytosis reported by Taylor. [117] More recently, a case complicating hereditary elliptocytosis has been reported; [71] the patient's serum contained IgM anti-i of high thermal amplitude, but the authors could not demonstrate increased agglutinability of the patient's red cells by anti-i, and they concluded that the elliptocytosis was coincidental.

Course: A majority of the reported cases of hemolytic anemia in infectious mononucleosis are associated with mild and self-limiting anemia, [120] and they usually resolve within several weeks. [117] Indeed, in a review published in 1970 of fatal cases of infectious mononucleosis, hemolytic anemia was not cited as a cause of death. [97] However, life-threatening episodes of hemolysis have been reported and, when the anemia is severe, it is logical to treat the patient with steroids, particularly since reported experience attests to their efficacy [65, 120] (see Chapter 11). Splenectomy has even been carried out, [129] but it would seem to be indicated rarely, if ever.

Occasionally the severity of the anemia may require blood transfusion. If an anti-i antibody of high thermal amplitude is demonstrated, it may be necessary to carry out compatibility testing strictly at 37°C, and, in such instances, it is logical to administer the blood using a blood warmer (see page 387).

Other Disorders Associated with High Titer Cold Agglutinins. The production of high titer cold agglutinins during influenza virus infection has been described [98] but is much less common than with *Mycoplasma pneumoniae* infections. A few occurrences of hemolytic anemia with high titer cold agglutinins in well documented cases of influenza virus infection have been reported. [98, 118]

Finally, in the early literature cold agglutinin syndrome has been reported in association with a wide variety of pathologic states, although the significance of the relationship is questionable. Included in this group have been trypanosomiasis, relapsing fever, cirrhosis, malaria, septicemia, pernicious anemia, and various forms of carcinoma.[98]

The Immunochemistry of Cold Agglutinins. Cold agglutinins are, with rare exceptions, IgM antibodies that exhibit a reversible, thermal-dependent equilibrium reaction with erythrocytes, association being favored at lower temperatures. The thermal maximum (i.e., the highest temperature at which agglutination is caused by undiluted serum) depends on the concentration and binding affinity of the cold agglutinin.

One or both types of light chains (kappa and lambda) may be present. Like other immunoglobulins, cold agglutinins are considered monoclonal when they possess a single light chain type *and* exhibit homogeneous electrophoretic mobility, and polyclonal when both light chains are present *and* the antibody exhibits normal electrophoretic heterogeneity.[77]

Cold agglutinins that occur after *Mycoplasma pneumoniae* infections are usually polyclonal, that is, electrophoretically and immunochemically heterogeneous. However, in a few patients monoclonal antibodies have been present, being homogeneous on electrophoresis and possessing only kappa chains. In other patients, "restricted polyclonal" proteins have been described, that is, antibodies that are monotypic (containing just one type of light chain) but electrophoretically heterogeneous *or* bytypic but electrophoretically homogeneous.[77] In contrast, in patients with chronic idiopathic cold agglutinin syndrome, monoclonal proteins are characteristically present and, when their concentration is high enough, they are evident as an M-component band on serum protein electrophoresis.[67] Cold agglutinins with anti-I specificity almost invariably have kappa light chains, whereas those with anti-i specificity usually have lambda light chains.[101]

The demonstration of the exclusive, or virtually exclusive, occurrence of κ-chains in anti-I cold agglutinins was the first example of a relation between antibody specificity and light chain type. Further restrictions have later been demonstrated. Three different variable region subgroups of κ-chains have now been delineated.[91] Amino acid sequence studies of light chains isolated from one cold agglutinin [46] and a study of the N-terminal amino acid in four other cold agglutinin light chains,[26] identified glutamic acid as the N-terminal amino acid in four of these five light chains, indicating that they belong to the subgroup V_{KII}, which probably accounts for only 13 percent of Bence-Jones proteins.[102] A restriction within the mu chains has also been demonstrated: [30] 13 out of 14 isolated cold agglutinins belonged to one mu subgroup, as shown by the lack of a particular peptide present in 40 percent of monoclonal M-globulins without known antibody activity.

Further immunochemical studies of the heavy chains of IgM cold agglutinins indicate that mu chains of different cold agglutinins share antigenic determinants not found on IgM molecules lacking cold-agglutinin activity. These specific antigenic determinants appear to be present on the heavy chains of monoclonal proteins of both anti-I and anti-i specificities,[130] and there is one report of similar structural characteristics of a restricted poly-clonal protein from a patient with *Mycoplasma pneumoniae* infection.[77] Fur-thermore, antisera specific for the heavy chains of IgM cold agglutinins cross-react with heavy chains of IgA cold agglutinins, which suggests that there is a common idiotypic specificity. Since the idiotypic determinants related to Ii specificity differ from those related to Pr specificity, it appears likely that the idiotypic determinants make up part of the antigen-binding site.

Although most cold agglutinins are IgM, some of IgA and IgG immuno-globulin class have been described. Cold agglutinins in some patients with infectious mononucleosis and angioimmunoblastic lymphadenopathy have been mixed IgG-IgM. Only occasionally are cold agglutinins cryoprecipitable. Rarely cryoprecipitable anti-I has been observed, but at least one third of anti-i cold agglutinins are cryoprecipitable.[101]

In 50 patients with cold agglutinin syndrome, the total concentration of IgM varied from 0.7 to 24.5 mg/ml.[67] In most of the patients, the cold aggluti-nin accounts for the entire elevation of serum IgM above normal levels. In two patients studied by Harboe,[67] a homogeneous protein remained in the serum after adsorption with red cell stroma in the cold. This finding was shown to be due to the presence of an additional monoclonal protein without cold aggluti-nin activity, thus indicating that these were instances of biclonal gammo-pathy.

The Relationship Between Cold Agglutinin Syndrome and Wal-denström's Macroglobulinemia. Waldenström, in 1944,[125] first described a disorder of insidious onset occurring in late adulthood with variable clinical manifestations and with an abnormal elevation of serum globulins, later iden-tified as macroglobulinemia. The term macroglobulinemia literally means the presence of macroglobulins in the blood, but, in modern usage, is applied only to indicate the presence of an IgM paraprotein.[21] Since patients with chronic cold agglutinin syndrome almost always have a monoclonal IgM protein in their serum, they may be said to have macroglobulinemia.

Many authors have noted similarities of laboratory findings in patients with cold agglutinin syndrome and patients who have monoclonal IgM pro-teins without cold agglutinin activity. In both instances, bone marrow findings may consist of increased numbers of abnormal lymphoid and plasma cells,[105] although Dacie[35] and Firkin et al.[56] reported no excess of plasma cells in patients with cold agglutinin syndrome. Schubothe[112] analyzed 14 patients with cold agglutinin syndrome and found that 9 had bone marrow lympho-cyte counts exceeding 25 percent; in 6 it exceeded 40 percent. In one patient, there was an impressive progression of lymphocytic infiltration of the marrow four years after the onset of the disease. On the basis of these similarities, some authors feel that a typical case of chronic cold agglutinin syndrome is probably a variant of Waldenström's macroglobulinemia in which the IgM M-component has cold agglutinin activity.[101]

However, it is also possible to catalogue an impressive list of differences between cold agglutinin syndrome and patients with macroglobulinemia without cold agglutinin activity. Physical findings in patients with cold agglutinin syndrome are notably absent, except for those directly related to the hemolytic anemia. Hepatomegaly and lymphadenopathy are infrequent findings in all reported series of patients. The more frequently noted modest degree of splenomegaly is most likely caused by "work hypertrophy" from chronic red blood cell destruction.[47] The course of the disease is usually stable, with gradual progression[133] or no progression over a period of years, and often with death due to unrelated causes. Dacie[35] reported 16 patients followed for at least a year, 10 of whom were still living after 5 years. In none did he note a progression of physical findings characteristic of malignant lymphoreticular disorders. Five patients died, the causes of death being carcinoma of the breast, tuberculosis, pulmonary embolism, pneumonia and "anemia." Similarly, Evans[53] reported close follow-up of a patient with cold agglutinin syndrome for 20 years, after which time the patient had continued evidence of mild hemolysis but refused additional examination. Throughout this period of time a monoclonal kappa chain IgM protein was present in the serum. The authors concluded that despite the fact that the cold agglutinin was monoclonal, the abnormal immunoglobulin production should be considered benign.

In contrast, findings in patients with typical Waldenström's macroglobulinemia syndrome include hepatosplenomegaly, lymphadenopathy, hypoproliferative anemia, and manifestations of hyperviscosity such as a bleeding diathesis, visual disturbances, and neurologic abnormalities.[25] Moreover, there is a statistically significant difference in survival rate ($p<.01$) between patients whose macroglobulin has cold agglutinin activity, compared with those patients without cold agglutinin syndrome.[21] The mortality rate in 204 patients with macroglobulinemia was reported as 16 percent at 12 months, 29 percent at 24 months, and 56 percent at 5 years.[21] It has been postulated that the presence of cold agglutinins causes clinical presentation at an earlier stage than in patients who have no hemagglutinin activity in the serum.[21] If this were true, progression of cold agglutinin syndrome would nevertheless be expected during ensuing years, but such a course is not frequently observed.[35, 53, 112]

Differences in the IgM monoclonal protein are also present. As noted above, mu chains of different cold agglutinins share antigenic determinants not found on IgM proteins lacking cold agglutinin activity. Further, 20 percent of IgM monoclonal proteins from patients with Waldenstöm's macroglobulinemia without serologic activity contain lambda chains, whereas almost all monoclonal cold agglutinins have kappa chains.[67]

On the basis of the preceding information, it is perhaps best to consider the cold agglutinin syndrome as being quite distinct from patients with typical Waldenström's macroglobulinemia without cold agglutinin activity, while recognizing that a minority of patients have similar clinical findings and course (Table 2-9).

Table 2-9. A COMPARISON OF WALDENSTRÖM'S MACROGLOBULINEMIA AND COLD AGGLUTININ SYNDROME

Cold Agglutinin Syndrome	Intermediate Cases	Typical Waldenström's Syndrome
Stable course	Progressive course	Progressive course
IgM monoclonal protein has cold agglutinin activity	IgM monoclonal protein has cold agglutinin activity	IgM monoclonal protein does not have cold agglutinin activity
No abnormal clinical symptoms and signs except manifestations of hemolytic anemia, cold sensitivity, and the presence of splenomegaly	Clinical manifestations overlap with cold agglutinin syndrome and Waldenström's syndrome	Clinical findings include hepatosplenomegaly, lymphadenopathy and manifestations of hyperviscosity

Paroxysmal Cold Hemoglobinuria

Historical Concepts. The history of paroxysmal cold hemoglobinuria is particularly interesting. Of all the hemolytic anemias, it was the first to be recognized.[35] Furthermore, the laboratory test for its diagnosis, the Donath-Landsteiner test, was the first immunohematologic test ever to be described.[11] This appears, at first, to be surprising since paroxysmal cold hemoglobinuria is the least common type of AIHA. Its early recognition is due to the fact that hemoglobinuria is a striking symptom, a fact that also explains the early recognition of march hemoglobinuria and paroxysmal nocturnal hemoglobinuria. It is also true that paroxysmal cold hemoglobinuria was much more common than it is at present since a majority of cases recorded in the early medical literature were associated with late syphilis or congenital syphilis.

There are many accounts of the disease in the nineteenth-century medical literature.[35] The relationship of acute attacks to exposure to cold was clearly described in accounts of the disease in 1865, as was the fact that the urine contained blood pigment but no blood corpuscles. A diagnostic test described in 1879 was based on the development of hemoglobinuria after immersion of the patient's feet in ice water. A test producing less discomfort to the patient was described in 1881 by Ehrlich, who showed that if a ligature was placed around a finger which was then chilled in ice-water, serum subsequently obtained from the finger would be hemolysed.

The greatest single step forward in understanding the pathogenesis of paroxysmal cold hemoglobinuria was the work of Donath and Lansteiner which was published in 1904. Excerpts from the original report of their work [43] are illustrated in Figures 2-1 and 2-2 on pages 51–53.

Aus der I. medizinischen Klinik in Wien (Prof. N o t h -
n a g e l) und dem pathologisch-anatomischen Institut in Wien
(Prof. W e i c h s e l b a u m).

Ueber paroxysmale Hämoglobinurie.

Von Dr. J u l i u s D o n a t h und Dr. K a r l L a n d s t e i n e r.

Zur Erklärung der Pathogenese der paroxysmalen Hämoglobinurie, jener eigentümlichen Erkrankung, bei der es anfalls-
weise, namentlich unter Einwirkung von Kälte, zu Hämoglobinurie und zur Ausscheidung von Blutfarbstoff durch den
Harn kommt, wurde bisher eine Reihe sehr verschiedenartiger
Theorien aufgestellt.

Einige ältere Erklärungsversuche lassen die Hämoglobinurie
durch Zerstörung der Blutkörperchen in der Niere zustande
kommen. Erst seit dem Nachweise einer während der Anfälle
bestehenden Hämoglobinämie [K ü s s n e r[1]] wurde die Ursache
der Erkrankung in das Blut verlegt. Die Hämolyse selbst
wurde von verschiedenen Faktoren abhängig gemacht. Der
ursprünglichen Annahme, dass die Kälte die bei dieser Erkrankung empfindlichen roten Blutkörperchen zerstört (H a b e r -
s o h n[2]), M u r r i[3]), E h r l i c h[4]) in seiner ersten Arbeit,
B o a s[5]), L e u b e[6]) u. a.) widerspricht die vielfach festgestellte
Tatsache [L i c h t h e i m[7]), E h r l i c h[8]), C h v o s t e k[9]), L u z -
z a t t i und S o r g e n t e[10]), D o n a t h[11])], dass das Blut dieser
Kranken in vitro gegen Kälteeinwirkung nicht empfindlicher ist
als normales Blut. Es musste darum nach anderen Ursachen des
Blutzerfalles geforscht werden. Natürlich haben die aus-
gedehnten Studien der letzten Jahre über Blutgifte die Ver-
mutung nahe gelegt, dass diese Erkrankung durch Haemolysine
hervorgerufen wird.

Für eine hämolytische Wirkung toxischer Substanzen haben
sich u. a. Wiltshire, Hayem[12]) und seine Schüler, Ehrlich[13]),
Chiaruttini[14]), Luzzatti und Sorgente[15]), Burck-
hardt[16]), Tedeschi und Mattirolo[17]), Kretz[18]) aus-
gesprochen. Trotz vielfacher Bemühungen ist es aber bisher nicht
gelungen, das toxische Agens sicher nachzuweisen, oder eine Versuchsanordnung zu finden, die ein Studium des während der Anfälle stattfindenden hämolytischen Prozesses gestatten würde.

*Figure 2-1. The original report published in 1904 by Dr. Julius Donath and Dr. Karl
Landsteiner describing their current theories of the pathogenesis of paroxysmal cold
hemoglobinuria and the development of the biphasic lysis test that remains the diagnostic
laboratory procedure for the disorder. A translation of the text follows.*

About Paroxysmal Hemoglobinuria

*Several different theories have been proposed to explain the pathogensis of paroxysmal
hemoglobinuria, an unusual disease characterized by paroxysms of hemoglobinuria under
the influence of cold and the secretion of blood pigment through the urine.*

*Some older reports explain the hemoglobinuria as caused by the destruction of blood
corpuscles in the kidneys. But after Küssner showed that hemoglobinemia is present
during such paroxysms, the cause was located in the blood. The hemolysis itself was
thought to be dependent on various factors. The original belief that cold would destroy the
red cells that are sensitive in this disease is in opposition to the commonly acknowledged
fact that the blood of these patients in vitro is not more sensitive to cold than the blood of
normal individuals. Therefore one had to look for other causes of the hemolysis. Recent
extensive studies on blood toxins have suggested that this disease is caused by hemolysins.
Authors have spoken for the hemolytic effect of these toxic substances, but despite numerous efforts it has not been possible to prove the presence of toxic agents, or even to find a
test system that allows one to study the hemolytic procedure during the attack of hemolysis.*

Serum	Blutkörperchen 3 Tropfen	Mischung durch ½ Stde. bei 5° gehalten, dann 2½ Stdn. bei 37°	Mischung durch 3 Stdn. bei 37° gehalten
Fall K. (Hämoglobinurik.) 4 Tropfen	Fall K. B. W. Ch. G. A. R.	rubinrot rot rot rot	0 0 0 0
Fall R. (Hämoglobinurik.) 10 Tropfen	Fall R. B. W. Ch. G. A. R.	rubinrot rubinrot rubinrot rubinrot	Spur Rötung Spur „ Spur „ Spur „
Fall N. (Hämoglobinurik.) 7 Tropfen	Fall N. B. W. Ch. G. A. R.	rubinrot rubinrot rot rubinrot	0 0 0 0
B. W. 6 Tropfen	B. W. Fall R. Fall N. Ch. G.	0 0 0 schwachrot	0 0 Spur Rötung deutlich rot
Ch. G. 7 Tropfen	Ch. G. Fall K. Fall N.	0 0 0	0 0 0
A. R. 6 Tropfen	Fall K. Fall N. Fall R. B. W. Ch. G.	0 0 0 0 0	0 0 0 0 0

Es zeigt sich somit, dass bei dieser Versuchsanordnung Blutkörperchen anderer Individuen von dem Serum der Hämoglobinuriker aufgelöst werden, wenn auch zum Teil in geringerem Masse als deren eigene Blutkörperchen; hingegen lösen sich bei der gleichen Versuchsanordnung die mit fremdem Serum abgekühlten Blutkörperchen der Hämoglobinuriker beim nachherigen Erwärmen nicht (Ser. B. W. hatte gegenüber Körperchen Ch. G. und N. gewöhnliche, durch Abkühlung nicht verstärkte isolytische Wirkung). Es kommt also die den Lösungsvorgang bedingende eigentümliche Beschaffenheit des Hämoglobinurieblutes dem Serum (resp. Plasma) zu, wenn auch die Blutkörperchen leichter lösbar sein können (wie dies deutlich bei unserem Fall K. zutraf). Das Serum (Plasma) des Hämoglobinurikers enthält eine lytische Substanz, die auf eigene und fremde menschliche Blutkörperchen wirkt. Dieses Lysin lässt sich direkt beim Zusammenbringen des Hämoglobinurikerserums mit den eigenen oder fremden Blutkörperchen nicht nachweisen, wohl aber bei Berücksichtigung der Abhängigkeit seiner Wirkung von der Temperatur.

Figure 2-2. The original protocol of the experiments performed by Donath and Landsteiner and their interpretation. A translation of the protocol is given on page 53.

Serum	Blood Cells 3 Drops	Held for ½ hr at 5°, then 2½ hrs at 37°	Held 3 hours at 37°
Patient K	Patient K	Ruby Red	0
(hemoglo-	B.W.	Red	0
binuria)	Ch.G.	Red	0
4 Drops	A.R.	Red	0
Patient R	Patient R	Ruby Red	Trace of Red
(hemoglo-	B.W.	Ruby Red	Trace of Red
binuria)	Ch.G.	Ruby Red	Trace of Red
10 Drops	A.R.	Ruby Red	Trace of Red
Patient N	Patient N	Ruby Red	0
(hemoglo-	B.W.	Ruby Red	0
binuria)	Ch.G.	Red	0
7 Drops	A.R.	Ruby Red	0
B.W.	B.W.	0	0
6 Drops	Patient R	0	0
	Patient N	0	Trace of Red
	Ch.G.	Red Tinged	Clear Distinct Red
Ch.G.	Ch.G.	0	0
7 Drops	Patient K	0	0
	Patient N	0	0
A.R.	Patient K	0	0
6 Drops	Patient N	0	0
	Patient R	0	0
	B.W.	0	0
	Ch.G.	0	0

It is shown with this sequence of experiments that the blood corpuscles of other individuals are hemolyzed by the serum of patients with hemoglobinuria, although to a lesser degree than their own blood corpuscles; however in the same series of experiments, the blood corpuscles of the hemoglobinuric patients which have been cooled with other serum do not lyse when they are warmed afterwards. (Serum B.W. had a normal isolytic activity against the red cells of Ch.G. and N which was not increased by cooling.) Therefore, the unusual composition of the blood of the hemoglobinuric patients which is causing the lysis lies in the serum (respectively plasma), although the red cells may be easier to lyse (as shown in our Case K). The serum (plasma) of the hemoglobinuric patients contains a lytic substance that is effective against the patient's and other human blood corpuscles. This lysis cannot be demonstrated directly by mixing the serum of the hemoglobinuric patient with his own or other red cells; however, one must consider the dependence of its effects on temperature.

Donath and Landsteiner demonstrated that hemolysis was due to an autolysin that reacted with the patient's red cells at low temperatures, and that labile serum factors (complement) caused lysis of the sensitized cells if the temperature was subsequently raised. This bithermic procedure remains the diagnostic test for the disorder (see Chapter 5 for technical details). The test is referred to as the Donath-Landsteiner test and the antibody thus detected as a Donath-Landsteiner antibody.

Their article describes further experiments in which two aliquots of a patient's blood were obtained. One aliquot was incubated at 0°C and the other was incubated at room temperature. Then the plasmas were removed and exchanged, mixed and incubated at 37°C. After two hours the aliquots that were cooled had undergone much lysis, but no lysis occurred in the other aliquot. "This finding indicates that red cells take up in the cold an effective substance from the plasma, and that neither red cells or white blood cells give hemolytic substance into the serum."

In an additional experiment "oxylative blood" of the patient was cooled in ice water, centrifuged in the cold, and then the plasma that had been removed in the cold was mixed with a new aliquot of red cells of the patient. This mixture was then cooled and subsequently incubated at 37°C. However, no hemolysis occurred, thus indicating that the hemolysin had been absorbed by the cells.

"Red cells that are cooled with serum or plasma of hemoglobinuric patients, whether the patient's own or other's red cells, take up substances that by this absorption develop the capability to hemolyze in the serum of hemoglobinuric patients and other human serum. The hemolysis is caused by the aid of factors in the serum described as complement (alexin, cytase, etc.)"

Incidence. Many reports emphasize that paroxysmal cold hemoglobinuria is a rare disease. Howard et al.[74] noted only two occurrences in 38 years and 298,878 admissions at the Montreal Hospital. Becker[7] noted that the diagnosis was made in only 1 patient in 20 years at the University of Chicago clinic, during which time 130,000 patients were admitted to the hospital and 382,792 patients were seen as out-patients. Pirofsky[98] encountered only 2 occurrences over a 15-year period at Bellevue Hospital in New York and at the University of Oregon hospitals and clinics.

Our own experience suggests that the preceding reports exaggerate the rarity of the disorder, since we have seen 6 occurrences of the disorder among our total of 347 patients for an incidence of 1.7 percent. The fact that the disorder is not quite as rare as some reports suggest is also indicated by the fact that Dacie and Worlledge[36] reported 15 cases out of a total of 295 patients with AIHA (5.1 percent), and van Loghem and his associates[123] reported an incidence of 10 percent in their 168 patients. Johnsen et al.[80] encountered 3 cases within a period of 7 months, and especially remarkable is the report of Bird et al.,[11] who diagnosed this disorder in 3 children within a period of just 16 days!

Race, Sex, and Age. There does not appear to be any particular racial distribution for the development of paroxysmal cold hemoglobinuria, nor is there any evidence that one sex is affected more frequently than the other. The disease affects patients of all ages, but is particularly common in children.

Idiopathic and Secondary Types. The relationship of paroxysmal cold hemoglobinuria to syphilis was described almost a century ago and, until the discovery of antibiotics, syphilis was considered an etiologic factor in a large majority of cases. Donath and Landsteiner's review of the literature from 1906 to 1925 revealed evidence of syphilis in 95 of 99 reported cases.[45] More recently, Becker [7] and Nabarro [94] also stressed this relationship and pointed out that, when related to syphilis, paroxysmal cold hemoglobinuria appeared only in congenital syphilis or in the quiescent stage of late syphilis. In these patients, the paroxysmal cold hemoglobinuria was a chronic comparatively benign disease with exacerbations related to cold exposure.

However, as early as 1908 Donath and Landsteiner suggested that the disease might be caused by infections other than syphilis,[44] and almost all recent reports describe an acute transient hemolytic anemia often associated with a viral disorder or a "flu-like illness." Cases have been reported in association with chicken-pox,[81] infectious mononucleosis,[49, 131] mumps,[27] *Mycoplasma pneumoniae* infection,[8] measles,[34, 96] and after prophylactic immunization against measles.[17] More commonly, however, a specific infectious disease is not present, but rather an upper respiratory infection of undefined etiology.[11, 124] Some patients have no history of an antecedent illness, and they appear healthy until the onset of the acute paroxysm.[11]

Symptoms and Signs. Acute attacks are characterized by the sudden onset of shaking chills, fever, malaise, abdominal distress, aching pains in the back or legs, and nausea. Usually, the first specimen of urine passed after the onset of symptoms contains hemoglobin. The extent of cold exposure may be surprisingly slight and, in some cases, a history of undue exposure to cold cannot be elicited. The requirement for cold exposure probably depends on the thermal amplitude of the Donath-Landsteiner antibody. In patients in which cold exposure is documented, the interval between chilling and the development of symptoms ranges from a few minutes to eight hours. The patient's temperature may rise to as high as 40°C (104°F). The acute constitutional symptoms and the hemoglobinuria may resolve within a few hours or persist for days. Splenomegaly and hyperbilirubinemia may develop and, if paroxysms recur, hemosiderinuria may result.

Not all the preceding findings are present in each patient or in each paroxysm occurring in a given patient. Hemoglobinuria may occur in some patients without other acute manifestations, and, conversely, constitutional symptoms in the absence of overt hemoglobinuria have been described.

Nelson and Nicholl [95] pointed out that constitutional symptoms associated with attacks of hemoglobinuria in paroxysmal cold hemoglobinuria are generally more severe than when patients suffering from the cold agglutinin syndrome develop hemoglobinuria in cold weather. This phenomenon is probably related to the sudden intensity of hemolysis in paroxysmal cold hemoglobinuria, which may result from the remarkable hemolytic potency of the Donath-Landsteiner antibody.

There are many descriptions in the older medical literature of Raynaud's phenomenon occurring in association with attacks of hemoglobinuria in probable cases of paroxysmal cold hemoglobinuria.[35] The fingers, toes, tip of the nose, lips, or ears may be blanched or become deeply cyanotic, and even gangrene has been described. However, acrocyanosis is not mentioned in more recent case reports,[11, 124] and it is possible that it occurs primarily in association with the chronic syphilitic form of paroxysmal cold hemoglobinuria.

Cold urticaria may occur as a prodromal manifestation, and Harris et al.[68] suggested that this occurrence might be due to an antibody, since they found that the serum of one patient, when injected intradermally into a nonsensitive subject, caused the formation of a pruritic erythematosis lesion that occurred when the site was chilled and then warmed. Becker[7] made similar observations in one patient. Such passive transfer of the ability to form a localized urticarical lesion on exposure to cold is also found in idiopathic cold urticaria.[73, 126] The relationship of the Donath-Landsteiner antibody to the serum factor resulting in cold urticaria has not been studied.

Hematologic Findings. Severe and rapidly progressive anemia frequently occurs. In the three patients reported by Johnsen et al.,[80] the hemoglobin of the least severely affected child was 9.8 gm/dl 1 day after onset of symptoms, with a drop to 6.8 gm/dl on the fourth day of the disease. A second child had a hemoglobin of 7.3 gm/dl 1 day after onset of hemoglobinuria; in spite of being kept warm, the hemoglobin fell to 4.7 gm/dl 2 days later. The third patient reported by these authors had a hemoglobin of 12.5 gm/dl 2 days after the onset of shaking chills, abdominal pain, vomiting, and passage of red-brown urine. Hemoglobinuria persisted and 3 days later the hemoglobin was 5 gm/dl, with a further drop to 4.2 gm/dl 4 days later.

The patient described by Weiner et al.[127] had a hemoglobin of 4.5 gm/dl when admitted to the hospital 2 weeks after onset of symptoms. Other reports also describe patients with an acute onset of severe anemia.

The presence of spherocytes, anisocytosis, poikilocytosis, fragmented red cells, basophilic stippling, polychromatophilia, erythrophagocytosis and nucleated erythrocytes have all been reported.[8, 80, 98]

Leukopenia may occur during a paroxysm being followed by a neutrophil leukocytosis with a shift to the left. Leukopenia was noted as early as 1913,[35] and remarkable drops in the white blood cell count have been recorded, particularly in the older medical literature. Uchida[122] found that maximum leukopenia occurred 5 to 20 minutes after chilling, the percentage fall being as much as 72 percent. After about two hours, leukocytosis developed. Similarly, Montagnani[92] described a reduction of leukocytes from 9,800 to 1,000/μl in an artificially produced attack. The modern literature usually describes normal white blood cell counts or leukocytosis during acute attacks.

Prognosis. Paroxysmal cold hemoglobinuria is rarely a cause of severe chronic anemia or death. However, acute attacks are frequently quite severe, as has been indicated. The acute illness characteristically resolves spontaneously within a few days to several weeks after onset and does not recur. The Donath-Landsteiner antibody may persist in low titer and with low thermal amplitude for longer periods of time. Indeed, Dacie reported the persistence of the Donath-Landsteiner antibody for eight years after a single episode of hemoglobinuria.[35] More commonly, the titer and thermal range of the antibody fall rapidly, so that two to three months later it is no longer detectable.[133]

Chronic paroxysmal cold hemoglobinuria has become an extreme rarity since almost all such cases were associated with congenital or late syphilis. However, occasional cases of chronic idiopathic paroxysmal cold hemoglobinuria do occur [5, 35, 104] (see case report, Chapter 9, page 341). Although a cause of some morbidity, no mortality has been recorded in the modern medical literature.

REFERENCES

1. Allgood, J. W., and Chaplin, H., Jr.: Idiopathic acquired autoimmune hemolytic anemia. Am. J. Med., *43:*254, 1967.
2. Ascensao, J., Kagan, W., Moore, M., Pahwa, R., Hansen, J., and Good, R.: Aplastic anaemia: Evidence for an immunological mechanism. Lancet, I:699, 1976.
3. Barcroft, H., and Edholm, O. G.: Temperature and blood flow in the human forearm. J. Physiol. (Lond), *104:*366, 1946.
4. Barry, K. G., and Crosby, W. H.: Auto-immune hemolytic anemia arrested by removal of an ovarian teratoma: review of the literature and report of a case. Ann. Intern. Med., *47:*1002, 1957.
5. Bastrup-Madsen, P., and Petersen, H. S.: Monoclonal gammopathy with the M-component behaving like Donath-Landsteiner haemolysin. Scand. J. Haemat., *8:*81, 1971.
6. Bean, R. H.: Haemolytic anaemia complicating infectious mononucleosis, with report of a case. Med. J. Australia *1:*386, 1957.
   chain-subclass in cold agglutinin heavy chains. Immunochemistry, 7:479, 1970.
7. Becker, R. M.: Paroxysmal cold hemoglobinurias. Arch. Intern. Med., *81:*630, 1948.
8. Bell, C. A., Swicker, H., and Rosenbaum, D. L.: Paroxysmal cold hemoglobinuria (P.C.H.) following mycoplasma infection: anti-I specificity of the biphasic hemolysin. Transfusion, *13:*138, 1973.
9. Bell, C. A., Zwicker, H., and Sacks, H. J.: Autoimmune hemolytic anemia: routine serologic evaluation in a general hospital population. Amer. J. Clin. Path., *60:*903, 1973.
10. Berman, L. B.: When the urine is red. Practical Nephrology. J.A.M.A., *237:*2753, 1977.
11. Bird, G. W. G., Wingham, J., Martin, A. J., Richardson, S. G. N., Cold, A. P., Payne, R. W., and Savage, B. F.: Idiopathic non-syphilitic paroxysmal cold haemoglobinuria in children. J. Clin. Path., *29:*215, 1976.
12. Blajchman, M. A.: Immunoglobulins in warm type autoimmune haemolytic anaemia. Lancet, *2:*340, 1969.
13. Bottiger, L. E., and Westerholm, B.: Acquired haemolytic anaemia. Acta Med. Scand., *193:*223, 1973.
14. Bowman, H. S., Marsh, W. L., Schumacher, H. R., Oyen, R., and Reihart, B. S.:

Auto-anti-N immunohemolytic anemia in infectious mononucleosis. Amer. J. Clin. Path., *61:*465, 1974.
15. Bowman, J. M.: Acquired hemolytic anemia. Use of replacement transfusion in a crisis. Amer. J. Dis. Child., *89:*226, 1955.
16. Bruyere, M. De, Sokal, G., Devoitille, J. M., and Fauchet-Dutrieux, M. C.: Autoimmune haemolytic anaemia and ovarian tumor. Brit. J. Haematol., *20:*83, 1971.
17. Bunch, C. F., Schwarz, C. M., and Bird, G. W. G.: Paroxysmal cold haemoglobinuria following measles immunization. Arch. Dis. Child., *47:*299, 1975.
18. Burston, J., Husain, O. A., Hutt, M. S., and Tanner, E. I.: Two cases of autoimmune haemolysis and aplasia. Brit. Med. J., *1:*83, 1959.
19. Calvo, R., Stein, W., Kochwa, S., and Rosenfield, R. E.: Acute hemolytic anemia due to anti-i; frequent cold agglutinins in infectious mononucleosis. J. Clin. Invest., *44:*1033, 1965.
20. Capra, J. D., Dowling, P., Cook, S., and Kunkel, H. G.: An incomplete cold reactive gamma G antibody with i specificity in infectious mononucleosis. Vox. Sang., *16:*10, 1969.
21. Carter, P., Koval, J. J., and Hobbs, J. R.: The relation of clinical and laboratory findings to the survival of patients with macroglobulinaemia. Clin. Exp. Immunol., *28:*241, 1977.
22. Casey, T. P., and Main, B. W.: Thrombocytopenia and haemolytic anaemia in infectious mononucleosis. New Zeal. Med. J., *66:*664, 1967.
23. Chaplin, H., and Avioli, L. V.: Autoimmune hemolytic anemia. Arch. Intern. Med., *137:*346, 1977.
24. Chertkow, G., and Dacie, J. V.: Results of splenectomy in autoimmune haemolytic anaemia. Brit. J. Haematol., *2:*237, 1956.
25. Cohen, R. J., Bohannon, R. A., and Wallerstein, R. O.: Waldenström's macroglobulinemia. Amer. J. Med., *41:*274, 1966.
26. Cohen, S., and Cooper, A. G.: Chemical differences between individual cold agglutinins. Immunology, *15:*93, 1968.
27. Colley, E. W.: Paroxysmal cold haemoglobinuria after mumps. Brit. Med. J., *1:*1552, 1964.
28. Cooper, A. G., and Hobbs, J. R.: Immunoglobulins in chronic cold haemagglutinin disease. Brit. J. Haematol., *19:*383, 1970.
29. Cooper, A. G., and Brown, M. C.: Serum i antigen: a new human blood group glycoprotein. Biochem. Biophys. Res. Commun., *55:*297, 1973.
30. Cooper, A. G., Chavin, S. I., and Franklin, E. C.: Predominance of a single
31. Crosby, W. H.: The clinical aspects of immunologic hemolytic anemia. Vox. Sang., *26:*3, 1955.
32. Crosby, W. H., and Rappaport, H.: Autoimmune hemolytic anemia. I. Analysis of hematologic observations with particular reference to their prognostic value. A survey of 57 cases. Blood, *12:*42, 1957.
33. Dacie, J. V.: The presence of cold haemolysins in sera containing cold haemagglutinins. J. Path. Bact., *62:*241, 1950.
34. Dacie, J. V.: The Haemolytic Anaemias, Congenital and Acquired. London, J. & A. Churchill, 1954.
35. Dacie, J. V.: The Haemolytic Anaemias. 2nd Ed., London, J. and A. Churchill Ltd., 1962.
36. Dacie, J. V., and Worlledge, S. M.: Auto-immune hemolytic anemias. Progr. Hematol. *6:*82, 1969.
37. Dacie, J. V.: Autoimmune hemolytic anemia. Arch. Intern. Med., *135:*1293, 1975.
38. Dameshek, W., and Komninos, Z. D. The present status of treatment of autoimmune hemolytic anemia with ACTH and cortisone. Blood, *11:*648, 1956.
39. Dausset, J., and Colombani, J.: The serology and the prognosis of 128 cases of autoimmune hemolytic anemia. Blood, *14:*1280, 1959.

40. Dawson, M. A., Talbert, W., and Yarbro, J. W.: Hemolytic anemia associated with an ovarian tumor. Amer. J. Med., *50:*552, 1971.
41. de Gruchy, G. C.: Clinical Haematology in Medical Practice. 4th Ed. Penington, D., Rush, B., and Castalde, P. Eds. Oxford. Blackwell Scientific Publications, 1978.
42. DeNardo, G. L., and Ray, J. P.: Hereditary spherocytosis and infectious mononucleosis, with acquired hemolytic anemia. Report of a case and review of the literature. Amer. J. Clin. Path., *39:*284, 1963.
43. Donath, J., and Landsteiner, K.: Über paroxysmale Häemoglobinurie. münch. med. Wschr., *51:*1590, 1904.
44. Donath, J., and Landsteiner, K.: Weitere Beobactungen über paroxysmale Haemoglobinurie. Abl. Bakt. (Abt I. Orig.), *45:*204, 1908.
45. Donath, J., and Landsteiner, K.: Über Kältehäemoglobinurie. Ergebn. Hyg. Bakt., *7:*184, 1925.
46. Edman, P., and Cooper, A. G.: Amino acid sequence at the N-terminal end of a cold agglutinin kappa chain. Fed. Europ. Biochem. Soc. Letters, *2:*33, 1968.
47. Eichner, E. R.: Splenic function: Normal, too much and too little. Amer. J. Med., *66:*311, 1979.
48. Eisemann, G., and Dameshek, W.: Splenectomy for pure red-cell hypoplastic and aregenerative anemia associated with autoimmune hemolytic disease; report of a case. New Engl. J. Med., *251:*1044, 1954.
49. Ellis, L. B., Wollenman, O. J., and Stetson, R. P.: Autohemagglutinins and hemolysins with hemoglobinuria and acute hemolytic anemia in an illness resembling infectious mononucleosis. Blood, *3:*419, 1948.
50. Ernstene, A. C., and Gardner, W. J.: The effect of splanchnic nerve resection and sympathetic ganglionectomy in a case of paroxysmal hemoglobinuria. J. Clin. Invest., *14:*799, 1935.
51. Evans, R. S., and Duane, R. T.: Acquired hemolytic anemia: relation of erythrocyte antibody to activity of the disease; significance of thrombocytopenia and leukopenia. Blood, *4:*1196, 1949.
52. Evans, R. S., and Weiser, R. S.: The serology of autoimmune hemolytic disease; observations on forty-one patients. Arch. Intern. Med., *100:*371, 1957.
53. Evans, R. S., Baxter, E., and Gilliland, B. C.: Chronic hemolytic anemia due to cold agglutinins: A 20-year history of benign gammopathy with response to chlorambucil. Blood, *42:*463, 1973.
54. Fagiolo, E.: Platelet and leukocyte antibodies in autoimmune hemolytic anemia. Acta Haematol., *56:*97, 1976.
55. Ferriman, D. G., Dacie, J. V., Keele, K. D., and Fullerton, J. M.: The association of Raynaud's phenomena, chronic haemolytic anaemia, and the formation of cold antibodies. Quart. J. Med., *20:* 275, 1951.
56. Firkin, B. G., Blackwell, J. B., and Johnston, G. A.: Essential cryoglobulinaemia and acquired haemolytic anaemia due to cold agglutinins. Aust. Ann. Med., *8:*151, 1959.
57. Fisher, J. A.: The cryptogenic acquired haemolytic anaemias. Quart. J. Med., *16:*245, 1947.
58. Frank, M. M., Atkinson, J. P., and Gadek, J.: Cold agglutinins and cold agglutinin disease. Ann. Rev. Med., *28:*291, 1977.
59. Fudenberg, H. H.: Immunologic deficiency, autoimmune disease, and lymphoma: Observations, implications, and speculations. Arthritis & Rheum., *9:*464, 1966.
60. Fudenberg, H. H.: Genetically determined immune deficiency as the predisposing cause of autoimmunity and lymphoid neoplasia. Amer. J. Med., *51:*295, 1971.
61. Fudenberg, H. H. Are autoimmune diseases and malignancy due to selective T-cell deficiencies? *In* Critical Factors in Cancer Immunology. New York, Academic Press, Inc., 1975.

62. Gaddy, C. G., and Powell, L. W., Jr.: Raynaud's syndrome associated with idiopathic cryoglobulinemia and cold agglutinins: report of a case and discussion of classification of cryoglobulinemia. Arch. Intern. Med., *102:*468, 1958.
63. Giblett, E. R., and Crookston, M. C.: Agglutinability of red cells by anti-i in patients with thalassaemia major and other haematological disorders. Nature (London), *201:*1138, 1964.
64. Goldberg, L. S., and Barnett, E. V.: The role of rheumatoid (antiglobulin) factors in hemolytic anemia. Ann. N.Y. Acad. Sci., *168:*122, 1969.
65. Green, N., and Goldenberg, H.: Acute hemolytic anemia and hemoglobinuria complicating infectious mononucleosis. Arch. Intern. Med., *105:*108, 1960.
66. Habibi, B., Homberg, J. C., Schaison, G., and Salmon, C.: Autoimmune hemolytic anemia in children. Am. J. Med., *56:*61, 1974.
67. Harboe, M.: Cold auto-agglutinins. Vox. Sang., *20:*289, 1971.
68. Harris, K. E., Lewis, T., and Vaughan, J. M.: Haemoglobinuria and urticaria from cold occurring singly or in combination; observations referring especially to the mechanism of urticaria with some remarks upon Raynaud's disease. Heart, *14:*305, 1929.
69. Hegde, U. M., Gordon-Smith, E. C., and Worlledge, S. M.: Reticulocytopenia and "absence" of red cell autoantibodies in immune haemolytic anaemia. Brit. Med., J., *2:*1444, 1977.
70. Hoagland, R. J.: Infectious Mononucleosis. New York, Grune and Stratton, 1967.
71. Ho-Yen, D. O.: Auto-immune haemolytic anaemia complicating infectious mononucleosis in a patient with hereditary elliptocytosis. Acta Haemat., *59:*45, 1978.
72. Horwitz, C. A., Moulds, J., Henle, W., Henle, G., Polesky, H., Balfour, H. H., Schwartz, B., and Hoff, T.: Cold agglutinins in infectious mononucleosis and heterophil-antibody-negative mononucleosis-like syndromes. Blood, *50:*195, 1977.
73. Houser, D. D., Arbesman, C. E., Ito, K., and Wicher, K.: Cold urticaria: Immunologic studies. Amer. J. Med., *49:*23, 1970.
74. Howard, C. P., Mills, E. S., and Townsend, S. R.: Paroxysmal hemoglobinuria with report of case. Amer. J. Med. Sci., *196:*792, 1938.
75. Iwai, S., and Mei-Sai, N.: Etiology of Raynaud's disease; a preliminary report. Jap. Med. World, *5:*119, 1925.
76. Iwai, S., and Mei-Sai, N.: Etiology of Raynaud's disease. Jap. Med. World, *6:*345, 1926.
77. Jacobson, L. B., and Longstreth, G. F.: Clinical and immunologic features of transient cold agglutinin hemolytic anemia. Amer. J. Med., *54:*514, 1973.
78. Janney, F. A., Lee, L. T., and Howe, C.: Cold hemagglutinin cross-reactivity with *Mycoplasma pneumoniae.* Infect. and Immunity, *22:*29, 1978.
79. Jenkins, W. J., Koster, H. G., Marsh, W. L., and Carter, R. L.: Infectious mononucleosis: An unsuspected source of anti-i. Brit. J. Haemat., *11:*480, 1965.
80. Johnsen, H. E., Brostrøm, K., and Madsen, M.: Paroxysmal cold haemoglobinuria in children: three cases encountered within a period of seven months. Scand. J. Haematol., *20:*413, 1978.
81. Kaiser, A. D., and Bradford, W. L.: Severe hemoglobinuria in a child, occurring in the prodromal stage of chickenpox; report of case. Arch. Pediat., *46:*571, 1929.
82. Keyloun, V. E., and Grace, W. J.: Acute hemolytic anemia complicating infectious mononucleosis. N.Y. State J. Med., *66:*273, 1966.
83. Krüger, J., Rahman, A., Mogk, K.-U., and Mueller-Eckhardt, C.: T-cell deficiency in patients with autoimmune hemolytic anemia (warm type). Vox. Sang., *31:*1, 1976.
84. Landsteiner, K.: Über Beziehungen zwischen dem Blutserum und den Körperzellen. Munchen. Med. Wschr., *50:*1812, 1903.

85. Leddy, J. P., and Swisher, S. N.: Acquired immune hemolytic disorders (including drug-induced immune hemolytic anemia). *In* Immunological Diseases. Samter, M., Ed. 3rd. Ed., Vol. I., 1187, 1978.
86. Lees, M. H., Fisher, O. D., and Sharks, J. M.: Case of immune aplastic haemolytic anaemia with thrombocytopenia. Brit. Med. J., *1:*110, 1960.
87. Lie-Injo, Luan Eng, and Pillay, R. P.: Idiopathic auto-immune haemolytic anaemia in Malaya. Acta Haemat. (Basel), *31:*282, 1964.
88. Logue, G. L., Rosse, W. F., and Gockerman, J. P.: Measurement of the third component of complement bound to red blood cells in patients with the cold agglutinin syndrome. J. Clin. Invest., *52:*493, 1973.
89. Meyer, R. J., Hoffman, R., and Zanjani, E. D.: Autoimmune hemolytic anemia and periodic pure red cell aplasia in systemic lupus erythematosus. Amer. J. Med., *65:*342, 1978.
90. Miescher, P. A., and Dayer, J. M., Autoimmune Hemolytic Anemias. In Textbook of Immunopathology. 2nd Ed. Miescher, P. A., and Müller-Eberhard, H. J., Eds. Grune and Stratton, 1976.
91. Milstein, C., and Pink, J. R. L.: Structure and evolution of immunoglobulins. Prog. Biophys. Molec. Biol., *21:*209, 1970.
92. Montagnani, M.: Crise hemoclassique et hemoglobinurie paroxystique. Presse Med., *29:*1017, 1921.
93. Mueller-Eckhardt, C., and Kretschmer, V.: Autoimmune hemolytic anemias. Blut, *25:*1, 1972.
94. Nabarro, D.: Congenital Syphilis. London, Arnold, 1954, 247–261.
95. Nelson, M. G., and Nicholl, B.: Paroxysmal cold haemoglobinuria. Irish J. Med. Sci. Sixth Series. *410:*49, 1960.
96. O'Neill, B. J., and Marshall, W. C.: Paroxysmal cold haemoglobinuria. Arch. Dis. Child., *42:*183, 1967.
97. Penman, H. G.: Fatal infectious mononucleosis: A critical review. J. Clin. Path., *23:*765, 1970.
98. Pirofsky, B.: Autoimmunization and the Autoimmune Hemolytic Anemias. Baltimore, Williams & Wilkins Company, 1969.
99. Pirofsky, B.: Clinical aspects of autoimmune hemolytic anemia. Seminars Hematol., *13:*251, 1976.
100. Pisciotta, A. V., and Hinz, J. E.: Occurrence of agglutinogens in normoblasts. Proc. Soc. Exp. Biol. Med., *91:*356, 1956.
101. Pruzanski, W., and Shumak, K. H.: Biologic activity of cold-reacting autoantibodies. New Eng. J. Med., *297:*538 and 583, 1977.
102. Quattrocchi, R., Cioli, D. D., and Baglioni, C.: A study of immunoglobulin structure. III. An estimate of the variability of human light chains. J. Exp. Med., *130:*401, 1969.
103. Rennert, O. M.: The hypogammaglobulinemias. Ann. Clin. Lab. Sci., *8:*276, 1978.
104. Ries, C. A., Garratty, G., Petz, L. D., and Fudenberg, H. H.: Paroxysmal cold hemoglobinuria: Report of a case with an exceptionally high thermal range Donath-Landsteiner antibody. Blood, *38:*491, 1971.
105. Ritzmann, S. E., and Levin, W. C.: Cold agglutinin disease: A type of primary macroglobulinemia: a new concept. Tex. Rep. Biol. Med., *20:*236, 1962.
106. Roelcke, D.: Cold agglutination, antibodies and antigens. Clin. Immunol. Immunopath., *2:*266, 1974.
107. Rørvik, K.: The syndrome of high-titre cold haemagglutination; a survey and a case report. Acta Med. Scand., *148:*299, 1954.
108. Rosenfield, R. E., Schmidt, P. J., Calvo, R. C., and McGinniss, M. H.: Anti-i, a frequent cold agglutinin in infectious mononucleosis. Vox. Sang., *10:*631, 1965.
109. Rosse, W. F.: Correlation of *in vivo* and *in vitro* measurements of hemolysis in hemolytic anemia due to immune reactions. Progr. Hematol., *8:*51, 1971.

110. Roth, G.: Paroxysmal hemoglobinuria with vasomotor and agglutinative features. Proc. Mayo Clin., *10:*609, 1935.
111. Schreiber, A. D., Herskovitz, B. S., and Goldwein, M.: Low-titer cold hemagglutinin disease. New Engl. J. Med., *296:*1490, 1977.
112. Schubothe, H.: The cold hemagglutinin disease. Seminars Hematol., *3:*27, 1966.
113. Seip, M.: Aplastic crisis in a case of immuno-hemolytic anemia. Acta Med. Scand., *153:*137, 1955.
114. Shashaty, G. G., Rath, C. E., and Britt, E. J.: Autoimmune hemolytic anemia associated with ulcerative colitis. Amer. J. Hemat. *3:*199, 1977.
115. Silverstein, M. N., Gomes, M. R., Elveback, L. R., ReMine, W. H., and Linman, J. W.: Idiopathic acquired hemolytic anemia. Survival in 117 cases. Arch. Intern. Med., *129:*85, 1972.
116. Stats, D., and Wasserman, L. R.: Cold hemagglutination—an interpretive review. Medicine, *22:*363, 1943.
117. Taylor, J. J.: Haemolysis in infectious mononucleosis: Inapparent congenital spherocytosis. Brit. Med. J., *4:*525, 1973.
118. Tanowitz, H. B., Robbins, N., and Leidich, N.: Hemolytic anemia: Associated with severe mycoplasma pneumoniae pneumonia. N.Y. State J. Med., *78:*2231, 1978.
119. Thurm, R. H., and Bassen, F.: Infectious mononucleosis and acute hemolytic anemia; report of two cases and review of the literature. Blood, *10:*841, 1955.
120. Tonkin, A. M., Mond, H. G., Alford, F. P., and Hurley, T. H.: Severe acute haemolytic anemia complicating infectious mononucleosis. Med. J. Aust., *2:*1048, 1973.
121. Troxel, D. B., Innella, F., and Cohren, R. J.: Infectious mononucleosis complicated by hemolytic anemia due to anti-i. Amer. J. Clin. Path., *46:*625, 1966.
122. Uchida, H.: Über die Erythrophagozytose der Leukozyten, besonders bei der paroxysmalen Häemoglobinurie. Mitt. med. Fak., *26:*503, 1921.
123. van Loghem, J. J., van der Hart, M., and Dorfmeier, H.: Serological studies in acquired hemolytic anemia. *In* Proceedings of the Sixth International Congress of the International Society of Hematology. New York, Grune and Stratton, 1958.
124. Vogel, J. M., Hellman, M., and Moloshok, R. E.: Paroxysmal cold hemoglobinuria of nonsyphilitic etiology in two children. J. Ped., *81:*974, 1972.
125. Waldenström, J.: Incipient myelomatosis or "essential" hyperglobulinemia with fibrinogenopenia—a new syndrome? Acta Med. Scand., *117:*216, 1944.
126. Wanderer, A. A., Maselli, R., Ellis, E. F., and Ishizaka, K.: Immunologic characterization of serum factors responsible for cold urticaria. J. Allergy, *48:*13, 1971.
127. Weiner, W., Gordon, E. G., and Rowe, D.: A Donath-Landsteiner antibody (nonsyphilitic type). Vox. Sang., *9:*684, 1964.
128. Wilkinson, L. S., Petz, L. D., and Garratty, G.: Reappraisal of the role of anti-i in haemolytic anaemia in infectious mononucleosis. Brit. J. Haemat., *25:*715, 1973.
129. Wilson, S. J., Ward, C. E., and Gray, L. W.: Infectious lymphadenosis (mononucleosis) and hemolytic anemia in a Negro; recovery following splenectomy. Blood, *4:*189, 1949.
130. Williams, R. C., Jr.: Cold agglutinins: Studies of primary structure serologic activity, and antigenic uniqueness. N.Y. Acad. Sci. Ann., *190:*330, 1971.
131. Wishart, M. M., and Davey, M. G.: Infectious mononucleosis complicated by acute haemolytic anaemia with a positive Donath-Landsteiner reaction. J. Clin. Path., *26:*332, 1973.
132. Wollheim, F. A., and Williams, R. C.: Studies on the macroglobulins of human serum. I. Polyclonal immunoglobulin class M (IgM) increase in infectious mononucleosis. New Engl. J. Med., *274:*61, 1966.
133. Worlledge, S.: Immune haemolytic anaemias. *In* Blood and Its Disorders. Hardisty, R. M., and Weatherall, D. J., Eds. Oxford, Blackwell Scientific, 1974, p. 714.

134. Worlledge, S. M., and Dacie, J. V.: Haemolytic and other anaemias in infectious mononucleosis. *In* Infectious Mononucleosis. Carter, H. G., and Penman, R. L., Eds. Oxford, Blackwell Scientific, 1969.
135. Yunis, J. J., and Yunis, E.: Cell antigens and cell specialization. I. A study of blood group antigens on normoblasts. Blood, *22:*53, 1963.
136. Zucker-Franklin, D., and Karpatkin, S.: Red-cell and platelet fragmentation in idiopathic autoimmune thrombocytopenic purpura. New Eng. J. Med., *297:*517, 1977.

3

Complement: A Review for the Immunohematologist

Immunohematologists have been interested in complement since the turn of the century when it was first described as a factor present in serum necessary for the lysis of red cells. Nowadays lysis of cells is not thought to be the primary function of complement. Müller-Eberhard [75] has defined complement as a multimolecular, self-assembling biological system that constitutes the primary humoral mediator of antigen-antibody reactions. The activation of this system may result in: membrane damage (e.g., lysis); the production of biologically active fragments of complement molecules (e.g., C3a and C5a anaphylatoxins); and membrane bound complement components that will interact with specific receptors on cells (e.g., red cell bound C3b will interact with the specific C3b receptor on macrophages). Complement is known to participate, together with antibody and cellular elements, in host defense against infection. Also, because of its potential to initiate inflammation and cell destruction, it may become involved in pathogenic processes, such as tissue injury.

Two pathways of complement activation have been described: the classical pathway, and the alternative (or properdin) pathway. [43] The biological consequences of complement activation (described in the preceding paragraph) are similar following the activation of either pathway. Eleven complement components have been described that participate in the classical pathway, and they are designated numerically: C1, C2, C3, C4, C5, C6, C7, C8 and C9; C1 is a trimolecular complex with the subcomponents designated C1q, C1r and C1s. They circulate throughout the extracellular compartment as inactive precursors until they are activated. This activation often involves limited proteolytic cleavage with the formation of fragments. One fragment often contributes to the inflammatory process and the other continues the complement sequence. Fragments of complement components are designated by a small letter; e.g., C3a and C3b. Activated complement components that have enzymatic activity are indicated by placing a bar over the numbered components; e.g., enzymatically active C1 is $\overline{\text{C1}}$. The bar may also be placed over a complex showing enzymatic activity; e.g., C3 convertase, $\overline{\text{C4b,2a}}$. C1, C2, and C4 do not participate in the alternative pathway of complement activation, but at least three other components, factor B, factor D and properdin, are necessary. In both pathways a series of inhibitors and inactivators operate; e.g., $\overline{\text{C1}}$ inhibitor

(C1INH) of the classical pathway, and C3b inactivator (C3bINA) that operates in both pathways.

THE CLASSICAL PATHWAY OF COMPLEMENT ACTIVATION

Physicochemical Properties of Proteins Participating in the Classical Pathway

All of the 11 proteins of the classical system have been purified. They are ·all glycoproteins and have all proven to be immunogenic when injected into animals, such as goats or rabbits. Their combined concentration in normal human plasma is approximately 300 mg/dl, or approximately 4 to 5 percent of the total serum proteins. Some of their properties are listed in Table 3-1.

Table 3-1. PROTEINS PARTICIPATING IN THE CLASSICAL PATHWAY OF COMPLEMENT ACTIVATION *

Protein	Molecular Weight	Number of Chains	Electrophoretic Mobility	Serum Concentration (μg/ml)
C1q	400,000	18	γ2	180
C1r	190,000	2	β1	100
C1s	85,000	1	α	80
C2	115,000	1	β1	25
C3	180,000	2	β2	1500
C4	206,000	3	β1	450
C5	180,000	2	β1	75
C6	128,000	1	β2	60
C7	121,000	1	β2	60
C8	154,000	3	γ1	80
C9	80,000	1	α	150

* Not including activated forms and reaction products.

C1. C1 exists in the plasma as a macromolecular complex of three separate molecules, C1q, C1r and C1s, bonded together by calcium (molecular weight of approximately one million daltons). C1q is chemically very similar to collagen. It has a molecular weight of 400,000 daltons and is composed of six subunits of identical molecular weight. Electron microscopy has revealed an ultrastructure of six peripheral subunits attached by string-like structures to one central unit (a bouquet-like appearance).[107, 120] It is thought that the six peripheral globular units may be the immunoglobulin binding sites of C1q, as six immunoglobulin molecules can bind to one C1q molecule. C1q recognizes immune complexes and thereby initiates the classical complement reaction. C1r and C1s are proenzymes, the natural substrate for C̄1̄r being C1s and the natural substrates for C̄1̄s being C4 and C2.

C2. C2 is a trace protein in normal human serum; its molecular weight is about 115,000 daltons.

C3, C4, C5. These three proteins have similar structures, and it has been suggested that they arise from a common ancestral molecule.[75] They have similar molecular weights; 180,000, 206,000 and 180,000 daltons respectively. They are β globulins with similar electrophoretic mobilities. C3 and C5 contain two chains (α and β) linked by disulfide bridges and noncovalent forces.[9,80] C4 contains three chains (α, β and γ).[103] Schematic drawings of the three molecules are shown in Figure 3-1. The three proteins are substrates for three enzymes: C3 is cleaved by $C\overline{4,2}$ (C3 convertase), into C3a (8,900 daltons) and

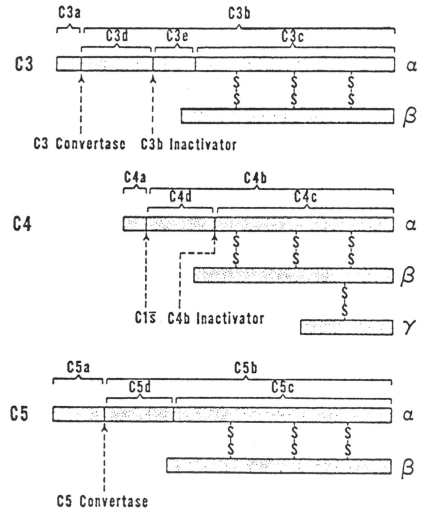

Figure 3-1. *Schematic representation of proposed polypeptide chain structure of C3, C4, and C5. The topological relationships between chains, fragments, functional sites, and enzymatic attack regions are indicated. (Müller-Eberhard, H.J.: Complement. Ann. Rev. Biochem., 44:697, 1975.).*

C3b (171,000 daltons); C4 is cleaved by C1s into C4a (8,000 daltons) and C4b (198,000 daltons); and C5 is cleaved by $\overline{C4,2,3}$ (C5 convertase) into C5a (17,000 daltons) and C5b (163,000 daltons). The enzymatic attack probably involves only a single peptide bond in the α chain. The release of the fragments endows the b fragment with *transient* activated binding sites through which the molecules may attach to cells (e.g., red cells). C3b and C4b have a second *stable* binding site which is responsible for immune adherence to a variety of cells and facilitates phagocytosis of complement sensitized cells.[76]

Bound C3b and C4b can, in turn, be acted on by a serum enzyme found in normal plasma, C3b inactivator (C3INA or KAF). In the presence of β1H (described later), this enzyme attacks the α chain in both molecules.[9, 16] The reaction produces the c and d fragments (see Fig. 3-1). The c fragment consists of the entire b chain and most of a 70,000-dalton fragment of the a chain. The d fragment consists of a single 25,000-dalton piece of the a chain. A further fragment, C3e (molecular weight 160,000 daltons), has recently been described as being released following fission of C3b [75]; this fragment might be the portion of the a chain which, in the intact molecule, connects the c and d portion (see Fig. 3-1).

C6, C7, C8, and C9. All these components have now been purified. Some of their properties are listed in Table 3-1. C8 appears to be another complement component with a three-chain structure.[75]

Reaction Mechanisms of the Classical Pathway

The activation of the classical pathway can be initiated by a number of substances (see Table 3-2). In immunohematology it is usually immunoglobulin that is the activating agent. Only one molecule of IgM on the cell membrane is necessary to activate the complement system; [11, 54] it is thought that two subunits have to attach to the membrane before activation occurs. In contrast, it is thought that IgG needs to form a "doublet," that is to say, two IgG molecules have to combine with antigens on the cell membrane as close together as 250–400Å before they are able to activate C1.[54] Only IgG1, IgG2 and IgG3 subclasses can activate complement. Their activity is in the order of IgG3 > IgG1 > IgG2.[3]

The interaction of antibody with antigen, as for example on an erythrocyte (the abbreviation EA is commonly used for the erythrocyte-antibody complex), leads to the activation of the complement system, often ending in cytolysis. This process involves a series of protein-protein interactions resulting in the generation of a series of cellular intermediates bearing bound complement components designated by numbers (e.g., EAC1, EAC1,4). The activation process is usually achieved by the cleavage of the next complement molecule into fragments. The activated products usually have enzymatic properties; thus, the whole pathway is an enzymatic cascade similar to the coagulation cascade. The system is held in check by the instability of the complexes formed and the naturally occurring inhibitors and inactivators present in normal plasma (e.g., C3b INA).

Table 3-2. ACTIVATORS OF THE CLASSICAL COMPLEMENT PATHWAY

Immunoglobulins	:	IgG3, IgGl, IgG2, IgM
Anions	:	DNA, RNA, dextran sulfate, polyinosinic, polyguanilic and polyuridilic acids
Enzymes	:	Trypsin, plasmin, lysosomal enzymes
Miscellaneous	:	Endotoxins, lymphocyte membranes, enveloped viruses, low ionic strength conditions

The pathway consists of three operationally defined functional units: the recognition unit (C1), the activation unit (C2, C3, C4), and the membrane attack unit (C5, C6, C7, C8, C9).

The Recognition Unit. C1q is a collagen-like protein with binding sites for IgG and IgM. When C1 collides with an antigen-antibody complex (e.g., EA) it is bound to the C_H2 domain of the Fc fragment of the immunoglobulin molecule (see Chapter 5) through the C1q subunit. This process activates C1r ($\overline{C1r}$) and subsequently C1s ($\overline{C1s}$) by the cleavage of a single polypeptide chain (Fig. 3-2). Two regulatory proteins are involved in this stage of the reaction.

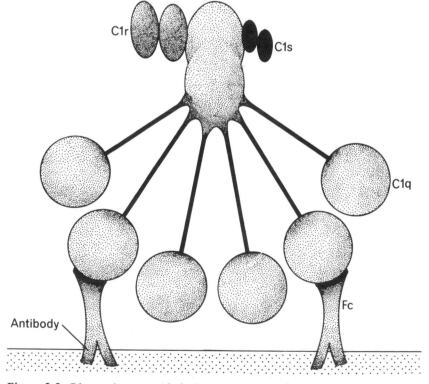

Figure 3-2. *C1q can interact with the Fc portion of immunoglobulin molecules (an IgG doublet is illustrated). Once a suitable interaction occurs, C1r is activated and finally C1s, which possesses esterase activity; its natural substrates are C4 and C2.*

C1q inhibitor (C1q INH) prevents the attachment of complement to the immunoglobulin molecule. C1 inhibitor (C1INH) abrogates the enzymatic activity of activated C1r and C1s (Fig. 3-3).

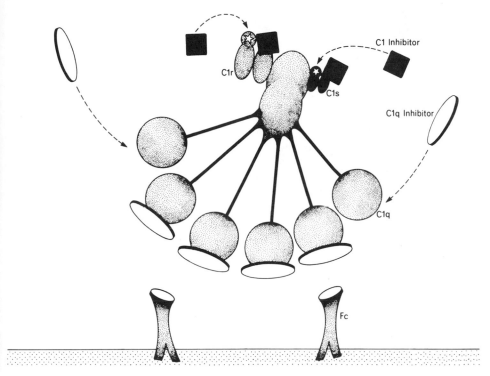

Figure 3-3. The interactions shown in Figure 3-1 can be inhibited by two regulatory proteins—C1q inhibitor, which prevents the attachment of complement to antibody, and C1 inhibitor, which abrogates the enzymatic activity of activated C1r and C1s.

The Activation Unit. This unit is assembled in two steps: activated C1 ($\overline{C1s}$) acts on native C4 by cleaving the molecule into C4a and C4b. The major fragment C4b binds to the cell membrane. A shower of fragments is produced by a single $\overline{C1s}$ enzyme, so that many C4b molecules may cluster around the EAC1 site on the cell. The binding site on C4b is short-lived and rapidly decays; if the C4b molecule does not attach to the membrane quickly it loses its ability to do so.

$\overline{C1s}$ also cleaves native C2 into two fragments. The major C2 fragment, C2a, combines with C4b on the cell membrane to form an active complex $\overline{C4b2a}$ (C3 convertase) that has enzymatic activity directed against C3. Magnesium ions are necessary for the formation of the $\overline{C4b2a}$ complex (Fig. 3-4).

C3 is cleaved by the $\overline{C4b2a}$ complex into two molecules, C3a and C3b. The smaller C3a molecule (MW 10,000) does not bind to the cell membrane but is released into the fluid phase as a mediator of inflammation (anaphylatoxin I).

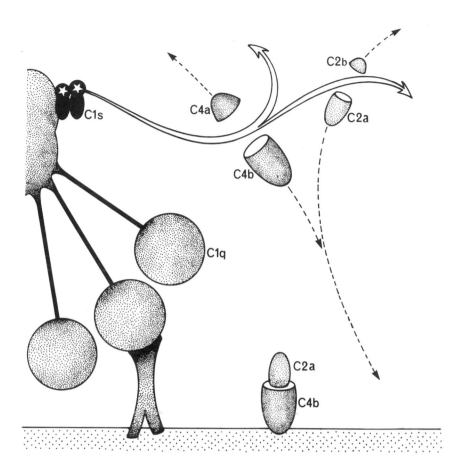

Figure 3-4. *If inhibition is overcome, then activated C1 ($C\overline{1}$) is capable of cleaving the C4 molecule into two fragments; C4a, which does not attach to cells and C4b, which can attach to cell membranes. $C\overline{1}$ also cleaves C2 molecules into C2b, which does not combine with membranes and C2a, which may combine with cell bound C4b to form a complex $C\overline{4b2a}$. This complex (C3 convertase) is enzymatic, having C3 as its natural substrate.*

The C3b molecule (MW 171,000) binds to the cell membrane and can also bind to its own activation enzyme, $C\overline{4b2a}$ (Fig. 3-5). As the $C\overline{4b2a}$ complex is an enzyme it can react more than once and produce a shower of C3b fragments each time. However, only the C3b fragments that become bound adjacent to the $C\overline{4b2a}$ enzyme are believed to participate in the next reaction, in which C5 is cleaved. Some of the C3b molecules combine with $C\overline{4b2a}$ to form $C\overline{4b,2a,3b}$ (C5 convertase), which will cleave the C5 molecule into C5a (anaphylatoxin II), and C5b (Fig. 3-6). This is the last enzymatic reaction in the pathway. During the enzymatic cascade only about 5 to 20 percent of C2, C3, C4, and C5 molecules become bound to the cell membrane.

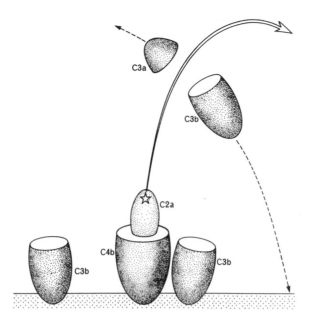

Figure 3-5. *C3 convertase (C4b2a̅) cleaves C3 into fragments, C3a anaphylatoxin, which circulates in the plasma and C3b, which can attach to cell membranes. Some C3b molecules will fall close to C4b2a̅ complexes and will form a new enzyme, C4b2a3b̅ or C5 convertase.*

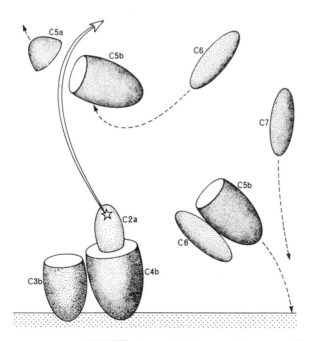

Figure 3-6. *C5 convertase (C4b2a3b̅) cleaves C5 into two fragments, C5a anaphylatoxin which circulates in the plasma and C5b that is capable of adsorbing C6 and C7. The trimolecular complex can attach to cell membranes, initiating the formation of the membrane attack complex (MAC).*

Membrane Attack Complex. C5b appears to bind C6 and C7 by absorption (Fig. 3-6). The resulting trimolecular complex attaches to the cell membrane and binds C8 and C9 (Fig. 3-7). Fully assembled, the membrane attack complex (MAC) consists of one molecule of C5b, C6, C7, and C8 and up to six molecules of C9. It has a molecular weight of about one million. The end result of the pathway is lysis of the cell.

Three regulatory proteins that function at the level of the MAC have been described: [76a] the MAC inhibitor (or S protein), antithrombin III and lipoprotein. These proteins are thought to be similar in structure to the biologic membrane and insert themselves into the complex as it is forming, competitively occupying a combining site and preventing the attachment of the complex to a target membrane surface (Fig. 3-8).

Electron microscopy shows that lesions start appearing in the cell membrane at the C8 stage, although the cell does not lyse until C9 is complexed. [55] Mayer [70] has proposed the so-called "doughnut" hypothesis; a stable hole is produced by the assembly of a rigid, doughnut-shaped structure in the lipid bilayer of the cell membrane. The hole forms a channel connecting the inside of the cell with the extracellular fluid. The outside of the doughnut could be composed of non-polar polypeptides, that is, protein chains that were hydrophobic; the interior would need polar peptides so that it could be hydrophilic. He suggests that C5b, C6, C7, C8, and C9 may be the proteins that form the doughnut or funnel shape, penetrating the lipid bilayer of the membrane. [70] The cell will then lyse either by direct egress of the hemoglobin or

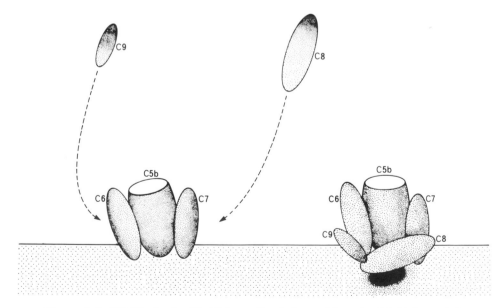

Figure 3-7. C5b67 absorbs C8. This complex is inserted into the bilipid layer of the membrane, forming a channel through the membrane. Finally C9 is absorbed, forming the final membrane attack complex (MAC), leading to lysis of the cell.

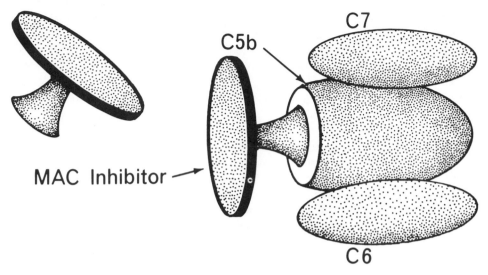

Figure 3-8. *Illustrated is one of the regulatory proteins that operates at the level of the membrane attack complex. The membrane attack complex (MAC) inhibitor (others are antithrombin III and lipoprotein) can insert itself into the complex as it is forming, competitively occupying a combining site and preventing the attachment of the complex to a target membrane surface.*

more commonly through colloid osmotic pressure.[45, 70] Water being attracted into the cell with resultant swelling, the membrane of the swollen cell becomes permeable to macromolecular substances, including intracellular proteins and nucleotides. Once intracellular contents have diffused out, the membrane seals again and effectively becomes an empty sac. The cellular remnant is removed from the circulation by phagocytosis.

THE ALTERNATIVE PATHWAY OF COMPLEMENT ACTIVATION

In 1954, Pillemer and his co-workers showed that a substance present in normal plasma, properdin, would react with a wide variety of naturally occurring polysaccharides and lipopolysaccharides to activate complement *without the presence of antibody.*[90] Several other factors present in normal plasma (e.g., C3, factor A and factor B) were found to be necessary for the reaction. They suggested that this might be an important defense mechanism *in vivo* in an unimmunized host. Few scientists accepted Pillemer's theories at this time, particularly when work emerged on the structure of immunoglobulins and the differences between different Ig classes in complement activation were described. Many workers believed that the *in vitro* complement activation that Pillemer had described due to zymosan (a yeast extract) was due instead to a naturally occurring IgM antibody to zymosan, and thus the complement activation was indeed antibody-dependent.[79] The theory of an antibody-independent complement activation mechanism lay fallow for about 10 to 15 years and then was gradually resurrected.

In 1968, Gewurz et al.[37] showed that endotoxin and immune complexes could consume C3-C9 without affecting C1, C2, or C4 levels. Schur and Becker[105] demonstrated that the F(ab)'2 fragments of rabbit antibody (i.e., rabbit IgG antibody that had the Fc fragment digested away but had both of its antigen combining sites intact) could fix complement. Sandberg et al.[102] showed that guinea pig immune complexes made with IgG1 or IgG2 antibodies would fix complement; this finding was of interest because guinea pig IgG1 antibodies are known not to activate C1 (i.e., they do not have a binding site for C1 on the Fc fragment). In addition, the IgG1 antibody-antigen complexes led to the preferential fixation of C3-C9 with very little fixation of C1, C4, and C2. Ellman and his co-workers[23] discovered a strain of guinea pigs that were genetically deficient in C4. This strain added to the evidence accumulating in support of Pillemer's original hypothesis, suggesting an alternative complement-activation pathway. The F(ab)'2 and endotoxin experiments could be duplicated by the addition of the appropriate antigen-antibody complexes or endotoxins to serum of animals totally deficient in C4. Bacterial endotoxins and immune complexes depleted the C4-deficient guinea pig sera of the later complement components, which seemed to prove without doubt that the alternative pathway must be operative.[30]

About this time Muller-Eberhard's group were studying the interaction of cobra venom and complement. In 1903, Flexner and Noguchi demonstrated that cobra venom would abolish the hemolytic activity of serum.[27] More recently it was shown that this factor could be isolated from cobra venom, and that it not only inactivated C3 but potentially activated the complement system at the C3 reaction step, leading to the formation of C5b-9. Studies on cobra venom led to the description of the C3 activator system, with its various factors, many of which could be equated with factors described originally by Pillemer. The C3 activator system has now been integrated with the properdin system, providing a basis for an alternative pathway of complement activation.[43] The alternative pathway leads to the formation of C5 convertase, and thus the self-assembling C5b-9 complex, with eventual cell damage, just as in the classical pathway.

Proteins Participating in the Alternative Pathway of Complement Activation

The components participating in the alternative pathway are listed in Table 3-3.

Properdin (P). Properdin has been purified and is one of the most cationic proteins of human serum; it has an isoelectric point of greater than 9.5. It is a tetramer with a molecular weight of approximately 212,000 daltons.

Table 3-3. PROTEINS PARTICIPATING IN THE ALTERNATIVE PATHWAY

Component	Symbol	Molecular Weight	Electrophoretic Mobility	Synonyms
Properdin	P	184,000	γ	–
Activated P	$\bar{\text{P}}$	184,000	γ	–
Proactivator	B	93,000	β	PA,GBG
Activated B	$\bar{\text{B}}$	63,000	γ	C3A, GGG, 2II, Bb
Proactivator Convertase	D	24,000	α	PAse, GBGase
C3	C3	180,000	β	Factor A, HSF
C3b	C3b	171,000	$\alpha2$	HSFa
C3b Inactivator	C3b INA	88,000	β	
β1H	β1H	180,000	β	

Factor B (Proactivator). Factor B is a β_r-glycoprotein consisting of a single polypeptide chain of 93,000 daltons. It exhibits genetic polymorphism with two common alleles, BfF (Gb^F) and BfS (Gb^S), and is genetically linked to the major HLA locus in man and monkey. Proteolytic activation of the molecule results in its cleavage into two fragments, Ba and Bb. The Bb fragment was originally called C3 activator (C3A) because it carries the active site of the enzyme.

Factor D (Proactivator Convertase). Human Factor D consists of a single polypeptide chain with a molecular weight of 24,000 daltons.

C3b Inactivator (C3bINA). C3bINA is a β-pseudo globulin with an approximate molecular weight of 88,000 daltons. It is composed of two nonidentical polypeptide chains. It acts on C3b as an endopeptidase, cleaving C3b into C3c and C3d fragments. It has sometimes been termed KAF (conglutinogen-activating factor). It has a serum concentration of approximately 50 μg/ml. Recently an additional protein β1H-globulin has been found to be necessary for full expression of C3bINA activity.

β1H-globulin. β1H-globulin was originally described as a contaminant of partially purified C3. It is a beta globulin with a molecular weight of 180,000 daltons. It has a serum concentration of approximately 500μg/ml. β1H is necessary for the efficient activity of C3bINA. It accelerates the decay of labile cell-bound C3bBb. Intrinsic and β1H-mediated extrinsic decay of Bb from C3bBb also serves to expose C3b for inactivation by C3bINA.[14a, 76b, 84a]

Reaction Mechanisms of the Alternative Complement Pathway

A number of substances have been described that activate the alternative pathway (see Table 3-4) but there is still controversy over the role of im-

Table 3-4. ACTIVATORS OF THE ALTERNATIVE COMPLEMENT PATHWAY

Immunoglobulins	:	IgA (aggregated)
		?IgG and IgE (see text)
Polysaccharides	:	Inulin, agar, endotoxin, yeast cell walls
Miscellaneous	:	Cobra venom factor, trypsin

munoglobulin. All workers agree that the alternative pathway can be activated without immunoglobulin (e.g., by endotoxin, inulin, zymosan). But whether non-aggregated immunoglobulin can activate the alternative pathway is still unsettled. Most workers agree that aggregated IgA can activate the pathway.[43] There are differing reports in the literature on the ability of aggregated IgG to activate the pathway.[43] One must be cautious in interpreting some of the data, as preparations of immunoglobulins can be contaminated with endotoxin, which alone can activate the pathway. IgG antibodies have been shown to participate in the activation of the alternative pathway by measles virus-infected cells,[61] and recently it was suggested that antibody may be involved in the lysis of rabbit red cells through the alternative pathway.[91] The exact sequence of events occurring in the alternative pathway is not yet elaborated; theories of alternative pathway activation are changing so fast that by the time this book is published the following theory may well have been modified!

Schreiber et al.[104] have recently suggested that the following may occur during the activation of the alternative pathway. Six proteins are responsible for alternative pathway activity of serum. Only five of these proteins are essential for initiation and amplification, because these events occur in the absence of properdin. Of these five proteins, three (C3, factor B, and factor D) are required for the generation of the initial enzyme and the amplifying enzyme of the pathway. The other two proteins (β1H and C3bINA) are regulators of the C3 convertase; they suppress C3 convertase formation in the fluid phase and confine enzyme formation to the surface of activators. Activation of the pathway consists of initiation and amplification.

Initiation is nonspecific, inasmuch as it does not require immunoglobulin or antibody-like recognition factor. Initiation appears to be a two-step process involving, first, random binding of C3b through its labile binding site to an activator and, second, discriminatory interaction of the bound C3b with surrounding surface structures. The random event is the result of the action of the initial C3 convertase, which is a fluid-phase enzyme. It is envisaged that native C3 and factor B form a reversible complex which, if activated by factor D, becomes the initial C3 cleaving enzyme C3,Bb. This complex constitutes a transient C3 convertase, splitting serum C3 into C3a and C3b, which can attach to the cell surface. Once on the surface, C3b can combine with more factor B and D, forming another C3 convertase (Fig. 3-9). The magnitude of the resultant C3b deposition is low due to the small amount of enzyme produced at any given time, and the low efficiency of binding that is characteristic for C3b deposition from the fluid phase.

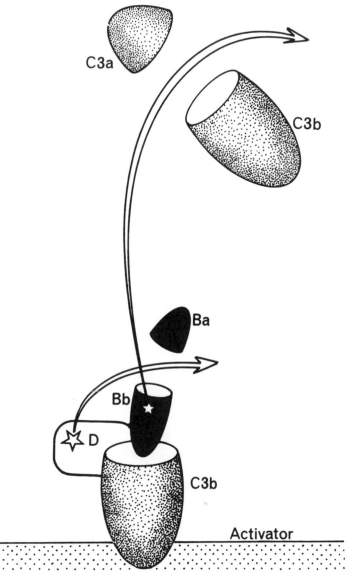

Figure 3-9. *C3b is formed through initial fluid phase cleavage of C3 (possibly by a C3, Factor B complex, which when activated by Factor D, becomes the initial fluid phase C3 convertase C3bBb). If C3b attaches to a surface containing structures capable of activating the alternative pathway then the C3b will combine with Factor B. Factor D will cleave Factor B, releasing a fragment Ba into the plasma. The resulting complex C3bBb will cleave more C3, resulting in the formation of additional C3b.*

The discriminatory interaction occurs after binding of C3b. When bound to a nonactivator, C3b is able to bind β1H and becomes inactivated through the combined effects of C3bINA and β1H (Fig. 3-10). When bound to an activator, control is restricted because β1H binding to C3b is decreased. As a consequence of the discriminatory phase of initiation, C3 convertase formation on the activator occurs, and amplification through the solid-phase C3 convertase commences. Through the additional enzymatic cleavage of C3, more C3b attaches to the membrane; receptor function is thought to reside in at least two critically oriented and closely spaced C3b molecules. Binding of activated factor B to the receptor results in the generation of the labile C5 convertase, $\overline{C3b,B}$, which also acts on C3. Upon the collision of native properdin (P) with the complex, P undergoes a transition to its bound form, $\overline{P}$. $\overline{P}$ confers an increased degree of stability on $\overline{C3b,B}$ converting it to the $\overline{C3b,B,P}$ enzyme. The $\overline{P}$-enzyme effects activation of C5 and self-assembly of the membrane attack complex C5b-9. Native C3 does not participate in this enzymatic reaction (Fig. 3-11).

Properdin itself does not seem to play the central role in the pathway it had once been assigned. It has been suggested that it is recruited late in the sequence rather than early as was previously assumed.[71] It greatly augments the cytolytic efficiency of the pathway, but its function is a non-essential one

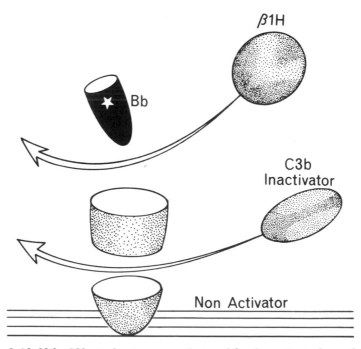

Figure 3-10. *If the C3b attaches to a non-activator of the alternative pathway, then β1H acts by dissociating the Bb fragment of Factor B from C3b, inactivating the alternative pathway C3 convertase, and rendering C3b vulnerable to cleavage by C3b inactivator (C3bINA). C3INA cleaves C3b, releasing C3c into the plasma, and leaving C3d bound to the membrane (see also Figure 3-11).*

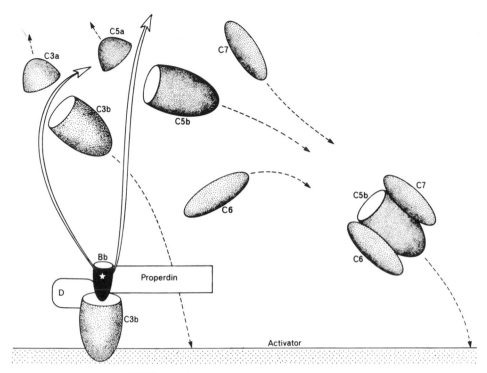

Figure 3-11. *The $\overline{C3b,Bb}$ complex (C3 convertase), by cleaving C3, will allow more C3b to accumulate on the surface. Properdin binds to the $\overline{C3b,Bb}$ complex, stabilizing the enzyme. The enzyme is also capable of cleaving C5 into C5a anaphylatoxin and C5b, which can combine with C6, C7, and attach to the membrane. Finally, C8 and C9 are absorbed, causing lysis of the cell.*

compared with that of the other components of the "Properdin" system.

Once C3 is activated in the alternative pathway, the molecular consequences seem to be identical to the classical pathway. The alternative pathway has not yet been incriminated in many immunohematologic problems; this may relate to the fact that it is very inefficient in the lysis of human red cells as compared with the classical pathway.[68] It is of interest to note that the red cells of patients suffering with paroxysmal nocturnal hemoglobinuria (PNH) can be shown to hemolyse through the alternative pathway as well as the classical pathway.[42] It is also of interest to note that activation of the alternative pathway by autologous red cell stroma has been described.[95]

BIOLOGICAL ACTIVITIES OF COMPLEMENT

Apart from the end result of cytolysis, the complement cascade is associated with other important biological activities. Most of these other activities, unlike cytolysis, do not need all the complement components to participate (Tables 3-5 and 3-6). Some of these activities are discussed briefly in the following paragraphs.

Table 3-5. BIOLOGIC ACTIVITIES OF COMPLEMENT COMPONENTS

C1	Increases association of Ag-Ab complexes
C4b	Virus neutralization
	Adherence via receptor on lymphocytes and phagocytic cells. ?Physiologic significance
C2 fragment	?C2 kinin
C3b	Adherence via receptor on lymphocytes and phagocytic cells—opsonin
	Activation of alternative pathway
	Triggers B lymphocytes to make mediators
	Triggers bone marrow leukocyte release
	Triggers release of Ag-Ab complexes from leukocyte surfaces
	Triggers more rapid division of tumor cells
C3d	Adherence via receptor on lymphocytes and macrophages opsonically active in association with IgG
C3a	Chemotactic factor, anaphylatoxin
C5a	Chemotactic factor, anaphylatoxin
C5b67	Chemotactic factor, may attack unsensitized cells
C8	Slow membrane damage
C9	Rapid membrane damage

Table 3-6. BIOLOGIC FUNCTIONS THAT CAN RESULT FROM ALTERNATIVE-PATHWAY ACTIVATION

Cobra-venom-mediated lysis of unsensitized erythrocytes
Erythrocyte lysis in paroxysmal nocturnal hemoglobinuria
Bactericidal activity
Phagocytosis
Anaphylatoxin production
Platelet histamine release, lysis, and promotion of blood clotting in animals
Leukotaxis
Mediation of Arthus vasculitis
Proteinuria of experimentally induced glomerulonephritis
Participation in renal damage of hypocomplementemic glomerulonephritis

Production of anaphylatoxins. Anaphylatoxins are substances of low molecular weight that are able to cause smooth muscle contraction, increased capillary permeability and systemic anaphylactic shock. Anaphylatoxin is derived from at least two distinct parent molecules, C3 and C5.[14] The C3a fragment (anaphylatoxin I) has a molecular weight of 10,000 and the C5a fragment (anaphylatoxin II) has a molecular weight of 12,000. These anaphylatoxins cause the release of histamine from mast cells and platelets.[60] Histamine increases the permeability of the blood capillaries, which enables leukocytes to penetrate the tissues where an infectious or allergic process is under way.[8, 121] The immediate effects seen following an ABO hemolytic transfusion reaction (e.g., flushing, pain in chest, headache, tingling along veins, etc.) probably result from the activation of the complement system with subsequent release of histamine.[74] More serious complications such as disseminated intravascular coagulation following incompatible blood transfusion may also be associated with activation of the complement cascade.

Chemotaxis. C3a, C5a and the trimolecular complex $\overline{C5,6,7}$ are chemotactic for granulocytes and monocytes, the C5a fragment being the more active one.[8, 121] Chemotactic factors cause the directed migration of leukocytes toward the chemotactic stimulus.

Immune adherence (IA). Immune adherence is based on the ability of antigen-antibody-complement complexes to adhere to the surface of non-sensitized particles such as red cells, leukocytes, platelets, and starch granules.[78] Immune adherence may be associated with phagocytosis *in vivo*. Sensitized bacteria or viruses that become attached to blood cells *in vivo* may be easier prey for phagocytes than highly mobile unattached organisms. In addition, the primary interaction (i.e., adherence) between monocytes/macrophages and C3b sensitized red cells (described in detail in Chapter 4) may be the *in vivo* equivalent of immune adherence. IA is usually dependent on bound C3b;[81] as a minimum for weak reactivity, more than 100 molecules per sheep red cell are necessary. Since only 10 to 20 percent of C3 is attached to red cells upon activation, an input of 1000 to 10,000 C3 molecules per red cell is required for efficient IA. EAC1,4b can produce IA, but many more molecules are needed (>3000/RBC).[15] Lymphocytes (B cells) have receptors for C3b and C4b; thus it is possible that immune adherence may play a role in the initiation of the immune response.[21, 64, 100]

Opsonization. Opsonins were described many years ago as substances present in normal plasma that enhanced bacterial destruction by making the organisms more "palatable" to phagocytes. Opsonization may be based on immune adherence. There is a receptor for C3b on macrophages. Thus, if cells escape cytolysis but have C3b on their surface (i.e., an opsonin) they may be engulfed and destroyed by macrophages (see Chapter 4). These end points can, of course, be reached through antibody initiating the classical pathway or, in the case of bacteria, initiation of the alternative pathway, by endotoxin.

Virus Neutralization. Complement has been shown to participate in antibody-mediated [19] and nonimmune viral inhibition. An extensive review of these mechanisms has been published recently.[16a]

Associations with Coagulation. The interactions between the complement and coagulation activation pathways are far from clearly understood. Some substances that activate the alternative pathway accelerate the clotting time of normal rabbits but not C6-deficient rabbits. Also, C6-deficient rabbits appear to have a prolonged clotting time and prothrombin consumption test that can be corrected by adding pure C6. In contrast, no defects in hemostasis have been mentioned in many reports of human inherited complement deficiencies. In fact, in a C6 deficient human family, no coagulation defects were observed.[49]

It has been suggested that Hageman factor (Factor XII) is the important link between immunologic reactions and clotting mechanisms.[97] Once activated, Hageman factor initiates three sequences. Firstly, Hageman factor initiates clotting by converting precursor plasma thromboplastin antecedent to its active form, starting the coagulation cascade, ending in fibrin formation. Secondly, Hageman factor acts in association with a co-factor to activate the fibrinolytic mechanism by converting plasminogen to its active proteolytic form, plasmin. Plasmin, once formed, not only digests fibrinogen, but it can activate C1 and cleave C3 directly. Finally, Hageman factor can directly activate prekallikrein to kallikrein. Kallikrein has the property of splitting off biologically active polypeptide fragments from an alpha globulin in plasma. These fragments, known as kinins (e.g., bradykinin), enhance vascular permeability, dilate small blood vessels, contract smooth muscle, and perhaps have chemotactic properties for leukocytes. These properties are similar to those of the anaphylatoxins (C3a and C5a) that are also released by the action of plasmin on C1 and/or C3.

In hereditary angio-edema (HAE), the affected individuals are heterozygotes for C1-esterase inhibitor (C1-INH) deficiency. Functional levels of the inhibitor are 5 to 30 percent of normal, but these fall to zero during acute attacks. The mechanism of edema seems to be related to the observation that C1-INH is a stoichiometric inhibitor, not only of C1-esterase, but also of enzymes released in their active form during triggering of the coagulation, fibrinolytic, and kinin cascades. These include FXIIa and its active fragments, FIXa, plasmin and kallikrein. C1-INH is consumed locally and systemically during the activation of one or more of these systems. The most likely candidate as a major substrate for the inhibitor is plasmin. As the C1-INH level falls to zero, C1 activates autocatalytically; a permeability-inducing kinin is liberated, probably from C2; and the increased vascular permeability leads to deep tissue edema.[12]

Rabbit platelets possess the C3b immune adherence receptor. Thus, these platelets may become involved in complement mediated reactions. Following immune adherence, platelet aggregation occurs, with release of vasoactive amines and ADP; in addition, platelet swelling, degranulation, and lysis may occur. It has been suggested that the C5b-9 complex is a likely candidate for conferring procoagulant activity on platelets.[132] So far, no such reaction has been demonstrated using the *immune-adherence negative* platelets of man.

Brown [12] has suggested that the most significant interaction between complement and coagulation may be in relation to vascular permeability. Anaphylatoxins, such as C3a and C5a, increase vascular permeability, causing neutrophils and monocytes to marginate on the walls of capillaries, arterioles and venules, leading to endothelial cell damage. The damage is caused by the released lysosomal enzymes, e.g., leucoprotease, collagenases, elastases and acid cathepsins D and E. Furthermore, the leucocytes may generate or release a leucocyte procoagulant with tissue thromboplastin-like activity. The effects may be reinforced by platelet aggregation on exposed subendothelial surfaces. In turn, the platelets also enhance leucocyte procoagulant activity, contributing further to local coagulation.

It has been suggested that disseminated intravascular coagulation associated with incompatible blood transfusion may be initiated by red cell stroma, which have a similar ultrastructure to endotoxin, activating the alternative complement pathway, which may interact with the coagulation cascade.[95]

Brown[12] has suggested that there is insufficient evidence at present to support the view that the complement and coagulation systems interact directly. Rather, during the activation of either cascade, biological functions are generated that may enhance the consumption of the other.

COMPLEMENT IN HUMAN DISEASE

Inborn Abnormalities

This type of complement abnormality is quite unusual. There are examples in the literature of individuals, or siblings in a family, lacking C1r, C1s, C4, C2, C3 (not total deficiency), C5, C6, C7 and C8 (Table 3-7).[28] The C1r,

Table 3-7. GENETIC COMPLEMENT DEFICIENCIES IN HUMANS

Deficient Component	Associated Clinical Findings
C1q (?)	SCID,* hypogammaglobulinemia
C1r	CGN,† SLE syndrome, frequent infections
C1s	SLE syndrome
C4	SLE syndrome, SLE ‡
C2	No disease, SLE syndrome, MPGN, § H-S purpura, ‖ dermatomyositis, discoid lupus, infections, chronic vasculitis, Hodgkin's disease
C3	Pyogenic infections, absence of expected neutrophilia
C5	Pyogenic infections, SLE
C5 dysfunction?	Infections, Leiner's disease
C6	No disease, meningococcal infections
C7	No disease, Raynaud's phenomenon, sclerodactyly, gonococcal infections
C8	No disease, gonococcal infections, SLE
C1-INH	Hereditary angioedema, SLE
C3b-INA	Pyogenic infections

* Severe combined immunodeficiency disease
† Chronic glomerulonephritis
‡ Systemic lupus erythematosus
§ Membranoproliferative glomerulonephritis
‖ Henoch-Schönlein purpura

C2, C3, C5 and C6 deficiencies have been shown to be inherited in an autosomal recessive fashion. Some of these patients have not been particularly sick. The C3 defective individuals did suffer from recurrent pyogenic infections but many patients with other defects deal with infections relatively well. An interesting finding has been an association of lupus-like syndrome with many of the inborn complement defects.[63]

The most common type of inborn defect is hereditary angioneurotic edema (HAE), which is transmitted as an autosomal dominant characteristic. This disease is associated with the defective synthesis of the C1 esterase inhibitor (C1-INH). Most patients have 5 to 30 percent of the normal inhibitor level. About 15 percent of the patients have a normal or elevated level; in these patients, the protein is nonfunctional. During acute attacks the C1-INH levels can fall to zero.[29]

Two patients with C3 inactivator deficiencies have now been reported.[1, 123] The patients had frequent infections, low levels of C3 and Factor B, and C3 inactivator was absent. The absence of C3 inactivator appeared to be associated with continuous fluid-phase activation of the alternative pathway, with resulting cleavage of C3. One interesting observation was that the cleaved C3b fragments attached to the patient's red cells, leading to a positive direct antiglobulin test but no *in vivo* hemolysis.

Acquired Abnormalities

Elevations. Elevated complement levels are usually associated with inflammatory conditions, e.g., acute rheumatic fever, rheumatoid arthritis, periarteritis nodosa, ulcerative colitis, sarcoidosis, diabetes, acute gout, Reiters syndrome and acute polyarthritis.

Depressions. *Increased utilization of complement.* This condition usually results from (a) fixation of complement by circulating or trapped antigen-antibody complexes, e.g., systemic lupus erythematosus (SLE), acute glomerulonephritis, bacterial endocarditis, cryoglobulinemia, or (b) fixation of complement to cells or tissue antibody, e.g., autoimmune hemolytic anemia, chronic glomerulonephritis.

Decreased synthesis: e.g., liver disease, progressive glomerulonephritis, and some cases of SLE.

MEASUREMENT OF COMPLEMENT ACTIVITY

Measurements of complement components are usually achieved by measuring the quantity of protein by an antigen-antibody reaction (e.g., precipitation) or by assays that measure the function of complement (e.g., hemolysis).[69, 96] The most commonly used method in the clinical laboratory is to measure the concentration of C3 (B1C/B1A) and/or C4 (B1E) in serum by the Mancini radial immunodiffusion technique.[66] The functional assay most commonly used is the "total" hemolytic complement assay. This assay expresses complement activity in CH_{50} units, which are defined as the reciprocal of the dilution of serum yielding 50 percent lysis of sheep erythrocytes sensitized with rabbit antibody (EA) under strictly controlled conditions. All nine components are necessary to cause cell lysis, and if any component is decreased to a limiting degree, an abnormal result will be obtained. In certain laboratories, specialized hemolytic assays have been developed to assess the functional activity of individual components. Further functional assays measure some of the biologic activities of complement, such as chemotaxis, enhancement of phagocytosis, or immune adherence.

In vivo fixed C3 and C4 may be located in tissues by the immunohistochemical analysis of biopsy or autopsy material, using a fluorescent or peroxidase technique with light microscopy or ferritin-conjugated antibody and electron microscopy.[51]

The number of molecules of C3 bound to human red cells can be measured by a technique based on the measurement of the inhibition of anti-C3 antibody after adding C3 sensitized red cells to a standard amount of the anti-C3 antibody.[10] The test may be standardized using known concentrations of C3 as determined immunochemically or radiochemically. We have applied this technique to study human erythrocytes that had been sensitized *in vitro* or *in vivo* with C3.[26] The amount of C3 on the red cells was measured with the quantitative assay, and this value was compared with results obtained using the antiglobulin test. Very weakly positive antiglobulin tests were noted when red cells were coated with 60 to 115 molecules of C3 per red cell. A highly significant correlation was demonstrated between the antiglobulin test titration scores and the quantitative assay of C3 sensitization. This correlation emphasizes that standard serologic tests utilizing antiglobulin test titration scores are very useful and simple means of obtaining information concerning the relative degree of sensitization of red cells by C3 (see Chapters 5 and 6).

The half-life of C3 and C4 in the circulation may be determined using radio-labelled, highly purified components. From these data can be computed the rate of destruction and synthesis of these proteins. Comparison of these data in normal subjects and patients have provided important evidence that complement plays a role in the pathogenesis of certain diseases.[86, 87] Petz et al.[86] showed that the fractional catabolic rate (FCR) of C3, in fifteen normal subjects, averaged 2.12 percent per hour and the normal range was from 1.56 to 2.68. The synthesis rate of C3 averaged 1.16 mg/kg/hr with a normal range of from 0.9 to 1.42. The mean serum level of C3 was 1.43 mg/ml (range 1.0–1.9 mg/ml).

The fractional catabolic rate and synthesis rate of C3 were at the upper limit of normal or were increased above normal in patients who had warm antibody autoimmune hemolytic anemia with complement on their erythrocytes and in patients with paroxysmal nocturnal hemoglobinuria studied during periods of active hemolysis. An increased C3 synthesis rate was also found in one patient who was hematologically normal but had an active peptic ulcer and elevated serum concentration of C3.

A normal fractional catabolic rate and C3 synthesis rate were found in patients with autoimmune hemolytic anemia associated with methyldopa administration, atypical cold antibody autoimmune hemolytic anemia, and in paroxysmal nocturnal hemoglobinuria during an asymptomatic interval.

In sixteen C3 protein turnover studies in patients with systemic lupus erythematosus (SLE), variable FCR and synthetic rates were noted, and these seemed related, at least in part, to the disease activity. Only patients with severe disease activity had a combination of abnormalities consisting of an increased fractional catabolic rate and a depressed rate of synthesis of C3 or, in one instance, a strikingly increased FCR. In all such patients, the serum concentration of C3 was strikingly reduced (0.50 mg/ml). Such patients were (with one exception) being treated with high doses of corticosteroids or immunosuppressive drugs.

Patients with less active disease characteristically had mildly to moderately elevated increased fractional catabolic rates. C3 synthetic rates were normal, mildly elevated or, in one case, reduced. Serum C3 concentrations were normal or somewhat reduced.

Patients with inactive disease had essentially normal metabolic studies. Three of these patients had end stage disease, although presently inactive SLE.

A patient with pathologic high titer cold hemagglutinin disease had an elevated FCR, with an elevated synthesis rate, and he maintained a serum C3 concentration that was at the lower limit of normal.

Two patients with paroxysmal nocturnal hemoglobinuria had essentially normal values of complement metabolism, borderline exceptions being a slightly low C3 concentration in one patient and a slightly elevated C3 synthesis rate in the other.

In a patient with hypocomplementemic nephritis, the fractional catabolic rate was strikingly increased at 11.3 percent per hour, and this finding was associated with a very low serum C3 concentration. The C3 synthesis rate was elevated, 1.85 mg/kg/hr.

In marked contrast, three patients with Laennec's cirrhosis of the liver with low serum C3 concentrations had fractional catabolic rates within normal limits and had borderline or very low C3 synthesis rates.

Such studies clarify aspects of the metabolism of C3 in selected disorders. They indicate that, in patients with SLE, the most acutely ill patients characteristically had a combined defect of increased catabolism and decreased synthesis, leading to a very reduced serum level of C3. Patients with less severe disease have moderate increases in fractional catabolic rate but still have borderline low or distinctly low serum C3 concentrations because of an apparent inability of such patients to compensate by adequately increasing their rate of synthesis of C3.

In contrast to patients with autoimmune disorders, hypocomplementemic patients with Laennec's cirrhosis of the liver had C3 synthetic rates that were strikingly reduced or at the lower limit of normal. This finding strengthens the concept that the liver is the primary site of synthesis of C3.

However, other investigators have reported that patients with another type of liver disease, i.e., acute viral hepatitis, may have a low serum concentration of C3 caused by activation of serum complement by immune complexes composed of hepatitis B antigen and antibody.

In summary, the latter studies extended previous observations concerning the metabolism of C3 in autoimmune disorders [86] and indicate that variable mechanisms may lead to low concentrations of serum complement, thus emphasizing that complement determinations must be cautiously interpreted in conjunction with clinical information.

THE ROLE OF COMPLEMENT IN IMMUNOHEMATOLOGY

Complement may be activated and sensitize red cells (without necessarily proceeding to lysis) through several different mechanisms.

Complement Activated by Antibodies

Complement may be activated by autoantibodies or alloantibodies of the IgM class, or IgG class, if they are of IgG1, IgG2, or IgG3 subclasses. It is not understood why some alloantibodies, such as anti-Rh, which are almost always IgG1 or IgG3, do not activate complement. It has been suggested that it might relate to the number of antigenic sites present on the red cell. [74] It has been calculated that 1000 IgG molecules would be necessary to form one IgG doublet on a red cell with 800,000 antigenic sites (e.g., A or B). There are only about 10 to 30,000 Rh sites per red cell, thus, the chance of two IgG molecules falling close enough together to form a doublet is remote. This explanation is hard to accept because: (a) some other antibodies (e.g., anti-K) can activate complement, [74, 85, 89] yet there are fewer K antigenic sites (approximately 3,000–6,000 per red cell) than Rh; (b) Rh antigens may be mobile in the membrane and cluster during the antigen-antibody reaction, [67] thus considerably increasing the chance of doublet formation; (c) IgM Rh antibodies do not activate complement; and (d) two examples of anti-Rh have been described that do sensitize red cells with complement. [4, 127]

Red cells may become sensitized with complement components without necessarily proceeding to lysis. The antiglobulin test has been used to show the presence of C3 (C3d), C4 (C4d), C5, C6, and C8 bound to the membrane of red cells that have not lysed. [34, 36, 46, 62, 94]

Some blood group alloantibodies commonly cause lysis of normal red cells, e.g., anti-A, -B, -Vel, -PP₁Pᴷ (Tjᵃ); others may sensitize the red cell with complement components, often not causing lysis of normal red cells unless they are enzyme-treated, e.g., some anti-Lewis, and -Kidd. Still other examples of anti-Lewis, -Kidd, -Kell, -Duffy, -S, -s, -I, -i, -H, -P, -Gyᵃ, and -Jr may sensitize red cells with complement components without causing lysis of untreated or enzyme-treated cells. It is not understood why some antibodies sensitize red cells with enough C3 to give strongly positive antiglobulin tests yet do not proceed to lysis; it cannot be explained in purely quantitative terms. Some of these antibodies are IgM and cause agglutination of the red cells, as well as complement sensitization detectable by the indirect antiglobulin test (e.g., anti-A, -B, -I, -i, -P_1 and some anti-Lewis). Other rare examples may be IgM and do not cause agglutination under normal conditions (e.g., some anti-Lewis, -Kell, -Duffy, and -Kidd) but may sensitize red cells with complement, detectable by the antiglobulin test. Still others are IgG (e.g., some anti-Kell, -Duffy, -Jr, -Gy[a], and most anti-Kidd); the IgG sensitization is usually readily detected by the antiglobulin test in addition to the complement sensitization, but in some cases (e.g., some anti-Kidd) the IgG sensitization is very weak and the complement sensitization very strong.[56, 59, 74, 89]

When blood group antibodies bind complement to the red cell membrane, the immunoglobulin responsible is demonstrable by the antiglobulin test sometimes and not other times. For instance, IgG complement binding alloantibodies (e.g., anti-K, -Fy[a], -Jk[a]) are usually detectable, in addition to bound complement, on the red cell membrane. IgG *auto*antibodies are detectable together with complement in 50 percent of autoimmune hemolytic anemia (AIHA) cases.

In some situations the immunoglobulin is not readily detectable by routine methods, or indeed, is no longer present on the red cell: (a) When IgM antibodies sensitize red cells without causing direct agglutination they are very difficult to detect by the antiglobulin test by using anti-IgM in the antiglobulin sera.[34, 53] Fortunately, these antibodies invariably bind complement and are detected by the anticomplement properties of the antiglobulin sera. This is theoretically a more sensitive method, as every IgM molecule will cause hundreds of C3 molecules to sensitize the red cell. (b) About 13 percent of the patients with warm autoimmune hemolytic anemia have positive direct antiglobulin tests due to sensitization with complement, with no IgG, IgM, or IgA being detected on the red cells by the antiglobulin test. Some of these patients are thought to have IgG present on their red cells, but it is present in amounts below the threshold of the antiglobulin test, as performed routinely. To obtain a positive antiglobulin test approximately 200 to 500 molecules of IgG per red cell must be present.[74] Gilliland et al.,[39] using an antiglobulin-consumption-complement-fixation assay, have shown that some of the patients described in this paragraph have IgG on their red cells, in the order of 50 to 200 molecules, which is not detectable by the regular antiglobulin test (see Chapter 9). (c) In cold agglutinin disease the patient's IgM autoantibody usually only reacts up to 30 to 32°C. Thus, the patient's red cells become sensitized with antibody in the peripheral circulation when the skin temperature drops to this range. The antibody usually binds complement to the red cells, and if conditions are optimal, hemolysis of the cells may occur. If the cells escape hemolysis they will recirculate to 37°C, and the cold autoantibody will elute back from the cell into the plasma, leaving complement components firmly bound to the red cell. Thus, when a positive direct antiglobulin test is obtained on these patients, it results from the anti-complement in the antiglobulin sera reacting with the red cell bound complement; IgM is usually not detectable on the red cell.

Complement Activation by Immune Complexes

Red cells can become sensitized with complement from the activation of the complement cascade by immune complexes. Sometimes these immune complexes are on the red cell, other times they may be remote from the cell. A good example of this is the formation of immune complexes by certain drugs, e.g., phenacetin or quinidine.[35] The drug-anti-drug complex can attach non-specifically to the red cells and cause activation of complement, with subsequent attachment of complement components to the red cell membrane (see Chapter 8). It is possible that other immune complexes such as DNA-anti-DNA, bacteria-anti-bacteria, and virus-anti-virus may also result in red cells becoming sensitized with complement.

Non-immune Sensitization of Red Cells with Complement

The cephalosporins can modify red cell membranes so that they can take up proteins non-immunologically, including complement components.[35] When incubated in normal plasma in vitro, cephalothin-sensitized cells become coated with numerous plasma proteins including albumin, IgG, IgA, IgM, α_1-antitrypsin, α_2-macroglobulin, C3, C4 and fibrinogen. This information is of significance in that one can generally determine whether the positive direct antiglobulin test has resulted from non-immunologic protein absorption or by antibody fixation. Non-immunologic absorption of proteins will result in the direct antiglobulin test being positive with antiglobulin sera raised to a variety of proteins (e.g., α, β, and γ globulins, albumin and fibrinogen). Hemolytic anemia has not been described as a result of non-immunologic protein absorption. These factors are discussed in detail in Chapter 8, page 283.

The Detection of Red Cell Bound Complement Components by the Antiglobulin Test. As discussed previously, complement components may be bound to the red cell membrane *in vitro* (e.g., by blood group alloantibodies, such as anti-Jk^a) or *in vivo* by alloantibodies (i.e., transfusion reactions), autoantibodies, or drug-induced antibodies. Usually the immunoglobulin responsible for the complement activation can also be detected on the cell surface, but occasionally the antiglobulin test detects the bound complement without detecting immunoglobulin.

It has been known for over 20 years that antiglobulin sera that contained antibodies to the "non-gamma" globulin fraction of human serum would react with red cell bound complement.[17] This finding was later shown to be due to the fact that C3 and C4, the predominant cell bound components, are both beta globulins (B$_{1C}$ and B$_{1E}$ respectively).[46, 94] Later work has shown that C5, C6, and C8 can also be detected on the red cells by the antiglobulin test.[36, 62]

As discussed earlier, it is the C3b, C4b and C5b fragments that attach to the cell membrane following an immune reaction. When C3b and/or C4b sensitized red cells are allowed to incubate in normal plasma or serum (circulating *in vivo* or prolonged incubation *in vitro*), they are acted on by a naturally occurring enzyme present in plasma/serum, C3b inactivator. Eventually (see reference 62 for *in vitro* conversion times), the C3b and C4b molecules are cleaved, releasing C3c and/or C4c into the plasma, leaving C3d and/or C4d on the red cell (Fig. 3-12). Antiglobulin sera will react with such cells only if they contain antibodies against determinants on the C3d and C4d molecules.[36, 89] Sometimes anti-C3 (anti-B$_{1C}$) or anti-C4 (anti-B$_{1E}$) reagents will only contain activity against determinants on the C3c (B$_{1A}$) or C4c molecule.[36, 57] Such reagents may react well with red cells sensitized with complement *in vitro*, as short incubations (e.g., 15 to 30 minutes) in serum are usually employed, but they will not react with red cells sensitized with complement *in vivo*.

In recent years, a major unresolved problem has been the definition of the optimal qualitative and quantitative characteristics of the anticomplement component of antiglobulin sera. It should be added that some uncertainties also remain in regard to antibodies against red cell bound immunoglobulins. In 1971, we evaluated commercially available antiglobulin sera with regard to their anticomplement activity.[34] This controversial subject is still unsettled. It is convenient to discuss the problems concerning the direct antiglobulin test and the indirect antiglobulin test separately.

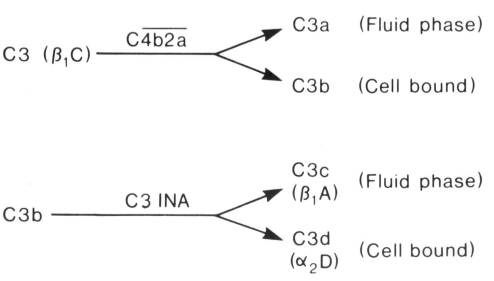

Figure 3-12. *Reaction products of C3. In vivo, or after prolonged incubation in vitro, the C3 inactivator (C3 INA) and β1H (see page 75) react with cell bound C3b so that only the C3d fragment remains on the cell surface.*[85]

The Role of Complement in the Antiglobulin Test *

Role of Complement in the Direct Antiglobulin Test. The direct anti-globulin test is used for the detection and differential diagnosis of immune hemolytic anemias, i.e., autoimmune hemolytic anemias, hemolytic transfusion reactions, and hemolytic disease of the newborn. It is well established that anti-IgG and anticomplement antibodies are essential components for a polyspecific ("broad-spectrum") antiglobulin reagent to be utilized for the direct antiglobulin test. Anti-IgG is essential, since most immune hemolytic anemias are caused by IgG antibodies that will be detectable on the patient's red cells by the direct antiglobulin test. Indeed, in regard to hemolytic disease of the newborn, there are only two patients described in the world literature in whom complement components but no IgG were detected on the cord red blood cells; the antibodies involved were anti-K and anti-Jk[a].[113] However, about one third of the patients with autoimmune hemolytic anemia will have a clinically misleading false negative direct antiglobulin test if the antiglobulin serum utilized contains only antibodies against IgG.[13, 25, 34, 36, 89] In all but a small minority of such instances, the use of an antiglobulin serum containing antibodies against C3d (a fragment of the third component of complement) will yield a positive reaction.[13, 25, 34, 36, 85, 88, 89] Although the red blood cells of patients with hemolytic transfusion reactions are commonly sensitized with IgG, cases are encountered in which the red blood cells react only with anti-globulin sera containing anticomplement. Stratton[111, 114] describes such a case due to anti-Jk[a] where the DAT was 4+ with a reagent containing anticomplement and negative with anti-IgG reagents. We have ourselves recently encountered a delayed transfusion reaction due to anti-Jk[a], where the DAT was positive with reagents containing anti-C3d but negative with anti-IgG; an eluate prepared from the patient's red cells was shown to contain anti-Jk[a].

Thus, there is agreement among all workers concerning the necessity for anti-IgG and anti-C3d antibodies in antiglobulin serum to be utilized for the direct antiglobulin test.

With regard to antibodies against other complement components in antiglobulin serum, we have occasionally found patients whose red blood cells are sensitized with C4d but not C3d. However, none of these patients have had hemolytic anemia.[36] Patients with immune hemolytic anemia frequently have C4d on their red blood cells in addition to C3d, but in testing literally hundreds of patients with acquired immune hemolytic anemia, we have not observed a single patient with hemolysis whose red blood cells were sensitized with only C4d.[36, 89] We know of no experience contrary to this in the literature. Therefore, anti-C4 antibodies appear to be superfluous in antiglobulin serum used for detection and differential diagnosis of immune hemolytic anemia. Similarly, although with less extensive data available, antibodies to other complement components in antiglobulin serum (C5,C6,C8) have not been proven to be of significant clinical value.[36, 62] Presently available data indicate that the

---

* Abbreviations in this text are as follows: DAT (direct antiglobulin test), IAT (indirect anti-globulin test), AGT (antiglobulin test), and AGS (antiglobulin serum).

optimal antibody specificities that should be required in antiglobulin serum for the direct antiglobulin test are anti-IgG and anti-C3d.

It is important to emphasize that, even though antibodies other than anti-IgG and anti-C3d may be generally superfluous, they are not detrimental in an antiserum that is to be utilized for the direct antiglobulin test. For instance, we know of no evidence to suggest that the presence of anti-IgA or IgM is detrimental and, indeed, their presence could be counted as a bonus. [40, 116, 130] From a practical standpoint, this is of importance to manufacturers because a pure anti-C3d antibody is difficult to produce, whereas an antiserum containing anti-C3d antibodies as well as antibodies to other antigenic determinants of C3 (e.g., C3c) and to other components of complement (e.g., C4) is much easier to produce. There is no evidence to suggest that anti-C3c is detrimental, but the question of anti-C4 activity has been debated. [36, 115] If one utilizes red blood cells from EDTA specimens (which are optimal since EDTA inhibits *in vitro* fixation of complement), the only possible disadvantage is the detection of a few clinically insignificant positive direct antiglobulin tests. This would not appear to be an important problem because many positive direct antiglobulin tests are also caused by red blood cell sensitization with C3d or IgG in patients who do not have immune hemolytic anemia. [13, 18, 36, 85, 88, 89]

For instance, we find 8 percent of hospital patients to have a positive DAT. Most of these positive results are due to red cell bound complement, and most are unassociated with anemia, although some are associated with possible autoimmune disease (e.g., SLE, RA). This finding emphasizes the fact that all positive results must be interpreted in conjunction with clinical and other serologic data.

The Role of Complement in the Indirect Antiglobulin Test. Prior to 1977, only polyspecific antiglobulin reagents (to be used for both the direct and indirect antiglobulin tests) were commercially available in the United States. As indicated in the preceding paragraphs, anti-complement antibodies are required for some uses of AGS, and there has been no doubt that for these uses AGS should contain anticomplement antibodies. In anticipation of the fact that monospecific reagents would become commercially available, we began to reassess the requirements for anticomplement antibodies in AGS with regard to compatibility testing. [85] Since all but a small percentage of AGS is used for compatibility testing, standards for this purpose are of great significance.

The central question in this regard is, "What are the incidence and clinical significance of red blood cell alloantibodies that are detectable, when using standard serologic techniques, only by the antiglobulin test and only by the anticomplement component of the antiglobulin serum?" To be more specific, we are referring to alloantibodies that are not detectable by direct agglutination in saline or albumin or by the anti-IgG component of antiglobulin serum, but are detected by the anticomplement component of antiglobulin serum. Also of importance are reports of antibodies whose reactivity in the indirect antiglobulin test is significantly enhanced because of the role of complement.

Polley and Mollison [92] reported six anti-Le[a] antibodies, two anti-Jk[a] antibodies, and one anti-Kell antibody which were predominantly incomplete, that is, nonagglutinating types of antibody. All these antibodies gave a positive IAT only when complement as well as antibody was absorbed onto the cells. In addition, these authors described one anti-Fy[a] antibody which gave positive indirect antiglobulin reactions in the absence of complement, although the presence of complement "greatly enhanced the reactions."

Stratton, Gunson, and Rawlinson [112] described enhancement of IAT results using anticomplement AGS with one example each of anti-Kell, anti-Jk[b] and anti-P₁ antibodies.

Polley, Mollison, and Soothill [93] described certain IgM antibodies that reacted as agglutinins only at temperatures up to 25 to 30°C but acted as incomplete antibodies at 37°C. Such antibodies were only weakly detected in the IAT using anti-IgM, and they were always easier to detect using anticomplement serum. Antibodies that reacted in this way included eight anti-Le[a] and single examples of anti-O(HI), anti-P₁ and anti-I (which was from an i donor). Unfortunately, there are no data to indicate the clinical relevance of such antibodies. The same workers also described three anti-Jk[a] antibodies that were warm incomplete IgM antibodies and that reacted more strongly in the indirect antiglobulin test when using anticomplement antiglobulin serum.

Adinolfi et al.[2] described IgM antibodies that did not cause agglutination at 37°C but that were detected in the IAT using anti-IgM (anti-β_2M) or anticomplement (anti-β_1) antiserum. Antibodies of anti-Jk[a], anti-P₁, anti-O(H) and anti-I specificities were reported, but it is not clear whether or not these were the same antibodies described by Polley, Mollison, and Soothill.[93]

Stratton, Gunson, and Rawlinson [113] reported two cases of hemolytic disease of the newborn caused by complement fixing antibodies; one associated with anti-K and the other anti-Jk[a]. The anti-Jk[a] antibody caused a 2+ IAT with anti-IgG, but 5+ reactions using antiglobulin sera containing anticomplement. In both cases the direct antiglobulin test performed on cord blood was positive only with anticomplement containing reagents.

Stratton, Smith and Rawlinson [118] described an anti-Jk[a] that was not detectable in the IAT using anti-IgG, gave weak reactions (2+) using anti-IgM, and gave strong reactions (5+) using anticomplement serum. In a further report, the same workers [117] reported an anti-Jk[a] and an anti-s that were nonagglutinating IgM antibodies and that were detectable in the IAT with anticomplement sera. The authors emphasized that they found it difficult to detect red blood cell sensitization with IgM antibodies in the IAT utilizing an anti-IgM antiserum. Similarly, Mollison [74] points out that "All incomplete IgM antibodies described (except for those with Rh specificity) have proved to be capable of binding complement, and in practice it is easier to detect complement components than to detect IgM on the red cells."

Stratton [111, 114] described a delayed hemolytic transfusion reaction due to anti-Jk[a]. The anti-Jk[a] reacted strongly by IAT when tested with AGS containing anticomplement, but no reactions were obtained with any anti-IgG reagents. Stratton commented that anticomplement antibodies are "an absolutely necessary ingredient" of AGS to be used for the IAT.

Sherwood, Haynes, and Rosse [108] reported a patient who had two symptomatic acute hemolytic transfusion reactions with hemoglobinemia and hemoglobinuria. Both suspect units were entirely compatible by routine crossmatch using commercial antiglobulin sera. However, both units were clearly incompatible using a potent anti-C3 antiserum (which was prepared in their laboratory) in the antiglobulin phase of the crossmatch. Subsequently, it was possible to predict *in vivo* compatibility using the potent anti-C3 antiserum.

Over a period of 20 years we have also seen examples of anti-Kell, anti-Duffy and anti-Kidd that are detectable using AGS containing anticomplement but do not react with AGS lacking anticomplement. Engelfriet [24] also reports seeing similar examples.

Issitt [56] and Issitt and Smith [59] have reported that 19 of 29 (65.5 percent) anti-Duffy and anti-Kidd antibodies gave a higher titer end-point in IAT titrations using an AGS containing anti-IgG and anticomplement compared with IAT titrations using a monospecific anti-IgG AGS. They emphasized that a stronger in vitro reaction will lessen the chance that a significant positive reaction will be missed in a compatibility test in the blood bank. We have also seen examples of anti-Kell, anti-Duffy and anti-Kidd that, although reacting with anti-IgG, give greatly enhanced reactions with AGS containing anticomplement.

In spite of such evidence indicating the need for anticomplement antibodies in AGS for the detection of clinically significant alloantibodies in the IAT phase of the compatibility test, there is justification for further study of this point. This is true because the total number of such antibodies reported in a period of more than 15 years is small and, in addition, techniques used in performing the compatibility test were frequently different than are presently utilized. Specifically, most early reports utilized antiglobulin tests performed on tiles rather than techniques involving centrifugation; some investigators did not include albumin in the incubation procedures; and it is possible that the anti-IgG present in modern reagents is better.

In 1976,[85] we presented data concerning 113 non-Rh alloantibodies including 94 of anti-Kell, anti-Duffy, anti-Kidd and anti-S specificities that were detectable in the indirect antiglobulin test. Although 29 percent of these antibodies fixed complement, only one (an anti-S) required the anticomplement component of AGS for detection in the IAT. Considering the incidence of anti-K, anti-Fy^a, anti-Jk^a, and anti-S antibodies (which are responsible for a vast majority of hemolytic transfusion reactions outside of the ABO and Rh systems) as about two in 1,000 patients,[74] we estimated that a blood transfusion service transfusing 6,000 units per year (about 2,000 patients per year) would require the anticomplement component of AGS for detection of such alloantibodies only once every 25 years, and that an average sized hospital in the San Francisco Bay Area would detect such antibodies only once every 107 years. Subsequently, Giblett [38] has indicated that the incidence of anti-K, anti-Fy, anti-Jk and anti-S antibodies has increased in recent decades and is 6.3 per 1,000 patients at the Puget Sound Blood Center. Using these data, a blood transfusion service transfusing 2,000 patients per year would require anticomplement antibodies in AGS about once every eight years to detect these antibodies if 1 percent of them required the anticomplement component of AGS for their detection.

We emphasized that such estimates are of some interest but, of course, could not be looked upon as definitive.[117] The study was done using sera that had been selected and stored because they were good typing sera. Thus, the sera may have been retained on the basis of being strong IgG antibodies. The sera used in the study had been stored at−20°C for months to years, and even though we added fresh complement to them, this may not have overcome anticomplementary properties that may have developed. We indicated that the data must be augmented by a carefully designed prospective study before a definitive conclusion could be reached. Indeed, we stated that "The reason for discussing the possible frequency of antibodies detected only with the anticomplement component of antiglobulin sera at this time when our data are so preliminary is to emphasize that we need more extensive data regarding this point."

Beck and Marsh [6] cited retrospective recollections of their own without supplying any information concerning methodology used, and cited our data without alluding to any of our qualifying comments, and concluded that "effective alloantibody detection is not dependent upon anticomplement activity of the antiglobulin reagents." Such a definitive statement does not appear warranted yet unless supported by the results of an extensive and carefully designed prospective study. Such a study must utilize well characterized anticomplement sera that are more potent than are presently available in polyspecific reagents. This is true because of the recent reports that question the *in vivo* significance of alloantibodies that are unreactive *in vitro* at temperatures less than 37°C.[38] The omission of a room temperature phase of the crossmatch may allow for significantly higher concentrations of anticomplement antibodies in AGS for compatibility testing. In addition, the limitations of utilizing sera from referring laboratories must be recognized. Information must be available concerning the anticomplement antibodies in AGS utilized in the referring laboratory, and the possibility of decay of complement in referred sera must be appreciated. The decay rate of serum complement in regard to activity in the IAT has previously been documented.[33] Studies designed to take into account the essential considerations previously indicated are in progress in several laboratories (including our own) and should furnish adequate data in order to develop valid conclusions in the near future. Our preliminary data support the arguments that clinically significant antibodies may be missed if the AGS used in the crossmatching procedure lacks anticomplement activity.

In 1977, the Bureau of Biologists (FDA) provided funds for a three-year study on the controversial role of anti-complement in antiglobulin reagents. As a part of that study, we have been collaborating with Stanford University in a prospective study to answer the question posed previously concerning the incidence and clinical significance of antibodies detected only or primarily by anticomplement. Eight hundred ninety-three antibodies were detected in testing sera from 18,445 patients using the antiglobulin technique. In six patients alloantibodies were detected only or primarily when the antiglobulin reagent contained anticomplement.

Four patients developed anti-Jk^a antibodies post-transfusion, two detectable only with antiglobulin sera containing anti-complement; the others reacting in such a way that they probably would have been missed without anticomplement. Two patients were found to have sustained delayed hemolytic transfusion reactions. In another patient, a ^{51}Cr survival of Jk(a+) red blood cells showed mild shortened survival. The fourth could not be evaluated. One patient, on initial compatibility testing, had a questionable weak anti-Jk^b reacting primarily with anti-complement. ^{51}Cr survival of Jk(b+) red cells showed a 10 percent survival at 24 hours. One patient was found on initial testing to have an antibody to a new low incidence antigen detectable only with anticomplement; its significance is uncertain. Without the use of antiglobulin sera containing anti-complement, most or all of these antibodies would not have been detected.[52]

Potential Detrimental Effect of Anticomplement Antibodies in Antiglobulin Sera. If anticomplement antibodies do prove to be of value only rarely in compatibility testing, an additional question that must be considered is whether such antibodies are in any way detrimental or whether their presence would, nevertheless, be advantageous. Several possible reasons have been proposed to support the concept that anticomplement antibodies are detrimental in AGS to be utilized for compatibility testing. Some workers firmly believe that AGS containing anticomplement antibodies cause numerous "false positive" reactions. There are several potential causes for such reactions. They may result from agglutination reactions caused by factors other than anticomplement antibodies, such as anti-species antibodies [56, 58, 59] or other nonspecific agglutinating components,[31]* or to be true but undesirable positive reactions resulting from complement fixation by clinically insignificant cold antibodies.

What is often meant in referring to such "false positive" reactions is that some weakly positive agglutination reactions are found in the IAT phase of compatibility testing that cannot be identified as being caused by any blood group antibody. Although such unwanted and clinically insignificant weakly positive reactions that occur with some batches of AGS are assumed by some to be caused by anticomplement antibodies, no data supporting this assumption have been published. In studying this problem, Issitt [56, 58, 59] performed a series of experiments that indicated that, with the products of certain American manufacturers, the incidence of unwanted positive reactions increased concomitantly with increases of anticomplement antibodies in those reagents. However, these "false positive" reactions were caused by the introduction of anti-species antibodies at the same time as the anticomplement levels were

* Garratty, G.: unpublished observations.

increased, and awareness of this fact allowed manufacturers to produce AGS with high concentrations of anticomplement antibodies without resulting in undesired "false positive" reactions.

Some inexplicable positive reactions may not be related to anti-species antibodies. Freedman, Chaplin, and Mollison [31] reported that two antiglobulin sera prepared in their laboratory continued to cause weak agglutination of normal red blood cells even after 12 absorptions with washed packed red blood cells of mixed A, B, and O groups. We have occasionally encountered similar results in antisera prepared in our laboratory, and we also find that such weak agglutination still occurs even using sera which may be considerably diluted.

Another potential cause of "false positive" reactions relates to the fact that clinically insignificant cold antibodies that are reactive at room temperature but not at 37°C are not infrequently encountered. It is common practice in the USA to incubate the mixture of serum and cells at room temperature before incubating at 37°C for the IAT. Some cold antibodies fix complement at room temperature, and the complement remains fixed to the red blood cells during incubation at 37°C. Although the antibody is not reactive at 37°C, anticomplement antibodies in AGS used in the IAT will detect the complement that had been fixed at room temperature. Such positive reactions would be caused by anticomplement antibodies in AGS reacting with complement sensitized red blood cells and therefore, would not be "false positive." Nevertheless, this terminology is usually applied when referring to such undesired positive reactions.

The detection and identification of such clinically insignificant antibodies is a waste of time. Most antibodies that are reactive at room temperature are detected because of agglutination, and there are no data available to indicate the frequency of clinically insignificant cold antibodies detected only with the anticomplement component of AGS. However, some are certainly detected only as a result of anticomplement antibodies in AGS, and the increased use of low ionic strength saline solutions in blood banks will probably increase the number detected. Nevertheless, what is likely to be more important in this regard is the fact that several investigators have suggested that the room temperature phase of the crossmatch is, in itself, a waste of time.[38] Giblett [38] states that it is unnecessary to be concerned with alloantibodies that do not react at 37°C since she has observed no instance of *in vivo* hemolysis associated with a cold reacting alloantibody (such as anti-A_1, anti-P, anti-M, anti-N, anti-Lu^a, etc.) during a 20-year period when over a million units of blood were transfused. If controlled prospective studies confirm such observations, the elimination of the room temperature phase of the crossmatch would eliminate the problem of detecting clinically insignificant cold antibodies. Further, the omission of the room temperature phase of the crossmatch and the use of red blood cells from anticoagulated specimens would make it practical to significantly increase the amount of anticomplement antibodies in AGS used for the indirect antiglobulin test.[24, 36, 111] Unfortunately, the increasing use of low ionic strength solution (LISS) in routine pre-transfusion testing has complicated the issue. Some weakly positive indirect antiglobulin tests due to bound complement are seen with clinically insignificant antibodies when LISS suspended red cells are used, even though the tests are carried out strictly at 37°C.*

Still another potential cause of "false positive" reactions is *in vivo* complement sensitization of the recipient's red blood cells by normal incomplete cold antibody during refrigeration. This is particularly true if clotted specimens are utilized as the source of red blood cells for the compatibility test, since most anticoagulants will inhibit such complement fixation. We have studied this problem in detail [36] and confirmed that potent anti-C3 and anti-C4 antisera containing high concentrations of antibodies to C3d and C4d respectively, prepared in our laboratory, did, indeed, cause numerous positive reactions when tested against refrigerated red blood cells from clotted and, to a lesser degree, anticoagulated (ACD and CPD) blood. This finding was particularly true using AGS containing anti-C4 (especially anti-C4d). However, we also emphasized that commercially available AGS that contained as high a concentration of anticomplement antibodies as any presently available at that time gave uniformly negative results when tested with samples obtained from clots and segments from 200 refrigerated donor units. Issitt and Smith [59] have similarly concluded that the concentration of anticomplement antibodies in commercially available AGS is insufficient to cause agglutination of red blood cells refrigerated in autologous serum or plasma. Thus, presently available data indicate that manufacturers have avoided this potential problem by avoiding excessively high concentrations of anticomplement antibodies in AGS.

The question of the existence of "false positive" reactions caused by anticomplement antibodies in AGS can and should be studied more extensively. This is a difficult problem to approach since two laboratories using the same AGS may disagree on the presence or absence of "false positive" reactions because of subtle technical differences in reading agglutination reactions (e.g., whether microscopic or macroscopic readings are made). Nevertheless, more extensive studies concerning the incidence of the various possible causes of these reactions would be important in clarifying this aspect of antiglobulin testing.

The three potential causes of "false positive" reactions are species antibodies, normal incomplete cold antibody, and other clinically insignificant cold antibodies. Species antibodies are unlikely to constitute a significant problem. If normal incomplete cold autoantibodies are responsible for complement fixation (even with the use of red blood cells from anticoagulated ACD or CPD) specimens and are thus the cause of "false positive" reactions, this would be a significant nuisance that could be tolerated only if balanced by benefit obtained from anticomplement antibodies in AGS. The detection of clinically insignificant cold antibodies at room temperature should be avoided. Eliminating anticomplement antibodies from AGS would eliminate the detection of only a portion of such antibodies since many are detected by direct

* Petz, L. and Garratty, G.: unpublished data.

agglutination. Eliminating the room temperature phase of the crossmatch might be the optimal approach. More data are necessary concerning the disadvantages (if any) of eliminating the room temperature phase of the crossmatch, and more data are also needed concerning the frequency with which clinically important alloantibodies are detected with the anticomplement component of AGS before the best solution to this problem can be reached. At the present time, a large majority of commercially prepared AGS manufactured in the USA contains a reasonable concentration of anticomplement antibodies, and such sera are used routinely for compatibility testing, so that the problem of "false positive" reactions does not appear to be of major significance.

COMPLEMENT RECEPTORS AND CELL ASSOCIATED COMPLEMENT COMPONENTS

Receptors for activated complement components are widely distributed amongst tissue cells of most mammalian species. In addition, the genetic control of certain complement components appears to be linked to the genes that code for the major histocompatibility complex (MHC). Many of these components are also present on the cell surfaces. In fact, it has been suggested that the functions of the complement system and the major histocompatibility complex may be related.[50]

C1q. Receptors for C1q have been reported on both T and B lymphocytes as well as on certain lymphoblastoid cells.[20, 109] Platelets have also been reported as having a C1q receptor.[119]

C3b. Receptors for C3b (immune adherence receptor) have been detected on the membrane of primate red cells, granulocytes, monocytes, macrophages, a subpopulation of lymphocytes, epithelial cells of normal renal glomeruli and non-primate platelets.[77] The C3b receptors have often been shown to also react with C4b, perhaps due to their structural similarity.[82]

C3d. Receptors for C3d are found on a small population of normal B lymphocytes and certain lymphoblastoid cells, but there are differences of opinion as to their presence on monocytes and macrophages; certainly, if they are present they appear to have very little, if any, biological activity in the process of immune red cell destruction by macrophages (see Chapter 4). The differences of opinion in the detection of C3d receptors on macrophages may relate to the fact that the workers who detected them were using purified complement components when preparing their target red cells (EAC3d), whereas the workers who could not detect them used whole serum to prepare their EAC3d;[7] one could argue that the use of whole serum would be the model closest to the *in vivo* situation. There is an association between the B lymphocyte receptor for the Epstein-Barr (E-B) virus and the C3d receptor.[131] Blocking of the C3d receptor produces blocking of the E-B virus receptor (and vice versa), and receptors co-cap on the lymphocyte surface, suggesting that the receptors are identical. It has been suggested that this finding may explain why E-B virus, unlike other viruses (e.g., measles virus) infects only B lymphocytes. [131]

It has been suggested that the complement receptors may be involved in three functions: control of the traffic of immune complexes and cells, control of the fate of immune complexes, and the triggering of cellular functions (e.g., the immune response). [7]

Cell Associated Complement Components. The genes controlling the serum expression of certain complement components, notably C2, C4, C8, and Factor B, are now known to be linked to the genes coding for the major histocompatibility complex. [50] Some of these components are also present on the cell membrane (e.g., C4, C8, and Factor B are present on lymphocytes). By contrast, genes controlling C1, C5, C6, and C7 are unlinked to the major histocompatibility complex, and none of these components are present on cells.

An exciting recent finding has been that Chido and Rodgers blood group antigens appear to be immunologically identical to determinants on the C4 complement component. [83] Chido (Ch[a]) and Rodgers (Rg[a]) were described as new blood group antigens in 1967 [47] and 1976 [65] respectively. The antibodies to these antigens were often termed nebulous by blood bankers because of their weak unreliable reactions with red cells. Both Ch[a] and Rg[a] were found to be present in plasma; in fact, the typing of patients was more accurately determined by using plasma in inhibition procedures than by using the red cells. Approximately 98 percent of random white donors were found to be Ch(a+) and Rg(a+). Neither of the antibodies appeared to be capable of destroying red cells *in vivo*. [124] The Chido and Rodgers loci were shown to be very close to HLA on chromosome 6. [73, 125] In 1978, O'Neill and his co-workers showed that Chido and Rodgers are distinct components of human complement C4. [83]

Using the techniques of immunofixation electrophoresis to study the polymorphism of C4 in EDTA plasma, O'Neill et al. [83] found three patterns defined by the number and position of the stained bands. In one pattern (C4F) there were four fast moving anodal bands; in another pattern (C4S) there were four slow moving cathodal bands; in the third pattern (C4FS) there were four fast moving bands and four slow moving bands. The C4S pattern occurred in about 1 percent of the donors; all were homozygous for HLA-B8; all were Rg(a−), Ch(a+). The C4F pattern occurred in about 5 percent of the donors; among these the HLA antigens B12, Bw35, B5, and B18 were common; all were Ch(a−), Rg(a+). Samples with the C4FS pattern were Ch(a+), Rg(a+). Further evidence was obtained by passing Ch(a+), Rg(+) plasma through an affinity column that would remove C4 specifically; after passage the plasma was found to have lost Ch[a] and Rg[a] activity. Purified C4 was found to inhibit anti-Ch[a] and anti-Rg[a]. Further studies have shown that both Ch and Rg antigens reside on the C4d fragment of C4. [125]

Other workers have also detected complement components on normal red cells. Graham et al.[44] showed that a high proportion of normal red cells had small amounts of C3d on their surface. Using a PVP-Augmented AutoAnalyzer System, Rosenfield and Jagathambal[98] recently showed that C3 and C4 (possibly in the form of C3d and C4d) are present on normal red cells; they suggested that this varied from <5 to 40 molecules per red cell, which would be below the threshold of the manual antiglobulin test.

THE STABILITY OF COMPLEMENT IN STORED HUMAN SERUM

A study by Garratty[33] was specifically designed to determine the effect of storage on the activity of complement with reference to the detection of blood group antibodies. In this study normal sera were stored at −90°C, −55°C, −20°C, 22°C, and 37°C from 24 hours to 3 months. Complement activity was assessed by a standard hemolytic assay, and also by an antiglobulin test assay that measured the ability of the stored sera to serve as a source of complement in the detection of blood group antibodies by the antiglobulin test. Hemolytic assays closely paralleled antiglobulin assays. At levels below 60 percent complement activity there was a danger of missing weak complement-binding antibodies. An average of these assays showed that at 37°C activity fell to 30 percent in 24 hours; at room temperature activity was 40 percent at 48 hours, zero at 72 hours; at 4°C it was 90 percent at 72 hours and 50 percent at 2 weeks. At −20°C activity was more than 60 percent for 2 months, at −55°C and −90°C activity was retained at 3 months (Fig. 3-13).

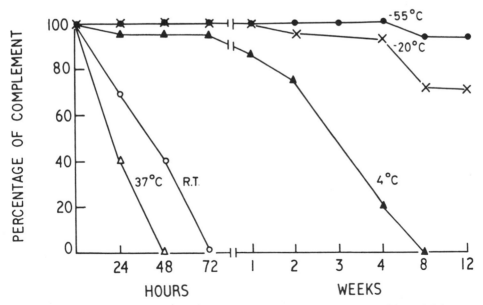

Figure 3-13. *Average complement activity of 12 normal sera as measured by antiglobulin test assay after storage at various temperatures.*[33] *(From Garratty, G.: The effects of storage and heparin on the activity of serum complement, with particular reference to the detection of blood group antibodies. Amer. J. Clin. Pathol., 54:531, 1970.)*

It should be stressed that these studies were carried out on normal sera, and that sera from hospital patients may be deficient in complement before storage, or they may develop anti-complement properties faster than the normal sera. In addition, it was found that at least a 60 percent complement level was needed in order to ensure that weak complement-dependent reactions were not missed.

THE EFFECT OF HEPARIN ON COMPLEMENT

Heparin was reported as being anticomplementary as early as 1931; [126] later papers confirmed this.[22, 33, 74, 99, 128, 129] How much this effect plays a role *in vivo* is controversial. A number of authors [48, 72, 84, 101, 110, 122] have suggested that heparin can be used to treat immune hemolytic anemia, and they have suggested that the "successful" results are due to the anticomplementary effect. Other authors have found heparin to be no value in treating immune hemolytic anemia [5, 32] (see Chapter 11).

Rosenfield et al.[99] transfused ^{51}Cr-labelled rat erythrocytes, sensitized in advance with IgG rabbit lysins, into rat recipients who had been injected with heparin previously. The rats were given a single intramuscular injection of 0.1 ml of sodium Heparin, 5,000 units per ml (500 units). The red cells were protected from rapid early destruction *in vivo*. The protective action of a single heparin dose lasted for less than four hours and only delayed cell destruction *in vivo*. As the cells were eventually destroyed, it was suggested that heparin had no effect on the antigen-antibody bond. These researchers further suggested the protection was associated with the anticomplementary effect of heparin, as the effect could be bypassed by applying lysins to the red cells in the presence of fresh serum, as a source of complement, *in vitro*.

The amount of heparin circulating in the plasma is obviously an important factor. In 1929 Ecker and Gross [22] reported that heparin neutralized complement *in vitro* at concentrations of 0.04 to 0.06 mg (4 to 6 units) of heparin per unit of complement.

Garratty [33] studied the effect of heparin on complement, both by a hemolytic assay and an antiglobulin test assay, that tested the ability of the serum to act as a source of complement in the indirect antiglobulin test. Heparin was confirmed as being anticomplementary. Some effects were noted when more than 5 units (0.05 mg) per ml of serum were present, but approximately 10 percent hemolytic activity was still observed in serum treated with 2500 units (25 mg) of heparin per ml.

The blood bank is sometimes faced with the problem of using heparinized blood for compatibility testing. Mollison [74] quotes that more than 1,000 units per ml of heparin are needed to completely prevent the taking up of complement components by Le^a-sensitized cells. The study by Garratty [33] confirmed this. However, smaller amounts of heparin significantly interfered with the detection of complement-binding antibodies. For instance, a weakly reacting anti-Le^a was barely detected when more than 50 units of heparin per ml of serum were present and, in fact, the reaction was measurably weaker when as few as 10 units of heparin per ml of serum were present. Patients receiving heparin anticoagulant therapy during dialysis or open heart surgery rarely, if ever, reach these levels.[33]

REFERENCES

1. Abramson, N., Alper, C. A., Lachmann, J., Rosen, F. S., and Jandl, J. H.: Deficiency of C3 inactivator in man. J. Immunol., *107*:19, 1971.
2. Adinolfi, M., Polley, M. J., Hunter, D. A., and Mollison, P. L.: Classification of blood group antibodies as B_2M or gamma globulin. Immunol., *5*:566, 1976.
3. Augener, W., Grey, H. M., Cooper, N. R., and Müller-Eberhard, H. J.: The reaction of monomeric and aggregated immunoglobulins with C1. Immunochem., *8*:1011, 1971.
4. Ayland, J., Horton, M. A., Tippett, P., and Waters, A. H.: Complement binding anti-D made in a D^u variant woman. Vox. Sang., *34*:40, 1978.
5. Bardana, E. J., Jr., Bayrakci, C., Pirofsky, B., and Henjyoji, H.: The use of heparin in autoimmune hemolytic disease. Blood, *35*:377, 1970.
6. Beck, M. L., and Marsh, W. L.: Complement and the antiglobulin test. Letter to the Editor. Trans., *17*:529, 1977.
7. Bianco, C.: Plasma membrane receptors for complement. *In* Good, R., and Day, S. B., Eds. Comprehensive Immunology. New York, Plenum Press, 1975.
8. Bokisch, V. A., Müller-Eberhard, H. J., and Cochrane, C. G.: Isolation of a fragment (C3a) of the third component of human complement containing anaphylatoxin and chemotactic activity and description of an anaphylatoxin inactivator of human serum. J. Exp. Med., *129*:1109, 1969.
9. Bokisch, V. A., Dierich, M. P., and Müller-Eberhard, H. J.: Third component of complement (C3): Structural properties in relation to functions. Proc. Nat. Acad. Sci. U.S.A., *72*:1989, 1975.
10. Borsos, T., and Leonard, E. J.: Detection of bound C3 by a new immunochemical method. J. Immunol., *107*:766, 1971.
11. Borsos, T., and Rapp, H. R.: Hemolysin titration based on fixation of the activated first component of complement: Evidence that one molecule of hemolysin suffices to sensitize an erythrocyte. J. Immunol., *95*:559, 1965.
12. Brown, D. L.: Complement and coagulation. Brit. J. Haemat., *30*:377, 1975.
13. Chaplin, H.: Clinical usefulness of specific antiglobulin reagents in autoimmune hemolytic anemias. Prog. Hemat., *8*:25, 1973.
14. Cochrane, C. G., and Müller-Eberhard, H. J.: The derivation of two distinct anaphylatoxin activities from the third and fourth components of human complement. J. Exp. Med., *127*:371, 1968.
14a. Conrad, D. H., Carlo, J. R., and Ruddy, S.: Interaction of β1H globulin with cell-bound C3b: quantitative analysis of binding and influence of alternative pathway components on binding. J. Exp. Med., *147*:1792, 1978.
15. Cooper, N. R.: Immune adherence by the fourth component of complement. Science, *165*:396, 1969.
16. Cooper, N. R.: Isolation and analysis of the mechanism of action of an inactivator of C4b in normal human serum. J. Exp. Med., *141*:890, 1975.
16a. Cooper, N. R.: Humoral immunity to viruses. *In:* Fraenkel-Conrat, H. and Wagner, R. R., Eds. Comprehensive Virology. New York, Plenum Press, 1979.
17. Dacie, J. V., Crookston, J. H., and Christenson, W. N.: "Incomplete" cold antibodies: Role of complement in sensitization to antiglobulin serum by potentially haemolytic antibodies. Brit. J. Haemat., *3*:77, 1957.

18. Dacie, J. V., and Worlledge, S. M.: Auto-Immune hemolytic anemias. Prog. Hematol., 6:82, 1969.
19. Daniels, C. A., Borsos, T., and Rapp, H. J.: Neutralization of sensitized virus by purified components of complement. Proc. Nat. Acad. Sci. U.S.A., 65:528, 1970.
20. Dickler, H. B., and Kunkel, H. G.: Interaction of aggregated γ-globulin with B lymphocytes. J. Exp. Med., 136:191, 1972.
21. Dukor, P., and Hartmann, K. U.: Hypothesis: Bound C3 as the second signal for B-cell activation. Cell Immunol., 7:349, 1973.
22. Ecker, E. E., and Pillemer, L.: Anti-coagulants and complementary activity. J. Immunol., 40:73, 1941.
23. Ellman, L., Green, I., and Frank, M. M.: Genetically controlled total deficiency of the fourth component of complement in the guinea pig. Science, 170:74, 1970.
24. Engelfriet, C. P.: C4 and C4 on red cells coated in vivo and in vitro. In International Symposium on "The Nature and Significance of Complement Activation." Pollack, W., Mollison, P. L., and Reiss, A. M., Eds. Raritan, New Jersey. Ortho Research Institute of Medical Sciences, 1977, 69.
25. Engelfriet, C. P., Pondman, K. W., Wolters, G., von dem Borne, A. E. G., Beckers, D., Broenveld, G., and van Loghem, J. J.: Autoimmune hemolytic anaemias. III. Preparation and examination of specific antisera against complement components and products and their use in serological studies. Clin. Exp. Immunol., 6:721, 1970.
26. Fischer, J., Petz, L. D., and Garratty, G.: Quantitation of erythrocyte bound C3 on human red cells sensitized in vitro or in vivo. Blood, 40:968, 1972.
27. Flexner, S., and Noguchi, H.: Snake venom in relation to hemolysis, bacteriolysis, and toxicity. J. Exp. Med., 6:277, 1903.
28. Frank, M. M., and Atkinson, J. P.: Complement in clinical medicine. Disease-a-Month. Chicago, Year Book Medical Publishers, January 1975.
29. Frank, M. M., Gelfand, J. A., and Atkinson, J. P.: Hereditary angioedema: The clinical syndrome and its management. Ann. Intern. Med., 84:580, 1976.
30. Frank, M. M., May, J. E., Gaither, T., and Ellman, L.: In vitro studies of complement function in sera of C4 deficient guinea pigs. J. Exp. Med., 134:176, 1971.
31. Freedman, J., Chaplin, H., and Mollison, P. L.: Further observations on the preparation of antiglobulin reagents reacting with C3d and C4d on red cells. Vox. Sang., 33:21, 1977.
32. Frimmer, D., and Creger, W. P.: Heparin and hemolytic anemia. Am. J. Med. Sci., 259:412, 1970.
33. Garratty, G.: The effects of storage and heparin on the activity of serum complement with particular reference to the detection of blood group antibodies. Am. J. Clin. Path., 54:431, 1970.
34. Garratty, G., and Petz, L. D.: An evaluation of commercial antiglobulin sera with particular reference to their anti-complement properties. Trans., 11:79, 1971.
35. Garratty, G., and Petz, L. D.: Drug-induced immune hemolytic anemia. Am. J. Med., 58:398, 1975.
36. Garratty, G., and Petz, L. D.: The significance of red cell bound complement components in development of standards and quality assurance for the anti-complement components of antiglobulin sera. Trans. 16:297, 1976.
37. Gewurz, H., Shin, H. S., and Mergenhagen, S. E.: Interactions of the complement system with endotoxin lipopolysaccharides: Consumption of each of the six terminal complement components. J. Exp. Med., 128:1049, 1968.
38. Giblett, E. R.: Blood group alloantibodies: An assessment of some laboratory practices. Transfusion, 17:299, 1977.
39. Gilliland, B. C., Baxter, E., and Evans, R. S.: Red-cell antibodies in acquired hemolytic anemia with negative antiglobulin serums test. New Engl. J. Med., 285:252, 1971.
40. Goldfinger, D., Sturgeon, P., Smith, L., Garratty, G., and Hurvitz, C.: Autoim-

mune hemolytic anemia associated exclusively with IgA of Rh specificity. American Association of Blood Banks 30th Annual Meeting, Atlanta, Georgia. 1977, 5 (abstract).

41. Götze, O., and Müller-Eberhard, H. J.: The C3-activator system: An alternate pathway of complement activation. J. Exp. Med., *134:*Suppl 90, 1971.
42. Götze, O., and Müller-Eberhard, H. J.: Paroxysmal nocturnal hemoglobinuria: Hemolysis initiated by the C3 activator system. New Eng. J. Med., *286:*180, 1972.
43. Götze, O., and Müller-Eberhard, H. J.: The alternative pathway of complement activation. Adv. Immunol., *24:*1, 1976.
44. Graham, H. A., Davies, D. M., Jr., and Brower, C. E.: Detection of C3b and C3d on red cell membranes. Proceedings of an International Symposium on "The Nature and Significance of Complement Activation." Pollack, W., Mollison, P. L., and Reiss, A. M., Eds. Raritan, New Jersey, Ortho Research Institute of Medical Sciences, 1977.
45. Green, H., Barrow, P., and Goldberg, B.: Effect of antibody and complement on permeability control in ascites tumor cells and erythrocytes. J. Exp. Med., *110:*699, 1959.
46. Harboe, M., Müller-Eberhard, H. J., Fudenberg, H. H., Polley, M. J., and Mollison, P. L.: Identification of the components of complement participating in the antiglobulin reaction. Immunol., *6:*412, 1963.
47. Harris, J. P., Tegoli, J., Swanson, J., Fischer, N., Gavin, J., and Noades, J.: A nebulous antibody responsible for cross-matching difficulties (Chido). Vox. Sang., *12:*140, 1967.
48. Hartman, M. M.: Reversal of serologic reactions by heparin. Therapeutic implications. II. Idiopathic acquired hemolytic anemia. Ann. Allerg., *22:*313, 1964.
49. Heusinkveld, R. S., Leddy, J. P., Klemperer, M. R., and Breckenridge, R. T.: Hereditary deficiency of the sixth component of complement in man. II. Studies of haemostasis. J. Clin. Invest., *53:*554, 1974.
50. Hobart, M. J., and Lachman, P. J.: Allotypes of complement components in man. Transpl. Rev., *32:*26, 1976.
51. Holborrow, E. J., and Reeves, W. G., Eds.: Immunology in Medicine. New York, Grune and Stratton, 1977.
52. Howard, J. E., Gottlieb, C. E., Hafleigh, E. B., Grumet, F. C., Petz, L. D., and Garratty, G.: Clinical importance of the anticomplement activity in antiglobulin antisera. Transfusion, abstract, *18:*631, 1978.
53. Hsu, T. C., Rosenfield, R. E., Burkart, P., Wong, K. Y., and Kochura, S.: Instrumented PVP-augmented antiglobulin tests. Vox. Sang., *26:*305, 1974.
54. Humphrey, J. H., and Dourmashkin, R. R.: Electron microscope studies of immune cell lysis, in CIBA Foundation Symposium. Complement. London, J. & A. Churchill, 1965.
55. Humphrey, J. H., and Dourmashkin, R. R.: The lesions in cell membranes caused by complement. Adv. Immunol., *11:*75, 1969.
56. Issitt, P. D.: The antiglobulin test and the evaluation of antiglobulin reagents. *In* Advances in Immunohematology. Oxnard, California, Spectra Biologicals, *4:*4, 1977.
57. Issitt, P. D., Issitt, C. H., and Wilkinson, S. L.: Evaluation of commercial antiglobulin sera over a two-year period. I. Anti-beta 1A, anti-alpha 2D, and anti-beta 1E levels. Trans., *14:*93, 1974.
58. Issitt, P. D., Issitt, C. H., and Wilkinson, S. L.: Evaluation of commercial antiglobulin sera over a two-year period. II. Anti-IgG and anti-IgM levels and undesirable contaminating antibodies. Transfusion, *14:*103, 1974.
59. Issitt, P. D., and Smith, T. R.: Evaluation of antiglobulin reagents. *In* A Seminar on Performance Evaluation. American Association of Blood Banks, 1976, 25.
60. Johnson, A. R., Hugli, T. E., and Müller-Eberhard, H. J.: Release of histamine

from rat mast cells by the complement peptides C3a and C5a. Immunol. *28*:1067, 1975.

61. Joseph, B. S., Cooper, N. R., and Olston, M. B. A.: Immunologic injury of cultured cells infected with measles virus. I. Role of IgG antibody and the alternative complement pathway. J. Exp. Med., *141*:761, 1975.

62. Kerr, R. O., Dalmasso, A. P., and Kaplan, M. E.: Erythrocyte-bound C5 and C6 in autoimmune hemolytic anemia. J. Immunol., *107*:1209, 1971.

63. Kohler, P. F.: Inherited complement deficiences and systemic lupus erythematosus: An immunogenetic puzzle. Ann. Intern. Med., *82*:420, 1975.

64. Lay, W. H., and Nussenzweig, V.: Receptors for complement on leukocytes. J. Exp. Med., *128*:991, 1968.

65. Longster, G., and Giles, C. M.: A new antibody specificity, anti-Rg[a], reacting with a red cell and serum antigen. Vox. Sang., *30*:175, 1976.

66. Mancini, G., Carbonara, A. O., and Heremans, J. F.: Immunochemical quantitation of antigens by single radial immunodiffusion. Immunochem., *2*:235, 1965.

67. Masouredis, S. P., Sudora, E. J., Mahan, L., and Victoria, E. J.: Antigen site densities and ultrastructural distribution patterns of red cell Rh antigens. Trans., *16*:94, 1976.

68. May, J. E., Green, I., and Frank, M. M.: The alternate complement pathway in cell damage: Antibody-mediated cytolysis of erythrocytes and nucleated cells. J. Immunol., *109*:595, 1972.

69. Mayer, M. M.: Complement. *In* Kabat, E. A., Ed. Experimental Immunochemistry. Springfield, Illinois, Charles C Thomas, 1961.

70. Mayer, M. M.: Mechanism of cytolysis by complement. Proc. Nat. Acad. Sci. U.S.A., *69*:2954, 1972.

71. Medicus, R. G., Schreiber, R. D., Götze, O., and Müller-Eberhard, H. J.: A molecular concept of the properdin pathway. Proc. Nat. Acad. Sci. U.S.A., *73*:612, 1976.

72. Miale, A.: Heparin therapy in autoimmune hemolytic anemia. Blood, *15*:741, 1960.

73. Middleton, J., Crookston, M. C., Falk, J. A., Robson, E. B., Cook, P. J. L., Batchelor, J. R., Bodmer, J., Ferrara, G. B., Festenstein, H., Harris, R., Kissmeyer-Nielson, F., Lawler, S. D., Sachs, J. A., and Wolf, E.: Linkage of Chido and HL-A. Tissue Antigens, *4*:366, 1974.

74. Mollison, P. L.: Blood Transfusion in Clinical Medicine. 5th Ed. Oxford, Blackwell, 1972.

75. Müller-Eberhard, H. J.: Complement. Annu. Rev. Biochem., *44*:697, 1975.

76. Müller-Eberhard, H. J.: Complement and phagocytosis. *In* Bellanti, J. A., and Delbert, H. D., Eds.: The Phagocytic Cell in Host Resistance. New York, Raven Press, 1975, 87.

76a. Müller-Eberhard, H. J.: Complement abnormalities in human disease. Hospital Practice, *13*:65, 1978.

76b. Nagaki, K., Iida, K., Okubo, M., and Inai, S.: Reaction mechanisms of $\beta 1H$ globulin. Int. Arch. Allergy Appl. Immun., *57*:221, 1978.

77. Nelson, D. S.: Immune adherence. Adv. Immunol., *3*:131, 1963.

78. Nelson, R. A., Jr.: The immune-adherence phenomenon. An immunologically specific reaction between microorganisms and erythrocytes leading to enhanced phagocytosis. Science, *118*:733, 1953.

79. Nelson, R. A.: An alternative mechanism for the properdin system. J. Exp. Med., *108*:515, 1958.

80. Nilsson, U. R., Mandle, R. J., Jr., and Mapes, J. A.: Human C3 and C5: Sub-unit structure and modifications by trypsin and $C\overline{4,2}-C\overline{4,2,3}$. J. Immunol., *114*:815, 1975.

81. Nishioka, K.. and Linscott, W. D.: Components of guinea pig complement. I.

Separation of a serum fraction essential for immune hemolysis and immune adherence. J. Exp. Med., *118:*767, 1963.

82. Nussenzweig, V.: Receptors for immune complexes on lymphocyte. Ad. Immunol., *19:*217, 1974.
83. O'Neill, G. J., Yang, S. Y., Tegoli, J., Berger, R., and Dupont, B.: Chido and Rodgers blood groups are distinct antigenic components of human complement C4. Nature, *273:*668, 1978.
84. Owren, P. A.: Acquired hemolytic jaundice. Scand. J. Clin. Lab. Invest., *1:*41, 1949.
84a Pangburn, M. K., Schreiber, R. D., and Müller-Eberhard, H. J.: Human complement C3b inactivator: isolation, characterization, and demonstration of an absolute requirement for the serum protein β1H for cleavage of C3b and C4b in solution. J. Exp. Med., *146:*257, 1977.
85. Petz, L. D.: Complement in immunohematology and in neurologic disorders. *In* International Symposium on "The Nature and Significance of Complement Activation." Pollack, W., Mollison, P. L., and Reiss, A. M., Eds. Raritan, New Jersey. Ortho Research Institute of Medical Sciences, 1977, 87.
86. Petz, L. D., Cooper, N. R., Powers, R., and Fries, J.: The metabolism of radiolabelled C3 (^{125}I-C3) in autoimmune disorders. *In* Protides of the Biological Fluids 22nd Colloquium. Peeters, H., Ed. Oxford, Pergamon Press, 1975, 547.
87. Petz, L. D., Fink, D. J., Letsky, E., Fudenberg, H. H., and Müller-Eberhard, H. J.: In vivo metabolism of complement. I. Metabolism of the third component (C3) in acquired hemolytic anemia. J. Clin. Invest., *47:*2469, 1968.
88. Petz, L. D., and Garratty, G.: Laboratory correlations in immune hemolytic anemia. *In* Laboratory Diagnosis of Immunologic Disorders. Vyas, G. N., Stites, D. P., and Brecher, G., Eds. New York, Grune and Stratton, 1975, 139.
89. Petz, L. D., and Garratty, G.: Complement in immunohematology. Prog. Clin. Immunol., *2:*175, 1974.
90. Pillemer, L., Blum, L., Lepow, I. H., Ross, O. A., Todd, E. W., and Wardlaw, A. C.: The properdin system and immunity. I. Demonstration and isolation of a new serum protein, properdin, and its role in immune phenomena. Science, *120:*279, 1954.
91. Platts-Mills, T. A. E., and Ishizaka, K.: Activation of the alternate pathway of human complement by rabbit cells. J. Immunol., *113:*348, 1974.
92. Polley, M. J., and Mollison, P. L.: The role of complement in the detection of blood group antibodies. Special reference to the antiglobulin test. Trans., *1:*9, 1961.
93. Polley, M. J., Mollison, P. L., and Soothill, J. F.: The role of 19S gamma globulin blood group antibodies in the antiglobulin reaction. Brit. J. Haemat., *8:*149, 1962.
94. Pondman, K. W., Rosenfield, R. E., Tallal, L., and Wasserman, L. R.: The specificity of the complement antiglobulin test. Vox. Sang., *5:*297, 1960.
95. Poskitt, T. R., Fortwengler, H. P., and Lunskis, B. J.: Activation of the alternative complement pathway by autologous red cell stroma. J. Exp. Med., *138:*715, 1973.
96. Rapp, H. J., and Borsos, T.: Molecular Basis of Complement Action. New York, Appleton-Century-Crofts, 1970.
97. Ratnoff, O. D.: The interrelationship of clotting and immunologic mechanisms. Hosp. Prac., *6:*119, 1971.
98. Rosenfield, R. E., and Jagathambal: Antigenic determinants of C3 and C4 complement components on washed erythrocytes from normal persons. Transfusion, *18:*517, 1978.
99. Rosenfield, R. E., Vitale, B., and Kochwa, S.: Immune mechanisms for destruction of erythrocytes in vivo. II. Heparinization for protection of Lysin-sensitized erythrocytes. Trans., *7:*261, 1967.

100. Ross, G. D., Polley, M. J., Rabellino, E. M., and Grey, H. M.: Two different complement receptors on human lymphocytes. One specific for C3b and one specific for C3b inactivator-cleaved C3b. J. Exp. Med., *138:*798, 1973.

101. Roth, K. L., and Frumin, A. M.: Effect of intramuscular heparin on antibodies in idiopathic acquired hemolytic anemia. Am. J. Med., *20:*968, 1956.

102. Sandberg, A. L., Oliveira, B., and Osler, A. G.: Two complement interaction sites in guinea pig immunoglobulins. J. Immunol., *106:*282, 1971.

103. Schreiber, R. D., and Müller-Eberhard, H. J.: Fourth component of human complement: Description of a three polypeptide chain structure. J. Exp. Med., *140:*1324, 1974.

104. Schreiber, R. D., Pangburn, M. K., Lesavre, P. H., and Müller-Eberhard, H. J.: Initiation of the alternative pathway of complement: Recognition of activators by bound C3b and assembly of the entire pathway from six isolated proteins. Proc. Nat. Acad. Sci. U.S.A., *75:*3948, 1978.

105. Schur, P. H., and Becker, E. L.: Pepsin digestion of rabbit and sheep antibodies. The effect on complement fixation. J. Exp. Med., *118:*891, 1963.

106. Shin, H. S., Synderman, R., Friedman, E., Mellors, A., and Manet, M. M.: Chemotactic and anaphylatoxic fragment cleaved from the fifth component of guinea pig complement. Science, *162:*361, 1968.

107. Shelton, E., Yonemasu, K., and Stroud, R. M.: Ultrastructure of the human complement component, C1q. Proc. Nat. Acad. Sci. U.S.A., *69:*65, 1972.

108. Sherwood, G. K., Haynes, B. F., and Rosse, W. F.: Hemolytic transfusion reactions caused by failure of commercial antiglobulin reagents to detect complement. Trans., *16:*417, 1976.

109. Sobel, A. T., and Bokisch, V. A.: Receptor for C1q on peripheral human lymphocytes and human lymphoblastoid cells. Fed. Proc., *34:*965, 1975.

110. Storti, E., and Vaccari, F.: Studies on the relationship between anticoagulants and hemolysis. I. Effect of anticoagulants on hemolysis and on the agglutination of red blood cells by antierythrocyte serum. Acta Haemat. (Basel), *15:*12, 1956.

111. Stratton, F.: Recent observations on the antiglobulin test. Wadley Med. Bull., *5:*182, 1975.

112. Stratton, F., Gunson, H. H., and Rawlinson, V. I.: The preparation and uses of antiglobulin reagents with special reference to complement-fixing blood group antibodies. Trans., *2:*135, 1962.

113. Stratton, F., Gunson, H. H., and Rawlinson, V. I.: Complement fixing antibodies in relation to hemolytic disease of the newborn. Trans., *5:*216, 1965.

114. Stratton, F., and Rawlinson, V. I.: C3 components on red cells under various conditions. *In* International Symposium on "The Nature and Significance of Complement Activation." Pollack, W., Mollison, P. L., and Reiss, A. M., Eds. Raritan, New Jersey, Ortho Research Institute of Medical Sciences, 1977, 113.

115. Stratton, F., and Rawlinson, V. I.: Observations on the antiglobulin tests. II. C4 components on erythrocytes. Vox. Sang., *31:*44, 1976.

116. Stratton, F., Rawlinson, V. I., Chapman, S. A., Pengelly, C. D. R., and Jennings, R. C.: Acquired hemolytic anemia associated with IgA anti-e. Trans., *12:*157, 1972.

117. Stratton, F., Smith, D. S., and Rawlinson, V. I.: 19S gamma M followed by 7S gamma G anti-Jk^a antibodies associated with pregnancy. Clin. Exp. Immunol., *3:*81, 1968.

118. Stratton, F., Smith, D. S., and Rawlinson, V. I.: Value of gel filtration on Sephadex G-200 in the analysis of blood group antibodies. J. Clin. Path., *21:*708, 1968.

119. Suba, E. A., and Csako, G.: C1q (C1) receptor on human platelets: Inhibition of collagen-induced platelet aggregation by C1q (C1) molecules. J. Immunol., *117:*304, 1976.

120. Svehag, S. E., Manhem, L., and Bloth, B.: Ultrastructure of human C1q protein. Nature (London) New Biol., 238:117, 1972.
121. Synderman, R., Phillips, J. K., and Mergenhagen, S. E.: Biological activity of complement in vivo. Role of C5 in the accumulation of polymorphonuclear leukocytes in inflammatory exudates. J. Exp. Med., 134:1131, 1971.
122. Ten Pas, A., and Monto, R. W.: The treatment of autoimmune hemolytic anemia with heparin. Am. J. Med. Sci., 251:63, 1966.
123. Thompson, R. A., and Lachmann, P. J.: A second case of human C3b inhibitor (KAF) deficiency. Clin. Exp. Immunol., 27:23, 1977.
124. Tilley, C. A. Crookston, M. C., Haddad, S. A., and Shumak, K. H.: Red-blood cell survival studies in patients with anti-Ch[a], anti-Yk[a], anti-Ge and anti-Vel. Trans., 17:169, 1977.
125. Tilley, C. A., Romans, D. G., and Crookston, M. C.: Localization of Chido and Rodgers determinants to a tryptic C4d fragment of human C4. Trans., 18:622, 1978.
126. von Falkenhausen, M.: Korpereigene (Antiprothrombin bzw. Heparin) und Korperfremde (Germainin, Salvarsan) gerinnungshemmende Substanzen in ihrer Beziehung zur Vorstufe des Gerinnungsferementes (Prothrombin). Ztschr. für die Gesamte Exper. Med., 79:18, 1931.
127. Waller, M., and Lawler, S. D.: A study of the properties of the rhesus antibody (Ri) diagnostic for rheumatoid factor and its application to Gm grouping. Vox. Sang., 7:591, 1962.
128. Wising, P.: The complement-fixing properties of heparin salts. Acta Med. Scand., 91:550, 1937.
129. Wising, P.: The identity of prothrombin and the midpiece of complement. Acta Med. Scand., 94:506, 1938.
130. Worlledge, S. M., and Blajchman, M. A.: The autoimmune haemolytic anaemias. Brit. J. Haemat., 23:61, 1972.
131. Yefenof, E., Bakacs, T., Einhorn, L., Ernberg, I., and Klein, G.: Epstein-Barr virus (EBV) receptors, complement receptors, and EBV infectibility of different lymphocyte fractions of human peripheral blood. I. Complement receptor distribution and complement binding by separated lymphocyte subpopulations. Cellular Immunology, 35:34, 1978.
132. Zimmerman, T. S.: The coagulation mechanism and the inflammatory response. In Miescher, P. A., and Müller-Eberhard, H. J., Eds. Textbook of Immunopathology. 2nd Ed. New York, Grune and Stratton, 1976.

4

Mechanisms of Immune Hemolysis

It has been obvious for most of this century that two distinct types of hemolysis seem to exist. Fairley [29] used the term intravascular to describe the type of hemolysis associated with the breakdown of red cells directly in the blood, which results in hemoglobinemia and sometimes in hemoglobinuria. The term extravascular was used to describe the destruction of red cells within the reticuloendothelial system without obvious signs of hemoglobinemia or hemoglobinuria, but rather with an increase in the later breakdown products such as bilirubin. Dacie [20] suggested that a sharp distinction does not always hold, as signs of intravascular hemolysis can be demonstrated in most, if not all, hemolytic anemias if sensitive enough tests are performed (e.g., haptoglobin determinations). We believe it is still convenient to use the terms intravascular and extravascular as a basis to discuss immune red cell destruction, and we will describe the areas in which the two may overlap later in this chapter.

INTRAVASCULAR IMMUNE RED CELL DESTRUCTION

This type of immune red cell destruction is complement-mediated. Not many antibodies destroy red cells intravascularly; among the alloantibodies that destroy red cells through this mechanism, anti-A and anti-B are the best examples; anti-Kidd, -Vel, -Tj[a] and anti-Le[a] can also sometimes activate the complement cascade and thus, on rare occasions, they are capable of causing the intravascular lysis of donor red cells. Intravascular hemolysis is also uncommon in autoimmune hemolytic anemia. When it occurs it is usually associated with paroxysmal cold hemoglobinuria, less commonly with cold agglutinin syndrome, and with rare cases of drug-induced hemolytic anemia due to immune-complex formation. Intravascular hemolysis does occur, but very rarely, in warm autoimmune hemolytic anemia.

Complement-mediated immune hemolysis usually occurs through the classical pathway of complement activation, which has been described in detail in the preceding chapter. Theoretically, any of the many substances that can activate the alternative pathway could cause intravascular hemolysis, but there is at present no evidence to suggest that immune (i.e., antibody-mediated) red cell lysis occurs through this pathway.

As was discussed in detail in Chapter 3, the classical pathway of complement activation can be activated by antibodies of the IgG and IgM class, but not by IgA. Only three of the four IgG subclasses activate complement; IgG1, IgG2, or IgG3. IgG4 does not activate complement. Only a single molecule of IgM is necessary to activate the first component of complement, but two molecules of IgG must fall close enough together on the red cell membrane (approximately 200 to 400 Å apart) to form a doublet before they can activate the cascade.

Once the red cell is sensitized with the appropriate complement-activating antibody, the first component of complement(C1) becomes activated (C$\overline{1}$); activated C1 cleaves the fourth component of complement, C4, into two fragments, C4a and C4b. The C4b fragment attaches to the red cell membrane. C$\overline{1}$ also cleaves the second component of complement, C2, into two fragments, C2a and C2b. The C2a fragment forms a complex with C4b, C$\overline{4b2a}$, which is also known as C3 convertase. This enzyme cleaves the C3 molecule into two fragments, C3a and C3b. C3b fragments attach to the red cell membrane and also forms a complex with C$\overline{4b2a}$ to form C$\overline{4b2a3b}$, an enzyme that cleaves the C5 molecule into C5a and C5b. The C5b fragment attaches to the red cell membrane and absorbs C6 and C7 to form a complex C5b,6,7. This complex combines with C8 and C9, a process that leads to defects in the red cell membrane. The membrane defects allow ions to enter the cell, causing the cell to swell and eventually rupture, thereby releasing hemoglobin into the plasma (hemoglobinemia).

When hemoglobin is released into the plasma, it rapidly combines with haptoglobin to form a complex that is cleared within a few hours by the reticuloendothelial system. When the haptoglobin system is saturated, free hemoglobin circulates in the plasma. Some of it is oxidized and bound to albumin as methemalbumin. Methemalbumin appears about 3 to 6 hours following a hemolytic episode and remains in the plasma for about 24 hours. This dark brown pigment may mix with free hemoglobin, leading to brownish colored plasma. When plasma contains about 20 mg of hemoglobin per 100 ml, it will appear slightly pink or light brown if examined in a thickness of about 1 cm. If present in the order of 100 mg per 100 ml, the plasma will appear red.[68] Both the hemoglobin-haptoglobin complex and the methemoglobin are broken down in the reticuloendothelial system to form bilirubin, which will then appear in the plasma. (Maximum concentrations are usually not attained for 3 to 6 hours after a hemolytic episode.) When the plasma hemoglobin level exceeds 25 mg per 100 ml, hemoglobin may be excreted in the urine, producing hemoglobinuria. During this process some hemoglobin may be absorbed by the renal tubules and after degradation, the iron may eventually (i.e., several days later) appear in the urine as hemosiderin.

EXTRAVASCULAR IMMUNE RED CELL DESTRUCTION

If red cells become sensitized with IgG, or if cells are sensitized with complement but do not proceed through the cascade completely to lysis, then they may be destroyed or damaged within the reticuloendothelial system. This system is capable of removing up to about 400 ml of red cells per day.[68]

It is believed that the sensitized red cells are destroyed within the reticuloendothelial system by interaction with mononuclear phagocytes. The most important phagocyte participating in immune red cell destruction is the macrophage. Macrophages arise primarily from bone marrow precursors, probably the promonocyte. After a short period of maturation in the bone marrow, monocytes are released into the blood. After spending a few days in the peripheral circulation they migrate to the tissues, and there they mature functionally and morphologically to become typical histocytic or exudative macrophages.[93] They are particularly prominent in the liver (Kupffer cells), lung (alveolar macrophages), spleen, and bone marrow (see Table 4-1). The survival time of mature tissue macrophages is thought to be several weeks, or even months.[92] Immune red cell destruction occurs predominantly in the spleen and the liver.

Table 4-1. THE MONONUCLEAR PHAGOCYTE SYSTEM

Development of Macrophages	Location of Cells
PRECURSOR CELLS ↓	bone marrow
PROMONOCYTES ↓	bone marrow
MONOCYTES ↓	bone marrow, blood
MACROPHAGES	connective tissue (histiocytes)
	liver (Kupffer cells)
	lung (alveolar macrophages)
	spleen (free and fixed macrophages)
	lymph node (free and fixed macrophages)
	bone marrow (macrophages)
	serous cavity (pleural and peritoneal macrophages)
	bone tissue (osteoclasts?)
	nervous system (microglial cells?)

(Van Furth, R., Cohn, Z. A., Hirsch, J. G., Humphrey, J. H., Spector, W. G., and Langevoort, H. L.: The mononuclear phagocyte system: A new classification of macrophages, monocytes, and their precursor cells. Bull. Wld. Hlth. Org., *46:*845, 1972.)

Macrophage Receptors

Macrophages have receptors on their membranes that specifically recognize certain classes of immunoglobulins (either free or in an immune complex) and certain complement components. The receptors are for IgG [48] (only

IgG1 and IgG3 subclasses [1, 49]) and C3b.[50] Some workers believe that there are also receptors for C3c,[77] C4,[17, 81] and C3d (described later). The IgG receptor is specific for the Fc portion of IgG1 and IgG3 molecules in a domain near the carboxyl terminus of the heavy chain.[103] There are thought to be approximately 1×10^6 IgG receptors on the membrane of each macrophage.[4] The number of receptor sites seems to increase during macrophage activation.[3] The attachment of appropriately sensitized red cells to macrophages can be visualized *in vitro* by so-called rosette formation; the macrophage becomes ringed by sensitized red cells, like petals on a flower (see Figure 4-1).[58] On attachment to the macrophage the red cells usually undergo considerable distortion and deformity in the region of attachments.[58] The sensitized red cell may become completely engulfed by the macrophage and destroyed internally (see Fig. 4-2), or a portion of the red cell may become internalized (see Figs. 4-3 and 4-4), resulting in loss of membrane protein and lipids. The portion of the red cell outside the macrophage may escape and circulate as a spherocyte [14] (see Fig. 4-5). The membrane of this spherocytic cell is rigid, due to the loss of protein and lipids, and thus the cell is unable to change its shape readily to traverse the fine channels of the spleen and is susceptible to early destruction.[18, 66, 99]

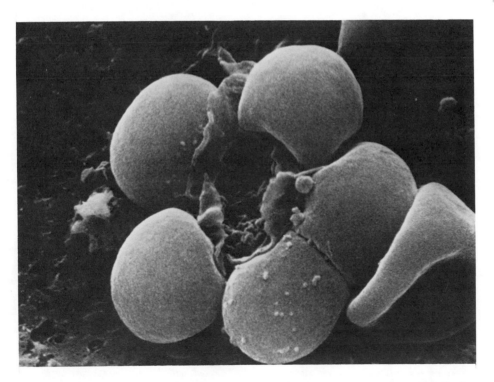

Figure 4-1. *Scanning electron micrograph illustrating the interaction of antibody coated red cells and a phagocytic white cell. The white cell is surrounded by sensitized red cells forming a rosette (courtesy of Dr. W. Rosse).*

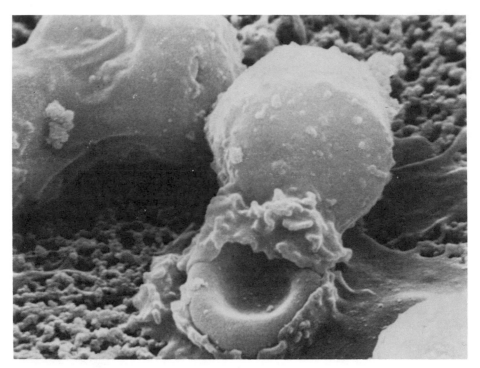

Figure 4-2. *Scanning electron micrograph illustrating the reaction of a phagocytic white cell with an antibody coated red cell. Only a small exposed area remains of a nearly ingested red cell. (Rosse, W. F., and de Boisfleury, A.: The interaction of phagocytic cells and red cells following alteration of their form or deformability. Blood Cells, 1:359, 1975.)*

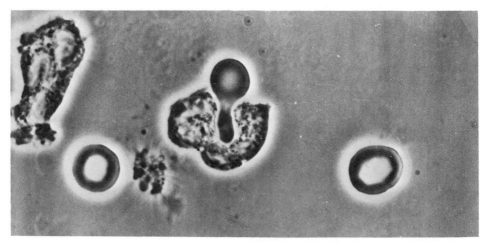

Figure 4-3. *Phase-contrast photomicrograph illustrating the interaction of an antibody coated red cell and a phagocytic white cell. The red cell, having been taken by the metapod, is deformed as the metapod flows along its sides. (Rosse, W. F., de Boisfleury, A., and Bessis, M.: The interaction of phagocytic cells and red cells modified by immune reactions. Comparison of antibody and complement coated red cells. Blood Cells, 1:345, 1975.)*

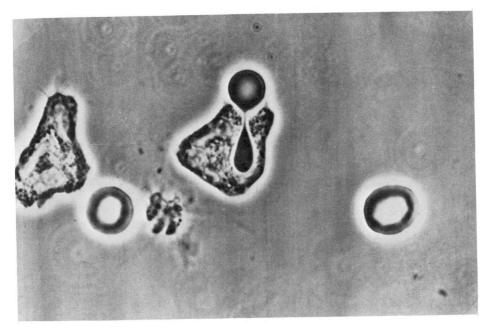

Figure 4-4. *Further interaction between the phagocytic white cell and the antibody coated red cell results in internalization of a portion of red cell. (Rosse, W. F., de Boisfleury, A., and Bessis, M.: The interaction of phagocytic cells and red cells modified by immune reactions. Comparison of antibody and complement coated red cells. Blood Cells, 1:345, 1975.)*

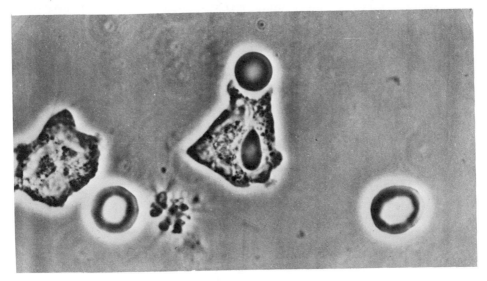

Figure 4-5. *The separation of the internal and external portions of the red cell is complete; the portion of the red cell outside the macrophage may escape and circulate as a spherocyte. (Rosse, W. F., de Boisfleury, A., and Bessis, M.: The interaction of phagocytic cells and red cells modified by immune reactions. Comparison of antibody and complement coated red cells. Blood Cells, 1:345, 1975.)*

Extravascular red cell destruction leads to the appearance in the plasma and urine of breakdown products of hemoglobin, such as bilirubin and urobilinogen. Occasionally, laboratory tests may show some results that are associated with intravascular lysis (e.g., hemoglobinemia and hemoglobinuria), even though no complement-mediated lysis has occurred. For instance, hemoglobinemia and hemoglobinuria have been reported following Rh incompatible transfusions,[68] and we have seen this ourselves. The Rh antibodies in these cases have never been shown to fix complement, thus it is believed that hemoglobin may be released into the blood following fragmentation of the red cells during extravascular phagocytosis, particularly when large amounts of blood are rapidly destroyed (e.g., several units.)[68] Recent evidence has suggested that macrophages (and possibly lymphocytes) may destroy sensitized red cells by extracellular cytotoxicity [35] in addition to phagocytosis; this phenomenon may be an alternative explanation for non-complement-mediated hemoglobinemia and hemoglobinuria associated with extravascular lysis.

Most alloantibodies (e.g., Rh, Kell, Duffy) other than Anti-A, Anti-B, or a few rare antibodies mentioned previously destroy red cells extravascularly. Most of the red cell destruction associated with autoimmune hemolytic anemia is extravascular (e.g., warm antibody autoimmune hemolytic anemia, which comprises almost 70 percent of all AIHA). In addition, almost all the drug-induced hemolytic anemias one commonly encounters (i.e., those caused by methyldopa or penicillin) are associated with extravascular red cell destruction.

Many factors may affect immune red cell destruction. Some are listed in Table 4-2.

Table 4-2. FACTORS POSSIBLY AFFECTING IMMUNE RED CELL DESTRUCTION

Number of antigen sites on red cell membrane
Mobility of antigens within membrane
Class of immunoglobulin
Subclass of IgG
Quantity of antibody sensitizing red cell
Equilibrium constant of antibody
Ability of antibody to activate complement
Thermal range of antibody
Activity of recipient's reticuloendothelial system (macrophages)

Effect of Type of Protein Causing Red Cell Sensitization

Some of the factors listed in Table 4-2 will be discussed relative to red cells sensitized with immunoglobulin alone and red cells sensitized with complement, with and without immunoglobulin present.

Destruction of Red Cells Sensitized with IgG Only. Red cells sensitized by IgG only are destroyed predominantly in the spleen. Although the liver is a much larger organ, it has been shown that the spleen is about 100 times more efficient at removing Rh (IgG) sensitized red cells.[68] About 20 to 30 μg of anti-Rh per ml of red cells will lead to complete clearance in a single passage through the spleen (half time 20 mins) but, in the absence of the spleen, the cells are removed by the liver with a half time of about 5 h.[68]

Lo Buglio and co-workers[58] showed that the reaction between the Fc receptor on human monocytes and macrophages with IgG sensitized red cells could be specifically inhibited with IgG or its Fc fragment in solution. They suggested that the soluble IgG of plasma competes with the IgG attached to the red cells for receptors on the monocyte/macrophage surface. At hematocrit levels in excess of 75 percent (comparable to those encountered in the splenic red pulp), plasma had little inhibitory effect. It was suggested that the entrapment of antibody-coated red cells *in vivo* is enhanced by plasma skimming; the fact that the spleen is notable for both erythroconcentration and for efficient trapping of IgG coated red cells supported this interpretation. Other workers[34, 35, 50] have confirmed the inhibitory effect of even small amounts of normal plasma or serum.

Fleer et al[34] recently published data supporting the thesis of Lo Buglio et al.,[58] that the efficiency of splenic destruction was related to the hemoconcentration (loss of plasma) that occurs in the spleen. They were able to show that the *in vitro* interaction between monocytes and IgG Rh sensitized red cells was completely inhibited by low concentrations of IgG (e.g., 30 to 100 μg/ml); however, the interaction with IgG anti-A sensitized red cells was not inhibited by IgG. Fleer and co-workers suggested that this difference was probably quantitative. The higher the number of IgG antibody molecules per sensitized red cell, the less the interaction between the sensitized red cell and monocyte is inhibited by IgG.

A second factor that had a strong influence on the inhibitory effect of IgG was the number of sensitized red cells per monocyte. When the number of sensitized red cells per monocyte was increased from 1 to 32, the percentage of inhibition by a fixed amount of IgG (50 μg/ml) decreased significantly. This *in vitro* effect was evident only when relatively weakly sensitized red cells were used, and the *in vivo* destruction of these weakly sensitized red cells is confined to the spleen. Since a considerable hemoconcentration occurs in this organ, it is conceivable that a high sensitized red cell to macrophage ratio is accomplished. A high ratio may allow interaction between weakly sensitized red cells and splenic macrophages despite the presence *in vivo* of a high concentration of IgG.

Not all workers accept this explanation. Scornik et al.[87] showed that IgG sensitized red cells are rapidly cleared from the circulation of patients with myelomas in spite of serum IgG concentrations several times higher than normal. They concluded that the current explanations derived from *in vitro* experiments are insufficient to explain the IgG-dependent clearance of red cells in the presence of free IgG.

Quantitative Factors. Generally speaking, there appears to be a direct relationship between the amount of IgG on the red cells and the amount of red cell destruction. This is generally true for alloantibodies, but there are many exceptions when autoantibodies are studied. Mollison [68] has clearly shown that if different quantities of a single example of an allo anti-Rh are used to sensitize red cells, there is a good relation between the amount of IgG sensitizing the red cell and the rate of clearance (see Fig. 4-6). Constantoulakis et al. [16] also showed this relationship, but in studying autoantibody sensitization, these workers were not able to make a close correlation among patients with AIHA between the amount of antibody on the red cell and the rate of destruction determined by ^{51}Cr. In contrast to this finding, Rosse [82] found that the amount of antibody detected on the red cell membrane was generally proportional to the rate of red cell destruction, although many exceptions could be found. In a given patient, the rate of destruction was closely related

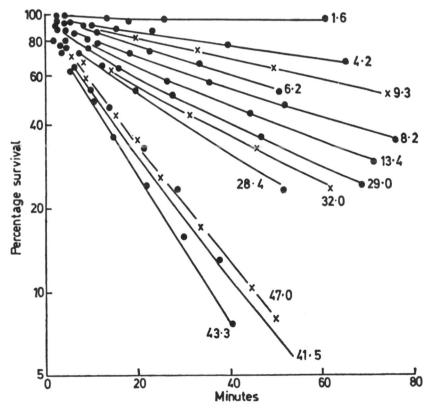

Figure 4-6. Survival of Rh-positive red cells sensitized in vitro *with varying amounts of a particular anti-Rh (Avg). Purified IgG, prepared from Avg serum, was used to sensitize the cells. The figures against each slope are the estimates of the amount of antibody on the red cells at the time of injection as μg antibody per ml red cells. In three cases (x) the estimates were made by using labelled anti-Rh. (From Mollison, P. L.: Blood Transfusion in Clinical Medicine. 6th Ed., London, Blackwell Scientific Publications, 1979.)*

to the concentration of IgG antibody detected on the membrane, and this observation is of some value in the "follow-up" of an individual patient during his response to therapy (see page 204). Our own data on several hundred patients with AIHA agree with that of Rosse.

It has been known for some time that red cells sensitized with the same amounts of IgG can have markedly different cell survival times. For example, Constantoulakis et al.[16] showed two different red cell samples with approximately $0.9\,\mu g$ IgG antibody N on each of them that had a half time of 45 mins and 11 days respectively. Most patients who have a positive direct antiglobulin test due to alpha-methyldopa (Aldomet) have normal red cell survival, although these cells can be extremely strongly sensitized with IgG (see page 205). Similarly, a small proportion of normal healthy blood donors have a strongly positive direct antiglobulin test (DAT) with normal red cell survival.[100] It is still not understood why this is so. When macrophages were found to have IgG1 and IgG3 receptors but not IgG2 or IgG4 receptors, it was thought this difference might explain the discrepancies. Although some rare cases can be explained by the subclass of IgG present on the red cell (e.g., IgG4 does not activate complement or have a receptor site for macrophages), this is not usually the answer. Not much work has been done in this area, as reliable subclass antisera are difficult to obtain; present results [26] would indicate that subclass differences are not the main explanation for this phenomenon.

There have been a few studies determining IgG subclass specificity of allo and auto red cell antibodies (see Table 4-3). Natvig and Kunkel [71] studied more than one hundred anti-Rh antibodies without finding any belonging to the IgG2 or IgG4 class. Abramson and Schur [2] studied 7 anti-D antibodies and found IgG1 and IgG3 predominated, although IgG2 was present occasionally in low titer. Two samples of anti-CD and one anti-c showed a predominance of IgG1 and IgG3; two samples of anti-S were shown to be IgG3, one had minimal quantities of IgG2; three samples of anti-K had small quantities of IgG1; two samples of anti-Kp^b were IgG1 and IgG3, respectively; one sample of anti-Jk^a appeared to be entirely IgG2. Frame, Mollison, and Terry [36]

Table 4-3. ALLOANTIBODY SUBCLASS

Natvig and Kunkel [71]	100 anti-Rh: all IgG1 or IgG3
Abramson and Schur [2]	10 anti-Rh: mainly IgG1 or IgG3 (occasionally IgG2)
	2 anti-S: IgG3 (one had ± IgG2)
	3 anti-K: IgG1
	2 anti-Kp^b: one IgG1, other IgG3
	1 anti-JK^a: IgG2
Frame, Mollison, and Terry [36]	41 anti-RH: mainly IgG1 or IgG3, but 4 contained IgG4
	11 anti-K ⎫
	1 anti-Fy^a ⎬ All IgG1 or IgG3
	1 anti-Jk^a ⎭

four examples of anti-D reacted by the indirect antiglobulin test with a potent anti-IgG4; 31 other anti-D, 5 anti-c, 1 anti-e, 11 anti-Kell, 1 anti-Duffy (Fy[a]), and 1 anti-Kidd (Jk[a]) were all negative. The anti-Rh molecules in the four IgG4 positive sera were not all of the IgG4 subclass. The authors suggested that these data might have some biological significance, because macrophages had receptors for IgG1 and IgG3 but not IgG2 or IgG4; thus red cells sensitized with IgG4 would not be ingested by macrophages.

Engelfriet et al.[26] studied 247 patients with positive direct antiglobulin tests due to IgG sensitization. Approximately 87 percent were found to have IgG1, 15 percent had IgG2, 13 percent IgG3, and 6 percent IgG4 on their red cells (see Table 4-4). Similar figures were obtained in a series of 57 patients with autoimmune hemolytic anemia studied by Dacie.[21] Engelfriet et al.[26] found that IgG3 sensitization was always associated with overt, often severe hemolytic anemia, whereas IgG1 sensitization was sometimes associated with hemolytic anemia, and sometimes the red cell donors had no evidence of increased red cell destruction. In two patients in whom only IgG4 was detected (reported in detail by Von Dem Borne, et al.[95]), no signs of increased red cell destruction were observed. Gergely, Fudenberg, and Van Loghem [37] also describe one case of IgG4 autoantibody eluted from red cells that was not associated with hemolysis. Approximately 15 to 20 percent of the patients receiving the hypertensive drug alpha-methyldopa develop a positive direct antiglobulin test due to IgG sensitization of the red cells. A maximum of 0.8 percent of the patients develop signs of hemolytic anemia (see Chapter 8). Engelfriet et al.[26] have found that, among this group of patients, those who have overt hemolysis and those with no observable signs of increased red cell destruction may have only IgG1 detectable on their red cells. Thus, there either appear to be two sub-populations of IgG1, one capable and the other incapable of adherence to the macrophage Fc receptor, or qualitative differences in the immunoglobulin are not the explanation of the *in vivo* reactions. It is possible that there are qualitative differences between those two groups that are not obvious by our regular antiglobulin testing. In both Engelfriet's and Dacie's series, approximately 20 percent of the patients whose red cells

Table 4-4. SUBCLASS SPECIFICITY ASSOCIATED WITH POSITIVE DIRECT ANTIGLOBULIN TESTS DUE TO IgG SENSITIZATION [26]

| | IgG Subclass Present on Patient's Red Cells | | |
| | Alone or | | Hemolytic |
Subclass	Mixed	Alone	Anemia
IgG1	87%	63%	Sometimes
IgG2	15%	0.8%	No, when IgG2 alone
IgG3	13%	2.0%	Always
IgG4	6%	0.4%	No, when IgG4 alone
No IgG1, 2, 3, or 4 Detectable	11%	–	Sometimes

were agglutinated strongly by anti-IgG serum did not react with any of the subclass-specific antisera. Absorption experiments with one such patient showed that none of the subclass-specific antisera were absorbed by these cells.[26] Although the routine direct antiglobulin test (i.e., using commercial antiglobulin serum undiluted), may not show significant quantitative differences between the hemolyzing and non-hemolyzing group, both our data and those of Worlledge suggest that there may be quantitative differences. This idea is discussed fully in Chapter 6.

At the other end of the spectrum are patients with negative direct antiglobulin tests who appear to have immune hemolytic anemia. These patients are discussed in detail in Chapter 9.

Destruction of Red Cells Sensitized with IgM Alone. This situation rarely arises *in vivo* in the normal human, as an IgM antibody usually activates complement when interacting with the red cell, and the red cells are then hemolyzed intravascularly or removed extravascularly through C3b/ macrophage interaction. Some interesting data have been published that suggest that red cells sensitized only with IgM survive relatively normally. This finding correlates well with the fact that macrophages have no receptor for IgM. Schreiber and Frank [84] utilized a strain of guinea pig genetically deficient in the fourth component of complement to show that red cells sensitized with IgM only showed no accelerated clearance whatsoever. Later experiments in humans with complement deficiencies yielded results similar to those of the guinea pig model.[85] In contrast, Cutbush and Mollison [19] and Burton and Mollison [15] have described examples of non-complement binding IgM alloantibodies that led to a shortened red cell survival of incompatible red cells. Mollison [68] has suggested that this observation might relate to agglutinates being trapped in small blood vessels and eventually suffering metabolic damage. It should be noted that Schreiber and Frank [84, 85] used relatively weakly sensitized red cells in their experiments.

Destruction of Red Cells Sensitized with IgA Alone. No one has been able to demonstrate IgA receptors on macrophages or monocytes, although they have been reported on neutrophils.[44] There are few experimental data on the survival of IgA sensitized red cells. Indeed, IgA serum alloantibodies and autoantibodies are uncommon, and for them to occur as the only immunoglobulin class is rare. Nevertheless, several examples of autoimmune hemolytic anemia in which IgA autoantibodies alone were shown to be present on the patient's red cells have been described.[89, 90, 97, 102] So far, no one has explained how the red cell destruction occurs in these cases. It is of interest to note that in one case we studied * we were able to show a small number of IgG molecules in addition to the IgA on the patient's red cells, but only when they were tested by the sensitive antiglobulin consumption complement fixation assay [38] (see Chapter 9).

---

* Garratty, G., and Petz, L. D.: Unpublished data.

Destruction of Red Cells Sensitized with IgG and Complement. In our series of immune hemolytic anemia, IgG and complement are found together on the red cells of 50 percent of the patients (67 percent of the warm AIHA). It is difficult to prove that the IgG present on the red cell is responsible for the presence of the bound complement. Often the IgG autoantibody present in the serum or present in an eluate made from the red cells will not sensitize normal red cells *in vitro* with complement. Sometimes complement sensitization can be demonstrated by the indirect antiglobulin test using an eluate, even when fresh complement is not added to the complement eluate; it has been suggested that this phenomenon can be explained by the eluted IgG antibody carrying the complement "piggyback." [55, 75] It is possible that the presence of IgG is sometimes coincidental to the complement sensitization; complement may be activated by immune complexes remote from the red cells, or small amounts of IgM (undetectable by the antiglobulin test) may also be present on the red cell surface and be responsible for the complement activation.

There is experimental evidence in the literature that suggests that extravascular red cell removal is enhanced considerably when complement is present on the red cells in addition to IgG. Mollison [68] showed that red cells sensitized with 7 to 9 μg/ml of a complement-binding IgG allo anti-Fy^a were cleared from the circulation with a half time of about 2 to 4 mins (indicating almost complete clearance of the cells at a single passage through the liver), whereas red cells sensitized with a similar amount of non-complement-binding IgG antibody were cleared with a half time of the order of 50 mins, indicating negligible clearance by the liver and only partial clearance at each passage through the spleen. Schreiber and Frank [85] injected normal guinea pigs and guinea pigs deficient in complement with IgG sensitized red cells. The red cells survived longer in animals lacking either C4 or C3 and the terminal components, which suggests that complement played a significant role in determining the rate of destruction.

Huber et al. [50] were the first to show that human monocytes have a receptor for C3 and that it may function independently of IgG, or cooperatively in the induction of phagocytosis. They showed that if the red cells were sensitized with complement in addition to IgG, then the inhibitory effect of free IgG described previously was diminished considerably. In fact, in experiments in which red cells sensitized with IgG only and IgG + C3 were added to monocytes in the presence of IgG in the fluid phase, it could be shown that only 100 molecules of bound C3 per red cell were sufficient to overcome the inhibitory effect of IgG on the monocyte sensitized red cell reaction. In addition, C3 sensitization of the red cells alone was found not to be sufficient to induce the ingestion of red cells by monocytes; when IgG antibodies were present, C3 appeared to initiate ingestion, suggesting a cooperative function in phagocytosis. Other workers have confirmed and extended these observations. [9, 24, 41, 61, 86]

Mantovani et al. [61] showed that at 10^4 molecules of IgG per red cell, binding of red cells sensitized with IgG and complement was sixfold higher, but ingestion was only 2 to 4 times higher than in red cells sensitized only with IgG. These workers suggested that the receptors for IgG and C3 on the macrophage membrane may not have the same function during phagocytosis, and that the C3 sites on the immune complexes are primarily involved in their attachment to the macrophage, although the ingestion phase may depend mainly on the cytophilic receptor. The first contact between a phagocyte and the immune complex is perhaps made through the C3 receptor, and the IgG receptor would be of primary importance only for interiorization.

Ehlenberger and Nussenzweig [24] studied the role of C3 and Fc receptors on human monocytes and neutrophils. Some of their findings were as follow.

Red cells sensitized with C3 but not IgG were bound and formed full rosettes with neutrophils. The rosettes frequently contained 10 or more red cells per leukocyte. However, no erythrocytes were ingested.

Neutrophils required large amounts of IgG on the red cells to be stimulated for ingestion. 6×10^3 molecules of IgG red cell, without C3, induced no ingestion, and even with 6×10^4 molecules of IgG per red cell, only 70 percent of the neutrophils ingested red cells.

C3 and IgG acted synergistically in opsonization. With C3 bound to an IgG sensitized red cell, ingestion occurred with less than 10 percent of the amount of IgG necessary for the ingestion of an IgG sensitized cell without C3. In experiments with ^{125}I-labeled C3, it was found that red cells bearing 10^3 molecules of C3 together with 2×10^3 molecules of IgG were ingested more effectively than red cells sensitized with 60×10^3 molecules of IgG alone. Similar results were obtained with monolayers of human monocytes; that is, IgG was 10 to 30 times more effective in inducing phagocytosis when red cells were sensitized with C3. Monocytes, however, showed a much greater sensitivity to opsonization with IgG alone. In many experiments, red cells sensitized with C3b and 10^2 molecules of IgG were ingested by 15 to 45 percent of the monocytes.

The authors [24] emphasized that the preceding experiments were carried out under conditions in which the phagocytes were saturated with red cells (overlay technique), and no shear forces existed between red cell and phagocyte. The effect of C3 is magnified if the red cells are kept in suspension (as they would be *in vivo*).

There is some evidence that C3d may play a synergistic role with IgG. Munn and Chaplin [70] showed that 1.5 to 5 times the amount of adherence (rosetting) occurred *in vitro* when Rh (IgG) sensitized red cells had C3d present in addition to IgG. Atkinson and Frank [7] also presented evidence to support this theory; Rh (IgG) sensitized red cells were infused into normal volunteers and patients with a low serum C4 (0.1 percent of normal). Each of six patients with low complement levels had a marked reduction in red cell clearance rates. Their observations on these patients suggested that complement participates in Rh antibody-mediated clearance, and these workers also demonstrated a synergistic role for C3d.

It appears that the ability of particle-bound C3 to enhance phagocytosis can be explained solely by its ability to bind the particle to the phagocyte. This phenomenon is also suggested by the observation that a variety of agents that induce contact between particle and phagocyte such as centrifugation, neuraminidase treatment of the red cells, and the presence of dextran or protamine in the incubation medium mimic the effect of C3. These experiments showed that, for efficient ingestion to occur (and sometimes for ingestion to occur at all), contact between particle and phagocyte must be "boosted" by some agent. It was suggested that this requirement may exist because most cells have an intrinsic negative charge and can be expected to repel each other over short distances; overcoming two such barriers may represent a considerable problem in the recognition of a membrane bound antibody molecule or of other surface moieties capable of triggering phagocytosis by the leukocytes. It was emphasized that, although C3 receptors serve to overcome this electrostatic repulsion, the effect of C3 is clearly not mediated by a reduction of the particle charge, since cells become even more negatively charged after C3 is added. The enhancement of phagocytosis by particle-bound C3 is specific; that is, it results from its interaction with C3 receptors of the plasma membrane of the phagocytes. One important consequence of this concept is that C3 may appear to trigger ingestion directly, because ingestion without C3 is negligible. Phagocytosis in these cases may actually be triggered, not by C3, but by other moieties of the particle surface which, in the absence of C3, are ineffective because of inefficient contact with the phagocyte. Such moieties as, for example, IgG in low doses, may function as "potential" or "hidden" triggers of phagocytosis.[24]

It has been suggested that the difference between IgG and C3 with respect to their capacity to promote binding or ingestion may be more apparent than real, and it may depend on their respective surface distribution on the red cell membrane. Large amounts of IgG combined with high density surface antigen are likely to be evenly distributed over the red cell membrane, whereas C3 deposits in clusters around C42 sites.[12] It has been hypothesized that the distribution of the opsonic stimulus over the large area of the red cell membrane determines the type of response by the phagocytic cell. It has been shown that the macrophage membrane can ingest one opsonized particle while failing to ingest a particle adjacent to it on the macrophage membrane, but attached to the macrophage by a non-opsonic linkage ($F(ab')_2$ anti-F $(ab')_2$), that is to say one lacking Fc.[40] Thus, a phagocytic stimulus does not appear to be propagated over the macrophage membrane but may remain a local event. Specificity of the red cell sensitizing antibody may also be important in determining the amount of macrophage interaction, as some red cell antigens may occur in clusters, whereas others may be more evenly distributed over the membrane.[62, 72, 94]

Schreiber and Frank[84, 85] have shown that although IgG is less efficient in initiating complement fixation, it appears to cause relatively more red cell damage than IgM. In their studies in guinea pigs, at least 60 molecules of IgM per red cell (60 complement-fixing sites) were required to initiate immune clearance, whereas although several thousand IgG molecules per red cell were needed to form one Cl-fixing site, as few as 1.4 IgG complement fixing sites per cell would effectively mediate clearance.

Complement sensitized red cells are destroyed mainly in the liver.[13, 68] In contrast to IgG, the complement receptor/complement sensitized red cell interaction is not inhibited by plasma or serum. This phenomenon can be explained by the fact that the receptor is specific for C3b, and normal plasma or serum does not contain C3b, which is, of course, an activation product of C3. As the liver is a much larger organ with a larger blood flow, proportionally more macrophage interactions will occur there, compared with the spleen.

Although all the experimental data suggest that patients with IgG and complement on their red cells should have more severe hemolysis than those with equivalent amounts of IgG but no complement, this is not always so. The relationship between the presence of complement on red cells and the severity of autoimmune hemolysis is not clear. Some patients with IgG but no complement on their red cells have more severe hemolysis than others with cells strongly sensitized with complement and IgG. Logue and Rosse [59] find that, in general, those patients with both IgG and complement on the red cell surface in large amounts have the greatest rates of hemolysis. When we analyzed data from our series, we found that there were many more patients with hemolytic anemia associated with weak IgG sensitization (i.e., DAT anti-IgG titers < 1024) if complement was present on the red cells than when it was absent.

We [30] have correlated the quantitative assay of red cell bound C3, serologic reactions and hemolytic anemia. The number of molecules of C3 on human red cells was determined using the method of Leonard and Borsos [56] based on the inhibition of anti-C3 antibody by cell bound C3. *In vivo* sensitized red cells were obtained from 25 patients who had a positive anti-C3 antiglobulin test. None of 14 patients with fewer than 1000 molecules of C3 per red cell had hemolytic anemia, whereas 8 of 11 patients with greater than 1000 molecules of C3 per red cell had overt hemolysis. The presence or absence of hemolysis was not explained by variations in the amount of IgG on these patients' red cells. Thus, the amount of C3 per red cell was found to be an important determinant of hemolysis *in vivo* (see page 199).

Destruction of Red Cells Sensitized with IgM and Complement (but no IgG). When red cells are sensitized with IgM and complement is activated, frank hemolysis (i.e., intravascular) often occurs. Sometimes the antibodies involved are not so readily hemolytic as, for instance, if group A blood is given to a group O hypogammaglobulinemic patient with no anti-A detectable *in vitro*. The half time of these cells may be from 2 to 20 days, with no gross signs of intravascular hemolysis.[68] Some other alloantibodies, such as anti-Le[a], may also give a similar pattern of destruction. [68] Although there is no IgM receptor on macrophages, there is a receptor for C3b [50]; thus, if cells do not go all the way through the complement cascade ending in lysis, they may be removed extravascularly if they have reached the C3 stage. But as discussed previously, this process is an inefficient one in the absence of IgG. All the factors discussed in the following paragraph concerning the destruction of red cells sensitized only with complement would also play a role in this situation.

Destruction of Red Cells Sensitized by Complement Components Only.
Sometimes red cells can be sensitized with complement components and no immunoglobulins. The complement cascade, once activated (e.g., by immune complexes remote from the red cell), may possibly cause complement sensitization and indeed, lysis of non-Ig sensitized "innocent bystander" red cells,[39] although as far as we know this action has been demonstrated only *in vitro* by using PNH red cells. Another case in which red cells can result with only complement components on the membrane is when the antibody elutes off the cell *in vivo*, as occurs in cold agglutinin syndrome. These patients have a powerful IgM cold autoantibody present in their plasma that reacts up to at least 30°C. When the patient is exposed to the cold and the peripheral circulation falls to this temperature, the IgM antibody is able to react with the patient's red cells. The antibody activates complement, sometimes causing direct intravascular lysis of some of the cells. The sensitized red cells that escape lysis recirculate, and at 37°C the cold antibody elutes from the cells into the plasma, leaving complement firmly bound to the membrane.

In 1960, Lewis et al.[57] showed that when complement-sensitized red cells from a patient with cold agglutinin syndrome were labeled with ^{51}Cr and reinjected into the patient, there was some immediate destruction of the cells, but most of the cells were sequestered by the liver and appeared later back in the circulation, and thereafter survived normally. Mollison[67] later obtained similar results after injecting volunteers with their own red cells sensitized with complement *in vitro* by such methods as incubation in low ionic strength solutions, etc. These red cells, although having strongly positive direct antiglobulin tests with anti-complement sera, survived relatively normally.

Brown et al.[13] elaborated on these experiments by using complement-deficient animals (C6-deficient rabbits). These workers again showed that if complement-sensitized cells (EC43) do not react all the way through the complement sequence to produce lysis, they become sequestered in the liver and are later released and survive normally. It was shown that complement-sensitized red cells attach to hepatic macrophages (Kupffer cells) in the liver, presumably through the specific C3b macrophage receptor, where some are immediately ingested. To activate the hepatic clearance mechanism, approximately 550 to 800 C3b molecules per red cell are required.[6, 51] With time, unphagocytized red cells returned to the circulation at a slow exponential rate (half time 25 to 100 mins). It was suggested that the return of the EC43 cells to the circulation from sites of attachment on fixed macrophages resulted from the progressive *in vivo* inactivation of fixed C3. The cell-bound C3b is acted on by the naturally occurring C3 inactivator in plasma; the molecule is cleaved into C3c and C3d, which remains attached to the red cell. The macrophage does not seem to interact efficiently, if at all, with C3d *in vivo*. Thus the red cell, although giving a strongly positive direct antiglobulin test due to bound complement (C3d), may now survive relatively normally. Schreiber and Frank [84, 85] confirmed these data by using C4 deficient guinea pigs and complement deficient humans. Evidence has also been presented in these publications that red cells sensitized only up to the C4 stage survive normally.

The presence of a C3d receptor on macrophages is controversial. Some workers [23, 70, 78, 101] have been able to detect a C3d receptor, and others have not.[6, 8, 9, 13, 41, 69] Bianco [8] makes the interesting observation that all the workers who have detected a C3d receptor used purified complement components to prepare their sensitized red cells, whereas the workers who could not detect a receptor were using whole serum as a source of complement. Bianco points out that the latter *in vitro* experiments would be closer to the *in vivo* situation; certainly, all *in vivo* evidence so far would suggest that the C3d receptor does not play an important role in the destruction of red cells sensitized with C3d but not IgG, although, as mentioned previously, recent reports have suggested that C3d may play a synergistic role to IgG.

C3b sensitization alone is a poor stimulus for phagocytosis.[9, 42, 83, 86] The adherence of complement-sensitized red cells to potentially phagocytic cells requires few C3b molecules on the membrane, but phagocytosis *in vitro*, even when splenic macrophages are used, is distinctly uncommon. Brown et al.[13] confirmed these *in vitro* findings but found that when such complement-sensitized red cells were injected into rabbits, evidence of phagocytosis occurred.

Rosse et al.[83] suggested that the number of complement molecules present on the membrane could affect the results. When more C3b molecules are present, engulfment is more likely to occur; however, the number of C3b molecules needed for this reaction approaches the number that leads to the direct lysis of the red cell, something in the order of 100,000 C3b molecules per red cell. Both Brown [12] and Rosse et al.[83] believe that the distribution of C3b and IgG molecules on the red cell membrane may explain the differences in their reaction with phagocytic cells. The distribution of C3b is apparently in spots of high concentration. Antibody, on the other hand, is probably distributed randomly over the red cell surface.[72] A more random distribution, as in the case of antibody, may serve as a greater stimulus to continued metapod activity in attempting engulfment, as compared with a more spotty distribution in the case of C3b.

An interesting observation is that if C3b is deposited on the membrane adjacent to the I blood group antigenic site and then cleaved to C3d, the C3d remains on the membrane in the form of an "immunologic scar." [7] That is to say, eventually C3d molecules occupy such a large number of sites in the proximity of the I antigen that newly formed C3b molecules are sterically prevented from binding, and the cells are protected from further damage mediated by C3b.[10, 25, 28] Such cells can be shown *in vitro* to be resistant to anti-I hemolysis, compared with non-sensitized red cells, but they are not resistant to lysis by other antibodies (e.g., anti-A). Jaffe et al.[51] performed red cell survival studies using [51] Cr labelled red cells that were (a) maximally sensitized with C3d using anti-I and then exposed to IgM anti-A *in vitro,* and (b) maximally sensitized with C3d using anti-I and then re-exposed to anti-I and complement. The cells sensitized in the second stage with anti-I + complement survived normally, but the cells sensitized with IgM anti-A were destroyed rapidly. These *in vivo* experiments confirmed the *in vitro* finding, suggesting that once red cells become sensitized with C3d by anti-I autoantibody, they are then protected against further lysis by auto anti-I. It also may explain why there are reports on transfused cells being destroyed more rapidly than the patient's own "protected" cells in patients with cold agglutinin syndrome.[27]

In summary, complement sensitization of red cells may result in (a) intravascular hemolysis; (b) sequestration in the reticuloendothelial system (e.g., liver) with ingestion by phagocytes; (c) sequestration with later return to the circulation, where the red cell may have normal survival; or (d) essentially normal survival.

Variation in Macrophage Activity

There are few data available correlating variations in macrophage activity with red cell destruction. However, this would seem to be an important area to study, as variation in macrophage activity may well explain some of the discrepant results we see in individual patients (e.g., patients with severe hemolysis associated with weakly sensitized red cells).

MacKenzie[60] found that monocytes from patients with autoimmune hemolytic anemia showed 40 to 80 percent ingestion of IgG sensitized red cells, compared with 10 to 15 percent when normal donors were used. Patients with non-hemolytic anemias and microangiopathic hemolytic anemia did not show such differences.

Kay and Douglas[53] also studied 21 patients with immune hemolytic anemia; 4 were studied sequentially. Fifteen of 17 patients showed enhanced monocyte activity (i.e., rosetting and phagocytosis) with autologous sensitized red cells, as compared with normal monocytes exposed to the same sensitized red cells. The most consistent elevation in monocyte activity occurred for cells from patients with both IgG and complement sensitized red cells. Of great interest was the finding that there seemed to be no difference in activity between monocytes from patients or normal donors when tested against sheep cells sensitized with IgG rabbit anti-sheep (Forssman) antibody or IgM antibody and complement. This observation contrasted strikingly with work by the same group showing increased IgG receptor activity for patients with sarcoidosis, Crohn's disease, and tuberculosis.[22] Kay and Douglas[53] suggested that there might be two explanations for these results: (a) there might be a subpopulation of monocytes that selectively bind the sensitized red cells, or (b) the patient's monocytes have an increased affinity for autologous immunoprotein or an increase in the number of Fc receptor sites that have developed a restricted specificity. They further speculated that the antigen-antibody complex that results when red cells combine with antibody in immune hemolysis effects a structured modification in the Fc portion of the IgG molecule; this binding could result in a unique conformation of that portion of the Fc that binds to the monocyte.

Munn and Chaplin [70] studied factors that affect donors of monocytes used in leukocyte monolayer activity testing involving [51] Cr-labelled IgG Rh sensitized red cells. Variation in rosette formation among monolayers obtained from 10 healthy donors was defined, as well as variation among 24 sequential monolayers obtained from one healthy donor and 8 sequential monolayers from a second healthy donor over a 4-month period. Rosette formation, expressed as eluate cpm per plate, averaged 220 (range 35 to 472) for the 10 donors; 24 determinations on one donor averaged 201 (range 59 to 420), 8 determinations on the second donor averaged 244 (range 69 to 395). Striking increases in rosette formation were observed employing monolayers from 4 of 4 normal subjects during the course of viral infections, with peak values exceeding 5,8,13, and 14 times the normal mean. Elevations were also observed with monolayers prepared fro.n blood of selected patients with hematologic disorders; a remarkable value 168 times the normal mean was repeatedly obtained for a patient with myeloid metaplasia whose monolayer consisted almost exclusively of mature granulocytic rosette-forming cells. The results emphasized the influence of monolayer donor variables on rosette formation.

There is considerable anecdotal evidence for the exacerbation of autoimmune hemolysis in relation to intercurrent viral infections; we have certainly seen examples of this ourselves. The findings of Munn and Chaplin [70] would be consistent with such exacerbations reflecting, at least in part, on activation *in vivo* of the macrophage system. Atkinson and Frank [5] showed increased clearance of IgG sensitized red cells in BCG-infected animals, hypothesizing that increased macrophage activation in such animals is responsible for the shortened *in vivo* red cell survival. A substantial increase of Fc receptors on circulating human monocytes has been shown to occur in individuals with solid malignant tumors (i.e., five times greater than normal). [79] Arend and Mannik [3] demonstrated an approximate doubling of IgG receptors and an increase in IgG association constants for rabbit alveolar macrophages following maximal stimulation with complete Freud's adjuvant. We and others [76, 82] have seen several patients with autoimmune hemolytic anemia following vaccination and immunization, and it is tempting to speculate that activation of the macrophage system may set off increased immune red cell destruction in patients whose red cells may already have been sensitized with small quantities of protein and have been surviving relatively normally up to the time of vaccination.

Bianco et al. [9] showed that both activated and non-activated macrophages ingest IgG coated red cells (activated cells ingested 1.5 to 2 times as many), whereas non-activated macrophages avidly bind C3 coated red cells but do not ingest them to a significant degree. Activated macrophages, on the other hand, bound and ingested C3 coated red cells.

It is also interesting to note that Zipursky and Brown [104] confirmed that normal neutrophils do not ingest IgG (Rh) sensitized red cells, but they were able to show neutrophils from patients with acute leukemia and leukocytosis readily ingested the sensitized red cells. Rosse et al.[83] also confirmed that normal granulocytes did not adhere to or phagocytose Rh (IgG) sensitized red cells, but they would adhere to and phagocytose red cells sensitized with IgG anti-B. These findings suggest that an IgG receptor is indeed present on granulocytes, but that the amount of IgG present on the red cells has to be considerable before an interaction with the macrophage occurs.

OTHER POSSIBLE MECHANISMS OF IMMUNE RED CELL DESTRUCTION

Possible Role of Lymphocytes in Immune Red Cell Destruction

The role, if any, of lymphocytes in immune red cell destruction is controversial. Lymphocytes are known to have receptors for IgG (Fc) and complement (C3b, C3d, and C4). They have been described as being capable of destroying sensitized nucleated cells (e.g., other lymphocytes, tumor cells, and chicken red cells).[74] The mechanism of cell destruction is cell-mediated cytotoxicity. Before the cell is damaged, contact between the lymphocyte and target cell has to occur; complement may or may not be involved. *In vitro*, cell mediated lysis requires several hours to occur, even under optimal conditions.

Cell mediated cytotoxicity can be independent of antibody. In this case, direct cell mediated cytolysis by presensitized lymphocytes occurs. The effector cells are thought to be cytotoxic T-lymphocytes, and these do not require IgG antibodies as specific recognition factors for target cell antigens. Cell mediated cytotoxicity can also be antibody dependent, where the target cells have to be sensitized with antibody. The effector cells for this reaction have been described as possibly being "null" lymphocytes (i.e., lacking sheep cell receptors and surface Ig, but having IgG and complement receptors),[11] or the so-called "killer" lymphocytes (K cells), which are non-phagocytic and non-adherent lymphocytic cells.[74] Brier et al.[11] believe that the "null" cells are a subset of B lymphocytes; Perlmann[74] believes that K cells represent a heterogenous family of effector cells (both B and T cells). Still another group of workers[88] believes that the effector cells are neither B nor T cells. All are agreed that the cells possess an Fc receptor.

Although chicken red cells were lysed by human lymphocytes, Holm[46] reported that human red cells were not directly lysed in the presence of anti-A or anti-Rh when the leukocyte preparation was more than 99 percent pure lymphocytes. Hinz and Chickosky,[45] using lymphocyte preparations containing less than 1 percent neutrophils and virtually no monocytes, were able to demonstrate cytotoxic reactions between lymphocytes and A and Rh positive red cells in the presence of anti-A and anti-Rh respectively. In the anti-A experiments, lymphocytes from group O, A or AB donors were equally active, but in the Rh experiments only lymphoctes from an Rh hyperimmune donor would cause lysis of the red cells. Normal lymphocytes from both Rh positive and Rh negative donors were completely without effect, even in the presence of a powerful anti-Rh. In contrast, Urbaniak [91] was able to show that normal or autologous lymphoid cells would lyse Rh sensitized red cells, and that killing occurred at a very low antibody concentration. Recently, other workers have also reported antibody dependent cell mediated cytotoxicity against human red cells, mediated by anti-A [73] and anti-Rh. [43, 54, 65, 73] It should be noted that some workers could demonstrate the reactions with anti-Rh only when the target red cells were enzyme-treated. [65]

The lymphocyte induced antibody dependent cell mediated cytotoxicity demonstrated with human blood group alloantibodies was almost as efficient as that obtained with monocytes. In addition, the lymphocyte mediated antibody dependent cell mediated cytotoxicity is not inhibited by free IgG (e.g., normal plasma), although it can be inhibited by aggregated IgG. Thus, it is possible that lymphocyte antibody dependent cell mediated cytotoxicity may play some role, sometimes, in immune hemolysis.

Macrophage/Monocyte Cytotoxicity

Since the incrimination of macrophages as the major effector cell in immune red cell destruction, the emphasis has been on the phagocytic properties of the cell. Recent studies have suggested that an extracellular mechanism is operative, and perhaps the cytotoxic properties of the macrophage may be more important than first thought.

Holm and Hammarstrom [47] showed that purified human monocytes were able to lyse red cells treated with hyperimmune anti-A. In fact, one monocyte was able to lyse 2 to 3 red cells within an 18-hour incubation period. Complement was not necessary for this reaction.

Actual lysis of the cell may result from a heat-labile cytotoxin designated by McIvor et al. [63] as specific macrophage cytotoxin. Most of the interactions are similar to those described previously for antibody dependent cell mediated cytotoxicity by lymphocytes: (a) specific recognition and cell adherence; (b) intimate contact stimulating membrane phagocytosis and triggering the release of specific macrophage cytotoxin; and (c) specific macrophage cytotoxin acts directly on the target cell membrane.

Kurlander et al. [54] were able to demonstrate monocyte mediated lysis *in vitro* of human red cells sensitized with IgG anti-Rh (D) and anti-A or B. Cells sensitized only with human complement components (even up to 80,000 molecules per red cell) were not lysed, but complement (C3b or C3d) sensitization augmented IgG-mediated lysis and reduced the amount of IgG necessary to produce lysis. Without complement, 1000 to 1500 molecules of anti-D per red cell were necessary for lysis; less than 1000 molecules were necessary when complement was present in addition to IgG on the red cell. IgG anti-A or -B were 5 to 10-fold less efficient in promoting phagocytosis or lysis per molecule of IgG bound; however, because of the greater antigen density of A or B, more than 100,000 molecules of IgG per red cell could be bound, producing equivalent lysis of anti-D sensitized cells. Even after degradation of C3b to C3d, complement augmentation persisted.

Fleer et al. [32, 33, 35] have suggested that cytotoxicity may play a more important role than phagocytosis in immune red cell destruction. Using ^{51}Cr labelled human red cells sensitized with anti-D, they were able to demonstrate cytotoxicity by monocytes, independent of phagocytosis. An interesting finding was that the cytotoxicity, but not the phagocytosis, was inhibited by hydrocortisone and colchicine. The release of lysosomal enzymes by the monocytes was also inhibited by hydrocortisone and colchicine; a significant correlation was found between lysosomal enzyme release and lysis. The authors concluded that lysosomal enzymes released by monocytes when incubated with Rh sensitized red cells were responsible for lysis of these red cells. The lysis occurred only over a short range, probably at the site of attachment of the red cell, because only red cells bound to the monocyte were lysed.

Unlike other workers [43, 45, 73, 91] Fleer et al. [32, 33, 35] were not able to demonstrate lysis of Rh sensitized cells by lymphocytes. Another important effect noted by Fleer et al. [31] was the development of an increased osmotic fragility of a considerable part of the non-lysed Rh sensitized red cells. In fact, they found that the osmotically more fragile cells considerably outnumbered lysed and ingested red cells. A correlation with increased osmotic fragility and severity of autoimmune hemolytic anemia has been described previously. [96] The presence of spherocytes has, for years, been said to be a hallmark of autoimmune hemolytic anemia; the spherocytes are now thought to be formed through fragmentation of the sensitized red cells by macrophages. [6] It has also been assumed that the increased osmotic fragility is due to the presence of spherocytes, but it may well be that the damage to the red cell membrane caused by cytotoxicity without fragmentation may also contribute to the increased fragility.

In Vivo Agglutination of Red Cells

Before the role of the macrophage was fully appreciated, the aggregation or agglutination of red cells *in vivo* was believed to play a major role in immune red cell destruction. [52, 98] It was commonly believed that red cells sensitized with non-agglutinating antibodies (e.g., IgG Rh) could be aggregated in the spleen where the protein concentration was high, and that these aggregates or agglutinates would be held up in the spleen and thus be more susceptible to destruction by macrophages. There is little evidence to support this theory as a major cause of immune red cell destruction, but it may play a role in some circumstances. Romano and Mollison [80] showed that red cells coated with as little as 110 to 190 IgG anti-A molecules/red blood cell would agglutinate if mixed with plasma and rocked on a tile, whereas the minimum amount of IgG anti-Rh required for agglutination under these conditions was about 19,000 IgG molecules/red blood cell. Complement binding by red cells coated with IgG anti-A could be demonstrated only when the amount of antibody on the cells was at least 5,134 IgG molecules/red blood cell. Since in ABO hemolytic disease the amount of antibody on the cells is frequently less than 0.6 μg/ml cells (approximately 200 IgG molecules per red blood cell), it seems that red cell destruction in this syndrome does not result from the activation of complement, but may result from the sequestration of agglutinated cells. Mollison [68] has also suggested that some non-complement binding IgM alloantibodies, active at 37°C (e.g., examples of anti-c and anti-M), may destroy red cells *in vivo* because agglutinates may become trapped in small blood vessels and eventually suffer metabolic damage.

REFERENCES

1. Abramson, N., Gelfand, E. W., Jandl, J. H., and Rosen, F. S.: The interaction between human monocytes and red cells. Specificity for IgG subclasses and IgG fragments. J. Exp. Med., *132:*1207, 1970.
2. Abramson, N., and Schur, P.: The IgG subclasses of red cell antibodies and relationship to monocyte binding. Blood, *40:*500, 1972.
3. Arend, W. P., and Mannik, M.: The macrophage receptor for IgG: Number and affinity of binding sites. J. Immunol., *110:*1455, 1973.
4. Arend, W. P., and Mannik, M.: Quantitative studies on IgG receptors on monocytes. *In* Mononuclear Phagocytes in Immunity, Infection, and Pathology. Van Furth, R., Ed. Oxford, Blackwell Scientific Publications, 1975.
5. Atkinson, J. P., and Frank, M. M.: The effect of Bacillus Calmette-Guérin-induced macrophage activation on the in vivo clearance of sensitized erythrocytes. J. Clin. Invest., *53:*1742, 1974.
6. Atkinson, J. P., and Frank, M. M.: Studies on the in vivo effects of antibody interaction of IgM antibody and complement in the immune clearance and destruction of erythrocytes in man. J. Clin. Invest., *54:*339, 1974.
7. Atkinson, J. P., and Frank, M. M.: Role of complement in the pathphysiology of hemotologic diseases. Progr. Hematol., *10:*211, 1977.
8. Bianco, C.: Plasma membrane receptors for complement. *In* Comprehensive Immunology. Good, R. A., and Day, S. B., Eds. New York, Plenum Press, 1977.
9. Bianco, C., Griffin, F. M., Jr., and Silverstein, S. C.: Studies of the macrophage complement receptor. J. Exp. Med., *141:*1278, 1975.
10. Boyer, J. T.: Complement and cold agglutinins. II. Interactions of the components of complement and antibody within the haemolytic complex. Clin. Exp. Immunol., *2:*241, 1967.
11. Brier, A. M., Chess, L., and Schlossman, S. F.: Human antibody-dependent cellular cytotoxicity. Isolation and identification of a subpopulation of peripheral blood lymphocytes which kill antibody-coated autologous target cells. J. Clin. Invest., *56:*1580, 1975.
12. Brown, D. L.: The behavior of phagocytic cell receptors in relation to allergic red cell destruction. Ser. Haemat., *VII:*3, 1974.
13. Brown, D. L., Lachmann, P. J., and Dacie, J. V.: The *in vivo* behavior of complement-coated red cells: Studies in C6-deficient, C3-depleted and normal rabbits. Clin. Exp. Immunol., *7:*401, 1970.
14. Brown, D. L., and Nelson, D. A.: Surface microfragmentation of red cells as a mechanism for complement-mediated immune spherocytosis. Brit. J. Haematol., *24:*301, 1973.
15. Burton, M. S., and Mollison, P. L.: Effect of IgM and IgG iso-antibody on red cell clearance. Immunol., *14:*861, 1968.

16. Constatoulakis, M., Costea, N., Schwartz, R. S., and Dameshek, W.: Quantitative studies of the effect of red blood cell sensitization in vitro hemolysis. J. Clin. Invest., *42:*1790, 1963.

17. Cooper, N. R.: Immune adherence by the fourth component of complement. Science, *165:*396, 1969.

18. Cooper, R. A.: Loss of membrane components in the pathogenesis of antibody-induced spherocytosis. J. Clin. Invest., *51:*16, 1972.

19. Cutbush, M., and Mollison, P. L.: Relation between characteristics of blood-group antibodies in vitro and associated patterns of red cell destruction in vivo. Brit. J. Haematol., *4:*115, 1958.

20. Dacie, J. V.: The Auto-Immune Haemolytic Anaemias. 2nd Edition. New York, Grune & Stratton, 1962, Part II.

21. Dacie, J. V.: Autoimmune hemolytic anemia. Arch. Intern. Med., *135:*1293, 1975.

22. Douglas, S. D., Schmidt, M. E., and Siltzbach, H. E.: Monocyte receptor activity in normal individuals and patients with sarcoidosis. Immunol. Commun., *1:*25, 1972.

23. Ehlenberger, A. G., and Nussenzweig, V.: Synergy between receptors for Fc and C3 in the induction of phagocytosis by human monocytes and neutrophils. Fed. Proc. *34:*854, 1975.

24. Ehlenberger, A. G., and Nussenzweig, V.: Immunologically-Mediated phagocytosis: Role of C3 and Fc receptors. *In* Clinical Evaluation of Immune Function in Man. Litwin, S. D., Christian, C. L., and Siskind, G. W., Eds. New York, Grune & Stratton, 1976.

25. Engelfriet, C. P., Borne, A. E. G. Kr. von dem, Beckers, D., Reynierse, E., and Van Loghem, J. J.: Autoimmune haemolytic anaemias. V. Studies on the resistance against complement haemolysis of the red cells of patients with chronic cold agglutinin disease. Clin. Exp. Immunol., *11:*255, 1972.

26. Engelfriet, C. P., Borne, A. E. G. Kr. von dem, Beckers, D., and Van Loghem, J. J.: Autoimmune haemolytic anaemia: Serological and immunochemical characteristics of the autoantibodies: Mechanisms of cell destruction. Series Hematologica, *VII:*328, 1974.

27. Evans, R. S., Turner, E., and Bingham, M.: Studies with radioiodinated cold agglutinins of ten patients. Am. J. Med., *38:*378, 1965.

28. Evans, R. S., Turner, E., and Bingham, M.: Chronic hemolytic anemia due to cold agglutinins: The mechanism of resistance of red cells to C′ hemolysis by cold agglutinins. J. Clin. Invest., *46:*1461, 1967.

29. Fairley, N. H.: The fate of extracorpuscular circulating haemoglobin. Brit. Med. J., *2:*213, 1940.

30. Fischer, J., Petz, L. D., Garratty, G., and Cooper, N.: Correlations between quantitative assay of red cell bound C3, serologic reactions, and hemolytic anemias. Blood, *44:*359, 1974.

31. Fleer, A., Koopman, M. G., Borne, A. E. G. Kr. von dem, and Engelfriet, C. P.: Monocyte-induced increase in osmotic fragility of human red cells sensitized with anti-D alloantibodies. Brit. J. Haematol., *40:*439, 1978.

32. Fleer, A., van der Hart, M., Borne, A. E. G. Kr. von dem, and Engelfriet, C. P.: (Abstract) Mechanism of antibody-dependent cytotoxicity by human blood monocytes towards IgG-sensitized erythrocytes. Europ. J. Clin. Invest., *6:*333, 1976.

33. Fleer, A., van der Hart, M., Borne, A. E. G. Kr. von dem, and Engelfriet, C. P.: Monocyte-mediated lysis of human erythrocytes. *In* Leucocyte Membrane Determinants Regulating Immune Reactivity. Eijsvoogel, V. P., Roos, D., and Zeijlemaker, W. P., Eds., New York, Academic Press, 1976, 675.

34. Fleer, A., Van Der Meulen, F. W., Linthout, E., and Borne, A. E. G. Kr. von dem, Destruction of IgG-sensitized erythrocytes by human blood monocytes: Modulation of inhibition by IgG. Brit. J. Haematol., *39:*425, 1978.

35. Fleer, A., Van Schaik, M. L. J., Borne, A. E. G. Kr. von dem, and Engelfriet, C. P.: Destruction of sensitized erythrocytes by human monocytes in vitro. Effects of Cytochalasin B, Hydrocortisone and Colchicine. Scand. J. Immunol., *8:*515, 1978.
36. Frame, M., Mollison, P. L., and Terry, W. D.: Anti-Rh activity of human γG4 proteins. Nature, *225:*641, 1970.
37. Gergely, J., Fudenberg, H. H., and Van Loghem, E.: The papain susceptibility of IgG myeloma proteins of different heavy chain subclasses. Immunochem., *7:*1, 1970.
38. Gilliland, B. C., Leddy, J. P., and Vaughan, J. H.: The detection of cell-bound antibody on complement-coated human red cells. J. Clin. Invest., *49:*898, 1970.
39. Götze, O., and Müller-Eberhard, H. J.: Lysis of erythrocytes by complement in the absence of antibody. J. Exp. Med., *132:*898, 1970.
40. Griffin, F. M., and Silverstein, S. C.: Segmental response of the macrophage plasma membrane to a phagocytic stimulus. J. Exp. Med., *139:*323, 1974.
41. Griffin, F. M., Jr., Bianco, C., and Silverstein, S. C.: Characterization of the macrophage receptor for complement and demonstration of its functional independence from the receptor for the Fc portion of immunoglobulin G. J. Exp. Med., *141:*1269, 1975.
42. Griffin, F. M., Jr., Griffin, J. A., Leider, J. E., and Silverstein, S. C.: Studies on the mechanism of phagocytosis. I. Requirements for circumferential attachment of particle-bound ligands to specific receptors on the macrophage plasma membrane. J. Exp. Med., *142:*1263, 1975.
43. Handwerger, B. S., Kay, N. W., and Douglas, S. D.: Lymphocyte-mediated antibody-dependent cytolysis: Role in immune hemolysis. Vox. Sang., *34:*276, 1978.
44. Henson, P. M., Johnson, H. B., and Spiegelberg, H. D.: The release of granule enzymes from human neutrophils stimulated by aggregated immunoglobulins of different classes and subclasses. J. Immunol., *109:*1182, 1972.
45. Hinz, C. F., Jr., and Chickosky, J. F.: Lymphocyte Cytotoxicity for Human Erythrocytes. Schwarz, M. R., Ed. In Leukocyte Culture Conference. Seattle, University of Washington, 1972.
46. Holm, G.: Lysis of antibody-treated human erythrocytes by human leukocytes and macrophages in tissue culture. Int. Arch. Allergy, *43:*671, 1972.
47. Holm, G., and Hammarström, S.: Haemolytic activity of human blood monocytes: Lysis of human erythrocytes treated with anti-A serum. Clin. Exp. Immunol., *13:*29, 1973.
48. Huber, H., and Fudenberg, H. H.: Receptor sites of human monocytes for IgG. Int. Arch. Allergy, *34:*18, 1968.
49. Huber, H., Douglas, S. D., Nusbacher, J., Kochwa, S., and Rosenfield, R. F.: IgG subclass specificity of human monocyte receptor sites. Nature (London), *229:*419, 1970.
50. Huber, H., Polley, M., Linscott, W., Fudenberg, H. H., and Müller-Eberhard, H.: Human monocytes: Distinct receptor sites for the third component of complement and for immunoglobulin. G. Science, *162:*1281, 1968.
51. Jaffe, C. J., Atkinson, J. P., and Frank, M. M.: The role of complement in the clearance of cold agglutinin-sensitized erythrocytes in man. J. Clin. Invest., *58:*942, 1976.
52. Jandl, J. H.: The agglutination and sequestration of immature red cells. Lab. Clin. Med., *55:*663, 1960.
53. Kay, N. E., and Douglas, S. D.: Monocyte-erythrocyte interaction in vitro in immune hemolytic anemias. Blood, *50:*889, 1977.
54. Kurlander, R. J., Rosse, W. F., and Logue, W. L.: Quantitative influence of antibody and complement coating of red cells on monocyte-mediated cell lysis. J. Clin. Invest., *61:*1309, 1978.

55. Leddy, J. P., Bakemeier, R. F., and Vaughan, J. H.: Fixation of complement components to auto-antibody eluted from human RBC. J. Clin. Invest., *44:*1066, 1965 (Abstr).
56. Leonard, E. J., and Borsos, T.: Effects of C3 inactivator on bound C3 antigen. J. Immunol., *108:*776, 1972.
57. Lewis, S. M., Dacie, J. V., and Szur, L.: Mechanisms of haemolysis in the cold-haemagglutinin syndrome. Brit. J. Hematol., *6:*154, 1960.
58. Lo Buglio, A. F., Cotran, R., and Jandl, J. H.: Red cells coated with immunoglobulin G: Binding and sphering by mononuclear cells in man. Science, *158:*1582, 1967.
59. Logue, G., and Rosse, W.: Immunologic mechanisms in autoimmune hemolytic disease. Seminars in hematol., *13:*277, 1976.
60. MacKenzie, M. R.: Monocytic sensitization in autoimmune hemolytic anemia. Clin. Res., *23:*132A, 1975 (Abstr).
61. Mantovani, B., Rabinovitch, M., and Nussenzweig, V.: Phagocytosis of immune complexes by macrophages. Different roles of the macrophage receptor sites for complement (C3) and for immunoglobulin (IgG). J. Exp. Med., *135:*780, 1972.
62. Masouredis, S. P., Sudora, E. J., Mahan, L., and Victoria, E. J.: Antigen site densities and ultrastructural distribution patterns of red cell Rh antigens. Trans., *16:*94, 1976.
63. McIvor, K. L., Piper, C. E., and Bell, R. B.: Mechanisms of target cell destruction by alloimmune peritoneal macrophages. *In* The Macrophage in Neoplasia. Fink, M. A., Ed. New York, Academic Press, Inc., 1976, 135.
64. Melewicz, F. M., Shore, S. L., Ades, E. W., and Phillips, D. J.: The mononuclear cell in human blood which mediates antibody-dependent cellular cytotoxicity to virus-infected target cells. II. Identification as a K cell. J. Immunol., *118:*567, 1976.
65. Milgrom, H., and Shore, S. L.: Lysis of antibody-coated human red cells by peripheral blood mononuclear cells. Altered effector cell profile after treatment of target cells with enzymes. Cellular Immunol., *39:*178, 1978.
66. Mohandas, N., and de Boisfleury, A.: Antibody-induced spherocytic anemia. I. Changes in red cell deformity. Blood Cells, *3:*187, 1977.
67. Mollison, P. L.: The role of complement in haemolytic processes in vivo. *In* Complement. Wolstenholme, G. E. W., and Knight, J. Eds. London, J. & A. Churchill, 1965, 323.
68. Mollison, P. L.: Blood Transfusion in Clinical Medicine. 5th Edition. Oxford, Blackwell Scientific Publications, 1972.
69. Müller-Eberhard, H. J.: Complement and phagocytosis. *In* Bellanti J. A., and Delbert, H. D. Eds.: The Phagocytic Cell in Host Resistance. New York, Raven Press, 1975.
70. Munn, L. R., and Chaplin, H., Jr.: Rosette formation by sensitized human red cells—Effects of source of peripheral leukocyte monolayers. Vox. Sang., *33:*129, 1977.
71. Natvig, J. B., and Kunkel, H. G.: Detection of genetic antigens utilizing gamma globulin coupled to red blood cells. Nature, *215:*68, 1967.
72. Nicholson, G. C., Masouredis, S. P., and Singer, S. J.: Quantitative two dimensional ultrastructural distribution of Rho (D) antigenic sites on human erythrocyte membranes. Proc. Natl. Acad. Sci., *68:*1416, 1971.
73. Northoff, H., Kluge, A., and Resch, K.: Antibody dependent cellular cytotoxicity (ADCC) against human erythrocytes, mediated by blood group alloantibodies: A model for the role of antigen density in target cell lysis. Z. Immun. Forsch., *154:*15, 1978.
74. Perlmann, P., and Holm, G.: Cytotoxic effects of lymphoid cells in vitro. Adv. Immunol., *11:*117, 1969.
75. Petz, L. D., Fink, D. J., Letsky, E. A., Fudenberg, H. H., and Müller-Eberhard,

H. J.: In vivo metabolism of complement. I. Metobolism of the third component (C3) in acquired hemolytic anemia. J. Clin. Invest., *47:*2469, 1968.
76. Pirofsky, B.: Autoimmunization and the Autoimmune Hemolytic Anemias. Baltimore, Williams & Wilkins Co., 1969.
77. Polley, M. J., and Ross, Gordon, D.: Macrophage and Lymphocyte Receptor Sites for Complement (C3) and for Immunoglobulin (IgG). Proceedings of an International Symposium on "The Nature and Significance of Complement Activation." Raritan, New Jersey, Ortho Diagnostics, 1976.
78. Reynolds, H. Y., Atkinson, J. P., Newball, H. H., and Frank, M. M.: Receptors for immunoglobulin and complement on human alveolar macrophages. J. Immunol., *114:*1813, 1975.
79. Rhodes, J.: Altered expression of human monocyte Fc receptors in malignant disease. Nature, *265:*253, 1977.
80. Romano, E. L., and Mollison, P. L.: Red cell destruction in vivo by low concentrations of IgG anti-A. Brit. J. Haematol., *29:*121, 1975.
81. Ross, G. D., and Polley, M. J.: Specificity of human lymphocyte complement receptors. J. Exp. Med., *141:*1163, 1975.
82. Rosse, W. F.: Correlation of in vivo and in vitro measurements of hemolysis in hemolytic anemia due to immune reactions. Progr. Hematol., *8:*51, 1973.
83. Rosse, W. F., De Boisfleury, A., and Bessis, M.: The interaction of phagocytic cells and red cells modified by immune reactions. Comparison of antibody and complement coated red cells. Blood cells, *1:*345, 1975.
84. Schreiber, A. D., and Frank, M. M.: Role of antibody and complement in the immune clearance and destruction of erythrocytes. I. *In vivo* effects of IgG and IgM complement fixing sites. J. Clin. Invest., *51:*575, 1972.
85. Schreiber, A. D., and Frank, M. M.: Role of antibody and complement in the immune clearance and destruction of erythrocytes. II. Molecular nature of IgG and IgM complement-fixing sites and effects of their interaction with serum. J. Clin. Invest., *51:*583, 1972.
86. Scornik, J. C., and Drewinko, B.: Receptors for IgG and complement in human spleen lymphoid cells. Preferential binding of particulate immune complexes through complement receptors. J. Immunol., *115:*1223, 1975.
87. Scornik, J. C., Salinas, M. C., and Drewinko, B.: IgG-Dependent clearance of red blood cells in IgG myeloma patients. J. Immunol., *115:*901, 1975.
88. Shore, S. L., Melewicz, F. M., and Gordon, D. S.: The mononuclear cell in human blood which mediates antibody-dependent cellular cytotoxicity to virus-infected target cells. I. Identification of the population of effector cells. J. Immunol., *118:*558, 1977.
89. Stratton, F., Rawlinson, V. I., Chapman, S. A., Pengelly, C. D. R., and Jennings, R. C.: Acquired hemolytic anemia associated with IgA anti-e. Trans., *12:*157, 1972.
90. Sturgeon, P., Smith, L. E., Chun, H. M. T., Hurvitz, C. H., Garratty, G., and Goldfinger, D.: Autoimmune hemolytic anemia associated exclusively with IgA of Rh specificity. Transfusion, *19:*324, 1979.
91. Urbaniak, S. J.: Lymphoid cell dependent(K-cell) lysis of human erythrocytes sensitized with rhesus alloantibodies. Brit. J. Haematol., *33:*409, 1976.
92. Van Furth, R.: Origin and kinetics of monocytes and macrophages. Seminars Hematol., *7:*125, 1970.
93. Van Furth, R., Cohn, Z. A., Hirsch, J. G., Humphrey, J. H., Spector, W. G., and Langevoort, H. L.: The mononuclear phagocyte system: A new classification of macrophages, monocytes, and their precursor cells. Bull. Wld. Hlth. Org., *46:*845, 1972.
94. Victoria, E. J., Muchmore, E. A., Sudora, E. J., and Masouredis, S. P.: The role of antigen mobility in anti-Rh (D) induced agglutination. J. Clin. Invest., *56:*292, 1975.

95. Von Dem Borne, A. E. G. Kr., Beckers, D., Van Der Meulen, W., and Engelfriet, C. P.: IgG_4 Autoantibodies against erythrocytes, without increased haemolysis: A case report. Brit. J. Haematol., *37:*137, 1977.
96. Von Dem Borne, A. E. G. Kr., Engelfriet, C. P., Beckers, D., and Van Loghem, J. J.: Autoimmune haemolytic anaemias. Biochemical studies of red cells from patients with autoimmune haemolytic anaemia with incomplete warm autoantibodies. Clin. Exp. Immunol., *8:*377, 1971.
97. Wager, O., Haltia, K., Rasauen, J. A., and Vuopio, P.: Five cases of positive antiglobulin test involving IgA warm type autoantibody. Ann. Clin. Res., *3:*76, 1971.
98. Wartiovaara, T. W.: Über die Entwicklung der Konglutinierenden Eigenschaft bei der Immunisierung. Acta Soc. Med., 'Duodecim' *14:*1, 1932.
99. Weed, R. I.: The importance of erythrocyte deformability. Am. J. Med., *49:*147, 1970.
100. Weiner, W.: "Coombs-positive" "normal" people. Proceedings of the 10th International Society of Blood Transfusion, Stockholm. 1964, p. 35.
101. Wellek, B., Hahn, H. H., and Opferkuch, W.: Evidence for macrophage C3d-receptor active in phagocytosis. J. Immunol., *114:*1643, 1975.
102. Worlledge, S. M., and Blajchman, M. A.: The autoimmune haemolytic anemias. Brit. J. Haematol., *23:*61, 1972 (Suppl.).
103. Yasmeen, D., Ellerson, J. R., Dorrington, K. J., and Painter, R. M.: Evidence for the domain hypothesis: Locations of the site of cytophilic activity toward guinea pig macrophages in the C_H3 homology region of human immunoglobulin G. J. Immunol., *110:*1706, 1973.
104. Zipursky, A., and Brown, E. J.: The ingestion of IgG-sensitized erythrocytes by abnormal neutrophils. Blood, *43:*737, 1974.

5

The Serologic Investigation of Autoimmune Hemolytic Anemia

In this chapter we review some aspects of the structure and function of immunoglobulins [18, 44, 72] and the role of albumin and enzymes in immunohematology as a basis for a better understanding of antibody detection. We then describe the laboratory tests that are of value in the diagnosis of autoimmune hemolytic anemias. The rationale for performance of the tests and the interpretation of the results are discussed briefly, and the methodology is described in detail. Each of these tests has a place in the diagnostic evaluation of at least some patients with acquired hemolytic anemia, but some of the procedures described in this chapter will be indicated only infrequently. The information in this chapter serves as a basis for the discussion in Chapter 6 of the differential diagnosis of autoimmune hemolytic anemias. In Chapter 6 no technical details are given, but instead, a more detailed narrative description of the step by step approach to diagnosis is presented. Additional technical procedures that are relevant to drug-induced immune hemolytic anemias, and to compatibility testing in autoimmune hemolytic anemias, are described in Chapters 8 and 10, respectively.

THE STRUCTURE AND FUNCTION OF IMMUNOGLOBULINS

Red cell autoantibodies, like alloantibodies, are usually IgM or IgG; on occasion they may be IgA. *In vitro,* the IgM antibodies will usually directly agglutinate saline suspended red cells (e.g., the IgM anti-I associated with cold agglutinin syndrome). Often they will hemolyse red cells if the conditions are right; for instance, one may have to use enzyme-treated red cells to demonstrate the reaction. IgG antibodies do not often cause direct agglutination of saline-suspended normal red cells, but they will almost always agglutinate enzyme-treated red cells; sometimes they will cause direct agglutination of albumin-suspended red cells. They rarely cause *in vitro* lysis of red cells (the IgG auto anti-P associated with paroxysmal cold hemoglobinuria is the best example of an IgG hemolysin), but they will often sensitize red cells and can be detected by the antiglobulin test (described later).

All immunoglobulins are oligomers of a basic four-chain structure. The monomer unit consists of two sets of identical polypeptide chains. One chain is shorter, with about 220 amino acid residues and is called the light (L) chain. The other has approximately 500 residues and is called the heavy (H) chain. The L chain is associated with the amino terminal half of the H chain, and it is usually linked to it by a disulfide bond (see Figure 5-1).

Throughout the H and L chains are interchain disulfide bonds. Each of these interchain disulfide loops encompasses approximately 60 amino acids.

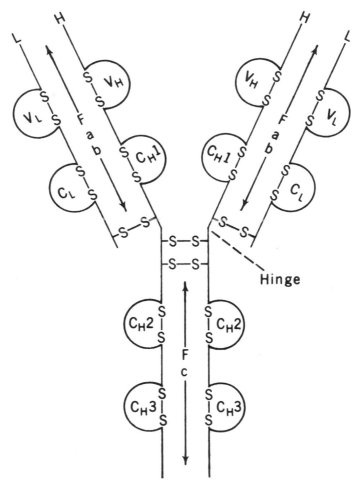

Figure 5-1. *Schematic diagram of an IgG molecule. The variable and constant regions of the light chain are represented by V_L and C_L, respectively. The variable and constant regions of the heavy chain are represented by V_H and C_H1, C_H2, and C_H3, respectively. Certain enzymes cleave IgG's in the vicinity of the "hinge" to form two Fab fragments and one Fc fragment. (Marx, J. L.: Antibody structure: Now in three dimensions. Science, 189:1075, 1975.)*

The H and L chains may be divided into structural domains of approximately 100 amino acids, each based on a single disulfide loop and surrounding amino acid residues. Each light chain has two domains, one called V_L (variable, light) and one called C_L (constant, light); each heavy chain of an IgG molecule has four domains; one in the variable region (V_H) and three in the constant region (C_H1, C_H2, C_H3). The heavy chains of IgA have domains similar to IgG, while IgM and IgE have an additional domain, C_H4, in the constant region of their heavy chains (see Figure 5-1).

The antigen binding properties of the immunoglobulin molecule are associated with the variable (V_H and V_L) domains. A high frequency of amino acid substitutions are observed in certain regions of the variable domains. These hypervariable regions, which also vary considerably in length, have been called "hot spots," as they appear to be the most important regions in controlling antibody specificity. The remaining amino acid residues may act to fold the chains in a suitable conformation to fit the three-dimensional antigenic complex, presenting the hot spots in an optimal position for reactivity. The C_H2 domain is involved in complement activation (i.e., C1q). The C_H3 domain mediates the Fc/macrophage interaction.

Classes and Subclasses of Human Immunoglobulins

Classes. Five distinct classes of human immunoglobulins have been described; these are IgG, IgM, IgA, IgE, and IgD (see Table 5-1). The immunologic differences between these classes are associated with the constant (C_H) region of the heavy chain. The heavy chains are designated gamma (IgG), mu (IgM), alpha (IgA), epsilon (IgE), and delta (IgD).

Light chains occur as two immunologically distinct types designated kappa and lambda. The H chain classes share kappa and lambda chains. Approximately 70 percent of light chains are kappa and 30 percent are lambda. Each antibody molecule possesses two light chains of the same type (i.e., two kappa or two lambda). Occasionally, a patient will produce a protein (e.g., an antibody) of only one light chain type; this occurence is thought to result from a single clone of lymphocytes producing antibodies. The protein is said to be monoclonal. For instance, the IgM anti-I produced in chronic idiopathic cold agglutinin syndrome is monoclonal, usually with only kappa chains present; in contrast, the IgM anti-I produced in cold agglutinin syndrome secondary to *Mycoplasma pneumoniae* appears to have the normal distribution of kappa (70 percent) and lambda (30 percent) light chains. This finding may be because the Mycoplasma have "I-like" determinants on their membranes, thus stimulating the naturally occurring anti-I present in most humans (naturally occurring anti-I has a normal distribution of kappa and lambda chains). In contrast, in the idiopathic case, a condition similar to Waldenströms macroglobulinemia and multiple myeloma occurs; here, for unknown reasons, an aberrant clone of lymphocytes produces an abnormal protein, and in this case it has antibody (e.g., anti-I) specificity.

Table 5-1. HUMAN IMMUNOGLOBULINS

Properties	IgG	IgM	IgA	IgD	IgE
Concentration mg%	700–1700	70–210	70–350	0.3–40	<0.06
Molecular weight (Daltons)	150,000	900,000 (and poly- mers)	160,000 (and poly- mers)	170,000	190,000
Sedimentation rate (S^o20^W)	6.6S	18S	7S (9S,11S, 13S)	6.5S	7.9S
Electrophoretic mobility	γ	$\gamma - \beta$	β	$\gamma - \beta$	$\gamma - \beta$
H chain class	γ	μ	α	δ	ϵ
Number of subclasses	4	1	2	?	?
L chain type	κ or λ	κ or λ	κ or λ	κ or λ	κ or λ
J chain	No	Yes	Yes	No	No
Synthesis rate mg/kg/day	20–40	3–55	3–17		
Placental passage	Yes	No	No	No	No
Activation of Cl	Yes	Yes	No	No	No
Monocyte/macrophage attachment	Yes	No	No	No	No
Blood group antibody activity described	Yes	Yes	Yes	No	No

Subclasses. Four distinct subclasses of human IgG have been described, and their relative percentages in composition of serum are: IgG1, 66 percent; IgG2, 23 percent; IgG3, 7 percent; and IgG4, 4 percent. Two subclasses of IgA have been described, IgA1 and IgA2. The structural homology among the IgG subclasses in the C_H region is high, approximately 90 percent. The majority of amino acid differences in the C_H region are in the hinge region of the IgG molecule.

Allotypic differences between the four IgG subclasses exist and have been termed Gm. In 1956, Grubb described the first genetic marker or allotype on IgG. It was not until 1964, when the subclasses of IgG were described, that the location of this genetic polymorphism was defined. Using purified myeloma proteins of different subclasses, it was possible to demonstrate that each allotypic marker was restricted to a single IgG subclass, that some molecules of a subclass simultaneously carried multiple allotypic markers, and that markers were located on different portions of the molecule. These serologic allotypic determinants have been localized to various C_H domains. In many instances, the responsible amino acid differences have been identified and have constituted only one or two residue changes.

The respective IgG subclasses differ considerably in their biological functions. IgG3 is the most efficient activator of C1q, followed by IgG1; IgG2 is inefficient, and IgG4 does not appear to activate complement. The complement binding site of IgG appears to be at the C_H2 region of the Fc fragment. IgG3 is also the most efficient in the reaction between the Fc receptor of macrophages and IgG; IgG1 is the next most efficient; IgG2 and IgG4 do not appear to react. The macrophage binding site of IgG seems to be at the C_H3 region of the Fc fragment. Finally, there appears to be a difference in subclass transport through the placenta; this difference seems to be a preferential transport of IgG1 across the placenta. By 20 weeks gestation, maternal IgG1 is detectable in cord serum, and by 26 weeks, cord levels of IgG1 equal or exceed maternal levels. In contrast, IgG3 does not reach maternal levels until 28 to 32 weeks gestation.

Differences between the Immunoglobulin Classes

IgG. IgG comprises about 75 percent of normal plasma immunoglobulins (plasma concentration of 700 to 1700 mg/dl). It usually exists in plasma in a monomeric 7S form with a molecular weight of approximately 150,000 daltons. It has a half-life of approximately 21 days (IgG3 appears to have a half-life of only 7 days).

IgM. IgM comprises approximately 5 to 10 percent of normal plasma immunoglobulins (plasma concentration of 20 to 210 mg/dl). It usually exists in plasma as a pentamer. Five 7S IgM monomeric units are covalently bonded together by intersubunit disulfide bonds into a 19S pentamer, of a molecular weight approaching one million daltons. In addition, a single polypeptide chain, termed J chain ("J" for joining), is covalently attached to one or two of the IgM monomeric units. The mu chain has been completely sequenced; it contains a total of 588 amino acid residues with five intrachain disulfide loops. The mu chain contains one V_H domain and four C_H domains in contrast to the three C_H domains of IgG and IgA. The main tissue distribution of IgM is intravascular, owing to its large molecular weight.

IgA. IgA is the predominant immunoglobulin of secretions. It comprises approximately 20 percent of the plasma immunoglobulins. In plasma, it exists primarily as a 7S monomer; in secretions, it is primarily an 11S dimer. In the dimeric form, a J chain is present and so is an additional polypeptide chain, secretory component (SC).

IgE and IgD. So far, no red cell antibodies have been found to be IgE or IgD. IgE is thought to be the immunoglobulin responsible for mediating immediate hypersensitivity reactions. This process involves an interaction with basophils and tissue fixed mast cells leading to the release of potent vasoactive amines (e.g., histamine, bradykinin). The function of IgD is not clear, although recently, it has been shown that IgD is extremely well represented as a membrane-bound immunoglobulin on B lymphocytes. IgD is present, either alone or with IgM on approximately 75 percent of all B lymphocytes. This is in contrast to the total plasma IgD, which represents only 1/500th of total plasma immunoglobulins.

ROLE OF ALBUMIN AND ENZYMES IN ANTIBODY DETECTION

In 1945, Cameron and Diamond [5] and Diamond and Denton [16] demonstrated that so-called "incomplete" antibodies that would not agglutinate saline-suspended red cells, would agglutinate these same cells in the presence of bovine albumin. In 1947, Morton and Pickles [43] showed that incomplete antibodies would react with red cells treated with trypsin. Other workers have shown the same effect using papain,[33] ficin,[71] and bromelin.[49] Enzyme-treated red cells are also much more susceptible to complement-mediated lysis.

The role of albumin and enzymes in agglutination is still controversial. The zeta potential theory of Pollack and his co-workers [52] has been the most favored to date. When red cells are in suspension they do not aggregate. The most important source of energy that opposes the aggregating force of surface tension results from the charge of the erythrocyte. This charge arises mainly by ionization of the carboxyl groups of surface sialic acid residues. Pollack et al.[52] suggested that agglutination of red cells would occur only when the balance of forces is such that the red cells can approach closely enough for antibody molecules to span the intercellular gap.

When charged bodies such as red cells are suspended in simple salt solutions, each red cell will be surrounded by a "cloud" of cations (mainly of opposite charge). This cloud extends outwards from the membrane with decreasing density and merges finally with the electrolyte of the bulk solution so that most of this diffuse cloud of ionized electrolyte will be so arranged as to maintain electrical neutrality. A double layer consisting of the negatively charged red cell membrane and the diffuse oppositely charged cation cloud extends outwards to a "slipping" or "shear" plane, at which the negative charge of the red cell is exactly neutralized by the positive charge of the surrounding diffuse cloud of cations. As the red cell moves, so does its cloud of cations. The potential at the shear plane is called the zeta potential, i.e., the electrical energy barrier at the kinetic surface of the diffuse atmosphere of ions surrounding the red cell. The magnitude of the zeta potential will depend on the volume net charge density of the surrounding cations, i.e., on the ionic strength. The magnitude of the zeta potential is thus directly proportional to the charge of the red cell and the thickness of the double layer. If the ionic strength is raised, more cations are packed around the red cell, thereby increasing the density of the double layer cloud, and the zeta potential becomes reduced. However, this process would also decrease the rate of association between antibody and the red cell. Another important factor affecting zeta potential is the dielectric constant. The dielectric constant is a relative measure of the electrical energy-consuming property of a solution; this property is directly atttributable to the molecules dissolved in it.[51]

Pollack et al.[51,52] suggested that both albumin and enzyme-treatment reduce the zeta potential. Albumin changes the dielectric constant of the solution; enzymes affect the negative charge of the membrane by removing sialic acid residues. Pollack et al.[52] found that the zeta potential of normal red cells was $-16mV$; when they reduced the zeta potential to about $-9mV$ the red cells would begin agglutinating in the presence of "incomplete" antibodies. Below $-7mV$ spontaneous aggregation of the red cells occurred without the presence of antibody. IgM antibodies can span distances between 285 and 350 Å,[51] and they are thought to be able to span between adjacent red cells when they are suspended in normal saline. On the other hand, IgG antibodies can only span 85 to 140 Å and are thought not to be able to span between adjacent red cells when suspended in normal saline, but they can do so if the zeta potential is reduced (i.e., allowing the red cells to come closer together).

Recently, some workers [60,61,64,67,68] have questioned the zeta potential theory. Some of the findings that have made them question the zeta potential theory are: (a) non-specific clumping of red cells occurs in low ionic strength media; this finding is difficult to explain, as the zeta potential should increase, leading to increased repulsion generated by stronger charged groups; (b) similarly, dextran and other high molecular weight colloids, although increasing zeta potential, cause aggregation (e.g., rouleaux) of normal red cells; (c) although polybrene (a positively charged macromolecule), causes aggregation of normal red cells, which fits with the zeta potential theory, it does not cause the aggregation of T and Tn red cells that are deficient in sialic acid—one would expect their charge repulsion to be more easily neutralized; (d) the addition of sialic acid *in vitro* causes aggregation of normal red cells, which does not seem to fit at all with the zeta potential theory; and (e) when red cells are treated with neuraminidase they do not react as efficiently with IgG antibodies as when treated with enzymes such as papain or ficin. For instance, Stratton et al.[62] found that, whereas the reduction in electrophoretic mobility of neuraminidase-treated red cells was almost 80 percent, a titer of only 10 was obtained with an IgG anti-D (from which anti-T had been removed). On the other hand, papainized red cells reacted to a titer of 5120 with the same antiserum, while the electrophoretic mobility exhibited only a 50 percent reduction.

Some alternative theories have been suggested to explain these anomalies. Steane [61] believes that, although charge and steric hindrance both play a role in agglutination, it is water at or near the antigenic sites that controls both antibody uptake and subsequent agglutination. He suggests the following.[61]

1. Red cell membrane glycoproteins, and especially the sialic acid terminal residues, bind water. This water is an integral part of the red cell membrane.

2. The balance of forces acting on the red cell membrane is such that cell separation is maintained. The negative charge of the terminal sialic acid groups and the steric hindrance associated with tightly bound water are the most significant forces opposing the natural cohesive forces. The removal of

the sialic acid, or the perturbation of the bound water layer, predisposes the cells to aggregation.

3. Aggregation probably represents an energy-conserving mechanism to maintain the water-binding requirements of the membrane. Significant reduction in membrane components decreases water-binding requirements (the membrane is markedly altered) and the cells are no longer predisposed to aggregate. Thus, neuraminidase-treated cells are not aggregated by Polybrene.

4. Antigen-antibody interaction at the cell surface is entropy controlled. That is, the degree of interaction depends upon the competition between the antigen-antibody reaction and the cell surface for the bound water of the membrane, water release providing the entropy component of the free energy change driving the reaction.

5. Antigen-antibody interaction at the cell surface is entropy limited. That is, the number of interactions occurring depends upon the number of antigen sites, the cell and antiserum concentrations, etc. If the number of antigen sites is small and the binding constant high, the cell is easily saturated, and free sites are unavailable because of entropy limitations. In addition, not enough water is released to push the cells to aggregate. It is the disturbance of bound water by proteolytic enzymes and potentiating media that makes available further sites permitting the potentiation of the second stage, agglutination, to occur.

6. Equilibrium is also affected by charge hindrance. Negatively charged sialic acid molecules probably repel antibody molecules. This repulsion is decreased following enzyme treatment, leading to increased antibody uptake.

7. The binding of antibody itself releases water, predisposing the cells to aggregation. Red cells with antigens that are present in large numbers (e.g., A and B) are easily agglutinated by 7S antibodies. Red cells with antigens present in small numbers (i.e., most others) require help in removing the water obstructions, or in making entropy available, before they can be agglutinated by 7S antibodies.

Stratton et al.[64] suggested the polypeptide stems on the red cell membrane may sterically hinder antibody from reacting with nearby antigenic sites. Proteolytic enzymes, such as papain and ficin, in contrast to neuraminidase, are known to cleave polypeptide stems, in addition to sialic acid, from the membrane. This finding may well be an alternative or additional explanation for the effect of enzymes on IgG-mediated agglutination.

Voak et al.,[68] using ferritin labelled anti-D, demonstrated clustering of Rh antigen sites on enzyme-treated red cells, but to a lesser extent on neuraminidase-treated red cells and none on untreated red cells. They suggested that the important factors for agglutination are antigen site density, antibody span, and antibody valency. The clustering of Rh antigens, which they suggest arise from membrane mobility, provides the high site density leading to large areas of cell to cell surface contact. They showed large areas of cell to cell contact when the cells are enzyme-treated and in the presence of bovine albumin, whereas neuraminidase only caused loose aggregation with small areas of cell to cell contact. It was suggested that albumin does not act by producing high localized site density, but has the effect of increasing the areas of cell to cell contact. Multiple bridges are needed for IgG agglutination to occur; the larger the areas of the cell to cell contact, the easier it will be to form multiple bridges. Brooks [3] has shown that dextran does not reduce the zeta potential but probably causes aggregation of normal red cells because of absorption of dextran molecules between adjacent cells (i.e., polymer bridging). These are relatively weak aggregates, and they are broken down by Brownian motion (e.g., if saline is added and the suspension agitated gently, the rouleaux disperses). Voak et al. [68] suggested that albumin works in a similar fashion, and that, in the presence of IgG antibody, sensitized red cells may be held together long enough for the rapidly reacting antibodies on adjacent cells to form sufficient bridges to support agglutination.

Van Oss et al. [66] support many of the previously described alternatives to the zeta potential theory, and they also suggest that the shape of the red cell, particularly in regard to spiculation of the red cell membrane, plays an important role. They confirmed Salsbury and Clarke's [59] findings that anti-A and anti-B but not anti-D caused strong spiculation of red cells (scanning electron microscopy was used). They speculated that the relative ease with which agglutination of group A and B cells is accomplished (even with IgG antibodies) and the difficulty of obtaining agglutination with IgG anti-D antibodies may be partly explained by the propensity of anti-A and anti-B to cause spiculation of their target cells, i.e., the A and B antigens would be extended from the surface of the membrane, thus cutting down the distance an antibody molecule has to span. They also noted that proteolytic enzymes and dextran caused spiculation of red cells. Polybrene and albumin (in concentrations as low as 1g/L) were found to cause the formation of stomatocytes (cup-shaped red cells). Van Oss et al. suggested that stomatocytes can approach one another closely with a considerably larger part of their surface than the usual biconcave disc.

We believe that, like most scientific theories, there are some aspects of hemagglutination that cannot be explained by the zeta potential theory, but that it plays an essential role in the process. Many of the other factors already mentioned probably play additional roles. We would be supportive of most of the additional theories previously discussed, but would be cautious in making too much of the theories based on changes in red cell shape, as judged by scanning electron microscopy, until more well controlled data appear in the literature. Longster and Tovey [39] pointed out that they could reproduce the results of Salsbury and Clarke [59] and Van Oss and Mohn [66] only if the antisera were contaminated with bacteria or chemicals (e.g., 0.1 percent sodium azide). Neither Salsbury and Clarke [59] nor Van Oss and Mohn [66] ran controls of red cells lacking the appropriate antigens (e.g., group 0 cells incubated with anti-A). Longster and Tovey [39] found similar spiculation on red cells lacking the antigens to the antibody used. The spiculations appeared to depend on the source of antiserum and thus were non-specific.

THE ANTIGLOBULIN TEST

In 1945, Coombs, Mourant, and Race [8] demonstrated the presence of so-called "incomplete" Rh alloantibodies in sera by the antiglobulin reaction.

In 1946, Boorman, Dodd, and Loutit [2] and Loutit and Mollison [40] reported that the red cells from a number of patients suffering from idiopathic acquired hemolytic anemia reacted with antiglobulin serum. The first application of the test became known as the indirect antiglobulin test (IAT) and the latter the direct antiglobulin test (DAT). Table 5-2 shows how these two tests can be applied in immunohematology.

Table 5-2. USES OF THE ANTIGLOBULIN TEST

Direct Antiglobulin Test
Valuable in diagnosis of:
    Hemolytic disease of the newborn
    Autoimmune hemolytic anemia
    Drug-induced immune hemolytic anemia
    Hemolytic transfusion reactions due to alloantibodies

Indirect Antiglobulin Test
Useful for:
    Detection of antibodies in serum
      Crossmatching
      Antibody screening
    Detection of antibodies in eluates prepared from sensitized red cells
    Determination of specificity of antibodies
    Typing of red cells
      D^u testing
      Using antiglobulin reactive typing reagents (e.g., anti-Fy^a, anti-Jk^a, etc.)
    Antiglobulin consumption test (e.g., complement fixation antiglobulin consumption test for measuring red cell-bound IgG)

Principles of the Antiglobulin Test

Red cell autoantibodies and alloantibodies are gamma globulins, usually IgM or IgG. If they are IgM they will usually directly agglutinate saline-suspended red cells. In contrast, IgG antibodies often will not agglutinate red cells, but will be adsorbed to the red cell membrane, giving a "sensitized" red cell. Thus, chemically speaking, the red cells are sensitized with gamma globulin.

If a rabbit is injected with human gamma globulin, the rabbit will form antibodies to the foreign protein, i.e., anti-human globulin. This anti-globulin serum ("Coombs" serum), after suitable treatment (outlined later) will react specifically with human globulin. Thus, if the human globulin, in the form of antibody, is attached to the red cell membrane, the antihuman globulin will combine with it, forming "bridges" until a lattice is formed and agglutination occurs (see Figure 5-2).

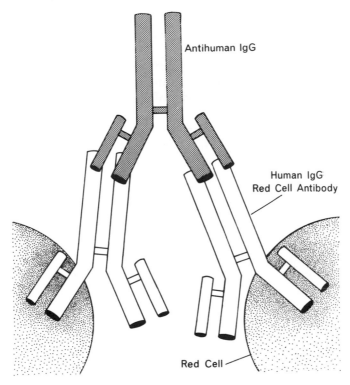

Figure 5-2. *The antiglobulin test. Antihuman IgG in the antiglobulin serum reacts with red cell bound IgG antibody, which causes the development of a lattice formation and agglutination. Although the reaction is illustrated with IgG sensitized cells, similar reactions can occur with red cells coated with other proteins (e.g., complement components), provided that appropriate antibodies are present in the antihuman serum.*

As shown in Figure 5-2, the anti-IgG reacts mainly with the Fc portion of the human IgG molecules (i.e., heavy chains). Antibodies to the light chains may be present as well. In a polyspecific antiglobulin serum, this finding has no disadvantages and theoretically may be an advantage by forming extra bridges across adjacent light chains. In a monospecific anti-IgG, the presence of antibodies to light chains can lead to false positive results as light chains are shared by IgG, IgM and IgA; only the heavy chains are specific for each class.

In 1947, Coombs and Mourant [9] showed that the component in antiglobulin serum (AGS) that reacted with Rh-sensitized red cells could be inhibited from reacting by the addition of small amounts of human gamma globulin; alpha and beta globulins did not inhibit the reaction. Dacie [12] reported that red cells from various patients with autoimmune hemolytic anemia reacted differently in the antiglobulin test. Some patients reacted better with high dilutions of the AGS (i.e., exhibited a prozone effect), whereas others reacted better with more concentrated AGS. Furthermore, the addition of purified gamma globulin to the AGS did not inhibit the reaction of the AGS with the red cells from some patients. The reactions that could be inhibited appeared to be those associated with warm autoantibodies. In contrast, those reactions not inhibited appeared to be associated with high titer cold autoagglutinins; it was suggested that the red cells from such patients were probably sensitized with antibodies that were non-gamma globulins. Further experiments [13] showed that the non-gamma globulin sensitizing the red cells was not antibody but complement, especially the C3d fragment of C3. The role of complement in immunohematology and the antiglobulin test in particular have been discussed in detail in Chapter 3.

Some immune hemolytic anemias are caused by immunoglobulins other than IgG. However, IgM sensitization of red blood cells is difficult to detect with the antiglobulin test,[4,22] and furthermore, IgM antibodies that cause immune hemolytic anemia characteristically, if not invariably,[42] fix complement which is much more readily detected. IgA antibodies only infrequently play a role in red cell sensitization and, in such cases, other immune globulins or complement components are almost always, although not invariably,[62,65,74] found on the cell surface as well. Thus, it does not seem reasonable to demand standards for manufacturers that would require the presence of anti-IgM and anti-IgA antibodies as a component of polyspecific antiglobulin serum, although we ourselves would prefer to have them present. Interested workers, especially those in research and reference laboratories, will continue to be concerned about the unusual instances in which they are of use, but such needs can usually be met by the use of monospecific antisera in selected cases.

To summarize, polyspecific antiglobulin sera used for the investigation of autoimmune hemolytic anemia must contain anti-IgG and anti-C3d and may contain antibodies to other C3 determinants (e.g., C3c) and C4; antibodies to other immunoglobulins (e.g., IgA or IgM) would be a bonus.

Monospecific Antiglobulin Reagents. Although it is reasonable and perhaps most convenient to perform the initial direct antiglobulin test with a polyspecific antiglobulin serum, it is advisable to perform further tests with monospecific reagents in all patients who have a positive DAT and who have hemolytic anemia. Such testing provides additional information that is helpful in determining the specific type of immune hemolytic anemia that is present.[7,47] For this purpose, the most important reagents are a monospecific anti-IgG and an anti-C3 antiserum containing anti-C3d activity (which may contain antibodies against other C3 determinants).[48] Such antisera, licensed in the United States by the Bureau of Biologics, are currently available for use in the DAT.

In the unusual instance in which a patient is suspected of having an immune hemolytic anemia but has a negative direct antiglobulin test with AGS containing anti-IgG and anti-C3d, the use of anti-IgM and anti-IgA antibodies is indicated. At present, antisera of such specificities have not been licensed for the DAT, but antisera of these specificities that are manufactured for immunodiffusion can be utilized for such unusual needs after appropriate absorption and standardization (described later).

The Significance of Positive Direct Antiglobulin Tests

The results of a DAT should reflect what is happening *in vivo,* not what has occurred *in vitro* through the use of inappropriate techniques. For instance, the red cells from refrigerated clots obtained from normal individuals will often have a positive DAT. This result is commonly due to the presence of a naturally occurring cold non-agglutinating autoantibody termed "normal incomplete cold antibody," which has anti-H specificity and binds complement to the red cells.[11] The commonly found low titer anti-I cold autoagglutinin may play an additional role in autocomplement sensitization at 4°C. Because of this phenomenon, the results of a positive DAT on cells from a cooled clotted sample should never be accepted without confirming the results on either freshly drawn blood kept at 37°C or, preferably, on red cells from a specimen that was obtained using EDTA anticoagulant (e.g., EDTA Vacutainer); the EDTA prevents any *in vitro* complement binding but does not interfere with any *in vivo* bound complement.

A positive direct antiglobulin test, even when due to *in vivo* sensitization, does not necessarily indicate autoimmune hemolytic anemia, or even that autoantibody has caused the positive reaction. Positive direct antiglobulin tests can be obtained (even when warm or EDTA-blood is used) for many reasons, some of which are listed below.

Causes of Positive Direct Antiglobulin Tests

1. Autoantibodies against intrinsic red cell antigens, leading to sensitization of the red cells with immunoglobulins or complement components. Hemolytic anemia may or may not be present (see Chapters 6 and 9).

2. Antibodies against drugs attached to red cell membrane, e.g., penicillin (see Chapter 8).

3. Immune-complex formation, e.g., anti-drug-drug complex (see Chapter 8).

4. Non-specific uptake of protein due to alteration of red cell membrane. An example of this is the positive DAT sometimes associated with cephalosporin administration (see Chapter 8). It is also possible that this is the cause of the positive DAT that has been described associated with some bacterial or viral illnesses and the rare families with weak MN antigens.[42]

5. Hemolytic transfusion reactions. Delayed hemolytic transfusion reactions can often be very difficult to differentiate serologically from AIHA (see Chapter 9). Alloantibodies present in the recipient can sensitize the donor's red cells, or alloantibodies present in the plasma of the donor can sensitize the recipient's red cells.

6. Hemolytic disease of the newborn. Maternal alloantibodies cross the placenta and sensitize the infant's red cells.

7. High reticulocyte count. Although there is one report in 1960 [31] indicating that high reticulocyte counts cause a false positive DAT due to anti-transferrin in the rabbit AGS, we have not found this to be a problem. Simi-

larly, Chaplin [7] and Worlledge [73] have not found this a cause of false positive results in their series.

8. Polyagglutinable red cells. When the T antigen is exposed on the red cell membrane (e.g., by bacterial infection), a false positive DAT can occur if sufficient anti-T is present in the rabbit AGS. [19, 73] Although we have found this to occur with low dilutions of our own AGS, we have not observed this in commercially prepared AGS, probably because the rabbit serum is diluted considerably or fractionated in the preparation of the AGS.

9. Silica, derived from glass, has been described as a cause of false positive DAT. [42] We have not encountered any examples of this.

10. Unknown causes. Approximately 8 percent of hospitalized patients whom we have tested have weakly positive DAT without an associated hemolytic anemia. The sensitization is usually caused by complement components. Worlledge has reported similar findings. [73]

Causes of False Negative Direct Antiglobulin Tests

1. Poor technique. (a) Insufficient washing of red cells will enable residual plasma globulin to inhibit the antiglobulin sera. To control this, known sensitized red cells must be added to every negative test and recorded as positive (i.e., indicating uninhibited antiglobulin sera to be present in the tube) before the negative test can be accepted as truly negative. (b) Use of saline or antiglobulin serum contaminated with human globulin (1 part in 4,000 of normal plasma/serum is often sufficient to completely inhibit the anti-IgG in an antiglobulin serum); this result can be controlled as in (a). (c) Resuspending centrifuged red cells too vigorously may disperse weak agglutination.

2. Antiglobulin serum does not contain appropriate antibody. As mentioned elsewhere, commerical polyspecific antiglobulin sera may have insufficient anti-C3d, [22] anti-IgA, [65] or anti-IgM [22] to detect these proteins sensitizing patient's red cells.

3. Antibody sensitizing a patient's red cells has a high dissociation constant. We occasionally encounter patients with red cells sensitized with autoantibody that does not seem to "fit" very well; i.e., it dissociates very easily, even during routine washing of the red cells for performing the DAT. More of the autoantibody is lost from the red cells when they are washed at 37°C than at room temperature or below, even though the patient has warm type AIHA. If we suspect that this is occurring we wash the red cells in ice-cold saline (preferably in a refrigerated centrifuge) with appropriate controls (e.g., after washing, centrifuge 1 vol of 2 to 5 percent washed cells in 2 vols of saline as well as 2 vols of antiglobulin serum to ensure that the cells are not agglutinated due to cold autoantibodies). We encountered one patient with acute AIHA whose DAT was negative when the cells were washed at 37°C; 1+ when washed at room temperature and 3+ when washed in ice cold saline. It is also important to add the antiglobulin serum to the washed cells immediately after washing and to read the antiglobulin tests immediately following centrifugation as these autoantibodies will elute from the red cells very rapidly following wash-

ing. It has been suggested that serum alloantibodies and autoantibodies that react only against enzyme-treated red cells are of such low affinity that they wash off the red cells during the washing process of the indirect antiglobulin test.[6] These may be similar in nature to the "poorly fitting" autoantibodies already discussed that have sensitized the patient's red cells *in vivo.*

4. IgG antibody present on the red cell membrane in a concentration too low to be detected by the antiglobulin test. In order for a positive antiglobulin test to occur, the red cells must be sensitized with about 150 to 500 molecules of IgG per red cell. [17,28] Sometimes, more sensitive techniques will show IgG to be present on the red cell (see Chapter 9 for full discussion).

METHODS FOR STANDARDIZATION AND EVALUATION OF ANTIGLOBULIN SERA

We are including methods in this section for standardization of raw antiglobulin sera (e.g., prepared in the reader's own laboratory or purchased in the raw state). Antiglobulin sera (for use with red cells) sold in the United States are already diluted "optimally" (i.e., checkerboard titrations have already been performed by the manufacturer and the AGS appropriately diluted). Once a manufacturer has diluted the AGS and it is licensed for sale, we would recommend that it is never further diluted for further standardization or comparative evaluations, but rather that the AGS as sold is tested against as wide a range as possible of very weakly sensitized cells. We would suggest that examples of weak antibodies (e.g., anti-Rh, K, k, Fy^a, Fy^b, Jk^a, Jk^b, S, s,) are kept frozen (below $-20°C$ preferably) for such evaluations, or that dilutions of such antibodies are made so that they react 1+ or less with a "standard" (i.e., an acceptable) antiglobulin serum. If the appropriate dilution is made in inert serum, the diluted antibody can be kept frozen at $-20°C$ or below for years with very little loss of activity.

The raw rabbit anti-human serum must first be inactivated by heating at 56°C for 30 minutes. If the antiglobulin serum causes agglutination of normal A, B, and O red cells, it is necessary to remove the heteroagglutinins or to dilute the serum until negative results are obtained. To absorb the antiserum [14,42] well-washed red cells of pooled A_1, B, and O groups should be used. The cells must be washed at least six times in a large volume of saline. The cell-serum suspensions should be left for at least 1 hour at 4°C before centrifuging. Usually one or two absorptions will suffice.

Anti-IgG Activity

1. Preparation of IgG-Sensitized Red Cells
   a. Prepare serial dilutions of an anti-D in 1 ml aliquots. Suitable dilutions should be made to finally achieve a range of IgG-sensitized red cells from negative to about 3+; if a commerical anti-D is used, 1:4 to 1:128 or 256 is usually adequate.

    b. Add 0.5 ml of 50 percent washed O Rh+ red cells.

    c. Incubate at 37°C for 15 minutes.

    d. Wash four times in isotonic saline.

    e. Resuspend red cells to 3 to 5 percent.

2. Determination of Optimal Dilution of Raw Antiglobulin Serum (Checkerboard Titration) (Table 5-3).

    a. Prepare serial dilutions of AGS in 1 ml aliquots (1:2 to 1:4096).

    b. Starting at highest dilution (e.g., 4096) place 2 drops each of the AGS dilutions into six 10 × 75 mm tubes.

    c. To the first row of 12 tubes (1:2 to 1:4096) add one drop of the washed red cells sensitized with 1:4 dilution of anti-D.

    d. Centrifuge the tubes at 1000 RCF and read the antiglobulin tests. Grade results carefully. Table 5-4 shows the agglutination grading and scoring we use throughout the text.

    e. Continue similarly with rows 2 to 6 tested against red cells sensitized with anti-D diluted 1:8 to 1:128.

Table 5-3. CHECKERBOARD TITRATION FOR DETERMINING OPTIMAL DILUTIONS OF ANTI-IgG

Dilutions of Anti-Rh Used to Sensitize O+ RBC	Dilutions of Antiglobulin Serum											
	1:2	4	8	16	32	64	128	256	512	1024	2048	4096
1:4	2+	2+	3+	3+	3+	3+	3+	2½+	2+	2+	2+	1+
1:8	(1+)	1+	1+	2+	3+	3+	2+	2+	1+	1+	1+	½+
1:16	½+	½+	(1+)	2+	2+	2+	2+	2½+	1½+	1+	1+	½+
1:32	0	0	0	½+	1+	1½+	1½+	2+	1+	(1+)	½+	0
1:64	0	0	0	0	(1+)	(1+)	(1+)	1+	(1+)	½+	0	0
1:128	0	0	0	0	0	0	0	½+	0	0	0	0

Agglutination reactions are graded as ½+ to 4+.

Table 5-4. AGGLUTINATION GRADING AND SCORES

Grading	Appearance of Red Cells	Score*
4+	No free cells	10
3+	Several large agglutinates, few free cells	8
2+	Large agglutinates in a sea of smaller clumps and some free cells	6
1+	Many small agglutinates (approximately 20 cells)	4
(1+)	Scattered small agglutinates in a sea of free cells; just visible macroscopically	3
½+	Small agglutinates visible only microscopically	1
0	No agglutinates seen	0

* Titration scores are developed by summing the score for agglutination obtained at each dilution.

The checkerboard titration is usually repeated using other IgG antibodies (e.g., anti-Fy^a and anti-Jk^a). Ideally, IgG autoantibodies should also be tested (e.g., eluates or sera from warm AIHA). Occasionally, differences in the optimal dilution are seen.

Table 5-3 shows a typical set of results obtained with one of our rabbits hyperimmunized with purified IgG. It is usual to see a marked prozone effect when the rabbits are hyperimmunized. This AGS would be diluted 1:256 for routine use in detecting IgG, as this dilution detected the smallest amount of cell bound IgG.

Anti-IgA and Anti-IgM Activity

At present in the United States, anti-IgA and anti-IgM are not available as licensed reagents for use with red cells. They are readily available as precipitating reagents for use in such techniques as immunoelectrophoresis, and they can often be used as long as they are carefully standardized and controlled (e.g., they often contain anti-species agglutinins that have to be removed either by dilution or absorption with non-sensitized human red cells). The quality control must be precise, as agglutination is a far more sensitive technique than precipitation; thus monospecificity by preciptitation techniques does not ensure monospecificity by the antiglobulin test (e.g., an anti-IgG that does not show any precipitin line may react 4+ with Rh-sensitized red cells).

Thus, anti-IgA must always be shown to be non-reactive by the antiglobulin test against red cells strongly sensitized with IgG, IgM, and complement; similarly, anti-IgM must not react with IgG, IgA, or complement-sensitized red cells.

It is difficult to find pure IgA and non-agglutinating IgM blood group antibodies; therefore, we "standardize" our AGS using a passive agglutination technique. We coat chromic chloride treated red cells with purified IgA or IgM and then test these coated red cells by a regular antiglobulin test.

1. Preparation of IgA or IgM Coated Red Cells
   Reagents required:
   1% Chromic Chloride Stock Solution (store in dark bottle at 4°C).
   Dilute 1:20 in *unbuffered* saline for use.
      Purified IgA 0.5 to 1 mg/ml
      Purified IgM 2 mg/ml
   Group O Human red cells (should be more than 24 hours old but less than 8 days old).
   Coupling procedure:
      a. In a test tube (good quality acid cleansed glass preferably—never plastic), mix 1 vol IgA or IgM solution and 1 vol packed washed red cells.
      b. Add 1 vol of 0.2% chromic chloride solution (1:20 dilution of stock solution).
      c. Mix well for 5 minutes at room temperature.

   d. Wash red cells four times in unbuffered saline. (Do not centrifuge
      longer than 30 seconds at 1000 RCF.)
   e. Reconstitute to 2 to 5 percent and use as in regular AGT.

Anti-Complement Activity

I. Preparation of Red Cells Sensitized with C3b and C4b.[24]
   1. Using Low Ionic Strength:
      a. Prepare 10 ml of 10 percent sucrose in water. (This can be done
         simply by adding sucrose to the 1 ml mark of a 10 ml graduated
         centrifuge tube and then adding water to the 10 ml mark.)
      b. Add 1 ml of whole blood. This can be fresh blood or ACD or CDP
         blood that has been stored at 4°C for less than three weeks.
      c. Mix and incubate at 37°C for 15 minutes.
      d. Wash four times.
      e. Resuspend to 2 to 5 percent.
   2. Using Anti-Lewis * (non-agglutinating):
      a. To 9 volumes of anti-Lewis antiserum, add 1 volume of neutral
         EDTA (4.5 percent K_2-EDTA + 0.3 percent NaOH).
      b. Add 1 volume of 50 percent washed Lewis-positive red blood cells.
      c. Incubate at 37°C for 30 minutes.
      d. Wash four times.
      e. To button of red blood cells, add 5 volumes of fresh normal serum,
         as a source of complement.
      f. Re-incubate at 37°C for 15 minutes.
      g. Wash four times.
      h. Resuspend to 2 to 5 percent.
   3. Using Anti-I *:
      a. Titrate an anti-I serum and select a dilution that agglutinates OI
         adult red cells approximately 2+ at 20 to 25°C. This should yield
         moderately strongly sensitized red cells.
      b. Dilute the anti-I appropriately in a source of complement (i.e.,
         "fresh" inert human serum). For instance, we routinely use serum
         from a patient with a cold agglutinin titer at 4°C of 4000; we dilute
         this anti-I, 1:1000 and 1:100 to prepare weakly and strongly C3b/
         C4b sensitized red cells respectively.
      c. Add $^1/_{10}$ volume of 50 percent washed red blood cells.
      d. Incubate at 20°C to 25°C for 10 to 15 minutes.
      e. Incubate at 37°C for approximately 5 to 10 minutes (to allow
         agglutination to disperse).
      f. Wash red blood cells four times at 37°C.
      g. Resuspend 2 to 5 percent.
II. Preparation of Red Cells Sensitized with C3b But Not C4b.
    Modification of method from reference 20, supplied by Dr. Hugh Chap-
    lin.

---

* The amount of complement on the red cells can be varied by using dilutions of the anti-Lewis or anti-I in fresh serum.

Diluent

Solution A: In a 250 ml flask containing approximately 125 ml distilled water, dissolve

23.1 g sucrose

173 *mg* Na H$_2$ PO$_4$ H$_2$O

395 *mg* Na$_2$ EDTA 2H$_2$O

q.s. to 250 with distilled water

Solution B: In a 250 ml flask containing approximately 125 ml distilled water, dissolve

23.1 g sucrose

178 *mg* Na$_2$H PO$_4$

395 *mg* Na$_2$ EDTA 2H$_2$O

q.s. to 250 ml with distilled water

Adjust solution A to pH 5.1 by addition of solution B (e.g., approximately 6.5 ml)

Coating Procedure

a. Whole ACD or CPD blood may be used equally well. Chill all reactants to ice-water temperature before combining.

b. Place 19 ml diluent in small flask in ice-water bath on magnetic stirrer in cold room.

c. With stirrer on, add 1.0 ml ACD or CPD blood dropwise, rapidly.

d. *Immediately* add 0.1 ml of 0.4M MgCl$_2$ (which is prepared by adding 810 mg MgCl$_2$-6H$_2$O to 10 ml distilled water).

e. Stir in ice bath 1 hour

f. Wash red blood cells four times with saline at 0°C.

III. Preparation of Red Cells Sensitized with C4b But Not C3b.[24]

Using Low Ionic Strength Method:

a. Add 10 ml of 10 percent sucrose in water to a 100 × 16 mm tube containing 12 or 15 mg K EDTA (e.g., Becton and Dickinson Vacutainer 427/3200 QS).

b. Add 1 ml of whole blood as previously described in section I1b.

c. Incubate at 37°C for 15 minutes.

d. Wash four times.

e. Resuspend to 2 to 5 percent.

IV. Preparation of Red Cells Sensitized with C3d/C4d, C3d, or C4d.[24]

a. Red cells sensitized with C3b/C4b, C3b or C4b can be prepared by any of the methods described previously.

b. Equal volumes of packed washed C3b/C4b, C3b or C4b red cells are incubated with 0.1 percent trypsin (pH 7.3) for 30 minutes, or inert fresh normal EDTA-treated serum (as a source of C3 inactivator), for 12 hours at 37°C. Non-complement sensitized red cells should also be incubated with the trypsin, or the normal serum, as a negative control.

c. The red cells are washed four times and resuspended to 2 to 5 percent.

Once prepared, any of the complement-sensitized cells can be stored frozen in liquid nitrogen. If the C3b or C4b-sensitized red cells are frozen immediately after preparation, they will not decay to C3d/C4d in storage.

Daily Quality Control of Antiglobulin Serum

For daily quality control, polyspecific AGS need only be tested against red cells weakly sensitized with IgG (e.g., anti-Rh). Testing against complement-sensitized red cells is unnecessary because daily quality control is primarily to ensure that the AGS has not become inactivated by contamination or improper storage. There is no evidence to suggest that the anti-complement activity can be selectively inactivated under the usual conditions of storage in blood banks; in our experience, when any inactivation occurs (e.g., contamination with human serum), the anti-IgG reaction will be a sensitive indicator as long as red cells weakly sensitized with IgG-sensitized red cells are used as indicator cells.

Preparation of IgG Weakly Sensitized Red Cells for Quality Control of AGS

a. To each of 12 tubes add 0.1 ml of saline.
b. To the first tube add 0.1 ml of an IgG anti-Rh_0 (D), e.g., a slide and rapid tube Rh_0 (D) commercial typing reagent, making a 1:2 dilution.
c. Prepare serial doubling dilutions by mixing saline and antibody, and then transferring 0.1 ml to the next tube. This process is repeated with each tube to the 12th tube, and the final 0.1 ml is discarded.
d. To each 0.1 ml of diluted anti-Rh_0 (D) add 1 drop of a 5 percent suspension of 0 Rh_0 (D)-positive red cells.
e. Incubate at 37°C for 15 minutes.
f. Wash red cells four times.
g. To each tube add 1 or 2 drops of antiglobulin serum (according to manufacturer's directions).
h. Centrifuge tubes and inspect for degree of agglutination, carefully noting the strength of reaction.
i. Select the dilution that shows 1+ macroscopic agglutination.
j. Prepare a quantity of diluted anti-Rh_0 (D) at this dilution, and freeze it in aliquots available for use each day in preparing fresh, sensitized cells. Alternatively, a batch of sensitized red cells can be prepared, washed, and stored in CPD or Alsevers solution at 4°C.

GENERAL SEROLOGIC INVESTIGATIONS IN AUTOIMMUNE HEMOLYTIC ANEMIA

The majority of cases of autoimmune hemolytic anemia can be correctly diagnosed simply by taking into account the clinical findings and results of the direct antiglobulin test (using anti-IgG and anti-C3 (C3d) antiglobulin sera), a cold agglutinin titer and a simple antibody screening procedure. However, such abbreviated evaluations lead to a surprising number of misinterpretations and erroneous diagnoses. Therefore, when we encounter a case of hemolytic anemia suspected of having an immune basis, we prefer, as a routine, to perform a panel of screening tests and then perform more specific tests to develop a more confident diagnosis. Technical details of the appropriate serologic tests are described below as is a brief rationale for their use and interpretation of the results. A more detailed description of the application of these tests in diagnosis of immune hemolytic anemias is given in Chapter 6.

Collection of Blood

We collect clotted blood to provide serum, and blood in EDTA to provide red cells for the direct antiglobulin test, grouping, and preparation of eluates. As a routine, we incubate all blood samples at 37°C for 10 to 15 minutes before we separate the serum (which is separated by centrifuging at 37°C), and perform the direct antiglobulin test.

Several problems can arise if the blood is not kept at 37°C from the time of bleeding and cold autoantibodies are present:

1. Autoagglutination of red cells occurs, leading to difficulties in grouping.

2. Loss of antibody from the serum by autoabsorption, leading to a false low agglutination titer.

3. Possible direct hemolysis of the red cells, utilizing antibody and complement, with possible misinterpretation of *in vitro* hemoglobinemia as being an *in vivo* occurrence. This result will only occur in the clotted sample, as EDTA will inhibit any *in vitro* complement-mediated lysis.

4. If EDTA blood is not used, then *in vitro* complement autosensitization may occur due to the presence of cold autoantibodies. This may lead to a false positive or increase in the strength of the direct antiglobulin test. EDTA will prevent any *in vitro* complement sensitization even if the blood is cooled, thus any complement detected on the red cells represents *in vivo* sensitization.

Nevertheless, we do not routinely bleed our patients into warmed syringes unless we know we are dealing with a severe case of cold agglutinin syndrome. We find that by always warming the samples before separation we can get reliable results in most cases.

ABO and Rh Grouping

ABO. There should be no problem in ABO and Rh typing patients with autoimmune hemolytic anemia if certain rules are followed; however, if these rules are not followed, serious errors can occur.

The blood samples should have been separated initially at 37°C. The cells should be washed at 37°C with warm saline. The cells are tested in the usual fashion with anti-A, anti-B, and anti-A,B, but a negative control of 5 to 10 percent albumin is also set up. This control should be compared with the tests and, if positive, indicates either nondispersed autoagglutination or spontaneous agglutination of heavily sensitized cells in albumin.

The patient's serum is tested against A₁, B, O, and his own cells as usual. If the patient is known to have or appears to have the cold agglutinin syndrome, the serum typing tests should be repeated strictly at 37°C. At this temperature, ABO agglutinins will usually react well, but the cold autoantibody will not react. These results may be confirmed (by the normal methods) after the cold autoantibody has been autoabsorbed from the patient's serum (see page 377). Problems in ABO typing patients with warm type autoimmune hemolytic anemia are rare.

Rh. It is useful to determine the Rh phenotype of patients with warm type autoimmune hemolytic anemia. If the cells have been separated and washed at 37°C, the main problem is that the cells are possibly strongly sensitized (perhaps with Rh autoantibodies) and will agglutinate spontaneously with the addition of albumin alone; therefore, if problems occur with the Rh control, then antisera for "saline tube test" should be used. Unfortunately, many commercial companies add a small amount of albumin (normally 5 to 10 percent) and/or other potentiating media to such sera, and therefore patient's cells should always be added to albumin (e.g., 10 percent) as a negative control. An ideal negative control is the actual diluent that the manufacturer has used to dilute the antisera, but this diluent is not readily available for "saline tube test" reagents. If the albumin antisera have been used (i.e., "slide and rapid tube" reagents), it is important that the diluent supplied by the same manufacturer of the antiserum be used as a negative control. If this diluent is not available, then 20 to 30 percent albumin should be used as a control.

If red cells are sensitized with complement but no IgG, as in cold agglutinin syndrome, the cells will not spontaneously agglutinate in the presence of albumin. Thus, the cheaper and more available slide and rapid tube reagents can usually be used safely, as long as the cells are washed at 37°C and the correct controls utilized.

Typing Red Cells for Antigens When Only Antiglobulin Reactive Antisera Are Available

Sometimes, only antiglobulin reactive antisera are available for typing red cells for certain antigens (e.g., Kell, Duffy, and Kidd). When patients have a strongly positive direct antiglobulin test, two approaches can be used:

Heating Patients' Red Cells to Dissociate Red Cell Bound Antibody. We have found that heating red cells for 5 to 30 minutes at 45°C, or for 3 to 10 minutes at 50°C, sometimes will dissociate enough bound antibody to allow the red cells to be typed by strongly reactive antisera. Occasionally, we have had to heat for 3 to 5 minutes at 51 to 56°C. The main disadvantage to this method, of course, is that red cell antigens become weaker if they are heated above 37°C. The degree of weakening depends on the antigens involved, the temperature, and the length of incubation. We try to heat the cells for the shortest time at the lowest temperature; unfortunately, heating at 45°C is not usually successful and one has to use at least 50°C, if the direct antiglobulin test is strongly positive. The direct antiglobulin test does not have to become completely negative, but if possible, we like to reduce it to 1+ to 1½+ at the strongest, to allow differentiation between weak positive typings and negatives when using antisera that are reacting 3 to 4+ with positive controls. It is imperative that heterozygote (i.e., weakly positive) controls are heated under exactly the same conditions as the test red cells. We would recommend trying 45°C first, and if the direct antiglobulin test is not reduced sufficiently, then trying 50°C and finally 51 to 56°C.

Differential Absorption Procedures. Equal aliquots of antisera and washed packed red cells, both positive (heterozygote and homozygote preferably) and negative for the appropriate antigen are incubated at 37°C, and the activity of the supernatant absorbed sera are compared with the absorbed sera from a similar mixture of the patient's red cells and the antisera. It is wise to titrate the absorbed serum against an appropriately positive red cell. If the patient's red cells contain the antigen, e.g., Jk^a, then the red cells will absorb antibody from the anti-Jk^a typing serum, leaving a lower titer. Heterozygote cells (Jk(a+b+)) will absorb some (or all) of the antibody, and homozygote cells (Jk(a+b−)) will be expected to absorb the antibody even more readily. Red cells lacking the appropriate antigen (i.e., Jk(a−)) will not absorb any anti-Jk^a; thus, the activity of the antibody would not be significantly changed after absorption. Titration scores of the absorbed sera from the control cells can be compared with those obtained using the patient's red cells for the absorption (see Table 5-5).

These methods can, of course, be used for Rh phenotyping if "saline tube test" antisera are not available and spontaneous agglutination is occurring using the "slide and rapid tube test" reagents.

Table 5-5. Jk^a TYPING OF PATIENT WITH POSITIVE DIRECT ANTIGLOBULIN TEST USING DIFFERENTIAL ABSORPTION

Red Cells used to Absorb Anti-Jk^a Typing Serum	Dilutions of Absorbed Anti-Jk^a Tested Against Jk (a+b+) Red Cells*						
	1	2	4	8	16	32	Score
Jk(a+b+)	2+	1+	1+	½+	0	0	16
Jk(a+b−)	1+	1+	0	0	0	0	8
Jk(a−b+)	3+	3+	2+	2+	1+	0	32
Patient's	2+	1+	0	0	0	0	10

* These results indicate that the patient is probably Jk(a+).

The Direct Antiglobulin Test

To diagnose the patient correctly, several questions have to be answered:

Question 1: Are the patient's cells sensitized with protein? To answer this question, the patient's washed red cells are first tested with a polyspecific antiglobulin reagent. Most commercial antiglobulin sera will detect IgG sensitization adequately, but approximately 20 to 30 percent of all patients with autoimmune hemolytic anemia have only complement (C3d and C4d) on their red cells, and rare patients have been described with only IgA or IgM on their cells. As mentioned previously, some commercial polyspecific antiglobulin sera will not detect IgA and IgM, and occasionally they will not detect C3d sensitization. Other cases exist in which sensitization of the cells with small numbers of IgG molecules, below the threshold of the antiglobulin test, explains the negative DAT in the presence of AIHA (see Chapter 9). Thus, if the DAT is negative and the patient has all they symptoms of AIHA, do not exclude the diagnosis on this one test.

Method

a. Red cells (preferably from EDTA-blood) are washed four times in large volumes of saline. We usually wash large quantities of red cells (e.g., 2ml packed RBC) and use the washed cells for preparing eluates following DAT and grouping. One can also wash 1 drop of 5 percent red cells in several tubes for DAT only.

b. One drop of 2 to 5 percent washed red cells is added to 2 drops of polyspecific AGS (or 2 drops of AGS are added to the dry button from 1 drop of 2 to 5 percent washed red cells).

c. Tubes are centrifuged at 1000 RCF for 15 to 20 seconds.

d. Tubes are inspected for agglutination (we prefer to check all macroscopically negative results for microscopic agglutination).

Controls

1. We always add 1 drop of the patient's washed red cells to 2 drops of the AGS diluent (or saline, if diluent is not available) and centrifuge this alongside the test. The DAT is truly positive only if the AGS reacts stronger than the diluent; ideally, of course, the tube containing diluent should be negative.

2. Red cells pre-sensitized with IgG (e.g., anti-Rh) "Coombs control cells" should always be added to all negative tests. After recentrifugation, the tests should now be positive, ensuring that the AGS has not been inhibited (e.g., by inadequate washing). No AGT should ever be called negative without this control.

Question 2: What proteins are present on the red cells? How much of each protein is present on the red cells?

The red cells are often sensitized with IgG and complement or IgG alone, and sometimes by complement alone. The presence of these proteins is best detected by performing antiglobulin tests using monospecific antiglobulin sera such as anti-IgG and anti-complement. IgA and IgM are sometimes detected, but they are usually present together with IgG and complement.

By testing the red cells of the patient with dilutions of the AGS (semi-quantitative DAT), one can obtain an estimate of the amount of protein sensitizing the red cells (Table 5-6). This estimate is particularly useful when making serial observations in a single patient (e.g., following treatment). For instance, the undiluted AGS may show similar results on two specimens, but the two may have very different agglutination scores on titration.

Agglutination scores correlated very well when compared with accurate assays of red cell bound IgG and C3 (see Chapter 6). Although we have previously emphasized that commercial antiglobulin sera should never be diluted when standardizing or evaluating (see page 153) such sera, it is acceptable to dilute these antisera when they are being used only to approximately quantitate cell bound IgG. We would stress once again that they must never be diluted when used for antibody detection or cross-matching.

Table 5-6. SEMI-QUANTITATIVE DIRECT ANTIGLOBULIN TEST (EXAMPLES OF THREE PATTERNS OBSERVED)

Proteins on RBC		Dilutions of Antiglobulin Serum					
		1:4	1:16	1:64	1:256	1:1024	1:4096
IgG & C3	Anti-IgG	4+	3+	3+	2+	2+	1+
	Anti-C3	3+	2+	1+	0	0	0
IgG (no C3)	Anti-IgG	4+	3+	3+	2+	2+	1+
	Anti-C3	0	0	0	0	0	0
C3 (no IgG)	Anti-IgG	0	0	0	0	0	0
	Anti-C3	3+	2+	1+	0	0	0

Agglutination reactions are graded as ½+ to 4+.

Determination of Type and Amount of Protein on Patient's Red Cells

1. Direct Antiglobulin Test Using Monospecific AGS
   a. Perform DAT exactly as in steps a through d described previously, but substitute monospecific AGS (e.g., anti-IgG and anti-C3) for polyspecific AGS in step b.
2. Semi-Quantitative DAT (Typical results obtained are shown in Table 5-6.)
   a. Serial dilutions of the AGS are prepared. When we are diluting our raw AGS, we prefer fourfold dilutions of the Anti-IgG (1:4, 1:16, 1:64, 1:256, 1:1024, 1:4096). Alternatively, we make doubling dilutions beginning with the previously determined optimal dilution (see page 153 and Table 5-3). We usually use doubling dilutions of the anti-complement reagents (1:4, 1:8, 1:16, 1:32, 1:64, 1:128). We would suggest doubling dilutions (1:1,1:2,1:4,1:8,1:16,1:32) if an already diluted commercial reagent is to be used.

b. Starting at the highest dilution, 2 drops of each dilution is placed in a 10 × 75 mm test tube.
c. One drop of a 2 to 5 percent washed red cell suspension from the patient is added to each of the 6 tubes.
d. Tubes are centrifuged at 1000 RCF for 15 to 20 seconds.
e. Inspect for agglutination as in the DAT.

Characterization of Antibodies in Serum and Eluate in Autoimmune Hemolytic Anemia

Question 3: Does the serum contain antibodies?
a. Are they agglutinins or "incomplete"?
b. Do they have hemolytic activity?
c. At what temperature do they react optimally?
d. What is their thermal range?
e. What is their specificity?
f. Are they autoantibodies or alloantibodies?

These questions can be answered by the usual serologic techniques (with a few minor additions) used in the blood bank for detection and identification of antibodies.

To aid in the visualization of hemolysis we use a 10 percent red cell suspension; to keep the antigen-antibody ratio in a similar ratio to usual, we add 1 volume of this cell suspension to 4 volumes of serum.

Because patients with autoimmune hemolytic anemia often have low serum complement levels, it is advisable to set up a duplicate set of tests to which an equal volume of fresh compatible inert serum has been added as a source of complement. We prefer the mixture of patient's serum and complement to be in the pH range 6.5 to 6.8 (i.e., add a one-tenth volume of 0.2N HCl to the serum), as this seems to be the optimal range for the detection of warm and cold hemolysins.[10,12] We usually set up, in addition, a tube containing the patient's acidified serum without added complement, but this tube rarely gives a positive result that is not detected in the other tubes.

Many warm and cold reacting autoantibodies give enhanced reactions with enzyme-treated red cells; thus it is useful to include such cells in the serum screening procedure. Hemolysis of enzyme-treated cells is much more commonly observed than hemolysis of untreated red cells.

It is extremely important that tests set up at 37°C are strictly at 37°C. In order to do this, the patient's serum, reagent red cells, and albumin are warmed to 37°C separately before mixing. The tests are then centrifuged at 37°C (see Chapter 10, page 376 and Figure 10-2) and the cells are washed at 37°C in 37°C saline for the AGT. If this is not done carefully (with careful control of the temperature at each stage) then positive results may be misinterpreted, leading to erroneous conclusions regarding the classification of the AIHA and to the clinical significance of the autoantibody.

The serum may contain: (a) no antibodies (they may all have been autoabsorbed onto the patient's red cells *in vivo*); (b) only autoantibodies; (c) autoantibodies plus alloantibodies; or (d) alloantibodies only.

Serum Screen to Determine Serum Antibody Characteristics.

a. Two sets of 8 (10 × 75 mm) tubes are labelled. Each set contains 2 tubes labelled "S" (patient's serum); 2 tubes labelled "AS" (acidified patient's serum)—the AS tubes are optional; 2 tubes labelled "ASAC" (acidified patient's serum and acidified complement); 2 tubes labelled "AC" (acidified complement). One of each pair is labelled "UC" (untreated red cells) and the other tubes are labelled "EC" (enzyme-treated cells). One set of 8 tubes will eventually be incubated at 37°C and the duplicate set at 20°C (or room temperature if a 20°C incubator is not available).

b. Approximately 1.5 ml of patient's serum and 1 ml of complement will be required for the full serum screen. The complement can be fresh normal serum that has been screened for antibodies and found to be negative, or the serum can be stored frozen for a period known to retain at least 60 percent complement activity. (See Figure 3-13, page 101 and Reference 21).

c. Four drops of patient's serum are placed into each of the four tubes marked S.

d. Thirty-six drops of patient's serum are placed in one of the tubes marked AS and 4 drops of 0.2N HCl are added (one-tenth volume). The pH is checked as being 6.5 to 6.8 and adjusted as necessary.

e. Four drops are put into the 4 tubes marked AS and 2 drops are put into each of the 4 tubes marked ASAC. The remaining drops in the pipette are kept in a separate tube or discarded.

f. To 1 of 4 tubes marked AC is added 18 drops of complement (fresh serum) and 2 drops of 0.2N HCl. The pH is checked and adjusted to 6.5 to 6.8 (a micro combination pH electrode is useful here).

g. Two drops of the acidified complement are added to the 2 drops of acidified patient's serum in the tubes marked ASAC. Two drops of the acidified complement are then added to the 4 negative control tubes marked AC. The remainder of the AC is stored in a separate tube or discarded.

h. One set of tubes is incubated in a 37°C water bath and the other set at 20°C. We use a water bath with cooling coil that maintains 20°C (available from Benco Grant, Dayton, Ohio). If a 20°C incubator is not available, room temperature will suffice. (Some blood banks now have platelet storage incubators operating at a constant 20 to 24°C which are useful for this purpose). The serum is allowed to equilibrate for about 10 minutes.

i. An aliquot of washed screening red cells (a pool of two) untreated and papain-treated, are resuspended to approximately 10 percent in saline and allowed to warm to the appropriate temperature by incubating them along with the sera.

j. When the sera and red cells have reached 20°C and 37°C respectively, 1 drop of untreated red cells is added to each tube marked UC and 1 drop of papain-treated red cells is added to each tube marked EC at each temperature.

k. The tests are allowed to incubate for 1 to 2 hours.
l. Following gentle mixing, the 20°C set is centrifuged at room temperature at 1000 RCF for 15 to 20 seconds and the supernatant immediately observed carefully for lysis. The button of cells is then gently resuspended and observed for agglutination. (If the room temperature is higher than 24°C, it would be wise to read the results following 2 hours sedimentation at 20°C with no centrifugation at room temperature.)
m. Following gentle mixing, the 37°C set is either centrifuged strictly at 37°C or observed for lysis and agglutination following 2 hours sedimentation at 37°C.
n. The 37°C set is then washed four times strictly at 37°C (i.e., in a heated centrifuge with warmed saline).
o. Two drops of polyspecific antiglobulin serum are added to the red cell buttons and the tubes centrifuged at 1000 rpm for 15 to 20 seconds and read for agglutination as described previously for the antiglobulin test.

Tables 5-7, 5-8, and 5-9 show typical findings in warm autoimmune hemolytic anemia, cold agglutinin syndrome, and paroxysmal cold hemoglobinuria.

Table 5-7. TYPICAL RESULTS OF SERUM SCREENING TESTS IN AUTOIMMUNE HEMOLYTIC ANEMIA

			Warm Type AIHA			**Negative Control**
			S	AS	AS+AC	AC
Untreated RBC	20°C	Lysis	0	0	0	0
		Agg	0	0	0	0
	37°C	Lysis	0	0	0	0
		Agg	0	0	0	0
		IAT	2+	2+	2+	0
Enzyme-treated RBC	20°C	Lysis	0	0	0	0
		Agg	1+	1+	1+	0
	37°C	Lysis	½+	1+	2+	0
		Agg	3+	3+	3+	0

S = Patient's serum
AS = Patient's serum + 1/10th vol. 0.2 NHCl
pH 6.5-6.8
AS+AC = Acidified serum + acidified complement
(normal inert fresh serum + 1/10th vol. 0.2 HCl)
pH 6.5-6.8

Table 5-8. TYPICAL RESULTS OF SERUM SCREENING TESTS IN AUTOIMMUNE HEMOLYTIC ANEMIA

Cold Agglutinin Syndrome

			S	AS	AS+AC	Negative Control AC
Untreated RBC	20°C	Lysis	1+	1+	3+	0
		Agg	4+	4+	. 4+	0
	37°C	Lysis	0	0	0	0
		Agg	0	0	0	0
		IAT	0	0	0	0
Enzyme-treated RBC	20°C	Lysis	2+	3+	4+	0
		Agg	4+	4+	X	0
	37°C	Lysis	0	0	0	0
		Agg	0	0	0	0

S = Patient's serum
AS = Patient's serum + 1/10th vol. 0.2 NHCl
    pH 6.5-6.8
AS+AC = Acidified serum + acidified complement
    (normal inert fresh serum + 1/10th vol. 0.2 HCl)
    pH 6.5-6.8

X = Not applicable; all cells lysed

Table 5-9. TYPICAL RESULTS OF SERUM SCREENING TESTS IN AUTOIMMUNE HEMOLYTIC ANEMIA

Paroxysmal Cold Hemoglobinuria

			S	AS	AS+AC	Negative Control AC
Untreated RBC	20°C	Lysis	0	0	0	0
		Agg	0	0	0	0
	37°C	Lysis	0	0	0	0
		Agg	0	0	0	0
		IAT	0	0	0	0
Enzyme-treated RBC	20°C	Lysis	0	0	2+ **	0
		Agg	1+ *	1+ *	1+ *	0
	37°C	Lysis	0	0	0	0
		Agg	0	0	0	0

S = Patient's serum
AS = Patient's serum + 1/10th vol. 0.2 NHCl
    pH 6.5-6.8
AS+AC = Acidified serum + acidified complement
    (normal inert fresh serum + 1/10th vol. 0.2 HCl)
    pH 6.5-6.8

* Found in 3 of 6 cases we studied
** Found in 4 of 6 cases we studied

Cold Agglutinin Titer/Thermal Range/Ii Specificity. We usually perform these tests only if agglutination is observed at 20°C in the serum screening. As indicated below, titrations may be performed using three types of red cells. Results of reactions using the patient's own cells are of particular significance if the autoantibody specificity is anti-i (see page 254). If only the cold agglutinin titer is required, the tests listed in the following paragraphs can be reduced to a single row of dilutions tested against group OI adult red cells incubated at 4°C. Precautions mentioned in step k still apply.

a. Serial dilutions of the warm (37°C) separated patient's serum are prepared in saline, 1:2 to 1:16,000 in 0.5 ml quantities. It is of prime importance that separate pipettes are used to transfer each 0.5 ml aliquot to the next tube when preparing each dilution, as "carry over" can give extremely inaccurate high titers if a single pipette is used. (See Table 5-10. The patient's correct titer was 8,000, not 128,000 as reported to us.)

Table 5-10. COLD AGGLUTININ TITER (PATIENT E.I.)

	Dilutions of Patient's Serum $\times 10^3$							
	1	2	4	8	16	32	64	128
Same pipette	4+	4+	4+	4+	3+	3+	2+	1+
Separate pipettes	3½+	3+	2+	1+	½+	0	0	0

b. Three rows of 10 × 75 mm tubes are placed in a rack. The first row is labelled "2I" through "16000I." the second row is labelled "2i" through "16000i," and the third row is labelled "2 auto" through "16000 auto."

c. Starting from the highest dilution (e.g., 16000), 2 drops of diluted serum are put into 3 tubes (e.g., 16,000I;16,000i and 16,000 auto).

d. Three 2 to 5 percent washed red cell suspensions are prepared from I adult group O cells (e.g., pool of two screening cells), i cord group O cells, and the patient's own 37°C washed red cells. It is useful, in addition, sometimes to test i adult ABO compatible red cells if they are available.

e. The tubes containing serum dilutions are incubated at 37°C until they reach 37°C (10 to 15 minutes).

f. Aliquots of the washed red cell suspensions are incubated at 37°C along with the serum dilutions and allowed to reach 37°C also.

g. When both cells and serum are at 37°C, 1 drop of cell suspension is added to each of the appropriate rows. The tubes are mixed and allowed to incubate for up to 2 hours.

h. The tubes are either centrifuged strictly at 37°C after 30 minutes to 1 hour or allowed to sediment at 37°C for 2 hours before reading for agglutination. If the tubes are centrifuged at 37°C, they must be put back in the 37°C water bath immediately after centrifugation and each tube read separately, as quickly as possible, so that no cooling ensues. Similar care must be taken if the cells are allowed to sediment.

i. Following reading, the tubes are moved to a 30°C water bath, incubated for 2 hours, and read for agglutination without centrifugation.

j. The tubes are then placed at 20°C or at room temperature. They may be centrifuged and read for agglutination after incubation for 30 to 60 minutes. (Again, if a 20°C incubator is used and if the room temperature is greater than 24°C, more accurate results will be obtained by reading for agglutination following sedimentation for 2 hours without centrifugation.)

k. Following reading, the tubes are incubated at 4°C. The tubes can either be centrifuged at 4°C (i.e., in a refrigerated centrifuge) after 30 minutes to 1 hour, or left for at least 2 hours (we often leave ours overnight) to sediment at 4°C before reading. When reading the test, it is important that the rack of tubes is placed in a melting ice bath (following centrifugation or sedimentation) and the tubes read rapidly, one at a time.

Using the above methods, the cold agglutinin titer, thermal range, and specificity within the Ii system are all determined simultaneously (see page 174 and Table 5-13).

If the patient has hemolytic anemia, and an abnormal cold autoagglutinin is detected (titer >64 at 4°C and/or thermal amplitude 20°C or higher), it may also be advisable to repeat the titrations substituting 30 percent albumin for saline, particularly if the cold agglutinin titer at 4°C in saline is not strikingly elevated (>2000). This is true because agglutination reactions at 30°C in albumin seem to correlate best with presence or absence of cold agglutinin syndrome (see page 214). Further, if the pathologic cold agglutinin reacts at 37°C in albumin but not in saline, one should consider omitting albumin in performing compatibility tests (see page 376). However, only infrequently are all of the above procedures indicated. The clinical significance of cold agglutinin titers at various temperatures in saline and albumin is discussed in detail in Chapter 6.

Titration of Hemolysins

a. Serial dilutions (1:2 to 1:512) of the patient's serum are made in "fresh" inert serum as a source of complement (stored serum may be used if appropriate storage conditions for complement activity are applied).[21] If the serum screen indicates lysis only in acidified complement, the fresh normal serum should be acidified to pH 6.5 to 6.8. A control tube of the complement alone should also be set up.

b. To 0.2 ml aliquots of each dilution is added 1 drop of 10 to 20 percent group O red cells in saline. If only the enzyme-treated red cells are hemolysed in the screening, these are substituted for the untreated red cells.

c. The tubes are mixed and incubated for 1 hour. If cold hemolysins are being quantitated, the tubes are incubated at 20°C. If warm hemolysins are being quantitated, the serum dilutions and red cells are warmed to 37°C separately for approximately 10 minutes, then the cells are added.

d. After incubation the tubes are mixed gently (this is important) and centrifuged at 1000 RCF for 2 minutes. If warm hemolysins are being measured, the centrifugation should be at 37°C.

e. The supernatants are examined for lysis and the results graded.

Note: If the patient's serum is already red due to *in vivo* lysis, it is a good idea to also take into account the size of the unlysed red cell button (i.e., to compare it with the tube containing complement only).

DETERMINING SPECIFICITY OF AUTOANTIBODIES

Question 4: What is the specificity of the antibody eluted from the patient's red cells and present in the patient's serum? Many interesting observations and concepts have been derived from detailed studies of the specificity of autoantibodies in autoimmune hemolytic anemia (see Chapter 7). However, such exhaustive studies are not required for diagnostic purposes. Nevertheless, we feel it highly advisable to perform at least limited specificity studies, especially in patients with suspected warm antibody AIHA. Diagnostic error is avoided by confirming that the patient's warm antibody is, indeed, an autoantibody. In some patients, alloantibody(ies) may be detected in addition to autoantibody, and it is helpful to have such information available since transfusion may be required. The specificity of the autoantibody may also be of significance in regard to transfusion. Delaying specificity testing until a decision is made that blood is needed for transfusion (at which time the need may be urgent) is not recommended. In still other patients, the initial impression of AIHA may not be substantiated. Antibodies found in initial screening tests of the patient's serum may be alloantibodies, and the direct antiglobulin test may be positive for any of the reasons listed on page 151. Finally, if the patient has been transfused recently, a distinction between delayed hemolytic transfusion reactions and AIHA may be difficult (see Chapter 9).

The following section describes techniques for determining autoantibody specificity. Techniques for the detection of alloantibodies present in association with autoantibodies are described in Chapter 10.

It is essential to prepare an eluate from the red cells in order to define the autoantibody. If the red cells have only complement components demonstrable on them by the DAT, no antibody is usually detectable in the eluate from the red cells, but if IgG is present on the cells, it can be eluted by simple methods such as using heat or ether. If the patient has not been transfused recently, the eluate should contain autoantibody only; if the specificity is obvious, one can confirm the presence of the matching antigen on the patient's red cells. If the DAT is positive due to IgG sensitization, and the eluate shows no activity against normal cells, an association with drugs should be strongly suspected. A good example of this phenomenon is penicillin-induced hemolytic anemia, in which the eluate from red cells that react strongly in the antiglobulin test will not react with untreated normal cells, but will react strongly with red cells treated with penicillin (see Chapter 8).

Heat Elution Method
a. Wash the cells from which the eluate is to be made 6 times in large volumes of saline.
b. Save some of last saline wash to run as a control to show absence of

antibody activity after washing. This test must be negative before it can be assumed that any eluate activity came from the red cells, rather than a contaminating antibody from the serum.

c. To the washed packed cells add an equal volume of saline (or AB serum or 6 percent albumin). The volume of saline added can be varied, depending on the strength of the DAT. A rough guide is 2 to 4 volumes for 4+, 2 volumes for 3+, equal volumes for 1 to 2+, and ½ volume for 1+ or less.

d. Mix well and place in a 56°C water bath for 5 to 10 minutes, agitating during incubation. If agitation is too vigorous, increased lysis will occur.

e. Immediately transfer the tube to pre-warmed centrifuge cups containing 56°C water.

f. Centrifuge at 1000 RCF for 5 minutes.

g. Immediately separate the hemoglobulin-tinted supernatant eluate.

h. The eluate should preferably be tested the same day, but it can be frozen, in which case it is preferable to elute into AB serum or 6 percent albumin.

Ether Elution Method [27,58]

a. In a glass tube add equal volumes of saline and washed * packed cells. (Use of less or no saline produces a more concentrated eluate in which antibody is liberated directly into the hemoglobin of the lysed cells.)

b. Add 2 volumes of diethyl-ether to the cells.

c. Stopper and mix by repeated inversion for one minute. (Care must be taken of pressure built up by ether. Do not use Parafilm to seal tube.)

d. Incubate at 37°C for 15 to 30 minutes.

e. Centrifuge at 1000 RCF for 10 minutes.

f. Three clearly defined layers will be visible: an upper layer of ether, a middle layer of stroma and proteins, and a bottom layer of hemoglobin-stained fluid, which is the eluate.

g. Carefully remove the eluate, without contaminating it with stroma.

Note: A modification of this technique is to remove the ether, then place the tube containing eluate and stroma at 56°C for 5 to 10 minutes. Agitate mixture periodically with applicator stick. (Be careful; mixture has a tendency to "boil over.") Centrifuge at 1000 RCF for 10 minutes and remove eluate.

Digitonin/Acid Method [1,32]

Principle

Red cells hemolyzed by digitonin produce intact stroma that is free of hemoglobin and will sediment readily. Stroma is then eluted with acid (pH 3.0, 0.1 M glycine buffer) to produce a clear eluate.

Reagents

---

* Control: Be sure to test an aliquot of the last cell wash in parallel with eluate.

a. Digitonin suspension. 5 mg/ml in saline. Stable at 4°C.
b. 0.1 M glycine buffer, pH 3.0 Prepare by mixing 3.754 gm glycine with 500 ml distilled water. Adjust pH (usually 34 drops of 12 N HCl).
c. 0.8m phosphate buffer pH 8.2:
   i. 0.8 M Na_2HPO_4 made by adding 113.57 gm Na_2HPO_4 to 1 liter of distilled water.
   ii. 0.8 M KH_2PO_4 made by adding 108.87 gm KH_2PO_4 to 1 liter of distilled water.
   iii. Make final solution by adding 0.35 ml 0.8M KH_2PO_4 to 9.65 ml 0.8 M Na_2HPO_4. Stable at 4°C.

Procedure
a. Warm phosphate buffer to room temperature.
b. Wash 1 volume of red cells six times in normal saline * and resuspend with 9 volumes of saline.
c. Invert to mix and add 0.5 volume of digitonin solution.
d. Invert several times until a clear hemolysate is visible.
e. Centrifuge at 1000 RCF for 5 minutes.
f. Remove and descard supernatant with Pasteur pipette.
g. Wash red cell stroma 4 times with normal saline or until stroma appears snow white.
h. Elute by adding 2 ml of 0.1 M glycine buffer, pH 3.0.**
i. Invert for 1 minute and centrifuge at 1000 RCF for 5 minutes.
j. Add 0.2 ml phosphate buffer to supernatant.
k. Mix and centrifuge at 1000 RCF for 2 minutes to remove any precipitate. The resulting supernatant is the final eluate.

Warm Type Autoimmune Hemolytic Anemia

Determination of Autoantibody Specificity: If the eluate reacts with all cells on a routine panel and no specificity is obvious, the most commonly recommended method is to test dilutions of the eluate (and/or serum) against rr, R_1R_1, and R_2R_2 red cells.[14, 41]

Dilution Technique
a. Prepare serial doubling dilutions of eluate (and/or serum) in saline from 1:1 to 1:512 (e.g., 0.2 aliquots).
b. Starting from highest dilution, transfer 2 drops to three 10 × 75 mm test tubes labelled rr, R_1R_1, R_2R_2.
c. Add 2 drops of 30 percent albumin to each tube. (This step is optional.)
d. Add 1 drop of 2 to 5 percent group O rr, R_1R_1, R_2R_2 red cells to each appropriate row of tubes.
e. Incubate at 37°C for 15 minutes.

---

* Control: Be sure to test an aliquot of last wash in parallel with eluate.
** Other elution methods (e.g., heat and/or ether) may be applied to the white stroma prepared in Step g.

f. Wash 4 times in isotonic saline.

g. Add AGS to button of washed cells.

h. Examine for agglutination.

Table 5-11 shows results of an eluate that would be interpreted as showing anti-e of "relative specificity" (some workers use the term "some anti-e" specificity).

The disadvantage of this method is that it assumes that the specificity is within the Rh system. We have often found that when eluates or sera showing results similar to those shown in Table 5-11 (i.e., anti-e of relative specificity) are tested with more red cells (e.g., more R_2R_2 cells), the specificity pattern is different. We recommend a modification of this technique;[23,41] i.e., a dilution of the eluate (and/or serum) is selected that gives an approximate 1 to 2+ reaction, and that dilution is tested against as many different phenotypes as possible. An additional advantage of this approach is that the results on the serum may indicate alloantibody specificity. Table 5-12 illustrates a case in which the undiluted eluate reacted with all cells and the serum appeared to have some anti-e specificity. A 1:64 dilution of the eluate showed some anti-e specificity, and a 1:4 dilution of the serum showed an allo anti-K to be present in addition to the anti-"e."

Table 5-11. ELUATE SHOWING ANTI-e OF "RELATIVE SPECIFICITY"

				Dilutions of Eluate				
	2	4	8	16	32	64	128	256
rr	4+	3+	3+	2+	2+	1+	0	0
R_1R_1	4+	3+	3+	2+	2+	1+	0	0
R_2R_2	3+	2+	1+	0	0	0	0	0

Table 5-12. SPECIFICITY TESTING OF RED CELL ELUATE AND SERUM

IAT on Pooled				Dilutions				
Screening Cells	2	4	8	16	32	64	128	256
Eluate	3+	3+	2+	2+	1+	1+	0	0
Serum	2+	1+	0	0	0	0	0	0

			Panel of Group O cells					
	rr	rr	r'r	R_1R_1	R_1R_1	R_1R_2	R_2R_2	r"r"
	K−	K+	K−	K+	K−	K−	K−	K−
Eluate 1:1	3+	3+	3+	3+	3+	3+	3+	3+
Eluate 1:64	1+	1+	1+	1+	1+	1+	0	0
Serum 1:1	2+	2+	2+	2+	2+	2+	0	0
Serum 1:4	0	1+	0	1	0	0	0	0

Cross Absorptions and Elutions. The patient's eluate can be absorbed with cells of known phenotype and the absorbed serum tested against a panel. In addition, an eluate is prepared from the absorbing red cells and tested against a panel. Such tests are time-consuming and need large quantities of red cells, but they have sometimes revealed interesting specificities. [69] Recent descriptions [29,30,53] of so-called mimicking autoantibodies have made the interpretations of this method complex. Issitt and Pavone [29] studied 48 autoantibodies with apparent "simple" Rh specificity (anti-e, -E, -d, -D, -C, -Ce, -G) by multiple absorption tests. The finding that 34 (70.8 percent) of these antibodies could bind to red cells lacking the antigens that the antibodies appeared to define indicated that the antibodies had different specificities than seemed to be the case in initial antibody identification tests. For instance, in contrast to allo anti-E, autoantibodies that appeared to have obvious anti-E specificity could be absorbed by E negative red cells. Those autoantibodies that at first appeared to be directed against the Rh antigens e, E, or c most often had anti-Hr or anti-Hr_0 specificity (see Chapter 7).

Cold Agglutinin Syndrome

Because the specificity in this disorder is almost always anti-I and less commonly anti-i, the specificity is usually obvious from the results of the cold agglutinin titer/thermal range technique described on page 168. As all adult cells contain some i and all cord cells some I, results are never clear-cut when determining specificity within the "Ii system." Often, at 4°C the i cells will react as strongly as the I cells, and only by performing a thermal range test will the specificity become obvious. (Table 5-13 shows the results of a typical anti-I.) The determination of the specificity of the cold agglutinin is often only of

Table 5-13. COLD AGGLUTININ TITER/THERMAL RANGE/Ii SPECIFICITY

Dilutions of Patient's Serum	RED CELLS USED/INCUBATION TEMPERATURE					
	4°C		25°C		30°C	
	Adult	Cord	Adult	Cord	Adult	Cord
2	4+	4+	4+	1+	1+	0
4	4+	4+	4+	1+	1+	0
8	4+	4+	4+	1+	1+	0
16	4+	4+	3+	(1+)	(1+)	0
32	4+	4+	2+	0	0	0
64	4+	4+	1+	0	0	0
128	4+	3+	(1+)	0	0	0
256	3+	3+	0	0	0	0
572	3+	2+	0	0	0	0
1024	2+	1+	0	0	0	0
2048	1+	0	0	0	0	0

Anti-I is present although the specificity is not evident at 4°C.

academic interest, as it is not recommended that the rare i adult blood is obtained for these patients, but rather that they are transfused with normal I adult blood at 37°C (see Chapter 10). If further confirmation of specificity is required (e.g., to determine whether the antibody is possibly anti-HI, etc.), then the titration/thermal range technique can be extended using more cells, e.g., I adult, i cord and/or i adult red cells of different ABO types and Oh (Bombay) red cells.

On rare occasions, another specificity is observed—anti-Pr. This antibody should be suspected if the I adult and i cord (and/or i adult) red cells react equally at all phases. The Pr antigens are destroyed by proteolytic enzymes. Thus, the cold agglutinin titer can be repeated comparing untreated red cells with enzyme-treated red cells (e.g., papain-treated). Both anti-I and anti-i react better with enzyme-treated red cells, but anti-Pr will give no reaction, or much weaker reactions. Other antibodies that react with antigens that are destroyed by enzyme-treatment (e.g., M and N) must be excluded by testing a panel of red cells; anti-Pr will react with all untreated human red cells on the panel. Further confirmatory tests can be performed using various animal red cells and neuraminidase-treated red cells.[25,55,56]

Paroxysmal Cold Hemoglobinuria

In our experience and in the experience of Dacie and Worlledge,[15] the specificity in PCH has always been anti-P. There are, however, isolated reports of anti-HI.[70] The specificity may be of clinical importance, as this is the only AIHA in which the specificity is clear-cut like an alloantibody. Some workers[54,57] have suggested that the rare p red cells have better survival and it is worth trying to obtain them for transfusing to patients with paroxysmal cold hemoglobinuria with severe acute hemolysis. Our limited experience has been that normal P positive blood, if given at 37°C, gives the expected rise in hematocrit level.

To determine specificity, the patient's serum should be tested against I adult, i cord (and/or i adult) and the rare p and/or P^k red cells by the Donath-Landsteiner test.

Donath-Landsteiner Test
1. Blood from the patient is allowed to clot undisturbed at 37°C and the serum separated (preferably by centrifugation at 37°C).
2. Pipette 10 volumes of patient's serum into two 10 ×75 mm tubes.
3. As patients with PCH may have low serum complement levels leading to false-negative results, it is recommended that tests with added complement be included. Pipette 5 volumes of fresh inert normal serum, as a source of complement, into two 10 ×75 mm tubes. Add 5 volumes of patient's serum to one tube. The tube containing complement alone acts as a negative control.
4. To all four tubes add 1 volume of a 50 percent suspension of washed normal group O, P positive red blood cells.

5. One of the tubes from step 2 and both tubes from step 3 are incubated in melting ice for 30 to 60 minutes.
6. The other tube from step 2 is incubated in a 37°C water bath to act as a negative control.
7. After 30 to 60 minutes, the tubes in the melting ice are gently mixed and moved to 37°C for 30 minutes.
8. All tubes are gently mixed and centrifuged.

Lysis visible to the naked eye indicates a positive test. The control tubes containing normal serum only and the tube left at 37°C (step 6) throughout the test should be negative.

The test can also be performed by placing samples of the patient's blood into tubes prewarmed to 37°C. One sample is left to clot at 37°C. The other is placed immediately in melting ice and left undisturbed for one hour. It is then moved to 37°C for 30 minutes, centrifuged, and inspected for hemolysis. This is a simple way of performing the test, but rather wasteful of blood.

Some additional comments about the Donath-Landsteiner test will be of assistance in some cases. The indication of a positive test is grossly evident hemolysis, so the presence of marked hemoglobinemia, which is common in the acute stages of paroxysmal cold hemoglobinuria, complicates the test. One way to observe for hemolysis when using a test serum that is already pink or red is to note the size of the cell button after centrifugation. A change in the color of the serum may not be evident, but only a small number of cells may remain, indicating that hemolysis has taken place. If a change in the size of the cell button is not readily apparent when compared with a control tube utilizing the same volume of red cells, additional variations on the theme should be performed as follow.

Since antibody is fixed to the red cells in the cold phase of incubation, and warming is necessary only to allow the complement cascade to proceed, the patient's serum may be replaced by fresh normal ABO compatible serum after the cold incubation. This technique is called a "two-stage" Donath-Landsteiner test and may be performed utilizing either the patient's serum or an eluate.[75] After incubation for an hour at 0°C, the supernatant serum or eluate is removed from the settled red cells (centrifugation is not necessary) and replaced with fresh normal ABO compatible serum. The tube is then incubated at 37°C and observed for hemolysis as previously described. Since a small amount of the patient's serum may remain in the original tube, a control tube utilizing the patient's inactivated serum followed by replacement with normal inactivated serum will be necessary.

It is also possible to test for the Donath-Landsteiner antibody by the indirect antiglobulin test, although this sometimes presents difficulties because of agglutination at 0°C caused by the Donath-Landsteiner antibody itself or by a coincidentally occurring IgM cold agglutinin. If direct agglutination after the cold incubation is absent or weak, the red cells may then be washed four times in ice-cold saline (to avoid elution of the antibody) and tested with monospecific anti-IgG antiglobulin serum.[75] Although it is advisable to do the indirect antiglobulin test in the cold for maximal reactivity, some antibody may

Table 5-14. CLASSIFICATION AND DIFFERENTIAL DIAGNOSIS OF THE AUTOIMMUNE HEMOLYTIC ANEMIAS

| | Cells | | Serum | |
	Direct Antiglobulin Test	Eluate	Immunoglobulin Type	Serologic Characteristics	Specificity
Warm AIHA (most common type); about 80% of our AIHA patients.	IgG (no complement) 20% IgG and complement 67% Complement (no IgG) 13%	IgG antibody	IgG (sometimes IgA or IgM present in addition, rarely alone)	Reacting by indirect anti-globulin test 57% Agglutinating enzyme treated cells (37°C) 90% Hemolyzing enzyme treated cells (37°C) 13% Agglutinating untreated cells (20°C) 35% Agglutinating or hemolyzing untreated cells (37°C) 5%	Usually within Rh system but often combined with a "non-specific" element. Other specificities include LW, U, Wr[b], En[a], I[T], K.
Cold agglutinin syndrome; about 18% of our AIHA patients	Complement alone	No activity	IgM	High titer cold antibody (usually >1024 at 4°C). Reacts up to 30°C. Monoclonal protein (κ light chain) in the chronic disease.	Usually anti-I but can be anti-i or anti-Pr (very rare)
Paroxysmal cold hemoglobinuria; about 2% of our AIHA patients	Complement alone (IgG cold antibody elutes off RBC at 37°C, e.g., in vivo, or even when RBC are washed at room temperature)	No activity	IgG	Potent hemolysin but will also agglutinate normal cells. Said to be biphasic (i.e., sensitizes cells in cold and then hemolyzes them when moved to 37°C). Usually only sensitized cells up to 15°C.	Anti-P (i.e., only negative with p or P[k] cells)

remain fixed to the cells even after incubation at 37°C.[12] This phenomenon is evidenced by the fact that the antiglobulin test is positive on unlysed cells remaining after performing the bithermic hemolysis test.

As a patient recovers from his illness and the antibody gradually weakens in reactivity, the indirect antiglobulin test may remain positive, indicating that this is a sensitive means of detecting the antibody. The specificity of the antibody as demonstrated by the indirect antiglobulin test will be the same as when tested by the classic bithermic hemolysis test.

A summary of serologic results in warm antibody AIHA, cold agglutinin syndrome, and paroxysmal cold hemoglobinuria is given in Table 5-14.

THE USE OF THE AUTOANALYZER FOR STUDYING AUTOIMMUNE HEMOLYTIC ANEMIA

Lalezari and co-workers [34-36] have applied the Autoanalyzer in studies on autoimmune hemolytic anemia in several different ways. They use a continuous flow system utilizing Polybrene (hexadimethrine bromide); the test is composed of three separate phases:

1. If the patient's serum is to be studied, an aliquot is mixed with washed normal screening red cells in a low ionic strength medium. If the equivalent of a direct antiglobulin test is to be performed, the patient's washed red cells are mixed in a low ionic strength milieu.
2. Polybrene is added, causing non-specific aggregation of the red cells. Polybrene is a synthetic positively charged polymer originally used as an anti-heparin agent.[50] It appears to cause non-specific aggregation of red cells by reacting with sialic acid and other negatively charged membrane components, thus reducing the "resistance" between cells and allowing them to come closer together. Under these conditions any antibody molecules on the red cells will be able to form cross-linkages between adjacent red cells; they are said to become "doubly bound." [45]
3. Hypertonic sodium citrate is now introduced into the flow system, to neutralize the Polybrene. Once the Polybrene is neutralized, non-sensitized red cells will resuspend easily, in contrast to sensitized red cells in which antigen-antibody bonds will prevent resuspension.

The aggregated red cells are allowed to settle, and the residual resuspended red cells are lysed and the color produced is measured by a colorimeter and recorded. A reduction in the hemoglobin optical density, which results from decantation of the aggregated cells, indicates antibody activity.

The test is said to be far more sensitive than the manual antiglobulin test; in fact, the claim is made that it can detect 1 molecule of IgG anti-Rh per red cell.[35]

Lalezari's group have used this system to make distinctions betwen warm, cold, and drug-induced immune hemolytic anemia. They subject the antigen-antibody bonds to temperature changes from 10°C to 60°C. The continuous recording of the results produces characteristic curves that were termed "temperature gradient dissociation curves." These curves reflect the process of antigen-antibody bond breaking caused by heat energy. A highly reproducible parameter of the curve was the temperature at which 50 percent of the aggregates dissociated (T 50 percent). The T 50 percent was found to depend both on the inherent thermal properties of the reaction system and the antibody concentration.[37]

In patients with AIHA the T 50 percent values obtained from testing red cell bound antibodies were arbitrarily divided into three groups: the majority of patients had a T 50 percent of greater than 60°C; the second group ranged between 30°C and 55°C; and the third group had a T 50 percent below 30°C. In the largest group of patients with warm antibody type AIHA the T 50 percent was near or greater than 60°C; similarly, patients with methyldopa-induced AIHA were near or greater than 60°C. In patients with SLE and related collagen diseases, the T 50 percent almost always was between 30°C and 55°C. Two types of antibodies were encountered in the majority of cases of cold agglutinin syndrome: a serum antibody with a T 50 percent value of 20°C to 34°C and a cell-bound antibody with T 50 percent of 30°C to 50°C (and on rare occasions greater than 60°C).

A very interesting finding was that the reaction slope for methyldopa-induced AIHA was consistently different than the slope seen with idiopathic warm antibody type AIHA.[70a] As the manual serology on these groups of patients is often identical and there are few reports of any differentiation between the two groups, this finding deserves more extensive investigations.

Two other areas studied by Lalezari have been quantitation and specificity of red cell antibody. He has not published much data on quantitating red cell-bound antibody yet, but the early results [35] suggest that the method may be very useful, especially in quantitating small amounts of IgG on the red cell. We will be interested to see if the method can be used to detect the "Coombs Negative" group of AIHA discussed in Chapter 9.

The work on determining specificity of red cell-bound antibody is very exciting, as it can be performed without eluting the antibody from the red cells. The results of such a procedure should be valuable, if only to compare with the results of the "classical" elution techniques we have used for years, where there is a real danger of possibly changing the characteristics of the autoantibody by the sometimes rather harsh procedures to which it is subjected (e.g., 56°C heat, ether, etc.). Lalezari uses a modification of the mixed agglutination reaction: washed antibody-sensitized red cells are mixed with each of a panel of red cells separately, and the mixtures then tested in the Polybrene-AutoAnalyzer system. If the added panel cells possess antigens that react with the cell-bound antibodies, they "coagglutinate" with the test cells. In contrast, if the panel cells lack the corresponding antigens, not only do they not react with the cell-bound antibodies, but, by interposing between the antibody-carrying test cells, they physically block their cross-linkage.

Using this technique Lalezari [34–36] has been able to not only demonstrate specificity of cell-bound auto-Rh antibodies, but also the specificity of *in vivo* red cell-bound anti-penicillin by utilizing *in vitro* penicillin-treated red cells in the system. Like the results obtained in manual testing (see Chapter 7), Lalezari was able to show clear differences between the results obtained with allo Rh and auto Rh antibodies. He suggested that blood group determinants that react with alloantibodies are composed of confined regions on the red cell membrane. The specificity of autoantibodies may include these determinants defined by alloantibodies, but the target area is usually larger and includes components that do not react with alloantibodies. Lalezari further commented that the difference between auto and alloantibodies may be the consequence of the duration of immunization, which could also explain why panagglutinins are often found together with specific autoantibodies.

None of the preceeding concepts are new, of course, but they do confirm similar conclusions reached by other workers using manual technology; these conclusions are discussed fully in other sections of this book (Chapter 7).

Hsu et al.[26] used an AutoAnalyzer to evaluate AIHA, but they used a PVP-augmented antiglobulin test system. They reported that the system used with red cells from patients with AIHA "provided a valuable body of information related to the presence or absence of specifice immunoglobulins and complement components on their erythrocytes. This was often of diagnostic importance and sometimes differed significantly from results of manual tests of the same cells."

They reported that 12 patients who had no clinical evidence of hemolytic anemia, despite positive direct antiglobulin tests due to IgG sensitization, by manual methods had neither C3 nor C4 on their red cells by either manual or automated procedures. Two patients had IgG and IgA, and of 10 with IgG alone on their cells, all had both kappa and lambda light chains, indicative of polyclonal IgG. Patients with active AIHA were quite different. Of 13 patients, 3 had "monoclonal" IgG on their red cells (i.e., only agglutinated by anti-kappa or anti-lambda antiglobulin sera). The other 10 patients had C3 on their red cells, and all but 3 had C4 present as well. (They suggested that the presence of C3 without C4 indicated activation of the alternative complement pathway.)

Nine other patients with active hemolytic anemia associated with warm autoantibodies disclosed a much more complex serologic picture. Eight cases demonstrated spontaneous agglutination in PVP. They all reacted in some fashion with anti-IgM, although only one was directly agglutinable manually with anti-IgM. They suggested that cell-bound IgM is associated with spontaneous agglutination, at least if PVP is present. The authors comment that red cell-bound IgM was not detected as readily as other red cell-bound immunoglobulins, even with the AutoAnalyzer. This has certainly been our experience also, especially with alloantibodies.[22] They made the interesting observation that the rabbit anti-human IgM appeared to remove the human IgM autoantibody, and they suggested that IgM may never be adequately detected directly, and the presence of IgM should be inferred when agglutination with both anti-C3 and anti-C4 is observed.

The final results of the studies by Hsu et al.[26] showed three patterns of warm antibody type AIHA: (1) monoclonal IgG without complement, (2) IgA or IgD with C3 but not C4, and (3) multiple immunoglobulins, C3 and C4; in this group, IgM appeared to be responsible for the complement fixation.

REFERENCES

1. American Association of Blood Banks: Digitonin elution technic. *In* Special Serological Technics Useful in Problem Solving. American Association of Blood Banks, Washington, D.C., Nov. 1977, 36.
2. Boorman, K. E., Dodd, B. E., Loutit, J. F., and Mollison, P. L.: Some results of transfusion of blood to recipients with 'cold' agglutinins. Brit. Med. J., *1:*751, 1946.
3. Brooks, D. E.: Effects of macromolecules on aggregation of erythrocytes. *In:* Human Blood Groups, Proceedings of the 5th International Convocation of Immunology, Buffalo, N.Y., 1976, Mohn, J. F., Plunkett, R. W., Cunningham, R. K., and Lambert, R. M., Eds. New York: S. Karger 1977, 27–35.
4. Burkart, P., Rosenfield, R. E., Hsu, T. C. S., Wong, K. Y., Nusbacher, J., Shaikh, S. H., and Kochwa, S.: Instrumented PVP-augmented antiglobulin tests. I. Detection of allogeneic antibodies coating otherwise normal erythrocytes. Vox. Sang., *26:*280, 1974.
5. Cameron, J. W., and Diamond, L. K.: Chemical, clinical and immunological studies on the products of human plasma fractionation. XXIX. Serum albumin as a diluent for Rh typing reagents. J. Clin. Invest., *24:*793, 1945.
6. Casey, F. M., Dodd, B. E., and Lincoln, P. J.: A study of the characteristics of certain Rh antibodies preferentially detectable by enzyme technique. Vox. Sang., *23:*493, 1972.
7. Chaplin, H., Jr.: Clinical usefulness of specific antiglobulin reagents in autoimmune hemolytic anemias. Progress in Hematology. *8:*25, 1973.
8. Coombs, R. R. A., Mourant, A. E., and Race, R. R.: A new test for the detection of weak and 'incomplete' Rh agglutinins. Brit. J. Exp. Path., *26:*255, 1945.
9. Coombs, R. R. A., Mourant, A. E., and Race, R. R.: In vivo iso-sensitization of red cells in babies with haemolytic disease. Lancet, *1:*264, 1946.
10. Dacie, J. V.: Hemolysins in acquired hemolytic anemia. Effect of pH on the activity in vitro of a serum hemolysin. Blood, *4:*928, 1949.
11. Dacie, J. V.: Occurrences in normal human sera of 'incomplete' forms of 'cold' autoantibodies. Nature (Lond.), *166:*36, 1950.
12. Dacie, J. V.: The Haemolytic Anaemias, Congenital and Acquired. 2nd Ed. Part II-The Auto-immune Haemolytic Anaemias. J. & A. Churchill, London, 1962.
13. Dacie, J. V., Crookston, J. H., and Christenson, W. N.: "Incomplete" cold antibodies: Role of complement in sensitization to antiglobulin serum by potentially haemolytic antibodies. Brit. J. Haemat., *3:*77, 1957.
14. Dacie, J. V., and Lewis, S. M.: Practical Haematology. 4th Ed. J. & A. Churchill, London, 1968.
15. Dacie, J. V., and Worlledge, S. M.: Auto-immune hemolytic anemias. *In* Progress in Hematology, *6:*82, 1969.
16. Diamond, L. K., and Denton, R. L.: Rh agglutination in various media with particular reference to the value of albumin. J. Lab. Clin. Med., *30:*821, 1945.
17. Dupuy, M. E., Elliot, M., and Masouredis, S. P.: Relationship between red cell bound antibody and agglutination in the antiglobulin reaction. Vox. Sang., *9:*40, 1964.
18. Edelman, G. M.: Antibody structure and molecular immunology. Science, *180:*830, 1973.

19. Fraser, K. B.: The formation of antibody: A study of the relationship between a normal and an immune haemagglutinin. J. Path. Bact., *70:*13, 1955.
20. Fruitstone, M. J.: C3b-sensitized erythrocytes (Letter). Transfusion, *18:*125, 1978.
21. Garratty, G.: The effects of storage and heparin on the activity of serum complement, with particular reference to the detection of blood group antibodies. Am. J. Clin. Path., *54:*531, 1970.
22. Garratty, G., and Petz, L. D.: An evaluation of commercial antiglobulin sera with particular reference to their anticomplement properties. Transfusion, *11:*79, 1971.
23. Garratty, G., and Petz, L. D.: The investigation of drug-induced problems in the blood bank. American Association of Blood Banks, Washington, D.C., 1974, 19.
24. Garratty, G., and Petz, L. D.: The significance of red cell bound complement components in development of standards and quality assurance for the anticomplement components of antiglobulin sera. Transfusion, *16:*297, 1976.
25. Garratty, G., Petz, L. D., Brodsky, I., and Fudenberg, H. H.: An IgA high-titer cold agglutinin with an unusual blood group specificity within the Pr complex. Vox. Sang., *25:*32, 1973.
26. Hsu, T. C. S., Rosenfield, R. E., Burkhart, P., Wong, K. Y., and Kochwa, S.: Instrumented PVP-augmented antiglobulin tests. II. Evaluation of acquired hemolytic anemia. Vox. Sang., *26:*305, 1974.
27. Hughes-Jones, N. C., Gardner, B., and Telford, R.: Comparison of various methods of dissociation of anti-D, using I-labelled antibody. Vox. Sang., *8:*531, 1963.
28. Hughes-Jones, N. C., Polley, M. J., Telford, R., Gardner, B., and Kleinschmidt, G.: Optimal conditions for detecting blood group antibodies by the antiglobulin test. Vox. Sang., *9:*385, 1964.
29. Issitt, P. D., and Pavone, B. G.: Critical re-examination of the specificity of auto-anti-Rh antibodies in patients with a positive direct antiglobulin test. Brit. J. Haemat., *38:*63, 1978.
30. Issitt, P. D., Zellner, D. C., Rolih, S. D., and Duckett, J. B.: Autoantibodies mimicking alloantibodies. Transfusion, *17:*531, 1977.
31. Jandl, J. H., and Simmons, R. L.: The agglutination and sensitization of red cells by metallic cations: Interactions between multivalent metals and the red-cell membrane. Brit. J. Haemat., *3:*19, 1957.
32. Jenkins, D. E., Jr., and Moore, W. H.: A rapid method for the preparation of high potency auto and alloantibody eluates. Transfusion, *17:*110, 1977.
33. Kuhns, W. J., and Bailey, A.: Use of red cells modified by papain for detection of Rh antibodies. Am. J. Clin. Path., *20:*1067, 1950.
34. Lalezari, P.: Direct determination of red cell bound antibody specificity. Brit. J. Haemat., *24:*777, 1973.
35. Lalezari, P.: Serologic profile in autoimmune hemolytic disease: Pathophysiologic and clinical interpretations. Seminars Hemat., *31:*291, 1976.
36. Lalezari, P., and Berens, J. A.: Specificity and cross reactivity of cell-bound antibodies. *In:* Human Blood Groups, Proceedings of the 5th International Convocation of Immunology, Buffalo, N.Y., 1976, Mohn, J. F., Plunkett, R. W., Cunningham, R. K., and Lambert, R. M., Eds. New York: S. Karger, 1977, 44.
37. Lalezari, P., and Oberhardt, B.: Temperature gradient dissociation of red cell antigen-antibody complexes in the polybrene technique. Brit. J. Haemat., *21:*131, 1971.
38. Landsteiner, K., and Miller, C. P.: Serological studies on the blood of the primates. II. The blood groups in anthropoid apes. J. Exp. Med., *42:*853, 1925.
39. Longster, G. H., and Tovey, L. A. D.: The effects of certain blood-grouping sera on the red cell surface as seen by the scanning electron microscope. Brit. J. Haemat., *23:*635, 1972.
40. Loutit, J. F., and Mollison, P. L.: Haemolytic icterus (acholuric jaundice) congenital and acquired. J. Path. Bact., *58:*711, 1946.

41. Miller, W. V. (Ed.-in-Chief): Technical Manual. 7th Ed., American Association of Blood Banks, Washington, D.C., 1977.
42. Mollison, P. L.: Blood Transfusion in Clinical Medicine. 6th Ed. London, Blackwell Scientific Publications, 1979.
43. Morton, J. A., and Pickels, M. M.: The proteolytic enzyme test in the detection of incomplete antibodies. J. Clin. Path., *4:*189, 1951.
44. Nisonoff, A., Hopper, J. E., and Spring, S. B.: The Antibody Molecule. Dixon, F. J., Jr., and Kunkel, H. G., Eds. New York, Academic Press, 1975.
45. Oberhardt, B. J., and Miller, I. F.: Kinetic studies of a doubly bound red cell antigen-antibody system. Biophys. J., *12:*933, 1972.
46. Oberhardt, R. J., Lalezari, P., and Jiang, A. F.: A physicochemical approach to the characterization of red cell antigen-antibody systems. Immunol., *24:*445, 1973.
47. Petz, L. D., and Garratty, G.: Laboratory correlations in immune hemolytic anemias. *In* Laboratory Diagnosis of Immunologic Disorders. Vyas, G. N., Sites, D. P., and Brecher, G., Eds. New York, Grune & Stratton, 1975.
48. Petz, L. D., and Garratty, G.: Antiglobulin sera—Past, present and future. Transfusion, *18:*257, 1978.
49. Pirofsky, B., and Mangum, M. E. J.: Use of bromelin to demonstrate erythrocyte antibodies. Proc. Soc. Exp. Biol. (N.Y.), *101:*49, 1959.
50. Preston, F. W., and Parker, R. P.: New antiheparin agent (Polybrene): Effect in peptone shock and in experimental radiation injury. A.M.A. Arch. Surg., *66:*545, 1953.
51. Pollack, W., and Reckel, R. P.: A reappraisal of the forces involved in hemagglutination. Int. Archs. Allergy Appl. Immunol., *54:*29, 1977.
52. Pollack, W., Hager, H. J., Reckel, R., Toren, D. A., and Singher, H. O.: A study of the forces involved in the second stage of hemagglutination. Transfusion, *5:*158, 1965.
53. Rand, B. P., Olson, J. D., Garratty, G., and Petz, L. D.: Coombs negative immune hemolytic anemia with anti-E occurring in the red blood cell eluate of an E-negative patient. Transfusion, *18:*174, 1978.
54. Rausen, A. R., LeVine, R., Hsu, T. C. S., and Rosenfield, R. E.: Compatible transfusion therapy for paroxysmal cold hemoglobinuria. Pediatrics, *55:*275, 1975.
55. Roelcke, D.: Serological studies on the Pr_1/Pr_2 antigens using dog erythrocytes. Vox. Sang., *24:*354, 1973.
56. Roelcke, D.: Cold agglutination. Antibodies and antigens. Clin. Immunol. Immunopath., *2:*266, 1974.
57. Rosenfield, R. E., and Jagathambal: Transfusion therapy for autoimmune hemolytic anemia. Seminars Haemat., *13:*311, 1976.
58. Rubin, H.: Antibody elution from red blood cells. J. Clin. Path., *16:*70, 1963.
59. Salsbury, A. J., and Clarke, J. A.: Surface changes in red blood cells undergoing agglutination. Rev. Franc. Etudes. Clin. Et Biol., *12:*981, 1967.
60. Steane, E. A.: The physical chemistry of hemagglutination. *In* A Seminar on Polymorphisms in Human Blood, Washington, D. C., American Association of Blood Banks, 1975, 105–125.
61. Steane, E. A., and Greenwalt, T. J.: Red cell agglutination. *In:* Human Blood Groups, Proceedings of the 5th International Convocation of Immunology, Buffalo, N.Y., 1976, Mohn, J. F., Plunkett, R. W., Cunningham, R. K., and Lambert, R. M., Eds. New York: S. Karger, 1977, 36–43.
62. Stratton, F., Rawlinson, V. I., Chapman, S. A., Pengelly, C. D. R., and Jennings, R. C.: Acquired hemolytic anemia associated with IgA anti-e. Transfusion, *12:*157, 1972.
63. Stratton, F., and Renton, P. H.: Effect of crystalloid solutions prepared in glass bottles on human red cells. Nature (Lond.), *175:*727, 1955.

64. Stratton, F., Rawlinson, V. I., Gunson, H. H., and Phillips, P. K.: The role of Zeta potential in Rh agglutination. Vox. Sang., *24:*273, 1973.
65. Sturgeon, P., Smith, L. E., Chun, H. M. T., Hurvitz, C. H., Garratty, G., and Goldfinger, D.: Autoimmune hemolytic anemia associated exclusively with IgA of Rh specificity. Transfusion. *19:*324, 1979.
66. Van Oss, C. J., and Mohn, J. F.: Scanning electron microscopy of red cell agglutination. Vox. Sang., *19:*432, 1970.
67. Van Oss, C. J., Mohn, J. F., and Cunningham, R. K.: Influence of various physicochemical factors on hemagglutination. Vox. Sang., *34:*351, 1978.
68. Voak, D., Cawley, J. C., Emmines, J. P., and Barker, C. R.: The role of enzymes and albumin in haemagglutination reactions. A serological and ultrastructural study with ferritin-labelled anti-D. Vox. Sang., *27:*156, 1974.
69. Vos, G. H., Petz, L. D., Garratty, G., and Fudenberg, H. H.: Autoantibodies in acquired hemolytic anemia with special reference to the LW system. Blood, *42:*445, 1973.
70. Weiner, W., Gordon, E. G., and Rowe, D.: A Donath-Landsteiner antibody (nonsyphilitic type). Vox. Sang., *9:*684, 1964.
70a. Wenz, B., and Lalezari, P.: Methyldopa: physicochemical characterization of the erythrocyte autoantibody. Blood, 42, 247, 1973.
71. Wiener, A. S., and Katz, L. J.: Studies on the use of enzyme-treated red cells in tests for Rh sensitization. J. Immunol., *66:*51, 1951.
72. Winkelhake, J. L.: Immunoglobulin structure and effector functions. Immunochemistry, *15:*695, 1978.
73. Worlledge, S. M.: The interpretation of a positive direct antiglobulin test. Brit. J. Haemat., *39:*157, 1978.
74. Worlledge, S. M., and Blajchman, M. A.: The autoimmune haemolytic anemias. Brit. J. Haemat., *23:*61, 1972 (Suppl.).
75. Worlledge, S. M., and Rousso, C.: Studies on the serology of paroxysmal cold haemoglobinuria (PCH) with special reference to its relationship with the P blood group system. Vox. Sang., *10:*293, 1965.

6

Differential Diagnosis of Immune Hemolytic Anemias

As indicated in Chapter 1, the laboratory evaluation of a patient who has an acquired hemolytic anemia should include the performance of a direct antiglobulin test which, if positive, allows a presumptive diagnosis of an immune hemolytic anemia. The physician must then differentiate among the multiple causes of immune hemolytic anemia which are listed in Table 2-1, page 27.

We begin the discussion of the differential diagnosis by emphasizing distinctive clinical and laboratory findings. The approach to the laboratory diagnosis of each kind of AIHA includes a narrative overview that omits technical details but explains the significance of the results of the tests described in Chapter 5. Included with the description of the essential points in diagnosis is a more detailed presentation of laboratory results in patients with immune hemolytic anemias of various types, including summaries of data from our own series of patients. In this chapter, we include the more common, classic types of AIHA. Cases that are unusual, atypical, and more difficult to classify are described in Chapter 9.

DISTINCTIVE CLINICAL AND ROUTINE LABORATORY FEATURES

Some of the clinical and routine laboratory findings in patients with immune hemolytic anemias are sufficiently distinctive as to strongly suggest the type of immune hemolytic anemia that is present. The following observations merit particular emphasis because they are most helpful.

Association With Exposure to Cold

A history of acrocyanosis and hemoglobinuria on exposure to cold in a patient with an acquired hemolytic anemia strongly suggests a diagnosis of cold agglutinin syndrome. Paroxysmal cold hemoglobinuria is another possible, albeit much less common diagnosis. The age of the patient is quite important in the diagnosis since cold agglutinin syndrome occurs primarily in the elderly, and paroxysmal cold hemoglobinuria is most common in young children.

However, neither acrocyanosis nor hemoglobinuria may be present in patients with cold agglutinin syndrome, and indeed, we find that a majority of patients lack these symptoms. Perhaps this finding is due to the fact that the cold agglutinin syndrome was the last type of autoimmune hemolytic anemia to be well characterized, and, initially, only those patients with the most striking findings were so diagnosed. A review of earlier serologic studies supports this impression. In Dacie's series of 26 patients, all but 2 had cold agglutinin titers of 4,000 or greater,[6] whereas in our present series, a majority of patients had a cold agglutinin titer of 1,000 or less (see page 223).

Association With Atypical Pneumonia

If a patient with autoimmune hemolytic anemia is convalescing from a pneumonia that satisfies the criteria for a diagnosis of "primary atypical pneumonia," and particularly if *Mycoplasma pneumoniae* can be identified as the causative agent, the cold agglutinin syndrome must be strongly suspected. Except for one case of paroxysmal cold hemoglobinuria,[1] all recorded cases of AIHA in association with *Mycoplasma pneumoniae* pneumonitis have been cold agglutinin syndrome.

Autoagglutination

Autoagglutination is a finding that should be noted by technologists in all sections of the laboratory, not just those in the blood transfusion or immunohematology laboratories. Indeed, cold agglutinins that react strongly at room temperature cause such striking findings that they are difficult to ignore. Autoagglutination visible to the naked eye occurring at room temperature is frequently found in patients with cold antibody AIHA. The autoagglutination caused by cold agglutinins is frequently very coarse (2+ to 3+) and almost always completely disperses after a few minutes of incubation at 37°C (Figure 6-1), whereas that caused by warm autoantibodies is much finer and will not disperse at 37°C. If the blood sample has been obtained from a patient known to have hemolytic anemia, such simple findings offer a clue to the correct diagnosis. However, the presence of cold agglutinins reactive at room temperature should not be over-interpreted, since many of these antibodies are clinically benign, albeit somewhat of a nuisance in the laboratory. The criteria for distinguishing clinically benign cold agglutinin from those pathologic cold agglutinin capable of causing cold agglutinin syndrome are discussed on page 213.

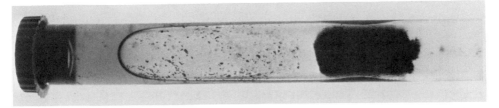

Figure 6-1. An anticoagulated blood sample from a patient with cold agglutinin syndrome. The cold agglutinin reacted to a titer of 2048 at 4°C and 512 at 20°C in saline. The figure shows a huge mass of agglutinated red cells in an anticoagulated blood sample that had been placed at 4°C. Such agglutination is often mistaken for a clot. However agglutination completely disperses after incubation at 37°C for 5 to 10 minutes.

Acute Intravascular Hemolysis in a Child

Many cases of paroxysmal cold hemoglobinuria reported in the recent medical literature have a characteristic clinical setting. The diagnosis should be suspected and a Donath-Landsteiner test performed whenever a child develops an acute hemolytic anemia with hemoglobinemia, hemoglobinuria, and severe anemia following a flu-like syndrome or other virus infection. Even in this setting, however, it should be emphasized that warm antibody AIHA is more frequently the diagnosis since it, too, occurs after viral syndromes and is far more common than paroxysmal cold hemoglobinuria.

Drug Ingestion

A history of drug ingestion may suggest the etiology of a patient's immune hemolytic anemia. Drug-induced autoimmune hemolytic anemia occurs in a small percentage of patients taking methyldopa (Aldomet, Aldoril, Aldoclor), and it is serologically indistinguishable from other warm antibody autoimmune hemolytic anemias. Other drugs that are well documented but much less frequent causes of autoimmune hemolytic anemia are L-dopa and mefenamic acid. These drugs have only been reported to cause warm antibody autoimmune hemolytic anemia. Other drug-induced immune hemolytic anemias can be distinguished from autoimmune hemolytic anemias by laboratory findings (see Chapter 8).

Alloantibody Induced Immune Hemolytic Anemia

Hemolytic disease of the newborn and hemolytic transfusion reactions occur in such distinctive clinical settings as to ordinarily make the diagnosis obvious. Even here, however, one must be aware of the fact that hemolytic disease of the newborn may occur as a result of maternal autoimmune hemolytic anemia caused by transplacental passage of the mother's IgG warm autoantibody, and that the differential diagnosis of a delayed hemolytic transfusion reaction and AIHA is difficult on occasion.[5, 40] These diagnoses are discussed further in Chapter 9.

LABORATORY DIAGNOSIS OF IMMUNE HEMOLYTIC ANEMIAS

Even in the presence of valuable clinical clues that may suggest a specific diagnosis, the confirmation of the precise diagnosis of the type of immune hemolytic anemia present depends on the laboratory. The serologic tests to be performed determine whether the patient's red cells are coated with immunoglobulin G (IgG), complement components, or both, and whether the red cells are weakly or strongly sensitized. The performance of the direct antiglobulin test supplies such information. Further tests must be performed to determine the characteristics of the antibodies in the patient's serum and in an eluate from his red cells.

The Significance of the Direct Antiglobulin Test in the Differential Diagnosis of Immune Hemolytic Anemias

The direct antiglobulin test utilizing polyspecific and monospecific antiglobulin reagents provides useful information in the evaluation of a patient with immune hemolytic anemia. However, the results must always be interpreted in conjunction with clinical and other laboratory data to avoid erroneous conclusions. As previously indicated (Chapter 5), a positive direct antiglobulin test occurs in situations other than immune hemolytic anemias. A positive direct antiglobulin test does not necessarily indicate the presence of autoantibody; furthermore, even if autoantibody is present, the patient may or may not have a hemolytic anemia. Thus, an independent assessment must be made to determine the presence or absence of hemolytic anemia, and the role of the direct antiglobulin test is to aid in the evaluation of the etiology of hemolysis when present.

Numerous complexities may be considered regarding the direct antiglobulin test, and highly detailed classifications of AIHA have been based on direct antiglobulin test results.[16, 17, 22] However, we believe that excessively detailed testing adds little to a clinically significant classification of immune hemolytic anemia. This belief is valid because prognosis and appropriate therapy cannot be correlated with classifications based on the results of the direct antiglobulin test even when it is performed with a large battery of antisera to immunoglobulins and complement components. Further, only a limited variety of monospecific antisera standardized for the antiglobulin test are readily available from commercial sources.

The following discussion begins with a consideration of the most important aspects of the interpretation of the direct antiglobulin test using antisera that are standardized for antiglobulin testing and that are commercially available in the United States. We then discuss additional aspects that are of significance less often and that may require special antisera (e.g., anti-IgA, anti-IgM).

Results Using Polyspecific and Monospecific Antiglobulin Reagents. It is convenient to first perform the direct antiglobulin test with a "polyspecific" antiglobulin serum, which is defined by the Bureau of Biologics of the United States Food and Drug Administration as one which must contain anti-IgG and anti-C3d and may contain antibodies of other specificities.[29] A positive result in a patient with acquired hemolytic anemia almost always indicates that the patient's red cells are coated with IgG, C3d, or both.

Using monospecific anti-IgG and anti-C3 sera, it is then a simple matter to determine which of these two proteins are coating the patient's red cells. The anti-C3 antiserum used in all direct antiglobulin tests must contain antibodies to C3d and may contain antibodies to other antigenic determinants on the C3 molecule. The significance of such results is outlined in Table 6-1 and may be described in more detail as follows.

In warm antibody AIHA, there is no diagnostic pattern of antiglobulin test reactivity. Most commonly positive reactions are obtained both with anti-IgG and anti-C3 antisera, but in a minority of cases, only IgG or C3 is found on the patient's red cells.

In contrast to the variable findings in warm antibody AIHA, the direct antiglobulin test in cold agglutinin syndrome is invariably positive when utilizing anti-C3 antiserum. Equally important is the fact that reactions are also invariably negative with anti-IgG antiserum; that is, a positive direct antiglobulin test with anti-IgG excludes cold agglutinin syndrome as the sole diagnosis (Table 6-2).

Paroxysmal cold hemoglobinuria [30] is caused by an IgG complement fixing antibody but, nevertheless, the direct antiglobulin test is usually positive only with anti-C3 antiserum (Table 6-2). The reactions may be only weakly positive, even during episodes of acute hemolysis. Negative reactions with anti-IgG antisera are probably caused by the fact that the Donath-Landsteiner antibody readily elutes from the red cell membrane during *in vitro* washing, whereas complement components remain fixed to the cell membrane. Dacie and Worlledge [7] report that if the patient's red cells are washed in saline at 10°C or below, the direct antiglobulin test may be positive using anti-IgG antisera as well as anti-C3. The direct antiglobulin test may be expected to be positive at the time of a paroxysm of hemoglobinuria and for a variable number of days thereafter.[7]

Methyldopa- and penicillin-induced immune hemolytic anemias are the most common causes of drug-induced immune hemolytic anemia, and the direct antiglobulin test in both instances is characteristically strongly positive with anti-IgG and is negative with anti-C3. Although this remains the most

Table 6-1. DIRECT ANTIGLOBULIN TEST RESULTS IN IMMUNE HEMOLYTIC ANEMIAS USING ANTI-IgG AND ANTI-C3 ANTISERA

	IgG	C3 *
Warm antibody AIHA		
(67%)	+	+
(20%)	+	0
(13%)	0	+
Cold agglutinin syndrome	0	+
Paroxysmal cold hemoglobinuria	0	+
Penicillin or methyldopa-induced †	+	0
Other drug-induced immune hemolytic anemias ‡	0	+
Warm antibody AIHA associated with systemic lupus erythematosus	+	+

* Such cells are primarily sensitized with the C3d component of C3 (see text).
† Weakly positive reactions with anti-C3 may occur; invariably, reactions are strongly positive with anti-IgG.
‡ The most common pattern of red cell sensitization is indicated, but occasionally IgG may be detected with or without C3 (see Chapter 8).

Table 6-2. DIRECT ANTIGLOBULIN TEST RESULTS IN COLD ANTIBODY HEMOLYTIC ANEMIAS USING ANTI-IgG AND ANTI-C3 ANTISERA

Cold Agglutinin Syndrome (54 Patients)	
IgG (no C3)	0%
IgG + C3	1.8%*
C3 (no IgG)	98.2%

* 1 patient who was receiving Aldomet

Paroxysmal Cold Hemoglobinuria (6 Patients)	
IgG (no C3)	0%
IgG + C3	0%
C3 (no IgG)	100%

common pattern of antiglobulin test reactivity, there are an increasing number of reports of the sensitization of red cells with complement components in penicillin-induced immune hemolytic anemia, and this trend agrees with our more recent experience (Table 6-3). The strength of the positive direct antiglobulin test using anti-C3d antiserum in all patients with methyldopa-induced immune hemolytic anemia was very weak and of questionable pathogenetic significance. The results in penicillin-induced hemolytic anemias were somewhat stronger, but in only 1 patient was the result stronger than 2+ (Table 6-4).

Table 6-3. DIRECT ANTIGLOBULIN TEST RESULTS IN PENICILLIN AND METHYLDOPA INDUCED IMMUNE HEMOLYTIC ANEMIAS USING ANTI-IgG AND ANTI-C3 ANTIGLOBULIN SERA

	IgG (no C3)	IgG + C3	C3 (no IgG)
Methyldopa (29 Patients)	82.8%	17.2%	0%
Penicillin (10 Patients)	60%	40%	0%

Table 6-4. STRENGTH OF DIRECT ANTI-GLOBULIN TEST RESULTS USING ANTI-C3 ANTIGLOBULIN SERUM IN IMMUNE HEMOLYTIC ANEMIAS CAUSED BY PENICILLIN OR METHYLDOPA

	Penicillin (10)	Methyldopa (29)
½ – 1+	0	5
1½ – 2+	3	0
2½ – 3+	1*	0
3½ – 4+	0	0
	4/10 = 40%	5/29 = 17.2%

* Reported as unique case showing *in vivo* intravascular hemolysis.[30]

The direct antiglobulin test in patients with hemolytic anemias caused by drugs other than methyldopa or penicillin is usually positive only with anti-C3, and the reactions are often only weakly positive. In some instances the drug-related antibody is of the IgM class, and in other cases the antibody (which may be IgG or part of an immune complex) apparently elutes from the red cell after fixing complement, or it is present on the red blood cell in concentrations too low to be detectable by the antiglobulin test. In a minority of patients, the direct antiglobulin test is positive using anti-IgG antiglobulin serum.

Systemic lupus erythematosus deserves particular consideration, since many patients with this disorder have C3 on their red cell even at times when no evidence of hemolysis exists. When patients with systemic lupus erythematosus do develop AIHA, their red cells are regularly coated with C3 and IgG. Indeed, Chaplin and Avioli report that only one or two patients with systemic lupus erythematosus and AIHA have been described in the literature as having only IgG on their red blood cells.[4]

One point that is evident from the preceding discussion but that must be emphasized is that the performance of the direct antiglobulin test with an antiglobulin serum that does not contain anti-C3d antibodies will frequently result in misleadingly negative results in patients with immune hemolytic anemias. This finding is true in all patients with cold agglutinin syndrome, 13 percent of patients with warm antibody AIHA, and essentially all patients with paroxysmal cold hemoglobinuria or drug-induced immune hemolytic anemia caused by drugs other than methyldopa or penicillin. Altogether, 26 percent of the patients in our series had positive direct antiglobulin tests caused only by complement sensitization of the red cells (Table 6-5). Other reported series of patients with autoimmune hemolytic anemias in which detailed antiglobulin testing was performed yielded comparable information. Indeed, Dacie and Worlledge [7] reported that 33 percent of 29 patients with autoimmune hemolytic anemia had red cells sensitized only with complement components.

Table 6-5. RESULTS OF DIRECT ANTI-GLOBULIN TEST WITH ANTI-IgG AND ANTI-C3 IN 347 PATIENTS WITH AIHA AND DRUG-INDUCED IMMUNE HEMOLYTIC ANEMIAS

	Percent*	
IgG (no C3)	23	73% have IgG on RBC
IgG + C3	50	76.4% have C3 on RBC
C3 (no IgG)	26.4	

* Two patients (0.6%) had only IgA present on their red blood cells.

Some immune hemolytic anemias are caused by immune globulins other than IgG. However, IgM sensitization of red blood cells is difficult to detect with the antiglobulin test,[14, 21, 36] and furthermore, IgM antibodies that cause immune hemolytic anemia characteristically, if not invariably,[11, 25] fix complement that is much more readily detected. IgA antibodies only infrequently play a role in red blood cell sensitization, and in such cases other immune globulins and/or complement components are almost always, although not invariably[3, 7, 18, 35, 36a, 41] found on the cell surface as well. Indeed, several percent of the patients with warm antibody AIHA have a direct antiglobulin test that is positive only with anti-IgA antisera.[41] Interested workers may wish to standardize anti-IgM and anti-IgA antisera for use in the antiglobulin test as described in Chapter 5.

In regard to antibodies against other complement components in anti-globulin serum, we have occasionally found patients whose red blood cells are sensitized with C4d but not C3d. However, none of these patients has had hemolytic anemia.[13, 27] Patients with immune hemolytic anemia frequently have C4d on their red blood cells in addition to C3d, but in testing literally hundreds of patients with acquired immune hemolytic anemia, we have not observed a single patient with hemolysis whose red blood cells had C4d but not C3d.[13] We know of no experience contrary to this in the literature. Therefore, anti-C4 antibodies appear to be superfluous in antiglobulin serum used for detection and differential diagnosis of immune hemolytic anemia. Similarly, although with less extensive data available, antibodies to other complement components in antiglobulin serum (C5, C6, C8) have not proven to be of significant clinical value.[13, 23]

Using anti-C4 antiglobulin sera, Stratton[34] demonstrated positive reactions in several patients with hereditary angioedema. This is not a consistent finding since we have obtained negative results in the several patients with this disorder that we have tested. The diagnosis of hereditary angioedema should be made on the basis of abnormalities in serum complement components (Chapter 3), and we do not recommend the antiglobulin test for this purpose.

We have performed the direct antiglobulin test with anti-IgG, -IgM, -IgA, and -C3 antisera in 104 of our patients with warm antibody AIHA. Although a wide variety of positive reactions was obtained (Table 6-6), such detailed

Table 6-6 DIRECT ANTIGLOBULIN TEST RESULTS IN 104 PATIENTS WITH WARM ANTIBODY AIHA USING SEVERAL MONOSPECIFIC ANTIGLOBULIN SERA

	Percentage
IgG only	18.3
C3 only	10.6
IgA only	1.9
IgM only *	0
IgG & C3	46.2
IgG & C3 & IgA	12.5
IgG & C3 & IgA & IgM	1.9
IgG & IgA	2.9
IgG & IgM	0
IgG & IgM & C3	3.9
IgG & IgA & IgM	0
C3 & IgA	1.9
C3 & IgM	1.9
IgG present alone or together with other proteins	85.6
C3 present alone or together with other proteins	78.9
IgA present alone or together with other proteins	21.2
IgM present alone or together with other proteins	7.7

* C3 is always present when IgM is present.

testing proved to be of little clinical value, and we do not recommend the routine performance of the direct antiglobulin test with monospecific antiglobulin sera other than anti-IgG and anti-C3.

Antiglobulin Test Titrations and Scores. It is useful to perform titrations of the monospecific antiglobulin reagents against antiglobulin test positive red cells in order to more accurately assess the relative strength of the reactions. For anti-IgG antisera, the use of doubling dilutions from 1:1 to 1:1024 is usually adequate. For anti-C3, doubling dilutions from 1:1 to 1:128 are usually optimal, although other dilutions may be chosen depending on the potency of the individual antiserum. Our experience indicates that commercially available monospecific antiglobulin reagents are suitable for this purpose. We make the dilutions in normal saline.

The strength of agglutination resulting with each dilution of the antiglobulin sera may then be used to develop an antiglobulin test titration score as discussed in Chapter 5. Scores are of value in more accurately assessing the strength of the antiglobulin test than is possible by the use of only a single dilution of antiglobulin serum.

Since the titration score obtained is arbitrary and is dependent on the antiglobulin serum utilized, each laboratory will need to develop experience in order to be able to recognize the range of scores that occur with the antisera used and then arbitrarily divide them into categories such as weak, moderate, strong, and very strong. Even before gaining experience on red blood cell samples from patients, a few simple experiments will be useful in devising such standards. Rh_0 (D) positive red cells may be sensitized with decreasing dilutions of a strong anti-D (e.g., commercial anti-D typing serum) and the range of scores obtained with various sensitized cells can serve as a useful basis for comparisons with results in patients. Similar experiments can be performed with complement sensitized red cells that may be obtained from patients with AIHA or prepared as described in Chapter 5. The results of some experiments of this type are listed in Table 6-7.

The relationship between antiglobulin test titration scores and quantitative measurements of red cell sensitization was particularly emphasized by the data of Fischer, Petz, Garratty, and Cooper regarding red cells sensitized with C3.[10] These investigators used an immunochemical method to quantitate the number of C3 molecules bound to human red cells *in vitro* or *in vivo*, and they compared these results with the antiglobulin test and the antiglobulin test titration score. The antiglobulin test using anti-C3 antiglobulin serum became weakly positive with 60 to 115 molecules of C3 per red cell, and it was strongly positive with 1,000 molecules of C3 per red cell. As illustrated in Figures 6-2 and 6-3, a wide range of cell bound C3 molecules may result in a 2+ to 4+ direct antiglobulin test using a single dilution of antiglobulin serum. In contrast are the data illustrated in Figures 6-4 and 6-5, which indicate that antiglobulin test scores correlated quite well with the immunochemical assessment of the number of molecules per red cell.

There is also a good correlation between the antiglobulin test titration

Table 6-7. COMPARISON OF COMMERCIAL MONOSPECIFIC ANTIGLOBULIN REAGENTS WITH REAGENTS MADE IN OUR LABORATORY IN ANTIGLOBULIN TEST TITRATIONS

Reciprocal of Dilutions of Anti-IgG Antiglobulin Serum	1	2	4	8	16	32	64	128	256	512	1024
				Red Cells Moderately Sensitized With Anti-Rh$_0$(D) In Vitro							
Commercial Serum A	3+	3+	3+	1½+	1+	½+	0	0	0	0	0
Commercial Serum B	2½+	3+	3+	2+	2+	1+	½+	0	0	0	0
Our Antiserum *	3+	3+	3+	1½+	1+	½+	0	0	0	0	0

Reciprocal of Dilutions of Anti-IgG Antiglobulin Serum	1	2	4	8	16	32	64	128	256	512	1024
				Red Cells From a Patient With Warm Antibody AIHA							
Commercial Serum A	4+	4+	4+	3+	2+	1½+	1½+	1½+	1½+	1+	0
Commercial Serum B	3½+	4+	4+	4+	3+	2½+	1½+	1½+	1+	1+	0
Our Antiserum*	4+	3+	3+	2½+	2½+	2+	1+	1+	½+	0	0

Reciprocal of Dilutions of Anti-C3 Antiglobulin Serum	1	2	4	8	16	32	64	128	256	512	1024
				Red Cells Sensitized In Vitro With C3d							
Commercial Serum A	4+	4+	4+	3+	3+	2+	1+	1+	0	0	0
Our Antiserum**	4+	4+	4+	4+	3+	3+	2+	1+	0	0	0

Reciprocal of Dilutions of Anti-C3 Antiglobulin Serum	1	2	4	8	16	32	64	128	256	512	1024
				Red Cells From a Patient With Cold Agglutinin Syndrome							
Commercial Serum A	3+	3+	3+	2+	1½+	½+	0	0	0	0	0
Our Antiserum **	3+	3+	2½+	2½+	2+	2+	1+	0	0	0	0

Agglutination reactions are graded as ½+ to 4+. * The initial dilution of our anti-IgG serum is 1:64 which was previously determined to be optimal by "checkerboard" titrations (see Chapter 5). ** The initial dilution of our anti-C3 serum is 1:4 which was previously determined to be optimal by "checkerboard" titrations (see Ch. 5).

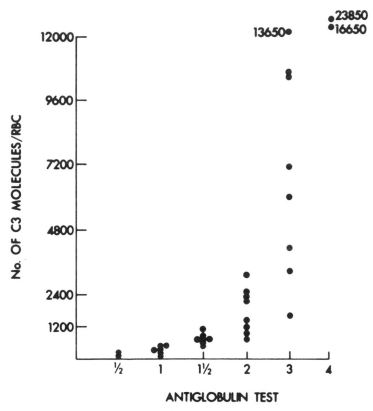

Figure 6-2. *The relationship between the number of C3 molecules per red cell and the antiglobulin test using a single dilution of anti-C3 antiserum. C3-sensitized red cells were prepared in vitro using Le*[a] *antibody in varying dilutions. (Fischer, J. T., Petz, L. D., Garratty, G., and Cooper, N. R.: Correlations between quantitative assay of red-cell bound C3, serologic reactions, and hemolytic anemia. Blood, 44:359, 1974.)*

scores and quantitative measurements of red cell bound IgG with red cells sensitized with less than 1,000 molecules of IgG per RBC as is illustrated in Figure 6-6.[28] Thus, a simple extension of the routine antiglobulin test affords useful data concerning the relative degree of sensitization of red cells by IgG or C3 without the necessity of performing sophisticated quantitative measurements.

Antiglobulin test titration scores are of significance in various ways in evaluating patients with AIHA, but, on the other hand, their significance must not be exaggerated. Although Rosse [32, 33] demonstrated that the amount of antibody detected on the red cell membrane was generally proportional to the rate of red cell destruction, exceptions to this correlation are frequent. Indeed, in an individual patient, it is impossible to state with certainty whether or not red cell life span is normal or is shortened on the basis of the direct antiglobulin test titration scores or other more quantitative measures of red cell bound IgG. This indicates that the *in vivo* significance of a given degree of red cell sensitization by autoantibodies varies greatly, even among antibodies of the same immunoglobulin class. Table 6-8 illustrates this point well since patient P.Y. had a high score but had no evidence of *in vivo* hemolysis, whereas patient M.W. had overt hemolytic anemia even though having a much lower score. The fact that only a small number of IgG molecules on the surface of red cells can cause clinically important hemolysis is most strikingly indicated by cases of AIHA in which the direct antiglobulin test is negative and the red cell sensitization is detectable only by the use of more sensitive techniques (Chapter 9). Thus, as a general rule, one does *not* use the strength of the direct antiglobulin test or the titration score to determine the presence or absence of hemolysis.

However, there are some exceptions to this rule and, with certain test results, tentative conclusions can be reached with a high degree of probability. For example, we find that very high direct antiglobulin test titers and titration

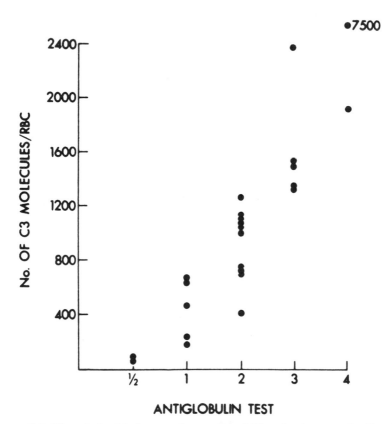

Figure 6-3. *The relationship between the number of C3 molecules per red cell and the antiglobulin test using a single dilution of anti-C3 antiserum. C3-sensitized cells were obtained from patients having a positive antiglobulin test caused at least in part by red cell sensitization by C3. (Fischer, J. T., Petz, L. D., Garratty, G., and Cooper, N. R.: Correlations between quantitative assay of red-cell bound C3, serologic reactions, and hemolytic anemia. Blood, 44:359, 1974.)*

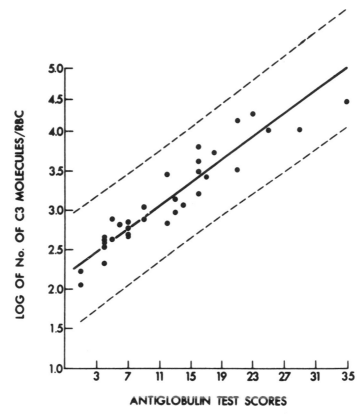

Figure 6-4. *Correlation between antiglobulin titration scores and the quantitative assay of cell-bound C3 (in vitro sensitized cells). The linear regression coefficient with 95 percent confidence limits is 0.071 ± 0.005. The coefficient of correlation by linear regression (r) = 0.83, significant at the 1 percent level. (Fischer, J. T., Petz, L. D., Garratty, G., and Cooper, N. R.: Correlations between quantitative assay of red-cell bound C3, serologic reactions, and hemolytic anemia. Blood, 44:359, 1974.)*

Table 6-8. ANTIGLOBULIN TEST TITRATIONS IN TWO PATIENTS
(Patient P.Y. had no evidence of hemolysis, whereas patient M.W. had overt hemolytic anemia.)

Reciprocal of Dilutions of our Anti-IgG Anti-globulin Serum	128	256	512	1024	2048	4096	Score
Patient P.Y.	4+	4+	4+	3+	1+	0	42
Patient M.W.	2+	1+	½+	0	0	0	13

Agglutination reactions are graded as ½+ to 4+.

scores merit immediate attention because of a high probability of the presence of AIHA. Using our anti-IgG antiglobulin sera, a titer of greater than 1,000 is frequently associated with clinical evidence of hemolysis. The most common exceptions to this rule occur in patients taking methyldopa who may have red cells heavily coated with IgG without having *in vivo* hemolysis.

In regard to the clinical significance of cell bound C3, Fischer, Petz, Garratty, and Cooper [10] obtained red cells from 25 consecutive patients discovered to have a positive direct antiglobulin test that was caused at least in part by red cell sensitization by C3. Only 2 of 14 patients with less than 1,100 molecules of C3 per red cell had hemolytic anemia, whereas 8 of 11 patients with at least 1,100 molecules of C3 per red cell did have overt hemolysis. The presence or absence of hemolysis was not explained by variations in the amount of IgG on these patients' red cells as assessed by the antiglobulin test using monospecific anti-IgG antisera (Table 6-9). This finding is well illustrated by patients 17, 19 and 23 to 25, who had hemolytic anemia without IgG

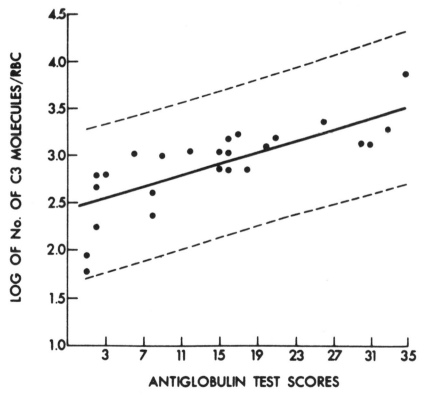

Figure 6-5. *Correlation between antiglobulin titration scores and the quantitative assay of cell bound C3 (cells sensitized in vivo). The linear regression coefficient with 95 percent confidence limits is 0.031 ± 0.012. The coefficient of correlation by linear regression (r) = 0.66, significant at the 1 percent level. (Fischer, J. T., Petz, L. D., Garratty, G., and Cooper, N. R.: Correlations between quantitative assay of red-cell bound C3, serologic reactions, and hemolytic anemia. Blood, 44:359, 1974.)*

on their red cells detectable by the antiglobulin test, in comparison with patients 5, 20, and 21, who did not have hemolytic anemia but had a strongly positive antiglobulin test using anti-IgG antisera.

Experiments by Logue et al.[24] further indicated that the *in vivo* significance of complement sensitization of red cells is related to the rate of addition of C3 to the membrane. When patients with cold agglutinin syndrome were subjected to acute cold stress, cell bound C3 rose abruptly and intravascular hemolysis occurred. Thus, although other studies have emphasized the role of red cell sensitization by IgG in relationship to red cell survival,[32, 33] it appears that C3 sensitization is an additional important determinant of hemolysis in human immune hemolytic anemias. The significance of red cell sensitization by complement components in regard to the mechanism of immune hemolysis is discussed in more detail in Chapter 4.

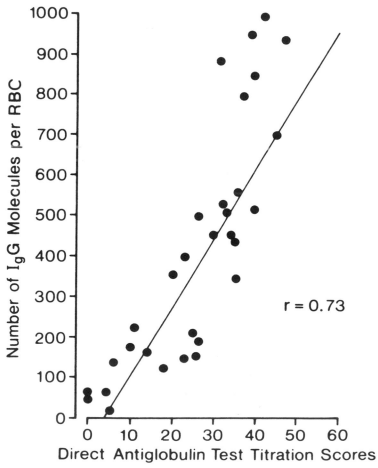

Figure 6-6. *Correlation between antiglobulin test titration scores and a quantitative immunochemical assay of red cell bound IgG.*

Table 6-9. RESULTS OF ASSAYS OF RED CELL-BOUND C3 IN 25 PATIENTS AND CORRELATION WITH CLINICAL AND SEROLOGIC DATA

Disease	Anti-C3 Antiglobulin Test (½+ to 4+)	No. C3 Molecules per Red Cell	Anti-C3 Antiglobulin Titration Score	Hemolytic Anemia	PCV	Hgb	Retic-ulocytes (%)	Anti-IgG Antiglobulin Test (½+ to 4+)
1 Systemic lupus erythematosus	½	60	1	No	41.7	14.8	–	1
2 Iron deficiency anemia	½	90	1	No	21.1	7.0	3	Neg.
3 Normal	1	180	2	No	39.8	14.0	–	Neg.
4 Systemic lupus	1	235	8	Yes	30.2	10.4	4.8	1
5 Hypertension	2	410	7	No	44.4	15.8	–	3
6 Drug-immune hemolysis (Aldomet)	1	465	2	Yes	37.5	12.6	3.1	4
7 Normal	1	625	2	No	42.0	–	–	Neg.
8 Systemic lupus erythematosus	1	630	3	No	41.5	13.4	–	Neg.
9 Vasculitis	2	700	16	No	40.0	14.1	2	Neg.
10 Systemic lupus erythematosus	2	720	18	No	44.0	14.7	–	2
11 Systemic lupus erythematosus	2	735	15	No	42.2	14.3	–	2
12 Systemic lupus erythematosus	2	1010	8	No	41.7	14.8	–	Neg.

Table 6-9. (CONTINUED)

Disease	Anti-C3 Antiglobulin Test (½+ to 4+)	No. C3 Molecules per Red Cell	Anti-C3 Antiglobulin Titration Score	Hemolytic Anemia	PCV	Hgb	Retic- ulocytes (%)	Anti-IgG Antiglobulin Test (½+ to 4+)
13 Autoimmune hemolytic anemia (warm antibody) (post-splenectomy)	2	1050	6	No	42.0	13.2	–	2
14 Chronic active hepatitis	2	1075	15	No	40.1	13.3	–	2
15 Drug-immune hemolysis (penicil- lin)	2	1100	16	Yes	11.0	3.6	26	2
16 Acute lymphatic leukemia	2	1125	11	Yes	17.0	4.5	0.3 *	3
17 Paroxysmal cold hemoglobinuria	3	1260	21	Yes	35.0	11.2	6.3	Neg.
18 Systemic lupus erythematosus	3	1335	30	No	26.7	8.5	2.1	1

19	Autoimmune hemolytic anemia (warm antibody)	3	1340	31	Yes	31.0	9.3	10.2	Neg.
20	Rheumatoid arthritis	3	1510	15	No+	34.0	10.0	2.0	3
21	Systemic lupus erythematosus	3	1560	21	No	38.0	12.9	0.8	4
22	Autoimmune hemolytic anemia (warm antibody)	2	1710	16	Yes	33.0	10.7	1.5	1
23	Cold agglutinin disease	4	1910	33	Yes	24.0	7.8	9.2	Neg.
24	Cold agglutinin disease	3	2375	19	Yes	20.5	7.1	4.4	Neg.
25	Cold agglutinin disease	4	7500	35	Yes	22.4	7.8	11.6	Neg.

* Hemolysis was present as indicated by an excessive transfusion requirement without evidence of blood loss. The patient's low reticulocyte response was presumably related to his acute leukemia.

† More recently this patient developed overt hemolytic anemia with the hematocrit level falling to as low as 10 percent and the reticulocytes increasing to a maximum of 30 percent.

(Fischer, J. T., Petz, L. D., Garratty, G., and Cooper, N. R.: Correlations between quantitative assay of red-cell bound C3, serologic reactions, and hemolytic anemia. Blood, 44:359, 1974.)

Another situation in which titers and scores are of some value is in follow-up of an individual patient during the response to therapy. Regardless of the strength of the antiglobulin test on presentation, remission of AIHA is frequently associated with a significant decrease in the strength of the antiglobulin test, as is illustrated in Table 6-10. In this table red cells from a patient with warm antibody AIHA in relapse gave a 4+ reaction with a 1:128 dilution of our anti-IgG antiglobulin serum, and red cells from the same patient in remission gave a 3+ reaction. Although the difference between a 4+ and 3+ reaction is unimpressive, the titration scores performed on red cells obtained while the patient was in remission indicated a markedly reduced value. Indeed, it is common for the direct antiglobulin test to remain positive in AIHA, even when the patient is in complete remission as assessed by other laboratory findings. The fact that the direct antiglobulin test score is often markedly reduced during remission is frequently missed. Chaplin has reported similar observations.[3, 4]

Patients with methyldopa-induced AIHA have direct antiglobulin test titers and scores that are quite characteristic. That is, the red cells are very heavily sensitized with IgG. Using anti-C3 antiglobulin serum, the results are generally negative, although very weakly positive reactions (1+ or weaker) were obtained in 17 percent of the patients in our series.

In 100 percent of the patients in our series with methyldopa-induced immune hemolytic anemia, the titer using anti-IgG was 1,000 or greater, and in 63 percent of the patients the titer was 2,000 or greater. In contrast, with warm antibody AIHA not associated with the administration of methyldopa the direct antiglobulin test was positive to a titer of 2,000 or more with anti-IgG and negative with anti-C3 in only 9.9 percent of the patients. Thus, the direct antiglobulin test titer and titration score may lead to a suspicion of methyldopa-induced hemolytic anemia (strong sensitization with IgG, negative with anti-C3), or may essentially exclude the diagnosis (negative or weak sensitization with IgG and/or strong sensitization with C3). Table 6-11 illustrates direct antiglobulin test titration scores in patients with warm antibody AIHA caused by methyldopa and in those cases not associated with methyldopa administration.

Table 6-10. ANTIGLOBULIN TEST TITRATIONS IN A PATIENT WITH WARM ANTI-BODY AUTOIMMUNE HEMOLYTIC ANEMIA IN RELAPSE AND AFTER REMISSION INDUCED BY CORTICOSTEROID THERAPY

Reciprocals of Dilutions of our Anti-IgG Antiglobulin Serum	128	256	512	1024	2048	4096	Score
Relapse	4+	4+	4+	3+	2+	1+	48
Remission	3+	2+	1+	0	0	0	18

Agglutination reactions are graded as ½+ to 4+.

Data reported by Dacie and Worlledge [7] and Worlledge [39] also indicate that patients receiving methyldopa only develop hemolytic anemia when the direct antiglobulin test is strongly positive using anti-IgG antiglobulin serum. Although others have reported a small number of patients with positive tests using anticomplement reagents,[9] Worlledge [39] reported that only 2 patients out of more than 80 who were thought to have methyldopa-induced hemolysis had positive reactions with anti-C3 as well as with anti-IgG. Both

Table 6-11. DIRECT ANTIGLOBULIN TEST TITRATIONS IN PATIENTS WITH METHYLDOPA INDUCED AIHA AND IN WARM ANTIBODY AIHA NOT ASSOCIATED WITH METHYLDOPA ADMINISTRATION

Maximum Dilution of Anti-IgG Giving 1+ Agglutination	Warm antibody AIHA Not Caused by Methyldopa							
	<1,000	1,000	2,000	4,000	8,000	16,000	32,000	64,000
Number of Patients with Direct Antiglobulin Test Positive with Anti-IgG Only	10	10	4	11	7	1	0	0
Number of Patients with Direct Antiglobulin Test Positive with Anti-IgG and Anti-C3	45	40	29	21	18	3	1	1
Dilutions of Anti-C3	**4**	**8**	**16**	**32**	**64**	**128**		
Number of Patients with Direct Antiglobulin Test Positive Only with Anti-C3	1	2	6	10	10	3		

Maximum Dilution of Anti-IgG Giving 1+ Agglutination	AIHA Caused by Methyldopa *							
	<1,000	1,000	2,000	4,000	8,000	16,000	32,000	64,000
Number of Patients with Direct Antiglobulin Test Positive with Anti-IgG Only	0	9	5	4	3	2	0	1
Number of Patients with direct Antiglobulin Test Positive with Anti-IgG and Anti-C3	0	0	2	0	3	0	0	0

* No patients with methyldopa-induced hemolytic anemia had a direct antiglobulin test that was positive only with Anti-C3.

patients continued to have hemolysis a year after stopping treatment with methyldopa, and they probably had the idiopathic variety of AIHA.

Tables 6-12 and 6-13 summarize the results of direct antiglobulin tests in patients in our series with methyldopa-induced hemolytic anemia and in warm antibody AIHA not associated with methyldopa administration.

Table 6-12. STRENGTH OF THE DIRECT ANTIGLOBULIN TEST USING A SINGLE DILUTION OF AN OPTIMALLY DILUTED ANTI-IgG ANTIGLOBULIN SERUM IN PATIENTS WITH METHYLDOPA-INDUCED WARM ANTIBODY AIHA, COMPARED WITH CASES NOT ASSOCIATED WITH THE ADMINISTRATION OF METHYLDOPA

Direct Antiglobulin Test Result Using Anti-IgG	Methyldopa-Induced AIHA (29 Patients)		Warm Antibody AIHA Not Caused by Methyldopa (210 Patients)	
	IgG (no C3) (25 Patients)	IgG + C3 (4 Patients)	IgG (no C3) (45 Patients)	IgG + C3 (165 Patients)
½ − 1+	0	0	1 (2.2%)	10 (6.1%)
1½ − 2+	0	0	7 (15.6%)	29 (17.6%)
2½ − 3+	8 (32%)	2 (50%)	13 (28.9%)	50 (30.3%)
3½ − 4+	17 (68%)	2 (50%)	24 (53.3%)	76 (46.1%)

Table 6-13. DIRECT ANTIGLOBULIN TEST SCORES AND TITERS USING ANTI-IgG ANTIGLOBULIN SERUM; WARM ANTIBODY AIHA CAUSED BY METHYLDOPA, COMPARED WITH CASES NOT ASSOCIATED WITH THE ADMINISTRATION OF METHYLDOPA

	AIHA Caused by Methyldopa (29 Patients)	Warm Antibody AIHA Not Caused by Methyldopa	
		IgG (45 Patients)	IgG + C3 (165 Patients)
Average Score	70.7	34.5	34.9
Range	27 to 81	12 to 71	4 to 71
Range of Titers	1024 to 64,000	256 to 16,000	64 to 64,000
Median Titer	2048	2048	1024

An Approach to the Characterization of Antibodies in Serum and Red Cell Eluate in Immune Hemolytic Anemias

Although the direct antiglobulin test provides useful information, the definitive diagnosis rests upon the characterization of the antibodies present in the patient's serum and red cell eluate. It is wise to initiate such studies with screening tests to develop a preliminary diagnosis and then to perform additional tests as are necessary for confirmation of the diagnosis and for the exclusion of alternative possibilities.

Although the differential diagnosis of immune hemolytic anemias appears lengthy (see Table 2-1, page 27) the initial evaluation can often be simplified in concept by keeping the following points in mind.

The differentiation between idiopathic and secondary AIHA is *not* based on serologic tests, but instead concerns the usual tests pertinent to the diagnosis of systemic lupus erythematosus, chronic lymphatic leukemia, lymphomas, etc.

Drug-induced immune hemolytic anemia may in some cases be excluded on the basis of the patient's history. If drug-induced immune hemolytic anemia is a plausible diagnosis, additional studies are often necessary to demonstrate the drug-related red cell antibody. These tests are discussed separately in Chapter 8. Even when drug-induced hemolytic anemia is suspected, it is pertinent to perform serologic studies relating to the diagnosis of AIHA for two reasons. First, some drugs cause AIHA that is serologically indistinguishable from idiopathic warm AIHA. Indeed, this is the most common type of drug-induced immune hemolytic anemia, with methyldopa being the prototype drug. Corroborative evidence may be obtained by observing resolution of the hemolytic anemia after cessation of the drug, but proof of the etiologic role of the drug can be obtained only by re-institution of the drug, a procedure no longer justifiable in the case of methyldopa.

Secondly, if a patient has an acquired immune hemolytic anemia with a positive direct antiglobulin test but no red cell antibodies are demonstrable in either the serum or red cell eluate, such findings lend weight to a diagnosis of a drug-induced hemolytic anemia. This is true since, with the exception of hemolytic anemias caused by methyldopa, L-dopa, and mefenamic acid, the presence of the drug in the *in vitro* test system is necessary in order to demonstrate the drug-related antibody.

Alloantibody-induced immune hemolytic anemias (hemolytic disease of the newborn and hemolytic transfusion reactions) can usually be reliably excluded by the clinical setting. Hemolytic transfusion reactions need be considered only if the patient has been transfused in recent weeks. Although AIHA has been reported in newborn infants, other causes of hemolytic anemia are very much more common. For convenience we discuss AIHA in infants and children, and the differentiation of AIHA and hemolytic transfusion reactions elsewhere (Chapter 9).

Thus, in spite of the lengthy list of diagnostic possibilities, it is usually optimal to perform the initial serologic tests with only three diagnostic considerations in mind: (1) warm antibody AIHA, (2) cold agglutinin syndrome, and (3) paroxysmal cold hemoglobinuria. If findings are not characteristic of any of these three syndromes, the patient may have a drug-induced immune hemolytic anemia (Chapter 8) or an atypical hemolytic anemia (Chapter 9).

Characterization of Antibodies in Serum and Red Cell Eluate in Warm Antibody AIHA

Essential Diagnostic Tests. If a patient has an acquired hemolytic anemia with a positive direct antiglobulin test and has not been transfused during the last four months, does not have a cold agglutinin of high thermal amplitude (see pages 213–216), and is not taking drugs, a tentative diagnosis of warm antibody AIHA may be entertained. However, as mentioned in Chapter 5, we find it highly advisable to perform additional serologic studies in order to make a more confident diagnosis. A reasonable number of tests to detect and characterize the antibody in the patient's serum and eluate can readily be performed. This will tend to avoid diagnostic error by confirming that the patient's warm antibody is, indeed, an autoantibody. In addition, alloantibody(ies) may be detected as well as autoantibody, and it is helpful to have such information available since transfusion may be required. The specificity of the autoantibody may also be of significance in regard to transfusion. In still other patients, the initial impression of AIHA may not be substantiated. Antibodies found in initial screening tests of the patient's serum may be alloantibodies, and the direct antiglobulin test may be positive for any of the reasons listed on page 151.

The screening tests utilized for the detection and initial characterization of warm antibodies in the serum and eluate in patients with immune hemolytic anemias are listed in Chapter 5. An example of screening test results is given in Table 5-7, and a summary of screening test results in our series of 244 patients with warm antibody AIHA is given in Table 6-14. The rationale for performing these screening tests and more definitive tests may be explained as follows.

The first objective is to perform tests to detect all red cell antibodies and to determine the optimal temperature of their reactivity. Since no single serologic test is capable of detecting all such antibodies, several screening tests are performed against group O red cells at 37°C. The donors of the red blood cells (RBC) are selected on the basis of detailed blood group typing so that as many red cell antigens as possible of the blood group systems other than the ABO system are represented. (Such group O red cells are commercially available and are a standard blood bank reagent.) For alloantibody testing, it usually is necessary to test against at least two cells for optimal representation of the various blood group systems. However, warm autoantibodies, except for those very unusual warm autoantibodies demonstrating clear-cut specificity, will react with all screening cells tested.

The screening tests previously described will determine whether or not any red cell antibodies are present in the patient's serum other than the anti-A and anti-B that may be "expected" depending on the patient's ABO blood group. Immunohematologists frequently refer to all other antibodies with the rather unsatisfactory terms "unexpected" or "irregular."

If tests are positive for "unexpected" serum antibodies that are optimally reactive at 37°C, further testing is indicated. Specificity is determined by test-

Table 6-14. RESULTS OF SERUM SCREENING IN 244 PATIENTS WITH WARM ANTIBODY AIHA

			Percent Reacting	
			Serum (% Positive Reactions)	Acidified Serum and Acidified Complement (% Positive Reactions)
20°C	Untreated RBC			
		Lysis	0.4	0.8
		Agglutination	34.8	34.8
20°C	Enzyme Treated			
		Lysis	1.6	2.5
		Agglutination	78.6	78.6
37°C	Untreated RBC			
		Lysis	0.4	0.4
		Agglutination	4.9	4.9
		Indirect Anti- globulin Test	57.4	57.4
37°C	Enzyme Treated			
		Lysis	8.6	12.7
		Agglutination	88.9	88.9

ing against a panel of red cells, usually from about 10 carefully selected persons. The donors are chosen so that the various red cell antigens are represented on some RBC samples but not others. (Again, such red cell panels are commercially available and are standard blood bank reagents.) For example, the antibody may demonstrate clear cut specificity by reacting only with red cells containing a particular Rh antigen (e.g., e or hr"). If that red cell antigen is absent from the patient's own red cells, the antibody is an alloantibody that has developed as a result of exposure to foreign antigens by blood transfusion or pregnancy. Such antibody may cause hemolytic transfusion reactions if the patient is transfused with red cells containing the antigen, but, since it cannot react with the patient's own red cells, it is not an autoantibody and is irrelevant in regard to a diagnosis of AIHA. However, if the antigen is present on the patient's own red cells, one has a clear demonstration of a red cell autoantibody. The finding of such clear cut specificity of a warm autoantibody does occur, but it is rare. More commonly, the antibody, while reacting with all cells on the panel, will consistently react more strongly with red cells containing a certain Rh antigen than with cells lacking this antigen. If the patient's own red cells contain this antigen, it is customary to consider that the antibody is an autoantibody with specificity, even though it reacts with all cells tested. We refer to autoantibodies that react with all red cells of common Rh phenotypes but that react to higher titer against red cells having a certain Rh antigen than with red cells lacking that antigen as demonstrating Rh "relative specificity."

The most common result obtained when testing for specificity of the antibody in warm antibody AIHA is that the antibody in the patient's serum and eluate will react about equally strongly with all red cells on the panel. It may not be possible to test the antibody for reactivity against the patient's own red blood cells because they are already coated with antibody. However, it is inferred from the reactivity with all normal red cells that the antigen with which the antibody is reacting is on the patient's own red cells as well; this theory may be further supported by finding that the antibody eluted from the patient's own red cells demonstrates a similar broad reactivity. Such an inference has been confirmed by freezing some of the serum and eluate and retesting against the patient's own red cells after a remission has been induced.

It is true that multiple alloantibodies, a combination of alloantibody(ies) and autoantibody, or a single alloantibody against a high incidence antigen may display broad reactivity against a panel of red cells and may be difficult to distinguish from autoantibody. However, if the patient has not been transfused within the last four months, alloantibodies cannot be causing either an acquired hemolytic anemia or a positive direct antiglobulin test. Patients who have been recently transfused may pose a significant diagnostic problem as discussed further in Chapter 9.

Although the testing described thus far may not have identified the specificity of the "unexpected" antibody found in the screening test, further studies utilizing rare donor cells and additional serologic tests such as absorption and elution will frequently demonstrate specificity of the autoantibody (see Chapter 7). However, such detailed tests are generally not considered essential for the diagnosis of warm antibody AIHA.[31]

Testing antibody that has been eluted from the patient's red cells also affords significant findings, and it is preferable to include such testing as a routine part of the diagnostic evaluation. Indeed, in some patients, autoantibody will not be found in the serum but will be detectable in the eluate. Further, positive reactions obtained with an eluate exclude drug-induced hemolytic anemias as a cause of the direct antiglobulin test (except in patients taking methyldopa, L-dopa, or mefenamic acid). Tests for specificity of the antibody in the eluate should be carried out against a routine panel of red cells in a manner similar to that for serum antibodies.

A diagnosis can usually be reached on the basis of the serologic tests described thus far. In spite of the seemingly complicated nature of the foregoing, the usual or "typical" essential diagnostic tests that lead to a reasonably confident diagnosis of warm antibody AIHA may be very simply summarized as follows: (a) the presence of an acquired hemolytic anemia, (b) a positive direct antiglobulin test, and (c) an "unexpected" antibody in the serum and eluate that reacts optimally at 37°C. The antibody usually reacts with all normal erythrocytes but, in some cases, it can readily be shown to react preferentially with antigens on the patient's own red blood cells.

An example of typical findings in a patient with warm antibody AIHA are given in the following case report with the serologic findings listed in Table 6-15.

Patient B.M., a sixty-six year old white woman, was admitted to hospital because of some weight loss, intermittent anorexia and nausea, jaundice, and left upper quadrant discomfort. A hematocrit reading performed when she was an out-patient revealed a value of 21 percent. Pertinent physical findings included jaundice, splenomegaly with the spleen palpable 3 cm below the left costal margin, and hepatomegaly with a liver palpable 3 cm below the right costal margin. The laboratory findings revealed a total bilirubin of 3.4 mg/dl with a direct reacting bilirubin being 1.2 mg/dl. The reticulocyte count was 50 percent. The total white blood cell count was $3,500/\mu l$. Serum LDH was 2,460 U and the serum SGOT was 127 U. Normal studies included total protein, albumin, amylase, electrolytes, BUN, creatinine, calcium, phosphorus, uric acid, rheumatoid factor, and antinuclear antibody test.

The patient was treated with 60 mg of prednisone daily, and over a two week period she experienced rapid resolution of her anemia. Her hemoglobin rose to 12.9 gm/dl with a hematocrit of 40 percent. Her white count rose to 22,000 with 81 percent segmented neutrophils, three bands, 12 lymphocytes, 2 monocytes, and 1 eosinophil. Reticulocytes decreased to 17.4 percent. The patient's prednisone therapy was complicated by mild hyperglycemia and glycosuria. The patient also developed oral moniliasis which was easily treated with topical therapy. Corticosteroid therapy was gradually decreased in subsequent weeks.

Additional Important Aspects of Serologic Tests. Several points concerning the preceding laboratory tests were made in Chapter 5 but merit emphasis here because they are particularly significant. Enzyme treated red cells are not routinely utilized in most blood transfusion laboratories for compatibility test procedures, but they should be used for adequate detection and characterization of autoantibodies in warm antibody AIHA. This is true because only 57 percent of the patients with warm antibody AIHA have antibody detectable in their serum when tests at 37°C are performed utilizing only "normal" red blood cells (i.e., non-enzyme treated). In contrast, autoantibodies are detectable in 89 percent of the patients when enzyme treated cells are utilized (Table 6-14).

Enzyme treated red cells are also essential for the demonstration of *in vitro* lysis by warm autoantibodies since these antibodies are only rarely capable of lysing untreated red blood cells. Warm hemolysins may occur in association with incomplete IgG autoantibodies, but in approximately 10 percent of the patients with warm antibody AIHA, the serum antibody will cause lysis of enzyme treated red cells but, when reacted against normal RBC will not cause lysis, agglutination, or a positive indirect antiglobulin test. The direct antiglobulin test in these patients is positive with anti-C3 and negative with anti-IgG antisera.[38] Almost all these warm hemolysins are IgM antibodies but, rarely, IgG antibodies have also been described. In contrast to autoantibodies

Table 6-15. SEROLOGIC FINDINGS IN A TYPICAL PATIENT WITH WARM ANTI-BODY AUTOIMMUNE HEMOLYTIC ANEMIA
(Patient B.M.)

Direct Antiglobulin Test: Polyspecific Antiglobulin Serum: 3+

Dilution of Anti-globulin Serum	64	128	256	512	1024	2048	4096	Score	Titer
Anti-IgG	3+	3+	2½+	2+	1½+	1+	0	38	2048
Anti-IgA	0	0	0	0	0	0	0	0	0
Anti-IgM	0	0	0	0	0	0	0	0	0

Dilution of Anti-globulin Serum	4	8	16	32	64	128	256	Score	Titer
Anti-C3	3+	2+	1+	0	0	0	0	18	16

Screening Tests For Serum Antibody:

			Serum	AS + AC *	Controls AC Alone	Auto **
20°C	Untreated Cells	Lysis	0	0	0	0
		Agglutination	0	0	0	0
	Papainized Cells	Lysis	0	0	0	0
		Agglutination	2+	2½+	0	2½+

			Serum Saline	Serum Alb†	AS + AC*	Controls AC Alone	Auto** with Alb†
37°C	Untreated Cells	Lysis	0	0	0	0	0
		Agglutination	0	1+	0	0	1+
		IAT	1+	2½+	1+	0	3+
	Papainized Cells	Lysis	0	NT	0	0	0
		Agglutination	3+	NT	2+	0	2½+

* AS = acidified serum; AC = acidified complement
** Auto = patient's own RBC
† Alb = Albumin

NT-Not tested
Agglutination reactions are graded 1+ to 4+.

Table 6-15. (CONTINUED)

Specificity of Antibody in Serum and Eluate:

Serum: No specificity evident with tests performed (1 to 2+ by indirect antiglobulin test and 3 to 4+ vs. enzyme treated cells of a panel)

Eluate: No specificity evident (1+ by indirect antiglobulin test vs. all cells of a panel)

Cold agglutinin Titer:
  Not performed (no agglutination in screening tests at 20°C)

Donath-Landsteiner Test: Not performed

Other data: All serum autoantibody removed by warm autoabsorptions (see Chapter 10)

Summary: Findings typical of warm antibody autoimmune hemolytic anemia

Follow-Up: Rapid improvement of anemia over two week period of prednisone therapy

---

reactive by the indirect antiglobulin test, specificity tests do not reveal specificity within the Rh system; they are maximally reactive at a pH of 6.5.[38]

When performing tests for lysis *in vitro,* one must keep in mind that the patient's serum is frequently deficient in complement, so it is advisable to add fresh complement. This is conveniently done by adding an equal volume of fresh [12] ABO compatible normal serum to the patient's serum.

It is logical and convenient to perform tests for specificity of the autoantibody utilizing the screening test that gave the strongest reactions. Usually this test is the indirect antiglobulin test or agglutination of enzyme treated red cells.

Characterization of Antibodies in the Cold Agglutinin Syndrome

Cold agglutinins that satisfy the "classic" characteristics described for antibodies in cold agglutinin syndrome often produce striking *in vitro* findings and make their presence known in several sections of the clinical laboratory. These cold agglutinins have a titer of 1,000 to 16,000 or higher in saline at 4°C (normal is <64) and cause *in vitro* agglutination of anticoagulated blood at room temperature that is grossly evident to the naked eye. Indeed, all the red cells may be bound in one huge agglutinate which may be mistaken by the uninitiated as a clot (Figure 6-1). Preparation of adequate blood smears at room temperature becomes impossible because of gross agglutination of red blood cells. Blood counts in Coulter counters produce nonsense numbers [8, 19, 26] and, if a sample is sent to the blood transfusion service for compatibility testing, the cold agglutinins are immediately apparent and special knowledge will be required to circumvent the problems that they produce.

For anyone who has observed just one similar case previously, the diagnosis of cold agglutinin syndrome comes immediately to mind.

However, other patients with an elevated cold agglutinin titer have no evidence of hemolysis. Even though these antibodies are clinically benign, they may react at room temperature, causing some of the *in vitro* problems previously described. The converse is also true, i.e., we frequently encounter patients who do not have striking increases in their cold agglutinin titer yet appear to have cold agglutinin syndrome since they have an acquired hemolytic anemia, an antiglobulin test that is positive only with anticomplement sera, a moderate elevation of cold agglutinin titer and thermal amplitude, and no other definable cause of hemolysis after extensive evaluation and long term follow-up. Further complicating the situation is the fact that about 30 percent of the patients with warm antibody AIHA also have a modest to moderate elevation of cold agglutinin titer and/or thermal amplitude and, especially if characteristic or "typical" serologic findings of warm antibody AIHA are not present, the patient may be erroneously diagnosed as having cold agglutinin syndrome.

Thus, when cold agglutinins are encountered, the task is to determine whether the patient has clinically insignificant albeit abnormal cold agglutinins, has warm antibody AIHA with an associated but probably insignificant elevation of cold agglutinin titer or thermal amplitude, or has cold agglutinin syndrome. Also, in rare patients, characteristic findings of both warm antibody AIHA and cold agglutinin syndrome occur simultaneously (see Chapter 9).

Development of Criteria to Distinguish Benign Cold Agglutinins from those Associated with *In Vivo* Hemolysis. In order to develop guidelines that may be of value in the diagnosis of cold agglutinin syndrome, we studied various characteristics of cold agglutinins in patients with cold agglutinin syndrome and in patients without hemolytic anemia. As with most red cell antibodies, it is difficult to predict the *in vivo* significance from *in vitro* tests, and it is obvious that the titer of an antibody when tested at 4°C is not a direct measurement of its clinical importance.

Our study characterized cold agglutinins by various techniques, but it emphasized the reactivity of the antibody at various temperatures against red cells suspended in saline or in 30 percent albumin medium.[15] The use of 30 percent albumin medium was based on the report of Haynes and Chaplin [20] who described an enhancing effect of albumin on cold agglutinins that was particularly striking in one patient. This patient had a hemolytic anemia associated with only a modestly elevated cold agglutinin titer of 128 at 4°C using saline-suspended red cells, but a titer of 131,000 in the presence of bovine albumin. We studied 32 patients who had elevated cold agglutinin titers and positive direct antiglobulin tests due to complement sensitization of their cells. Twenty-eight of these patients had an associated hemolytic anemia.

We found that testing for cold hemolysis did not differentiate clinically important antibodies from benign cold agglutinins. Although sera from all patients with cold agglutinin syndrome caused lysis of enzyme treated cells at 20°C, sera from 3 of the 4 patients without hemolytic anemia also caused *in vitro* lysis.

The cold agglutinin titer at 4°C, when performed in saline or albumin, did not correlate with the presence or absence of hemolysis, but determination of the thermal range did prove helpful. Table 6-16 shows the comparative titrations using saline and albumin at 4°C, 30°C and 37°C in the 32 patients that were divided into 4 groups. Patients 1–12 all had hemolytic anemia associated with high titer cold agglutinins at 4°C, and all sera reacted at 30°C with saline suspended red cells. The sera of two patients (M.C. and E.T.) reacted at 37°C with saline suspended red cells, and all 12 reacted at 37°C in the presence of albumin.

Patients 13–21 all had hemolytic anemia associated with cold agglutinins of high titer at 4°C, but none of the sera from these 9 patients reacted at 30°C unless albumin was present in the incubation mixture. In the presence of albumin all 9 reacted at 30°C, and 5 of the 9 reacted also at 37°C.

Patients 22–28 all had hemolytic anemia but normal to moderately increased cold agglutinin titers at 4°C (i.e., not more than about 2 tubes above our upper limit of normal). Three of the 7 sera reacted at 30°C with saline suspended red cells, and all 7 reacted in the presence of albumin. Two of the 7 (J.W. and M.E.) reacted at 37°C in the presence of albumin.

Patient 28 (M.E.) is of considerable interest because he had severe hemolytic anemia associated with a cold agglutinin titer of only 8 at 4°C when saline suspended red cells were tested (normal cold agglutinin titers at 4°C range up to 64 in our laboratory). In the presence of albumin the cold autoantibody reacted to a titer of 128 at 4°C and up to 37°C. Moreover, these tests were reproducible even with very strict control of temperature. This patient had a strongly positive direct antiglobulin test due to complement sensitization of the red cells. In addition to the cold agglutinin, the serum contained a cold hemolysin, reacting optimally at 20°C against enzyme treated red cells. The Donath-Landsteiner test was negative. The reactions at 30°C and 37°C in the presence of albumin showed anti-I specificity, and the reactions were inhibited by 2-mercaptoethanol. No other antibody activity at 37°C could be demonstrated in the serum or in an eluate prepared from the patient's red cells. Thus, it appeared that all reactions were due to the IgM cold autoantibody with a high thermal maximum and that no additional warm autoantibodies optimally reactive at 37°C were present. No other cause of hemolysis was found in this patient.

Patients 29–32 all had increased cold agglutinin titers at 4°C but no associated hemolytic anemia. None of these sera reacted at 30°C or 37°C, even in the presence of albumin. Thus all patients with hemolytic anemia had cold agglutinins that reacted at 30°C in albumin in contrast to negative reactions in patients without hemolytic anemia. Based on the empiric findings in this report, it appears that reactivity of a cold agglutinin at 30°C in albumin may be the optimal means for distinguishing clinically insignificant cold agglutinins from those associated with *in vivo* hemolysis.

An additional point of significance in this study was that we excluded IgG antibody activity in 22 of the 28 sera that reacted at 30°C in the presence of albumin by treating them with 2-mercaptoethanol. It was concluded that IgG antibodies were not causing the original agglutination reactions observed at 30°C or 37°C.

Table 6-16. TITERS AND THERMAL RANGES IN 32 PATIENTS WITH ABNORMAL COLD AGGLUTININS

Patient	Hemolytic Anemia	4°C		30°C		37°C	
		Saline	Albumin	Saline	Albumin	Saline	Albumin
1. M.W.	yes	2560	5120	1	640	0	320
2. A.B.	yes	5120	10240	1	640	0	160
3. F.Br.	yes	2560	5120	4	320	0	80
4. D.W.	yes	2560	5120	20	320	0	20
5. M.C.	yes	1280	1280	10	160	1	1
6. R.D.	yes	10240	10240	1	40	0	1
7. E.F.	yes	640	1280	1	20	0	1
8. H.L.	yes	640	5120	10	160	0	10
9. J.Sc.	yes	640	2560	1	40	0	1
10. E.C.	yes	2560	5120	1	10	0	1
11. S.F.	yes	1280	1280	1	10	0	1
12. E.T.	yes	8192	4096	128	128	8	16
13. F.Bc.	yes	1024	256	0	1	0	0
14. C.D.	yes	1024	2048	0	2	0	1
15. M.J.	yes	640	2560	0	10	0	1
16. V.W.	yes	640	1280	0	40	0	1
17. O.M.	yes	1280	5120	0	20	0	1
18. M.P.	yes	1024	256	0	4	0	2
19. W.W.	yes	640	640	0	1	0	0
20. L.U.	yes	640	640	0	1	0	0
21. E.Sc.	yes	2048	1024	0	8	0	1
22. F.M.	yes	320	320	0	10	0	0
23. E.St.	yes	320	320	0	1	0	0
24. J.W.	yes	256	1024	1	4	0	1
25. D.S.	yes	256	512	1	2	0	0
26. E.D.	yes	256	512	0	4	0	0
27. E.Sh.	yes	128	1024	1	1	0	0
28. M.E.	yes	8	128	0	1	0	1
29. M.B.	no	320	320	0	0	0	0
30. G.H.	no	320	640	0	0	0	0
31. J.S.	no	1280	2560	0	0	0	0
32. C.W.	no	320	20	0	0	0	0

(Garratty, G., Petz, L. D., and Hoops, J. K.: The correlation of cold agglutinin titrations in saline and albu haemolytic anaemia. Brit. J. Haematol., *35:* 587, 1977.)

Essential Diagnostic Tests for Cold Agglutinin Syndrome. On the basis of the preceding findings we offer the following approach to the diagnosis of cold agglutinin syndrome. The diagnosis must be considered in all patients with acquired hemolytic anemia who have a positive direct antiglobulin test using anti-C3 serum and a negative direct antiglobulin test using anti-IgG (Table 6-2). A practical initial serum screening procedure is to test the ability of the patient's serum to agglutinate saline suspended normal red cells at 20°C after incubation for 30–60 minutes (Chapter 5). This recommendation is based on data illustrated in Table 6-17, namely, that the sera of essentially all patients in our series who had cold agglutinin syndrome caused agglutination of saline suspended red cells at 20°C. If this screening test is negative, cold agglutinin syndrome is extremely unlikely; if positive, further studies are necessary to determine the thermal amplitude of the antibody.

When cold agglutinin syndrome appears to be a possible diagnosis on the basis of the preceding evaluation, studies of the thermal range of reactivity of the antibody in saline and albumin are indicated. It is also convenient to determine possible Ii blood group specificity of the antibody simultaneously (see Chapter 5). The titer of the cold agglutinin in cold agglutinin syndrome is invariably highest at 4°C and progressively decreases at higher temperatures. Of particular note are the reactions at 30° and 37°C. If the former is positive in albumin, the antibody may well be of pathogenetic significance, i.e., it may be causing short red blood cell survival *in vivo*. If the reaction at 37°C is also

Table 6-17. RESULTS OF SERUM SCREENING IN 57 PATIENTS WITH COLD AGGLUTININ SYNDROME

		Percent Reacting	
		Serum (% Positive Reactions)	Acidified Serum and Acidified Complement (% Positive Reactions)
20°C	Untreated RBC		
	Lysis	2.0	14.3
	Agglutination	98	98
20°C	Enzyme Treated		
	Lysis	24.5	93.8
	Agglutination	100	100
37°C	Untreated RBC		
	Lysis	0	0
	Agglutination	10.7	10.7
	Indirect Anti-globulin test	5.4	5.4
37°C	Enzyme Treated		
	Lysis	12.2	22.5
	Agglutination	28.6	28.6

positive in albumin (as was true in 19 of the 28 patients in Table 6-16) or in saline (2 of 28 patients or 7.1 percent) the antibody will cause particular problems in the compatibility test (see Chapter 10).

Utilizing clinical information, the results of the direct antiglobulin test, and the preceding screening tests, a reasonably confident assessment of the presence or absence of cold agglutinin syndrome may be made. Cold agglutinin syndrome may be diagnosed if the following are present: (1) clinical evidence of acquired hemolytic anemia; (2) a positive direct antiglobulin test caused by sensitization with C3; (3) a negative direct antiglobulin test using anti-IgG antiglobulin serum; and (4) the presence of a cold autoagglutinin with reactivity up to at least 30°C in albumin.

An alternative diagnosis must be sought for patients who do not satisfy all these criteria.

An example of typical findings in a patient with cold agglutinin syndrome are given in the following case report with serologic findings listed in Table 6-18.

Case Report: Mrs. V. W.,* a 52-year-old woman, sought medical attention in November, 1970 because she noted that her fingers turned blue on exposure to cold. This sign was associated with mild discomfort under her fingernails and a sensation of tingling. The findings resolved quickly upon warming. She had no other complaints and, in particular, had no symptoms of fatigue. She worked daily as an office manager in a law firm. Approximately one year previously her hematocrit level was 35 percent. There was no history of blood loss. She appeared neither acutely or chronically ill, and a physical examination revealed no abnormal findings.

Laboratory data revealed a hemoglobin level of 9.6 gm/dl, hematocrit level of 25 percent, white cells 7,700/μl with a normal differential, platelets 392,000/μl and reticulocytes 15.6 percent. Total bilirubin was 1.2 mg/dl; direct reacting bilirubin 0.21 mg/dl, serum iron 107, and total iron binding capacity was 199 mcg/dl. Urinalysis revealed a specific gravity of 1.009, and there was no proteinuria or glycosuria; a test for Bence-Jones protein was negative. Tests for occult blood in the stool were negative. Antinuclear antibody was negative. Total protein was 7.6 gm/dl; serum electrophoresis revealed that the albumin was 59.2 percent (4.5 gm/dl), α_1-globulin 2.9 percent, α_2-globulin 6.2 percent, β globulin 10.1 percent and γ globulin 21.6 percent. No M component was detected.

The laboratory technologists noted that 4+ agglutination occurred at room temperature (23°C), and that there was no agglutination at 37°C. Hemolysis was present in serum samples collected at room temperature. The direct antiglobulin test was positive. Smears of aspirated bone marrow revealed gross clumping and were inadequate for interpretation. Sections revealed normoblastic erythropoiesis and no evidence of an infiltrative process, although an occasional focus of mature lymphocytes was seen.

Her serologic findings are indicated in Table 6-18. Although the antibody was only minimally reactive at 30°C without albumin, it caused 4+ agglutination at that temperature in the presence of 30 percent albumin and reacted against adult OI red cells even at 37°C. The clinical and serologic findings were considered diagnostic of cold agglutinin syndrome.

* Patient referred by Thomas Kilbridge, M.D.

Table 6-18. SEROLOGIC FINDINGS IN A TYPICAL PATIENT WITH COLD AGGLUTININ SYNDROME (PATIENT V.W.)

Direct Antiglobulin Test: Polyspecific Antiglobulin Serum: 4+

Dilution of Antiglobulin Serum	64	128	256	512	1024	2048	4096	Score	Titer
Anti-IgG	0	0	0	0	0	0	0	0	0

Dilution of Antiglobulin Serum	4	8	16	32	64	128	256	Score	Titer
Anti-C3	4+	4+	4+	3+	2+	1½+	1+	47	256
Anti-C4	4+	4+	3+	2+	1½+	1+	0	41	128

Screening Tests For Serum Antibody

		Serum	AS + AC*	Control AC
20°C	Untreated Cells			
	Lysis	0	2+	0
	Agglutination	4+	4+	0
	Papainized Cells			
	Lysis	0	4+	0
	Agglutination	4+	4+	0

		Serum	AS + AC	Control AC
37°C	Untreated Cells			
	Lysis	0	0	0
	Agglutination	0	0	0
	IAT	0	0	0
	Papainized Cells			
	Lysis	0	0	0
	Agglutination	0	0	0

* AS = Acidified serum; AC = acidified complement

Table 6-18. (CONTINUED)
Titer, Thermal Range and Specificity of Cold Agglutinin
i. Using Saline Suspended Red Cells

Dilution	Patient Serum	1	2	4	8	16	32	64	128	256	512	1024	2048	4096	Titer
4°C	Adult OI	4+	4+	4+	4+	4+	4+	4+	4+	2½+	1+	1+	(1)+	0	2048
	cord Oi	4+	4+	4+	4+	4+	4+	3½+	2+	2+	1+	1+	0	0	1024
	Adult Oi	4+	4+	4+	4+	3½+	3½+	2½+	2+	1+	1+	0	0	0	512
25°	Adult OI	4+	4+	3+	2½+	2+	1½+	1+	(1)+	0	0	0	0	0	128
	cord Oi	3+	1+	0	0	0	0	0	0	0	0	0	0	0	2
	Adult Oi	2+	0	0	0	0	0	0	0	0	0	0	0	0	1
30°C	Adult OI	1+	0	0	0	0	0	0	0	0	0	0	0	0	1
	cord Oi	0	0	0	0	0	0	0	0	0	0	0	0	0	0
	Adult Oi	0	0	0	0	0	0	0	0	0	0	0	0	0	0
37°C	Adult OI	0	0	0	0	0	0	0	0	0	0	0	0	0	0
	cord Oi	0	0	0	0	0	0	0	0	0	0	0	0	0	0
	Adult Oi	0	0	0	0	0	0	0	0	0	0	0	0	0	0

ii. 30% Bovine Alumin Added

Dilution	Patient Serum	1	2	4	8	16	32	64	128	256	512	1024	2048	4096	Titer
4°C	Adult OI	4+	4+	4+	4+	4+	4+	3+	2½+	2+	1+	1+	1+	(1)+	4096
	cord Oi	4+	4+	4+	4+	3½+	3½+	3+	2½+	1+	1+	1+	0	0	1024
	Adult Oi	4+	4+	4+	4+	3+	3+	3+	2+	1+	1+	0	0	0	512

25°C	Adult OI	4+	4+	4+	4+	4+	3+	3+	2+	1+	(1)+	0	0	1024
	cord Oi	4+	3+	3+	3+	2+	1+	(1)+	0	0	0	0	0	64
	Adult Oi	4+	3+	3+	2+	1+	1+	0	0	0	0	0	0	32
30°C	Adult OI	4+	2+	1½+	1+	0	0	0	0	0	0	0	0	8
	cord Oi	2+	0	0	0	0	0	0	0	0	0	0	0	1
	Adult Oi	0	0	0	0	0	0	0	0	0	0	0	0	0
37°C	Adult OI	2+	0	0	0	0	0	0	0	0	0	0	0	1
	cord Oi	0	0	0	0	0	0	0	0	0	0	0	0	0
	Adult Oi	0	0	0	0	0	0	0	0	0	0	0	0	0

Specificity of Serum and Eluate:

Serum: Anti-I

Eluate: not tested

Cold Agglutinin Titer: 2048 vs. adult OI red cells at 4°C

Cold Agglutinin Thermal Amplitude: up to 30°C in saline and 37°C in albumin

Donath-Landsteiner Test: not performed

Other Data: Total hemolytic complement < 10 CH_{50} units

Normal = 114 to 210 CH_{50} units

Summary: Findings characteristic of cold agglutinin syndrome

Follow-up: Chronic moderately severe anemia with no change in serologic reactions in seven years

Agglutination reactions are graded as ½+ to 4+

She has been treated with folic acid and her course initially was quite stable, although she had exacerbations in cold weather, particularly when also developing an upper respiratory infection. In February of 1976 she developed a sore throat, malaise, chilly sensations, and a fever of 101°F. Her hematocrit level dropped to 16 percent and reticulocytes dropped to 3.5 percent. She was admitted to hospital and placed in a warmed room, and she wore gloves and warm stockings continuously. A bone marrow aspiration revealed striking erythroid hyperplasia with normal megakaryocytes and granulocytic precursors. Occasional plasma cells were present, but there was no lymphocytic infiltration. Her hematocrit level reached a low of 14 percent, but then gradually improved. She was discharged from the hospital when the hematocrit reached 20 percent, and a progressive increase to 31 percent was noted as she continued as an outpatient.

In subsequent years her usual hematocrit level has become somewhat lower, usually in the range of about 24 percent. In September 1976, therapy with chlorambucil was initiated at a time when her hematocrit had dropped to 18 percent. A bone marrow biopsy at this time revealed multiple nodules of mature lymphocytes; the biopsy was interpreted as indicating the presence of a lymphoma. However, no abnormal physical findings were present and, in particular, there was no hepatosplenomegaly or lymphadenopathy. Her hematocrit level improved to 24 percent during therapy with 8 mg of chlorambucil daily, during which time she was also more meticulous about avoiding cold. Chlorambucil was gradually increased to 10 mg per day in December 1976, after which date she developed pancytopenia and reticulocytopenia. Her hematocrit level in January 1977 was 12.5 percent; white cells 2,500/μl with 67 neutrophils, 4 bands, 24 lymphocytes, and 4 monocytes; platelets 88,000/μl; and reticulocytes 2.0 percent. She was treated with transfusions of 2 units of packed red cells on three occasions to keep her hematocrit level at about 20 percent, after which her marrow function spontaneously improved. Her pancytopenia resolved and her hematocrit level remained stable at about 24 percent. A repeat bone marrow examination revealed marked improvement, and nodules of lymphocytes were no longer apparent, although the total number of lymphocytes was increased above normal.

As of July 1979 her disease had remained stable and she had received no transfusions since January 1977. Her hematocrit level has remained about 24 to 26 percent, she was being treated only with folic acid, and she continued to work daily. She still noticed acrocyanosis on exposure to mild cold. There were no new physical findings.

Serologic evaluations performed at intervals throughout her course revealed a minimal diminution in the strength of the direct antiglobulin test using anti-C3 antiserum. In September 1976 the titer was 128 and the score was 36. The cold agglutinin titer and thermal amplitude were essentially unchanged.

Additional Comments Regarding Serologic Tests. A few final comments are necessary concerning the diagnostic tests that have been described. We recognize that the characterization of cold agglutinins is not commonly performed in blood transfusion laboratories, and that taking time from the more usual tasks of compatibility testing and alloantibody identification to set up unfamiliar and infrequently performed tests in order to evaluate a possible case of autoimmune hemolytic anemia is disruptive of schedules. Nevertheless, we feel that characterization of the patient's cold agglutinin, at least to the degree described above, is crucial in order to avoid diagnostic errors. We rather frequently encounter cold agglutinins that are reactive at room temperature and are noticed because they cause difficulty in compatibility testing, and cause agglutination visible to the naked eye in an anticoagulated blood sample as well as other of the *in vitro* phenomena previously described. Commonly it is assumed that such cold agglutinins must be potent enough to cause *in vivo* shortening of red blood cell survival and, if the patient has a hemolytic anemia, an erroneous diagnosis of cold agglutinin syndrome is made without further characterization of the antibody.

Although we have pointed out that the titer of the cold agglutinin at 4°C is not a direct measurement of its *in vivo* significance, nevertheless we find such information is usually of distinct value. We have observed only 1 patient with a titer greater than 1,000 at 4°C in saline who did not have hemolytic anemia, and we have not observed a patient with a titer of 2,000 without hemolytic anemia. Thus, for patients with very high titers at 4°C (>2,000 in saline) (assuming proper technique using separate pipettes for each dilution to avoid "carry-over"), and who otherwise satisfy the criteria for the diagnosis of cold agglutinin syndrome, a diagnostic error is unlikely to result from failure to determine the thermal amplitude. However, many cold agglutinins in patients with the cold agglutinin syndrome have a titer in the range of 1,000 or less at 4°C in saline (see Tables 6-16 and 6-19), and it is in these patients that determination of thermal amplitude is extremely important.

The specificity of the antibody in 54 patients with cold agglutinin syndrome in our series is indicated in Table 6-19. Although such specificity results are of interest, they are not essential either for diagnosis or for the selection of blood for transfusion.

As we have already indicated, the ability of cold antibodies to cause lysis at 20°C was a characteristic of essentially all antibodies from patients with cold agglutinin syndrome, but it was also a characteristic of antibodies from some patients with no evidence of in vivo hemolysis. Thus, positive tests for lysis at 20°C are not diagnostic of cold agglutinin syndrome. What is more important is that cold antibodies will cause a decreasing amount of lysis at progressively higher temperatures. If results for lysis are more strongly positive at 37°C than at 20 or 30°C, a warm hemolysin that may be a separate antibody must be suspected (see p. 211).

Laboratory Diagnosis of Paroxysmal Cold Hemoglobinuria

Essential Diagnostic Tests. The diagnosis of paroxysmal cold hemoglobinuria or the exclusion of that diagnosis in the laboratory is usually considerably easier than that of either warm antibody AIHA or cold agglutinin syndrome. The essential laboratory test is the Donath-Landsteiner test, which is described in detail on page 175. A positive test is illustrated in Figure 6-7. A negative test excludes the diagnosis of paroxysmal cold hemoglobinuria and a positive test is, with rare exceptions (described later in this chapter) diagnostic of the disorder.

TABLE 6-19. THE COLD AGGLUTININ TITER (AT 4°C IN SALINE) AND SPECIFICITY IN 54 PATIENTS WITH COLD AGGLUTININ SYNDROME

Cold Agglutinin Titer	
Titer	No. of Patients
Less than 1000	23
1000–2000	7
2000–4000	13
4000–8000	4
8000	3
32,000	3
256,000	1

Autoantibody Specificity	
Specificity	No. of Patients
Anti-I	49 (90.7%)
Anti-i	4 (7.4%)
Unidentified *	1 (1.9%)

* Not anti-I, -i, -H, -HI, or Pr (but mixtures of these were not excluded)

Since paroxysmal cold hemoglobinuria is quite rare, one may justifiably question the advisability of performing a Donath-Landsteiner test routinely in patients with acquired hemolytic anemia. Our own attitude is to be liberal with the indications for performance of the test since it is simple to perform and its inclusion avoids diagnostic errors and gives us a greater sense of security. If preferred, only a one tube test need be performed initially and, if positive, this can be repeated with appropriate controls. We certainly feel that the performance of the test is indicated in any child, any patient with hemoglobinuria, patients with a history of hemolysis exacerbated by cold, and in all cases with "atypical" serologic findings. If, however, our tests for warm antibody AIHA or cold agglutinin syndrome quickly lead us to perfectly characteristic findings for these disorders, we may omit the Donath-Landsteiner test as superfluous. If positive results are obtained in the Donath-Landsteiner test, determination of the specificity of the autoantibody is indicated. In all six of our patients and in almost all patients reported in the literature, the autoantibody reacts with clear-cut anti-P specificity. This finding is of some diagnostic significance since autoantibodies of this specificity have not been reported in any other type of AIHA. Red cells necessary for determining anti-P specificity are rare but, with the assistance of reference laboratories, specificity testing can be carried out. Typical findings in a patient with paroxysmal cold hemoglobinuria are presented in the following case report and in Table 6-20.

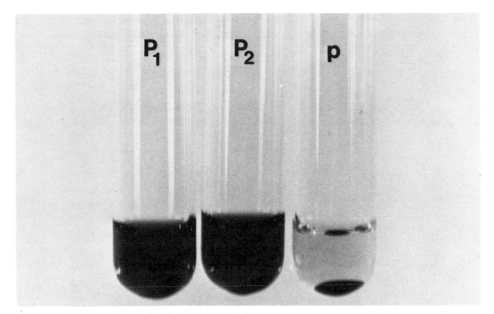

Figure 6-7. *A positive Donath-Landsteiner test. All three tubes contained the patient's serum and were incubated at 0°C in crushed ice for 30 minutes and then placed in a 37°C water bath for 30 minutes. All red cells were group O. Red cells in the two tubes with hemolysis were of group P₁ and P₂, whereas the red cells in the tube with no lysis were of the rare type p. As is illustrated here, the Donath-Landsteiner antibody characteristically demonstrates anti-P specificity.*

Case Report: K. B.,* a 4½-year-old boy, was in good health until 10 days prior to admission to the hospital, at which time he developed a cough and sore throat. Three days prior to admission, he developed a fever of 102°F, headache, myalgia, abdominal pain, vomiting, and diarrhea. He was treated with oral penicillin. Two days prior to admission he began passing dark urine, and the next day he was noted to be jaundiced. His parents noted that his urine output was scanty.

On admission to the hospital he was in no acute distress. Temperature was 37°C, pulse 120, respirations 30, and blood pressure 110/50 mm Hg. Physical examination was unremarkable. The hematocrit level was 31.9 percent, bilirubin 2.4 mg/dl total and 0.2 mg/dl direct reacting, glutamic oxalacetic transaminase (SGOT) was 206, and the lactic dehydrogenase (LDH) 2868 units. The urine was brown, specific gravity 1.017, pH 5.5, hemoglobin test 3+, protein 3+, bilirubin negative and only 2 red blood cells were present per high-power field. The creatinine was 2.6 mg/dl; the sodium was 132 meq, potassium 5.9 meq, chloride 102 meq, and the carbon dioxide 8 meq per liter.

During the next 24 hours he was anuric. At this point his hemoglobin level was 7.0 gm/dl, the hematocrit level 19.6 percent, reticulocytes 1.1 percent, the white cell count was 17,400 with 59 percent neutrophils, 2 percent bands, 29 percent lymphocytes, 8 percent monocytes, and 2 percent monocytes. The platelet count was 214,000. The peripheral blood film showed moderate numbers of spherocytes

* Patient referred by Marian A. Koerper, M.D.

Table 6-20. SEROLOGIC FINDINGS IN PATIENT K.B.

Direct Antiglobulin Test: Dilution of Antiglobulin Serum	Polyspecific Antiglobulin Serum: 3+								
	64	128	256	512	1024	2048	4096	Score	Titer
Anti-IgG	0	0	0	0	0	0	0	0	0
Anti-IgA	0	0	0	0	0	0	0	0	0
Anti-IgM	0	0	0	0	0	0	0	0	0

Dilution of Antiglobulin Serum	4	8	16	32	64	128	256	Score	Titer
Anti-C3	3	2	1½	1	1	½	0	28	128

Screening Tests for Serum Antibody

			Serum	AS + AC*	Control AC Alone
20°C	Untreated cells	Lysis	0	0	0
		Agglutination	0	0	0
	Papainized cells	Lysis	0	1+	0
		Agglutination	1+	1+	0

			Serum Saline	AS + AC	Control AC Alone
37°C	Untreated cells	Lysis	0	0	0
		Agglutination	0	0	0
		IAT	0	0	0
	Papainized cells	Lysis	0	0	0
		Agglutination	0	0	0

Specificity of Serum and Eluate:
  Serum: Anti-P
  Eluate: not done

Cold Agglutinin Titer: Negative

Donath-Landsteiner Test: Positive; titer = 2

Summary: Findings diagnostic of paroxysmal cold hemoglobinuria.

Follow-up: Rapid improvement in anemia and in renal function after initial episode of intravascular hemolysis and renal failure. Two months later the direct antiglobulin test was weakly positive with anti-C3 (titer 16, score 7) and the Donath-Landsteiner test was negative.

* AS=acidified serum; AC=acidified complement.

and poikilocytes. The blood urea nitrogen was 192 mg, and the creatinine 6.0 mg/dl. The sodium was 136 meq, potassium 6.9 meq, chloride 100 meq, and carbon dioxide 9 meq per liter. Total bilirubin was 2.3 mg, and haptoglobin 20 mg/dl. The direct antiglobulin test was 3+. Cultures of blood, urine, throat, stool, and cerebral spinal fluid failed to reveal pathogenic bacteria.

Serologic findings are summarized in Table 6-20 and were diagnostic of paroxysmal cold hemoglobinuria.

The hospital course was marked by 10 days of oliguria necessitating peritoneal dialysis twice. Thereafter the urine output was normal (greater than 60 ml/kg/day), and his creatinine level decreased from a high of 12.9 to 1.9 mg/dl at the time of discharge. Therapy with prednisone was begun on the fourth hospital day at a dose of 2 mg/kg/day for one week, after which it was gradually decreased and then discontinued. The patient's hemoglobin level dropped to 4.3 gm/dl on the day after admission, and he was transfused with 95 ml of P positive red cells without clinical symptoms of a reaction and with transient benefit. Two days later his hemoglobin had again dropped to 4.8 gm/dl and he received 160 ml of red cells, which raised his hemaglobin to 8.6 gm/dl. The following day his reticulocyte count was 5.1 percent and thereafter his hemoglobin level remained stable and he required no further transfusions.

Follow-up examination two months later revealed a hemoglobin level of 13.3 gm/dl, hematocrit 38.6 percent, reticulocytes 0.6 percent, creatinine 0.4 mg/dl, urinalysis normal, and a 24 hour protein excretion of 50 mg.

Comparison of Paroxysmal Cold Hemoglobinuria and the Cold Agglutinin Syndrome. The cold agglutinin syndrome and paroxysmal cold hemoglobinuria are generally quite distinct disorders, and typical findings in each syndrome are compared in Table 6-21. A few similar features may result in the blurring of the distinction between the two disorders, especially in some unusual cases. Clinically, similarities result from the fact that Raynaud's phenomenon and hemoglobinuria may develop in either disorder after exposure to cold. In addition, both syndromes have been reported to occur after *Mycoplasma pneumoniae* infection, although paroxysmal cold hemoglobinuria following infection with this organism is rare.[1]

Table 6-21. COMPARISON OF TYPICAL CHARACTERISTICS OF THE ANTIBODY IN COLD AGGLUTININ SYNDROME WITH THE DONATH-LANDSTEINER ANTIBODY OF PAROXYSMAL COLD HEMOGLOBINURIA

	Cold Agglutinin Syndrome	Donath-Landsteiner Antibody
Titer (4°C)	high (> 500)	moderate (< 64)
Thermal range	high (> 30°C)	moderate (< 20°C)
Bithermic lysis (Donath-Landsteiner test)	negative	positive
Immunoglobulin class	IgM	IgG
Specificity	anti-I or i	anti-P

In the laboratory, some exceptions to the typical findings listed in Table 6-21 occur. For example, patients with the cold agglutinin syndrome may have a cold agglutinin titer less than 500 (Table 6-16). The thermal range of the Donath-Landsteiner antibody has been reported as high as 32°C in 1 exceptional case [30] and there are several reports of Donath-Landsteiner antibodies reactive at temperatures of 18°C to 25°C.[2, 37] These antibodies will therefore not require incubation at 0°C as in the Donath-Landsteiner test and they will cause "monophastic" lysis. Also, the specificity of the Donath-Landsteiner antibody in rare instances may be anti-I or anti-HI, similar to that found in cold agglutinin syndrome. Finally, some antibodies from patients with cold agglutinin syndrome have been reported to give a positive Donath-Landsteiner test. This finding is perhaps not surprising, since some cold antibodies from patients with the cold agglutinin syndrome cause lysis at room temperature (Table 6-17).

During the performance of the Donath-Landsteiner test, there is a brief period of time when cells and serum are at room temperature after being moved from the ice bath to a 37°C water bath. Dacie [6] has reported slight hemolysis in the Donath-Landsteiner test using 2 sera containing high titer cold agglutinins (titers of 4,000 and 64,000 respectively). We have attempted to duplicate these results using two sera with high titer cold agglutinins from patients with cold agglutinin syndrome. One serum had a cold agglutinin titer of 8,000 at 4°C in saline and caused lysis of pre-papainized red cells to a titer of 128 at 22°C, but it did not cause lysis of non-papainized erythrocytes. The other serum had a cold agglutinin titer of 16,000 in saline at 4°C, caused lysis of pre-papainized red cells at 22°C to a titer of 4,000, and lysis of normal red cells at 22°C to a titer of 256. The Donath-Landsteiner test was negative using each of these sera even when pre-papainized red cells were used. Nevertheless, it appears that the Donath-Landsteiner test must be interpreted with caution when the serum contains a high titer cold agglutinin, particularly if it is a potent hemolysin.

Although the preceding findings may seem to add an air of uncertainty to the differentiation between the two disorders, it is rare that the distinction is actually difficult, either on clinical grounds or in the laboratory. Clinically, paroxysmal cold hemoglobinuria is an acute hemolytic anemia associated with marked constitutional symptoms; modern case reports describe the disorder almost exclusively in children or young adults, and it is almost always transient. In contrast, when the cold agglutinin syndrome occurs in middle-aged or elderly persons, the patient's symptoms are frequently just those of anemia, and the disorder is chronic except in the minority of patients who have transient anemia following *Mycoplasma pneumoniae* infection or other infectious diseases.

In the laboratory, a positive Donath-Landsteiner test should be considered diagnostic of paroxysmal cold hemoglobinuria unless a cold agglutinin that is of high thermal amplitude and is a potent hemolysin is present. Such antibodies will cause weakly positive reactions in the Donath-Landsteiner test and maximum lysis after "monophasic" incubation at 20°C.[6] These reactions should be interpreted as a "false-positive" Donath-Landsteiner test in a patient with cold agglutinin syndrome.

Opposite findings occur in patients with paroxysmal cold hemoglobinuria. That is, even if the thermal range of a Donath-Landsteiner antibody is high enough to result in monophasic lysis, maximal lysis will occur if an incubation at 0°C precedes incubation at 37°C. Also, specificity tests are usually of value in separating the two disorders and, finally, the antibody in paroxysmal cold hemoglobinuria is invariably of the IgG immunoglobulin class, in contrast to the IgM antibody of cold agglutinin syndrome.

REFERENCES

1. Bell, C. A., Zwicker, H., and Rosenbaum, D. L.: Paroxysmal cold hemoglobinuria (P.C.H.) following mycoplasma infection: Anti-I specificity of the biphasic hemolysin. Transfusion, *13:*138, 1973.
2. Bird, G. W. G., Wingham, J., Martin, A. J., Richardson, S. G. N., Cole, A. P., Payne, R. W., and Savage, B. F.: Idiopathic non-syphilitic paroxysmal cold haemoglobinuria in children. J. Clin. Pathol., *29:*215, 1976.
3. Chaplin, H.: Clinical usefulness of specific antiglobulin reagents in autoimmune hemolytic anemias. Prog. Hematol., *8:*25, 1973.
4. Chaplin, H., and Avioli, L. V.: Autoimmune hemolytic anemia. Arch. Intern. Med., *137:*346, 1977.
5. Croucher, B. E. E., Crookston, M. C., and Crookston, J. H.: Delayed haemolytic transfusion reactions simulating autoimmune haemolytic anaemia. Vox. Sang., *12:*32, 1967.
6. Dacie, J. V.: The Haemolytic Anaemias. 2nd Ed. London, J. & A. Churchill Ltd., 1962.
7. Dacie, J. V., and Worlledge, S. M.: Auto-immune hemolytic anemias. Progr. Hematol., *VI:*82, 1969.
8. de Lange, J. A., Eernisse, G. J., and Veltkamp, J. J.: Cold agglutinins and the Counter counter model S. Amer. J. Clin. Pathol. (correspondence) *58:*599, 1972.
9. Eyster, M. E., and Jenkins, D. E., Jr.: γG erythrocyte autoantibodies: Comparison of *in vivo* complement coating and *in vitro* "Rh" specificity. J. Immunol., *105:*221, 1970.
10. Fischer, J. T., Petz, L. D., Garratty, G., and Cooper, N. R.: Correlations between quantitative assay of red-cell bound C3, serologic reactions, and hemolytic anemia. Blood, *44:*359, 1974.
11. Frank, M. M., Schreiber, A. D., Atkinson, J. P., and Jaffe, C. J.: Pathophysiology of immune hemolytic anemia. Ann. Intern. Med., *87:*210, 1977.
12. Garratty, G.: The effects of storage and heparin on the activity of serum complement with particular reference to the detection of blood group antibodies Amer. J. Clin. Pathol., *54:*531, 1970.
13. Garratty, G., and Petz, L. D.: The significance of red cell bound complement components in development of standards and quality assurance for the anti-complement components of antiglobulin sera. Transfusion, *16:*297, 1976.
14. Garratty, G., and Petz, L. D.: An evaluation of commercial antiglobulin sera with particular reference to their anticomplement properties. Transfusion, *11:*79, 1971.
15. Garratty, G., Petz, L. D., and Hoops, J. K.: The correlation of cold agglutinin titrations in saline and albumin with haemolytic anaemia. Brit. J. Haematol., *35:*587, 1977.

16. Gerbal, A., Homberg, J. C., Rochant, H., Perron, L., and Salmon, C.: Les autoanticorps d'anémies hémolytiques acquises. I. Analyse de 234 observations. Nouv. Rev. Franc. Hémat., 8:155, 1968.
17. Gerbal, A., Homberg, J. C., Rochant, H., Perron, L., and Salmon, C.: Les autoanticorps d'anémies hémolytiques acquises. II. Nature, spécificité, interêt clinique et méchanisme de formation. Nouv. Rev. Franc. Hemat., 8:351, 1968.
18. Goldfinger, D., Sturgeon, P., Smith, L., Garratty, G., and Hurvitz, C.: Autoimmune hemolytic anemia associated exclusively with IgA of Rh specificity. Presented at the American Association of Blood Banks 30th Annual Meeting, Atlanta, Georgia, 1977.
19. Hattersley, P. G., Gerard, P. W., Caggiano, V., et al.: Erroneous values on the model S Coulter counter due to high titer cold autoagglutinins. Amer. J. Clin. Pathol., 55:442, 1971.
20. Haynes, C. R., and Chaplin, H., Jr.: An enhancing effect of albumin on the determination of cold hemagglutinins. Vox. Sang., 20:46, 1971.
21. Hsu, T. C. S., Rosenfield, R. E., Burkart, P., Wong, K. Y., and Kochwa, S.: Instrumented PVP-augmented antiglobulin tests. II. Evaluation of acquired hemolytic anemia. Vox. Sang., 26:305, 1974.
22. Jeannet, M.: Specificity of the antiglobulin test in "autoimmune" hemolytic anemias. Helv. Med. Acta, 33:151, 1966.
23. Kerr, R. O., Dalmasso, A. P., and Kaplan, M. E.: Erythrocyte-bound C5 and C6 in autoimmune hemolytic anemia. J. Immunol., 107:1209, 1971.
24. Logue, G. L., Rosse, W. F., and Gockerman, J. P.: Measurement of the third component of complement bound to red blood cells in patients with the cold agglutinin syndrome. J. Clin. Invest., 52:493, 1973.
25. Mollison, P. L.: Blood Transfusion in Clinical Medicine. 5th Ed. Oxford, Blackwell, 1972.
26. Petrucci, J. V., Dunne, P. A., and Chapman, C.: Spurious erythrocyte indices as measured by the model S Coulter counter due to cold agglutinins. Amer. J. Clin. Pathol., 56:500, 1971.
27. Petz, L. D., and Garratty, G.: Complement in immunohematology. Prog. Clin. Immunol., 2:175, 1974.
28. Petz, L. D.: Complement in immunohematology and in neurologic disorders. In The Proceedings of an International Symposium on "The Nature and Significance of Complement Activation." Raritan, New Jersey, Ortho Research Institute of Medical Sciences, September 1–3, 1976.
29. Petz, L. D., and Garratty, G.: Antiglobulin sera—Past, present and future. Transfusion, 18:257, 1978.
30. Ries, C. W., Garratty, G., Petz, L. D., and Fudenberg, H. H.: Paroxysmal cold hemoglobinuria: Report of a case with an exceptionally high thermal range Donath-Landsteiner antibody. Blood, 38:491, 1971.
31. Rosenfield, R. E., and Jagathambal: Transfusion therapy for autoimmune hemolytic anemia. Seminars Hematol., 13:311, 1976.
32. Rosse, W. F.: Quantitative immunology of immune hemolytic anemia. I. The fixation of C1 by autoimmune antibody and heterologous anti-IgG antibody. J. Clin. Invest., 50:727, 1971.
33. Rosse, W. F.: Quantitative immunology of immune hemolytic anemia. II. The relationship of cell-bound antibody to hemolysis and the effect of treatment. J. Clin. Invest., 50:734, 1971.
34. Stratton, F., and Rawlinson, V. I.: Observations on the antiglobulin tests. II. C4 components on erythrocytes. Vox. Sang., 31:44, 1976.
35. Stratton, F., Rawlinson, V. I., Chapman, S. A., Pengelly, C. D. R., and Jennings, R. C.: Acquired hemolytic anemia associated with IgA anti-e. Transfusion, 12:157, 1974.
36. Stratton, F., Smith, D. S., and Rawlinson, V. I.: Value of gel filtration on Sephadex G-200 in the analysis of blood group antibodies. J. Clin. Pathol., 21:708, 1968.

36a. Sturgeon, P., Smith, L. E., Chun, H. M. T., Hurvitz, C. H., Garratty, G., and Goldfinger, D.: Autoimmune hemolytic anemia associated exclusively with IgA of Rh specificity. Transfusion, *19:*324, 1979.

37. Vogel, J. M., Hellman, M., and Moloshok, R. E.: Paroxysmal cold hemoglobinuria of nonsyphilitic etiology in two children. J. Ped., *81:*974, 1972.

38. von Dem Borne, A. E. G. Kr., Engelfriet, C. P., Beckers, D., Van Der Kort-Henkes, G., Van Der Giessen, M., and Van Loghem, J. H.: Autoimmune haemolytic anaemias. II. Warm haemolysins—serological and immunochemical investigations and ^{51}Cr studies. Clin. Exper. Immunol., *4:*333, 1969.

39. Worlledge, S. M.: Immune drug-induced hemolytic anemias. Seminars Hematol., *10:*327, 1973.

40. Worlledge, S. M.: The interpretation of a positive direct antiglobulin test. Brit. J. Haematol., *39:*157, 1978.

41. Worlledge, S. M., and Blajchman, M. A.: The autoimmune haemolytic anaemias. Brit. J. Haematol., *23:*61, 1972.

7

Specificity of Autoantibodies

SPECIFICITY OF AUTOANTIBODIES ASSOCIATED WITH WARM-ANTIBODY TYPE AUTOIMMUNE HEMOLYTIC ANEMIA

Early Observations

Up to 1953 autoantibodies were generally considered to be "non-specific;" that is to say, they reacted with all human red cells tested, although some variation in reaction had been observed.[23] Some workers had obtained negative results with red cells from other species (e.g., rhesus monkey, sheep, mouse, guinea pig, rabbit, fowl, and horse).[23] Some similarities to Rh antibodies had been observed [23] and in 1953, Wiener and Gordon [129] and Wiener, Gordon, and Gallop [130] suggested that the autoantibodies might be directed against the "nucleus of the Rh-Hr substance." Their hypothesis was based mainly on the similarity in reactions seen with red cells of other species and the similarity in reactions with antiglobulin sera. Pirofsky and Pratt,[90] in 1966, compared the reactions of allo anti-Rh and warm autoantibodies with the red cells of a large variety of primates and non-primates and essentially agreed with Wiener's findings. Neither allo anti-Rh nor autoantibodies reacted with non-primate red cells or certain primates (e.g., tree shrew, fulvus lemur, and woolly monkey), but both reacted with other primates (ringtail lemur, squirrel monkey, celebes ape, rhesus monkey, baboon, and chimpanzee). Allo anti-c was found to react strongly with squirrel monkey, celebes ape, rhesus monkey, and chimpanzee; anti-D reacted strongly with chimpanzee. The authors concluded that the data strongly suggested that warm autoantibodies have specificity for an Rh antigen.

The first convincing data suggesting an association with Rh were presented by Race, Sanger, and Selwyn in 1951.[91] Using red cells from the recently discovered rare phenotype $-D-$, they showed the so-called "non-specific" autoantibodies could be subdivided into two groups; one that reacted with the $-D-$ cells, and the other that did not. The first case of a clearly specific autoantibody was an auto anti-e in an R_1R_1 patient described by Weiner et al. in 1953; [127] others soon followed. Hollander [50] described an auto anti-c in an R_1r patient and showed that an additional "non-specific" element was also present in the eluate made from the patient's red cells. In 1953 and 1954, Dacie [22] and Dacie and Cutbush [25] reported specificities on ten patients with warm-antibody type autoimmune hemolytic anemia: one R_1r patient had auto anti-C+e; the other nine patients had "non-specific" autoantibodies, but three also had clearly demonstrable auto anti-e, and one patient auto anti-e and D (at different times). In the next decade, many other workers confirmed and extended these findings.[23]

With the exception of an anti-Jk[a][117] and two examples of anti-K,[27, 36] all the specificities reported during this time were associated with Rh. Auto anti-e specificity was the most common reported specificity; it has been pointed out [23] that the reported relative incidence of different specific Rh autoantibodies corresponds well with the incidence of Rh antigens in the population (i.e., e is present on the red cells of approximately 98 percent of the population).

In 1963 Weiner and Vos [126] expanded the work of Race et al.[91] who used red cells of the rare phenotype −D− to demonstrate "Rh" specificity. Weiner and Vos studied sixty red cell eluates that were initially thought to be nonspecific; these eluates were tested against red cells of common phenotypes and rare phenotypes such as −D−, cD−, and the recently discovered Rh_{null} (− − −/− − −). Absorptions, elutions (i.e., eluates made from red cells incubated *in vitro* with eluates prepared from patients' red cells sensitized *in vivo*), and titrations were performed, utilizing saline, albumin, enzymes, and indirect antiglobulin tests.

Fifty-three percent of the eluates failed to react with Rh_{null} red cells, and 18 percent reacted weaker than with red cells of common phenotypes. Thus, almost 70 percent of the eluates appeared to be reacting with antigens at the Rh locus. The patterns of reactivities obtained suggested three different autoantibody types that could be present separately or in combination. They were termed anti-nl, anti-pdl, and anti-dl. The nl determinants were said to be present on red cells of common phenotypes, but not −D−, Dc− or Rh_{null}; the pdl determinants present on red cells of common phenotypes, −D−, Dc−, but not Rh_{null}; the dl determinants present on red cells of common phenotypes, −D−, Dc−, and Rh_{null} (see Table 7-1).

Thus, if an autoantibody reacts with all red cells of common phenotype

Table 7-1. AUTOANTIBODIES IN ACQUIRED HEMOLYTIC ANEMIA AND THEIR SEROLOGIC REACTIVITY FOR SELECTED RED CELLS [126]

	Anti-nl	Anti-pdl	Anti-dl	Suggested Antigenic Make-up of Red Cells
"Normal" cells CDe/cde, cDE/cde, cde/ cde, etc.	+	+	+	nl, pdl, dl
"Partially deleted" cells −D−/−D− or cD−/cD−	−	+	+	pdl, dl
"Fully deleted" cells − − −/− − − (Rh_{null})	−	−	+	dl

but not "partially deleted" or "fully deleted" red cells, the autoantibody would be classified as having anti-nl specificity. If the autoantibody(ies) reacts with all cells, it may be anti-dl, but selective absorptions may reveal a mixture of anti-dl + pdl, anti-dl + nl, or anti-dl + pdl+nl. In other words, absorption of a "non-specific" autoantibody with Rh$_{null}$ red cells may reveal an antibody only reacting with red cells of common phenotype. We have confirmed these findings in our own laboratory and have collaborated with Vos in recent years to extend the original observations.[121-123]

In 1967, Celano and Levine[19] demonstrated anti-LW activity in all six cases of warm antibody type AIHA they studied: all six showed "non-specific" reactions when first tested against a panel of common phenotypes, but when the panel included Rh$_{null}$ and Rh positive and/or Rh negative LW negative red cells, one serum exhibited clear anti-LW specificity. Further absorption studies on the other cases revealed the presence of anti-LW together with a "non-specific" element. The authors pointed out that the primate red cells that reacted with autoantibodies in the studies of Pirofsky and Pratt[90] (mentioned previously) are known to contain LW antigens.

Observations During the Last Decade

In a detailed review in 1969, Dacie and Worlledge reviewed results on their series of patients with autoimmune hemolytic anemia seen since 1947.[26] Specificity testing of eluates from ninety-eight patients with warm antibody-type AIHA were reported. When tested against a panel of red cells with common phenotypes, approximately 30 percent showed obvious Rh specificity (23 anti-e, 4 anti-c, 1 C+D, 1 D+e). When −D− red cells were added to the panel, a further 17 percent could be classified as "Rh" specific (47 percent of the total), and if Rh$_{null}$ cells were added, then a further 5 percent could be added, giving a total of 52 percent showing some "Rh" specificity.

An interesting further analysis of these results showed that if the specificities were calculated according to whether the eluates were prepared from red cells sensitized with IgG but no complement and red cells sensitized with IgG and complement, the results were very different. For instance, 38 percent of the "IgG alone" group showed clear cut Rh specificity when tested against a panel of common phenotypes, compared with only 10 percent in the "IgG + complement" group. When −D− and Rh$_{null}$ cells were included, 68 percent of the "IgG only" group showed "Rh" specificity, in contrast to only 14 percent of the "IgG + complement" group.

Other workers, including ourselves, have also found a marked difference in specificity when the eluates from "IgG only" direct antiglobulin tests are compared with "IgG + complement." Eyster and Jenkins[33] studied eluates from 37 patients. (One showed anti-e specificity, another failed to react with some cells, but no specificity was obvious; the other 35 reacted with all cells tested.) Of the 35 eluates that reacted with all red cells, 6 of 12 eluates from red cells having an "IgG only" positive direct antiglobulin test showed "Rh" specificity, whereas only 6 of 23 "IgG + complement" eluates showed specificity. They also confirmed the experiments of Weiner and Vos [126] by showing that if the "non-specific" eluates were absorbed with Rh_{null} cells, the absorbed serum sometimes demonstrated "Rh" specificity with red cells of common phenotypes.

Leddy et al. [66] studied eluates prepared from 46 patients with warm antibody type AIHA. They used a panel of rare human red cells including Rh_{null}, −D−, LW negative, and Ko red cells as well as monkey red cells (rhesus and stump tailed monkeys). Sixteen of 20 eluates derived from patients whose red cells were sensitized with both IgG and complement reacted with all cells. Conversely, 12 of 26 eluates from "IgG only" red cells did not react with Rh_{null} red cells, suggesting "Rh" specificity. Leddy et al. [66] found four patterns of reactions (see Table 7-2) that suggested a working classification: Group I reacted with red cells of common phenotype but were negative with Rh_{null} and monkey red cells, no complement was fixed *in vivo;* group II reacted with red cells of common phenotype and weaker with Rh_{null}, about 25 percent reacted with monkey red cells; group III reacted with red cells of common phenotype and Rh_{null} cells equally strongly, but did not react with monkey cells; group IV reacted equally strongly with red cells of normal phenotypes, Rh_{null} and monkey red cells.

Vos et al. [121] studied 24 sera and red cell eluates from patients with warm antibody type AIHA. They showed that the indirect antiglobulin test often showed different specificities than tests using ficin. As found by previous workers, they reported that the eluates from red cells sensitized only with IgG showed clearer specificity than the "IgG + complement" group; 72 percent of the "IgG only" group did not react with Rh_{null} red cells, in contrast to 100 percent of the "IgG + complement" group reacting with Rh_{null} cells in addition to common phenotypes. Additional studies using red cell eluates revealed that no direct correlation could be established between the presence of complement components on the patient's red cells, as determined by direct antiglobulin testing, and the intensity of the indirect antiglobulin test using anti-IgG serum. On the other hand, the simultaneous presence of anti-nl and anti-dl autoantibodies was often associated with the presence of complement

Table 7-2. WORKING CLASSIFICATION OF MAJOR
SPECIFICITIES OF IgG AUTOANTIBODIES
SUGGESTED BY LEDDY ET AL., 1970 [66]

| Group | Number of Cases | Reactions with Human RBC | | Reactions with Monkey RBC |
		Common Phenotype	Rh_{null}	
I	12	4+	0	0/12
II	12	4+	2+	3/12
III	12	4+	4+	0/12
IV	10	4+	4+	10/10

in the red cell eluates. They suggested that the presence of complement components in association with anti-nl and anti-dl may be analogous to complement fixation by multiple Rh alloantibodies as described by Rosse.[105] The formation of anti-nl with anti-dl, which tends to result in complement components being fixed by the antibody, may be considered a natural progression of antibody synthesis with an advanced state of autoimmunization comparable to the development of Rh alloantibodies in which, as a rule, anti-D is more often noted in the early stages of alloimmunization than anti-CD.

In a later publication [122] the same group of workers showed that the presence of complement on red cells, in addition to IgG, seemed to be associated exclusively with antoantibodies of multiple immunoglobulin classes, as well as multiple red cell specificities. They postulated that the variability encountered in multiple antibodies may reflect continuous differences in the inciting stimulus resulting from altered configuration of red cell antigenic determinants.

The observed pattern of serologic and immunologic findings does not readily support the concept that the red cell autoantibodies are homogenous populations of immunoglobulins, at least not in the same sense that myeloma globulins are products of monoclonal proliferation.

Bell et al.[11] reported specificity studies on 38 patients with warm antibody type AIHA. In approximately 60 percent of 35 reactive eluates, no specificity was obvious; approximately 17 percent showed obvious Rh specificity (anti-e (2), anti-e + "non-specific" (1), anti-e + other "Rh" specificities (4), anti-E (2)). Forty percent demonstrated "Rh" specificity based on their non-reactivity with Rh_{null} red cells.

In 1972, we collaborated with Vos to study in depth eight eluates made from patients with warm antibody type AIHA.[123] We used a panel of red cells containing very rare phenotypes and performed selected absorption and elution studies. We were able to demonstrate autoantibody specificities not definable without the rare cells and further defined heterogeneity of the LW antigen. Six of the eluates contained anti-LW, two anti-nl, five anti-pdl, three anti-dl, and one anti-e.

The pdl autoantibody described by Weiner and Vos [126] is often found in AIHA eluates and is known to react with all human red cells except Rh_{null}. This antibody previously could not be classified as anti-LW because it sensitized LW-negative red cells. Of particular interest in our study was the observation that some LW-negative red cells could separate anti-pdl into anti-pdl plus anti-LW. Absorption and elution studies using the rare Rh positive LW negative cells (Mrs. Bigelow), showed that anti-pdl may, in fact, represent anti-LW + LW_1 and that Mrs. Bigelow may represent a weak variant of LW rather than being LW negative. The absorption studies were confirmed by injecting Mrs. Bigelow's red cells into guinea pigs and demonstrating the presence of anti-LW after absorption with Rh_{null} cells.

It is tempting to suggest an analogy to the ABO system and postulate that Rh-positive cells represent LW_1, Rh-negative cells represent LW_2 (as suggested by Levine),[67] and Mrs. Bigelow represents LW_3. Rh_{null} appears to be the true

LW-negative. It will be interesting to see if studies of Rh-negative, LW-negative samples will show them to have a weaker form of LW than Mrs. Bigelow, who is Rh-positive. An apparent criticism of this analogy is that if Mrs. Bigelow represents LW_3, comparable to A_3 in the ABO system, then the anti-LW in her serum should react with only LW_1 (i.e., Rh-positive) red cells, comparable to the anti-A_1 found in the sera of some A_3 individuals. However, the anti-LW reacted strongly with Rh-positive (LW_1) cells and weakly with LW_2 (Rh-negative) cells. It is possible that the results were simply reflecting a quantitative difference rather than a qualitative difference. Even though anti-A_1 usually does not agglutinate A_2 cells, some workers have reported that anti-A_1 found in A_x individuals reacts with both A_1 and A_2 cells.[52] We know there is a quantitative effect, as anti-A_1 can be removed by several absorptions with A_2 cells. This demonstrates that anti-A_1 does indeed react with A_2 cells. By analogy, anti-LW_1 reacts with LW_1 strongly and LW_2 weakly. The only difference between the LW_1 reactions and the reactions of anti-A_1 with A_1 and A_2 cells is that LW reactions are demonstrated by strong agglutination versus weak agglutination, whereas the A_1, A_2 reactions are demonstrated by agglutination versus absorption. The overall results of our studies suggested that LW represents a spectrum of variations; LW_1, LW_2, LW_3, and maybe LW_4. Rh_{null} cells may be the only true LW-negative cells.

In 1975 Dacie[24] reported further data on 121 patients with warm antibody type AIHA. "Rh" specificity could be demonstrated in 68 percent of the patients and was as high as 83 percent if only patients with IgG but no complement on their red cells were considered; only 37 percent of patients with IgG + complement on their red cells showed "Rh" specificity.

In an extensive study published in 1976, Issitt et al.[56] found "obvious" anti-Rh specificity (specificities seen included anti-D, -C, -E, -c, -e, -f, -Ce, and anti-G) to be present alone in 3 of 87 cases (3.5 percent). Autoantibodies of these specificities, together with autoantibodies of other specificities, such as anti-nl, -pdl, -dl and anti-Wr^b (described later) were found in 23 of 87 cases (26 percent). Overall, 73.6 percent of the autoantibodies reacted as well with $-D-$ and Rh_{null} red cells as with common phenotypes. This study also confirmed our earlier studies[122] in terms of the immunoglobulin class of the autoantibodies and the fact that complement fixation *in vivo* generally occurs only when autoantibodies with complex specificity, such as anti-pdl or anti-dl are produced.

Autoantibody Specificity Not Associated with Rh

In early reports, isolated examples of autoantibodies with specificity other than Rh were described, but the evidence presented was incomplete, or very unconvincing. In 1954, Van Loghem et al.[117] listed an auto anti-Jk^a as being associated with acquired hemolytic anemia, and in 1955 and 1957, Flückiger et al.[36] and Dausset et al.,[27] respectively, described examples of auto anti-K being associated with autoimmune hemolytic anemia. A single case of auto anti-Xg^a has been described,[137] but although the patient was anemic, no evidence was presented concerning the clinical significance of this antibody; indeed, no evidence for hemolytic anemia was presented.

The first undisputed obvious specificity, other than Rh, in patients with warm antibody type AIHA was described in 1971 when Nugent and co-workers [85] described a patient with an autoantibody with U blood group specificity. Because of the observations of Schmidt et al. [108] that Rh_{null} red cells also have aberrant U antigen, together with some degree of abnormality of the Ss antigens, Marsh et al. [79] thought autoantibodies that were being called "Rh" specific because they failed to react with Rh_{null} red cells should be re-examined. They studied eluates from 50 patients that reacted with all red cells of common phenotypes; 24 of these eluates reacted significantly weaker with Rh_{null} red cells, and in some of these cases, well-defined specificity for known Rh antigens could be demonstrated (e.g., anti-e). Three of the cases showed autoantibodies that reacted with all red cells but more weakly with both U-negative and Rh_{null} red cells. In two of these, absorption and elution studies resulted in the separation of anti-e and anti-U with an additional "non-specific" component reacting with Rh_{null} red cells. Absorption and elution studies in a third case yielded anti-U and "non-specific" antibody only. Thus, in 50 eluates, 3 (6 percent) showed auto anti-U specificity. Other workers since have also demonstrated auto anti-U specificity associated with warm-antibody type AIHA [123] and in patients with a positive direct antiglobulin test and no hemolytic anemia. [5] In our study with Vos [123] described previously, we used the only Rh_{null} U+ red cell sample so far described, [51] in addition to an Rh_{null} U negative sample, to study 8 selected red cell eluates from patients with warm antibody-type AIHA. We were able to demonstrate autoantibodies with U specificity in 3 of the 8 eluates (38 percent), but they were always present with autoantibodies of other specificity (e.g., anti-LW, -nl, -pdl, -dl, and anti-e). Without the rare Rh_{null} U positive cells, it would have been difficult to demonstrate the presence of the anti-U, and this probably accounts for the much higher incidence of auto anti-U detected compared with other series (e.g., Marsh et al. [79]).

As mentioned previously, there were two early reports of patients with warm antibody AIHA who had autoantibodies associated with the Kell system. [27,36] In 1972, another case was intensively studied in Warsaw and London. [109] A 17-year-old boy developed severe hemolytic anemia and was treated with steroids and blood transfusion without effect. His direct antiglobulin test was initially negative, but during his hospitalization it became weakly positive. During the next several weeks he was treated with steroids, azathioprine, and blood transfusion without much success. During the fourth week of the disease, he had a severe hemolytic transfusion reaction following 500 ml of red cells. During the fifth week of his disease his red cells were found to lack K, Kp^a, and Js^a antigens, while the antithetical antigens k and Kp^b were only weakly expressed. His serum now contained anti-Kp^b (titer of 256 by albumin technique). Following transfusion of Kp(b−) red cells, the patient began to improve (^{51}Cr half-life of transfused red cells was 19 days). Serologic tests performed six weeks after this first compatible Kp(b−) blood transfusion revealed a very low level of anti-Kp[b] in the serum and a weakly positive direct antiglobulin test; anti-Kp[b] could be eluted from the cells. The patient's red cells now reacted strongly with a sample of his serum collected six weeks previously, although the cells were compatible with current serum, unless the red cells were ficin-treated in which case they reacted weakly. The ⁵¹Cr half-life of the patient's red cells at this time was still short—8.5 days, with most of the cells being destroyed in the spleen. During the eighth week of his illness more Kp(b−) red cells were transfused; although he had an excellent hematologic response, the ⁵¹Cr half-life of his own cells was only 8.5 days. The patient was discharged in excellent condition after four months of hospitalization. By the sixteenth week, although the direct antiglobulin test was still weakly positive (only complement was present on his red cells), the anti-Kp[b] in the serum was undetectable; the Kell phenotype was now normal, K(−), Kp(a−), Js(a−), with normal expression of k and Kp[b]. After seven months, the ⁵¹Cr half-life of his own cells was 26 days. The authors suggested that, although blocking of the Kp[b] antigen could have occurred during the acute phase of the disease, the structure of the antibody molecule must have differed from that which normally has anti-Kp[b] specificity, because antiglobulin sera reacted with it only weakly (i.e., very weak direct antiglobulin test). An alternative and more probable explanation, they thought, was that during the acute stage of the disease, an unknown exogenous factor such as a virus disturbed the synthesis of Kell antigens by inhibiting the action of transferases which are necessary for the full expression of these antigens on red cells. Another case closely resembling this case has recently been described.[7]

In 1973,[43] we described another association of anti-K with warm antibody type AIHA. The patient was a 49-year-old white woman who presented in 1971 with intermittent fevers of unknown origin. She was found to have granulomas of the lung and liver, and to be anemic. She was treated with tetracycline, INH, and pyridoxine. In December 1972 she was admitted to hospital with fever and hemolytic anemia. Her direct antiglobulin test was found to be strongly positive. Her hemolysis cleared spontaneously, and by January 1973 she was hematologically normal and has remained so since. When we first studied her serologically at the end of 1972, her direct antiglobulin test was found to be strongly positive due to sensitization with IgG, IgM, and complement. The eluate prepared from her red cells contained an IgG and IgM anti-K. No reactions were obtained against Kell negative red cells. Ether, heat, and acid elution methods yielded identical results. The patient's serum contained IgG and IgM anti-K, reacting by indirect antiglobulin test at 37° C. Enzyme-treated homozygote Kell positive cells were completely hemolyzed. The serum also contained another IgG antibody reacting by indirect antiglobulin test at 37° C, against 93 percent of 183 Kell negative samples, including Ko, McLeod, Chido negative and York negative red cells; positive reactions ranged from ½–3+. The serum placed known weak, moderate, and strong Bg[a] + red cells in order, when tested blind and a tail of weak agglutination reactions was observed on titration (high titer, low avidity). The patient's serum also contained anti-HLA-A2, -B7, and -A28, which have been shown to react with the Bg blood groups on red cells.[83, 84]

The patient's red cells typed as AB, K−k+, Kp(a−b+), Js(a−b+) Ku+ and Kl+. As Seyfried and co-workers [109] had described an apparent depression of Kell antigens associated with autoimmune hemolytic anemia, the patient's cells were tested by titration against several different anti-K, -k, and Js^b reagents. No depression of any Kell antigens was noted. Her lymphocytes typed as HLA-A3, -A11, -B5, and -B8. Her lymphocyte auto-cytotoxicity was negative.

When the patient's serum was incubated at 4° C or 37° C with Kell negative cells, it was possible to elute anti-Kell from these cells. The reaction was always weaker than the eluate obtained from Kell positive cells. Eluates from these *in vitro* sensitized cells and from the patient's own red cells were also tested for anti-HLA activity with negative results.

In 1971, Giblett and co-workers [47] described a possible association between the rare sex-linked chronic granulomatous disease and the Kell system, in that there appeared to be a high incidence of the rare Ko phenotype. As our patient presented with granulomas and an unusual serologic phenomenon involving Kell, we investigated the family history carefully. We found that Mrs. Sh had one living healthy son 26 years of age, but that another boy had died at the age of nine. His case history and autopsy findings in retrospect were classic for chronic granulomatous disease, although it was not recognized as such at that time. Mrs. Sh's leukocytes were tested for their ability to kill Staphylococci and Serratia. The killing effect was intermediate between leukocytes from a normal individual and a patient with chronic granulomatous disease. The leukocytes were also tested by the nitroblue tetrazolium dye reduction test. Once again, the results obtained were intermediate between normal and chronic granulomatous disease. Both sets of test results are diagnostic for a carrier state of chronic granulomatous disease.

Marsh and co-workers [78] have shown that anti-KL contains an antibody anti-K$_x$ that reacts with an antigen present on Ko cells. They have further described a difference in the Kell antigens on leukocytes from patients with chronic granulomatous disease, in that they appear to lack the K$_x$ antigen. Marsh kindly tested the leukocytes from Mrs. Sh and showed that they absorbed anti-K$_x$ from an anti-KL serum much less efficiently than normal leukocytes.

The patient's direct antiglobulin test became progressively weaker, and when last tested, it was negative. The anti-K had also diminished in strength, as had the other antibodies reacting against the Kell negative red cells. In contrast, the HLA-A2 and -B7 titers had not weakened. The ability of the serum to sensitize Kell negative cells *in vitro* with anti-K appeared to diminish in direct relationship to the other red cell antibodies in the serum. To summarize: Mrs. Sh was a female carrier of chronic granulomatous disease who presented with hemolytic anemia associated with red cell sensitization due to anti-K. The patient was Kell negative and we were unable to explain why the anti-K sensitized Kell negative cells *in vivo* and *in vitro*. The antibody may be an autoantibody mimicking an alloantibody [43] (see below) or its reactivity could be explained on the basis of the Matuhasi-Ogata phenomenon.[43] Although another antibody was present in the serum, we were unable to demonstrate the presence of this antibody together with anti-K in eluates from Kell negative red cells, so we were unable to prove this as an example of the Matuhasi-Ogata phenomenon,[80, 86, 87] but it is of interest to note that Wilkinson et al.[133] have described *in vitro* absorption of anti-D onto D negative red cells in the presence of anti-Bg, and that anti-Bg is highly suspect in our patient's serum.

In 1974, we reported a new specificity to be associated with warm antibody type AIHA, i.e., anti-I^T.[42] Anti-I^T had previously only been reported as a cold autoagglutinin in Melanesians [14] and Yanomana Indians in Venezuela,[65] except for one case of an IgG antibody we described in a Caucasian with Hodgkin's disease; [40] neither this case nor the cold autoantibodies were associated with hemolytic anemia. Anti-I^T reacts more strongly with cord red cells than with adult red cells. In contrast to anti-i, anti-I^T reacts even more weakly with i adult red cells than normal I adult red cells. If only I adult red cells and cord red cells are used, then anti-i and anti-I^T may appear the same; i adult red cells must be tested to differentiate the two (see Table 7-3).

Table 7-3. RELATIVE STRENGTH OF REACTIONS SEEN WITH ANTI-I, ANTI-i AND ANTI-I^T

	I ADULT	i CORD	i ADULT
Anti-I	4+	1+	(+)
Anti-i	1+	3+	4+
Anti-I^T	1+	4+	(+)

In our 1974 study, four patients with warm antibody type AIHA associated with Hodgkin's disease were described. Three of the four had autoantibodies that demonstrated anti-I^T specificity. No further examples of auto anti-I^T were found in 50 cases of Hodgkin's disease with no hemolytic anemia (47 cases had negative direct antiglobulin tests and 3 had positive direct antiglobulin tests but no hemolytic anemia). In addition, no further examples were found in 70 cases of warm type AIHA, either idiopathic or secondary to other diseases of the reticuloendothelial system. It should be noted that, as with the cold auto agglutinins showing anti-I^T specificity, the I^T specificity only becomes obvious when the eluates and/or serum were titrated against I adult, i cord, and i adult red cells and antiglobulin agglutination scores compared (see Table 7-4). In 1977, Freedman et al.[37] described a patient with AIHA with no history of Hodgkin's disease, associated with an IgM complement-binding anti-I^T reacting optimally at 37° C. Levine et al. (personal communication, 1979) have submitted for publication a report of four further cases of Hodgkin's disease associated with positive direct antiglobulin tests due to IgG auto anti-I^T.

Table 7-4. ELUATE FROM RED CELLS OF AIHA PATIENT SHOWING ANTI-I[T] SPECIFICITY

Red Cells	Dilutions of Eluate								Agglutination Score
	2	4	8	16	32	64	128	256	
I adult	1+	1+	1+	½+	0	0	0	0	18
i adult	2+	1+	½+	0	0	0	0	0	12
i cord	3+	3+	2+	1+	1+	½+	0	0	32

Two cases of autoimmune hemolytic anemia due to IgG auto anti-N have been described. The first, described by Dube et al.[28] occurred in a 7-year-old boy who had a severe hemolytic anemia that responded dramatically to treatment with prednisone (and a one unit transfusion) within 10 days. His serum and an eluate from his red cells contained an IgG autoantibody that reacted with only N+ red cells by the antiglobulin test. His serum also contained a saline-reactive cold antibody that reacted more strongly with N+ red cells, but also reacted weakly with all N negative red cells.

We recently described a similar case.[20] A 21-year-old white woman with severe hemolytic anemia and thrombocytopenia was found to have strong auto anti-N in her serum. The antibody agglutinated only N+ red cells at 30° C and 37° C, but reacted weakly with N-negative cells at 22° C and 4° C. The indirect antiglobulin test (IAT) at 37° C was negative. The patient's red cells were strongly sensitized with both IgG and complement (C3). An ether eluate from her cells reacted strongly with N+ red cells by direct agglutination and IAT with anti-IgG. Some N-negative cells reacted weakly by IAT. The IgG nature of the antibody was confirmed by showing that 2-mercaptoethanol did not inhibit its reactivity. The patient's red cells typed as M−N+ and yielded agglutination scores similar to homozygous N cells. They showed weak spontaneous agglutination when centrifuged in various media including saline. The patient had a positive ANA and strong antibody to double stranded DNA, and an LE test was negative. The patient's anemia and thrombocytopenia resolved completely following steroid treatment and splenectomy.

A very unusual case of fatal fulminant intravascular hemolysis associated with an anti-A autoantibody was described by Szymanski et al.[111] A group A_1 patient experienced severe bilateral lumbar pain associated with generalized weakness, jaundice, and lethargy and was admitted the next day semi-comatose. The patient was grossly icteric, had splenomegaly, and was severely oliguric. Eighteen hours later acute tachycardia developed, followed by respiratory and cardiac arrest. On admission, the patient was found to have a strongly positive direct antiglobulin test (IgG but no complement). The patient's serum contained antibody(ies) that agglutinated all red cells tested (A_1, A_2, O adult and O cord cells) at 22° C and reacted by indirect antiglobulin test at 37° C; type O red cells reacted much more weakly. When the patient's serum was diluted 1:5, A_1 and A_2 red cells still reacted (2+ at 4° C) and O red cells were negative; the reactions with group A cells could be inhibited by the addition of porcine A substance. A heat eluate prepared from the patient's IgG sensitized red cells demonstrated anti-A specificity by indirect antiglobulin test at 37° C. It is interesting to note that the patient's former medical history was non-contributory until 7 years previous when he was hospitalized for myocardial infarction associated with hypotension. Subsequently, clinical gout, obstructive lung disease, glomerulonephritis, and cirrhosis developed. An additional finding of extramedullary hematopoiesis indicated a long-standing hemolytic process. The authors speculated that during this period anti-A autoantibodies may have combined with A antigen of tissue cells, and that such a phenomenon could have contributed to the multisystem disease in a similar way to the humoral antibodies that have been suggested for Goodpasture's syndrome, some cases of glomerulonephritis, fibrosing alveolitis and chronic active hepatitis.

Another extraordinary recent report concerned an auto-anti-Jk^a associated with autoimmune hemolytic anemia, that appeared to be induced by Aldomet.[89]

Recently, some fascinating new specificities have been described. These specificities were discovered when, once again, red cells of very rare phenotypes were employed, namely the rare En(a−) phenotype and the unique Wr(a+b−) phenotype.

In 1972, Worlledge reported that approximately 33 percent of anti-dl autoantibodies failed to react with En(a−) red cells. She also noted that those anti-dl autoantibodies most likely to fail to react with En(a−) red cells were the same ones that reacted less strongly with enzyme-treated red cells than untreated red cells.[134] A series from the same department in a later report found 44 percent of 23 "non-specific" eluates to react more weakly, or not at all, with En(a−) red cells.[24]

In 1975, Goldfinger et al.[48] reported a case of warm antibody type AIHA associated with an autoantibody of Wr^b specificity. The antibody was initially noticed to react with all red cells tested (including many cells lacking high frequency antigens), but it gave weaker reactions with heterozygous Wr(a+b+) red cells than with the common Wr(a−b+) red cells. The specificity was confirmed by finding a negative reaction against the only known example of Wr(a+b−). The same authors, and Issitt et al.[55] found that the antibody reacted weakly with En(a−) red cells. The En(a−) red cells, when tested with the only known example of anti-Wr^b, were found to type Wr(b−). It was suggested that the anti-En^a specificity reported earlier by Worlledge[134] may perhaps be anti-Wr^b instead. The only known example of Wr(a+b−) typed as En(a+), thus, anti-Wr^b and anti-En^a do not have the same specificity.

In a detailed study, Issitt et al. reported on anti-Wr^b and other autoantibodies responsible for positive direct antiglobulin tests in 150 individuals.[56] Of 87 patients with AIHA, 64 eluates (73.6 percent) had autoantibodies reacting with all red cells including Rh$_{null}$. Of these 64 anti-dl autoantibodies, 34 contained auto anti-Wr^b (53.1 percent). Of 33 patients being treated with alpha-methyldopa who had developed positive direct antiglobulin tests, 23 had anti-dl autoantibodies (69.7 percent), 4 of which contained auto anti-Wr^b (17.4 percent). Of 30 hematologically normal donors with positive direct antiglobulin tests, 23 eluates contained anti-dl autoantibodies (76.7 percent) and 8 eluates contained auto anti-Wr^b (34.8 percent).

If autoantibodies not reacting with Rh$_{null}$ red cells were included, a total of 46 examples of auto anti-Wr^b were encountered. The incidence of auto anti-Wr^b in each group was: 39.1 percent in AIHA; 12.1 percent in alpha methyldopa-induced positive direct antiglobulin tests, and 26.7 percent in normal blood donors with positive direct antiglobulin tests. These workers commented that auto anti-Wr^b can cause gross red cell destruction *in vivo* or can be benign on occasions; it occurs with a higher frequency in AIHA and "normal" donors with positive direct antiglobulin tests than in patients with alpha methldopa-induced positive direct antiglobulin tests. We would like to comment that if the group of patients with AIHA with only IgG on their red cells (i.e., 38 patients) is analyzed, the percentage associated with anti-Wr^b is lower, 28.9 percent (11 of 38 patients), compared with 39.1 percent of the total number of patients with AIHA. If this group is compared with the alpha methyldopa group (who also have only IgG on their red cells), the difference is not as marked (i.e., 28.9 percent versus 12.1 percent, instead of 39.1 percent versus 12.1 percent); the difference is then similar to that seen with the normal donors (70 percent of whom had only IgG on their red cells), compared with the alpha methyldopa group (i.e., 26.7 percent versus 12.1 percent) (see Tables 7-5 and 7-6).

Issitt et al.[56] also commented on Worlledge's report concerning auto anti-En^a and the weaker reactions seen with enzyme-treated red cells. Issitt et al.[57] had already shown that the Wr^b antigen was partially denatured by ficin, which would seem to support the concept that the antibodies Worlledge reported might be anti-Wr^b. However, in tests on the unabsorbed eluates from 110 individuals with auto anti-dl, Issitt et al.[56] found only four (3.6 percent) that failed to react with En(a−) red cells, a very different incidence than the 33 percent Worlledge reported. Issitt et al. believe this difference may just reflect

Table 7-5. AUTOANTIBODIES FOUND IN THE 87 PATIENTS WITH AIHA [56]

Specificity	Found as the Only Autoantibody Present	Found with Other Autoantibodies Simultaneously Present
"Simple" anti-Rh	4 *	33 †
Anti-nl	4	20
Anti-pdl	3	29
Anti-dl	13	49
Anti-Wr^b	2	32
Anti-U	1	1

* In three patients.
† In 23 patients.
(Issitt, P. D., Pavone, B. G., Goldfinger, D., et al.: Anti-Wr^b and other autoantibodies responsible for positive direct antiglobulin tests in 150 individuals. Brit. J. Haematol., 34:5, 1976.)

Table 7-6. THE INCIDENCE OF ANTI-dl, "PURE" AUTO-ANTI-Wr[b] AND AUTO-ANTI-Wr[b] AS A COMPONENT OF ANTI-dl IN 150 PATIENTS WITH POSITIVE DATs *

	Total No. of Cases Tested	No. (and Percent of All Cases Tested) in Which Anti-dl Was Present	No. (and Percent of All Cases Tested) in Which Anti-dl was Pure Anti-Wr[b]	No. (and Percent of All Cases Tested) in Which the Anti-dl Present Contained Anti-Wr[b]	Percent of Cases in Which anti-dl Was Present in Which the Anti-dl Was or Contained Anti-Wr[b]
AIHA	87	64 (74)	2 (2)	32 (37)	53
Aldomet-induced positive DAT †	33	23 (70)	0	4 (12)	17
"Normal" donors with positive DATs ‡	30	23 (77)	2 (7)	6 (20)	35

* All eluates and sera containing anti-dl were absorbed with Wr(a+b−) red cells to determine whether auto-anti-Wr[b] was present. Anti-nl and anti-pdl did not contain auto-anti-Wr[b] since the D− − and Rh_null cells used (one or both of which failed to react with these antibodies) were shown to be Wr(b+).
† The majority of these patients showed no evidence of increased rates of red cell destruction in vivo.
‡ As far as could be determined, none of these donors was undergoing an increased rate of red cell destruction in vivo.
(Issitt, P. D.: Autoimmune hemolytic anemia and cold hemagglutinin disease: Clinical disease and laboratory findings. Prog. Clin. Path., 7:137, 1977.)

a difference in technique, as they were able to show that in one case an ether eluate contained anti-Wr[b] + anti-dl, whereas a heat eluate from the same red cells contained only anti-Wr[b]. When the anti-dl were absorbed with Wr(a+b−) red cells, then anti-Wr[b] could be demonstrated in 41.8 percent of them, which is much closer to the 33 percent figure of "anti-En[a']" described by Worlledge.[134] Issitt et al.[56] believe that similar technical differences may account for the fact that 73.6 percent of the 87 AIHA patients had anti-dl, while the incidence in 55 patients studied by Vos et al.[122] was 40 percent.

More recent studies by Bell and Zwicker [8] have confirmed that autoantibodies may have anti-Wr[b], anti-En[a], or a mixture of both specificities.

Autoantibodies Mimicking Alloantibodies

Occasionally, the specificity of the antibody eluted from the patient's red cells does not match the phenotype of the red cells (i.e., the "wrong" antibody is eluted). We previously mentioned a K negative patient in whom anti-K was eluted from the red cells, but more commonly the "wrong" antibodies have specificity within the Rh system. In our experience, anti-E eluted from E negative red cells is by far the most common "wrong" antibody seen.

In the first report by Fudenberg et al.[38] in 1958, it was suggested that the antibody might be reacting with all antigens containing the basic Rh structure, but which preferentially reacted with one or more specific Rh antigens. In a series of papers (1959–1964) Matuhasi [80] and Ogata [86,87] showed that the "wrong" alloantibody can be adsorbed onto cells lacking its particular antigen if another specific antibody present in the serum is adsorbed onto the cells. They showed that if a mixture of anti-B and anti-D were present in a serum and this serum were incubated with group B, D negative cells, then an eluate prepared from the B cells could be shown to contain anti-D as well as anti-B. In 1967, Svardel et al.[110] reported the absorption of anti-e, f, and -Ce to the cells of a cDE/cDE individual who had auto anti-I present in addition. They suggested that this finding was due to the Matuhasi-Ogata phenomenon. During the next decade, the "Matuhasi-Ogata" phenomenon became a popular term to use when immunohematologists had no other explanation for a particular phenomenon, and, in our opinion, the term has been greatly overused in the field by workers who usually had very little, if any, evidence to support their hypothesis.

One paper appearing in 1969 [2] did offer data to suggest that the "Matuhasi-Ogata" phenomenon may be responsible for the absorption of the "wrong" antibody in autoimmune hemolytic anemia. Later studies by Bove et al.[16] seemed to exclude this explanation and, indeed, one of the authors (P. D. Issitt) of the 1969 publication [2] has also rejected his own earlier hypothesis.[54] In 1976, we presented data at the annual meeting of the American Association of Blood Banks, and in 1978 [92] published a report on an unusual patient who not only had the "wrong" antibody eluted from his red cells, but also was classified as having "Coombs negative" AIHA (see Chapter 9).

A previously untransfused 20-year-old man presented with a seven-day

history of malaise, fatigue, jaundice, dark urine, and splenomegaly. Hemolytic anemia was indicated by a hemoglobin level of 8.7 g/dl, reticulocyte count
8 percent, bilirubin 4.3 mg/dl (direct 0.1 mg/dl), and undetectable serum
haptoglobin. Tests for nonimmunologic mediated hemolytic anemia were
negative. The direct antiglobulin test (DAT) was repeatedly negative with
polyspecific, anti-IgG, -IgA, -IgM and anti-C3 antisera. The patient's serum
contained a weak anti-I, anti-E strongly reactive by indirect antiglobulin test
(IAT), and an antibody reactive against all cells tested. The latter antibody
reacted weakly by the IAT but strongly against enzyme-treated cells (titer
160). Eluates from the patient's red blood cells reacted only with E+ red blood
cells. The patient typed E negative.

The results of serum absorptions with group O rr(cde/cde), R_1R_1(CDe/
CDe), and R_2R_2(cDE/cDE) cells are illustrated in Table 7-7. Following the first
and second absorptions, the sera reacted only with the R_2R_2 cells, and following three absorptions with either rr, R_1R_1, or R_2R_2 cells, there was no detectable antibody. These data indicate that the serum antibody could be absorbed
to exhaustion by a variety of Rh phenotypes, although the serum reacted only
with E positive cells.

The results of ether eluates prepared from the group O rr, R_1R_1 and R_2R_2
red blood cells used for the absorptions which were titered against group O rr,
R_1R_1, and R_2R_2 cells by the indirect antiglobulin test are presented in Table
7-8. Regardless of the Rh phenotypes used for absorption, all eluates reacted
only with E positive cells. This finding was confirmed by repeated testing with
cells of varying Rh phenotypes. A possible anti-c previously detected in the
patient's serum was apparently too weak to be detected after the absorption-
elution procedures. Similar absorption and elution procedures were attempted with an eluate prepared from red blood cells of the original patient

Table 7–7. ANTIBODY TITERS (37°C INDIRECT ANTIGLOBULIN TEST)
OF SERUM FROM PATIENT WITH "MIMICKING" ANTI-E[92]

Serum (Admission)	Red Cells Tested*		
	rr	R_1R_1	R_2R_2
Unabsorbed	1	1	64
Absorbed with rr Cells			
X1	0	0	8
X2	0	0	2
X3	0	0	0
Absorbed with R_1R_1 Cells			
X1	0	0	8
X2	0	0	2
X3	0	0	0
Absorbed with R_2R_2 Cells			
X1	0	0	8
X2	0	0	1
X3	0	0	0

* rr = cde/cde; R_1R_1 = CDe/CDe; R_2R_2 = cDE/cDE.

Table 7-8. ANTIBODY TITERS (37°C IAT) OF ELUATES PREPARED FROM THE RED CELLS USED FOR ABSORPTION IN TABLE 7-7 [92]

| | Red Cells Tested | | |
Eluate From	rr	R_1R_1	R_2R_2
Absorbing rr Cells	0	0	4 *
Absorbing R_1R_1 Cells	0	0	4 *
Absorbing R_2R_2 Cells	0	0	8 *

* Anti-E specificity identified by panel.

specimen, but the reactions were too weak to interpret with any certainty. We believe, as first suggested by Fudenberg et al.,[38] that the antibody in the patient's serum, although appearing like an allo anti-E in an E negative individual, was in fact an autoantibody reacting with a more "basic" Rh antigen but reacting preferentially with E positive red cells.

The patient was treated with high doses of prednisone. By the twelfth day his response allowed the medication to be tapered, and by one month from the onset of treatment results of laboratory studies had returned to normal. The DAT remained negative; however, following recovery, anti-E could not be eluted from the red blood cells. Anti-E remained in his serum, but the titer of the enzyme reactive antibody had decreased to 16. Of particular significance is the decrease of the serum anti-"E-like" antibody titer. In our experience, true alloantibodies usually are not affected during steroid treatment, although autoantibodies do decrease in titer. This finding suggests that the serum anti-"E-like" antibody in this patient behaved more like an autoantibody than an alloantibody.

Issitt et al.[54, 58] made some interesting observations on this phenomenon. In 1977, [58] they described a patient with serologic findings similar to those in the patient described above, except that their patient had a positive direct antiglobulin test. They suggested that the anti-"E" might represent auto anti-Hr rather than anti-E. They state that some Rh alloantibodies are known to show marked preferences for red cells of certain phenotypes when indirect antiglobulin tests are performed, but that absorption studies reveal that some weakly, or even nonreactive, red cells carry small amounts of the antigens against which the antibodies are directed. For example, Rosenfield [103] has observed that anti-hr[s] reacts better with red blood cells from individuals who have ce cis genes than with those from individuals who have Ce cis genes. In spite of this, almost all CDe/CDe bloods are hr[s]-positive. This means, of course, that in initial studies anti-hr[s] might well mimic anti-c or anti-f, but that in absorption studies CDe/CDe red blood cells (which are c-negative, f-negative) invariably absorb anti-hr[s] to exhaustion. A similar situation exists with anti-hr[B], which "prefers" red blood cells from individuals with Ce cis genes to those from individuals with ce cis genes. Such was the preference of anti-hr[B] for C-positive red blood cells that the original "Bastiaan" serum was believed to contain anti-C until it was found that this specificity could not be isolated by absorption.

In working with the sera from a series of individuals with highly exotic Rh phenotypes (Shabalala, Davis, Santiago, Ellington, and Fentry), Rosenfield observed some reactions that were very similar to those described above regarding our patient with "anti-E." Although these observations have never been published in full, they were mentioned briefly in a 1962 paper by Rosenfield et al.[104] In several of the sera studied, there were antibodies that showed marked preferences for E or e. These antibodies were shown not to be anti-E or anti-e by absorption studies with red blood cells of appropriate phenotypes. It was shown that an antibody with a preference for E could be readily absorbed with E+, e− or E+, e+ red blood cells, but that E−, e+ samples would eventually totally absorb the antibody as well. In several instances the antibody-makers were Hr-negative, so that their antibodies resembled the anti-Hr that is often made as an alloantibody by D− − /D− − or Dc−/Dc− individuals. Thus, Issitt et al.[54, 58] feel that since auto anti-nl (i.e., autoantibody that reacts with all red cells of common phenotypes but not -D- or Rh_{null} phenotypes) reacts similarly to allo anti-Hr, then the autoantibodies previously discussed that appear to be anti-E may, in fact, be auto anti-Hr (anti "Hr" or anti-"Hr-like"). We support this hypothesis. Data obtained from experiments on specificity of warm antibodies utilizing the AutoAnalyzer [63] would also seem to support this concept.

Issitt et al.[58] also studied 48 autoantibodies with apparent "simple" anti-Rh specificity (anti-e, -E, -c, -D, -C, -Ce, -G) by means of multiple absorption tests. They showed that 34 (70.8 percent) of these antibodies could be absorbed by red cells lacking the antigens the antibodies appeared to define. These autoantibodies, that at first appeared to be directed against e, E or c antigens, most often had anti-Hr or anti-Hr_0 specificity. Anti-"C-like" autoantibodies may represent auto anti-Rh 34, rather than anti-Hr or anti-Hr_0. Issitt et al.[58] also comment that this new interpretation of the Rh-associated specificity does not change the philosophies (discussed in Chapter 10) for the selection of blood for transfusion. We would agree with this. If one believes (as we do) that a patient with an autoantibody showing some auto anti-E specificity should receive E negative blood (see Chapter 10 for exceptions and a fuller discussion), then it makes no difference if we now call this autoantibody auto anti-Hr, anti-"Hr," anti-"E," or anti-"E-like." As E negative red cells are reacting so much more weakly than E positive red cells (e.g., E negative red cells are sometimes negative by indirect antiglobulin test), we would expect these cells to survive better *in vivo* than more strongly reacting E positive red cells.

From a practical point of view, it is sometimes important to differentiate whether antibody present in the serum of a patient with a positive direct antiglobulin test is an alloantibody (e.g., anti-E) or autoantibody (e.g., anti-"E"). One used to rely mainly on Rh phenotyping the patient's red cells and the comparison with the eluate and serum specificities, but we now know that even in an E negative patient the anti-E present in the serum could be alloantibody, autoantibody, or a mixture of both. The best way of determining the difference is to perform absorptions with red cells of different phenotypes (e.g., E negative and E positive red cells). An allo anti-E should be absorbed only by E positive red cells and not E negative red cells, whereas, as discussed previously, the auto anti-"E" will probably be absorbed by E negative as well as E positive red cells.

Changes in Specificity of Autoantibodies

We have observed the specificity of warm autoantibodies to change during the course of a patient's disease. Other authors have also commented on this phenomenon.[6,12,44] In our experience it has usually been a broadening of specificity. For instance, a patient will start with an autoantibody of "simple" Rh specificity and, as the disease progresses, the antibody will show more "non-specific" characteristics until it reacts with all cells tested, even by indirect antiglobulin test. Other authors have described other patterns. For instance, Beck et al.[6] described a patient whose autoantibody over a five-year period changed from "non-specific" to specific; furthermore, the specificity varied from anti-e to anti-c and anti-f. The authors wisely comment on the fact that the treatment the patient was receiving (prednisone and methotrexate) may have affected the specificity patterns seen. They suggest that particular clones of immunocytes may have been selectively destroyed or suppressed.

We have also seen patients who first make a single alloantibody following transfusion, then make more alloantibodies, and then eventually make autoantibodies. (see Chapter 9).

SPECIFICITY OF AUTOANTIBODIES ASSOCIATED WITH COLD AGGLUTININ SYNDROME

Non-specific cold autoagglutinins were first reported by Mino in 1924.[81] The story of the unravelling of their specificity closely parallels the history of the Ii blood group "System."

Ii Blood Group "System"

In 1956, Wiener and co-workers [131] studied an unusual patient with cold agglutinin syndrome who had severe transfusion reactions, even if the donor blood was kept warm. They were energetic enough to screen over 22,000 donors with the patient's serum, finding five to be compatible (four blacks, one white). No correlation was found with the Lewis, Lutheran, Duffy, Kidd, P, Vel, or ABO systems. The authors concluded they were dealing with a new blood group specificity which they designated I (to indicate its high degree of individuality). The antibody was thus anti-I, and the rare individuals whose red cells were compatible with the serum (containing anti-I) were designated i, or "I negative." Although red cells from the five donors did not react at room temperature when untreated, they all reacted at 4° C and at room temperature when ficin-treated. A feature of Wiener's case that we find hard to understand is that the patient's own washed red cells were not agglutinated by his own serum at room temperature, unless the red cells were enzyme-treated; in fact, they reacted similarly to the so-called i donors!

In 1960, Jenkins et al.[60] found that 50 sera containing weak cold autoagglutinins that had previously been called "non-specific cold agglutinins" had anti-I specificity; none of these donors had hemolytic anemia. Later in the same year, Marsh and Jenkins [73] and in 1961, Marsh [72] described the first two examples of anti-i; antibodies that appeared to react antithetically to anti-I. Using anti-I and anti-i, Marsh was able to show that, unlike other blood group systems so far described, cord red cells were rich in i antigen and possessed very little I antigen. The I antigen slowly developed at the expense of i until at least 18 months of age, at which time adult status was reached. Adult red cells normally are rich in I antigen, but they have only small amounts of i antigen present. Some adults are found to give intermediate reactions, I_{INT} (i.e., weaker I antigen). Rare adults are found whose red cells have less I antigen and more i antigen than cord red cells; these are the rare i adult; i_1 subjects are usually white and i_2 are usually black. Marsh [12] suggested the following order of increasing strength of I: i_1, i_2, i_{cord}, $I_{(INT)}$, I.

Although cord cells react much more weakly than adult red cells at all temperatures when tested with a low titer cold agglutinin, the results can be very confusing when the pathologic high titer cold agglutinins are tested; very little difference in titer is noticed at 4° C, but the specificity becomes more obvious as the temperature is raised. (Table 7-9 shows typical reactions of adult and cord red cells with a pathologic high titer anti-I.) It should also be

Table 7-9. REACTIONS OF A TYPICAL ANTI-I ASSOCIATED WITH COLD AGGLUTININ SYNDROME

Dilutions of Patient's Serum	4°C		25°C		30°C	
	Adult OI	Cord Oi	Adult OI	Cord Oi	Adult OI	Cord Oi
2	4+	4+	4+	1+	1+	0
4	4+	4+	4+	1+	½+	0
8	4+	4+	3+	½+	0	0
16	4+	4+	3+	0	0	0
32	4+	4+	3+	0	0	0
64	4+	4+	2+	0	0	0
128	4+	3+	1+	0	0	0
256	3+	3+	½+	0	0	0
512	3+	2+	0	0	0	0
1024	2+	1+	0	0	0	0
2048	1+	0	0	0	0	0
4096	0	0	0	0	0	0

noted that various examples of cord red cells can show marked differences in reactivity with some anti-I.[77]

In 1970,[31] a powerful anti-I was described that was strongly inhibited by hydatid cyst fluid and inhibited to a varying extent by all of the 181 human saliva samples tested; previously, saliva had been reported not to inhibit anti-I.[72] Infants at birth and i adults were also found to have high concentrations of I substance in their saliva. This investigation suggested that I antibodies are of two kinds—those inhibitable by saliva and those not inhibited. This finding confirmed an earlier suggestion by Marsh who had termed the two types I^a and I^b. Marsh et al.[76] found that human milk contained a high concentration of water soluble I blood-group substance. Tests with 24 different anti-I showed that to a variable extent, all of them could be inhibited by milk, and some could be inhibited by strong I secretor saliva. This susceptibility to inhibition was not related to titer, and the results suggested that qualitative differences in the antigen-antibody reactions were responsible.

In 1971, Marsh et al.[77] described two components of the I antigen which they named I^F (fetal) and I^D (developed). The I^F component was found to be present on all human red cells, including those of i_{cord}, i_{adult}, and also on rhesus monkey red cells. The I^D component develops slowly on the red cells before birth, and to a greater extent 18 months after birth (see Table 7-10). Inhibition studies with human milk showed that strongly-inhibitable anti-I were of the anti-I^D variety, but only a minority of such sera were inhibitable. Naturally occurring low titer cold autoagglutinins were found mainly to be anti-I^D, whereas the high titer cold autoagglutinins associated with AIHA were found commonly to contain anti-I^F, either alone or together with anti-I^D; rarely, anti-I^D was encountered exclusively. This pattern suggests an explanation for the strong reaction of high titer anti-I associated with AIHA, with cord red cells (see Table 7-9), which are rich in I^F but have little, if any, I^D. Marsh et al.[77] also discussed the possible place of I^F and I^D in the development of the I antigen (see Table 7-11).

Dzierzkowa-Borodej et al.[30] have suggested that the anti-I that are inhibitable are different from anti-I^D. Although they act similarly serologically, they can be differentiated by their capability to precipitate in gel at 4° C. Saliva, colostral IgA, and desialized glycoprotein from red cells gave strong precipitin lines with inhibitable anti-I but not with other anti-I. They suggested that the inhibitable anti-I be called anti-I^S. In an extensive study on 12 anti-I cold autoantibodies (one of normal titer 32, the others ranging from 256 to

Table 7-10. RELATIVE STRENGTH OF i, I^F AND I^D ANTIGENS ON Red Cells

Red Cells	i	I^F	I^D
i_{cord}	3+	3+	½+
i_{adult}	4+	2+	0
I_{adult}	½+	3+	4+
Rhesus Monkey	4+	3+	0

2×10^6), they found that only 4 of 12 sera demonstrated single specificity (1 anti-I^S, 3 anti-I^F) and that the others demonstrated two or more specificities (1 anti-I^D + anti-I^S, 1 anti-I^D + anti-I^F, 3 anti-I^D + anti-i, 2 anti-I^D + anti-I^F + anti-I^S). These differences could not be easily determined by using I_{adult}, i_{cord}, and i_{adult} cells, but they became more obvious when the red cells from a rare adult having only I^F were used (these red cells failed to react with anti-I^D and anti-i, but they were agglutinated by anti-I^F). It is interesting to note that the same authors have shown that desialization of red cells enhanced their agglutinability by anti-I^D and anti-I^S but had no effect on their reaction with anti-I^F [70].

Table 7-11. POSSIBLE PATHWAYS FOR
DEVELOPMENT OF I ANTIGEN [77]

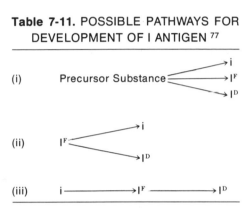

It has been clear over the years that auto anti-I can exist in two forms: (1) a low titer autoantibody occurring in almost all normal human serum as a naturally occurring cold agglutinin, reacting optimally at 0 to 4° C and rarely reacting above room temperature; and (2) a high titer autoantibody often associated with cold agglutinin syndrome, reacting optimally at 0 to 4° C, often reacting up to 30 to 32° C and rarely to 37° C when saline suspended red cells are used (Table 7-12). It is by far the most common antibody to be associated with cold agglutinin syndrome (both the chronic idiopathic cases and those secondary to *Mycoplasma pneumoniae* infection). In our own series, 49 of 54 cases (91 percent) were associated with anti-I. Other workers have reported similar findings. [23]

Anti-i is not commonly detected in normal serum as is anti-I, but it has been reported to be present in as high as 70 percent of sera from patients with infectious mononucleosis. When it is detected in other cases, it is often associated with diseases of the reticuloendothelial system. When it is present in high enough titer and its reactivity is of high thermal range, it can cause AIHA. Of 54 cases of cold agglutinin disease in our series, four were associated with anti-i.

Although the clinical histories are limited, there is a suggestion that one of the first two patients to be described as having anti-i had AIHA. [73] This patient came under investigation for suspected reticulosis and moderate anemia. An anti-i reacting to a titer of 256,000 with i_{adult} red cells was present in his serum,

Table 7-12. TYPES AND SOURCES OF ANTI-I

1. Auto
   a. Naturally occurring, low titer cold antibody.
   b. High titer, cold antibody associated with cold agglutinin syndrome.
2. Allo
   a. Antibody in sera of i_1 adult reacts with i_2, cord and adult cells.
   b. Antibody in sera of i_2 adult reacts with cord and adult, not i_1 cells.

reacting strongly at room temperature and weakly at 37° C. The anti-i reacted only to a titer of 16 with I_{adult} red cells. Often even strong anti-i (i.e., high titers against i_{adult} and i_{cord} red cells) will not react or react only weakly at room temperature with normal adult red cells, including the patient's own. Thus, hemolytic anemia is rare even when a powerful anti-i is present. Sometimes the i antigenic status of the patient's red cells is increased,[18, 46] thus making the patient's red cells more reactive than normal adult red cells. When performing cold agglutinin titers and thermal ranges, etc., it is always useful to include tests against the patient's own red cells.

Since the original description of anti-i, many cases of cold agglutinin syndrome caused by anti-i have been described.[18, 116, 132, 135]

Chemistry of Ii Antigens

Evidence has been accumulating to suggest that the Ii antigens are closely related to the ABH Lewis blood group substances. A number of antibodies have been described that will react only when I is present together with other antigens from the ABH, Lewis and P system (e.g., anti-IA, -IH, iH, HI, IB, IP, IP$_1$, iP$_1$, -I^{T}P$_1$ and anti-ILe^{bH}). These antibodies appear to react with complex antigens distinct from the separate antigens, e.g., anti-IB will react only with red cells containing both I and B antigens, and not with red cells containing I but not B or B but not I. The amount of IB on red cells is not related to the amount of I or B on the red cells,[82, 112] thus appearing to be a completely separate antigen. In 1971, Feizi et al.[35] analyzed the I-active antigen extracted from human milk. The sugar composition of this material closely resembled the chemistry associated with ABH blood group substances; however, its content of fucose was unusually low. In this respect, it resembled blood group precursor-like substances that had been isolated from human ovarian cyst fluid lacking ABH and Lewis substances as reported by Vicari and Kabat[118] and Watkins and Morgan.[125] Feizi et al.[35] suggested that I specificity was concealed in interior structures of the blood A, B, H, Le^a and Le^b substances and may be exposed by stepwise periodate oxidation and Smith degradation of ABH substances. Thus, I substance would seem to be a precursor for the biosynthesis of ABH. In a later study,[34] the same workers studied 11 anti-I sera and found they could be divided into at least six groups based on their reactions with human milk, ovarian cyst fractions (containing "ABH" precursor blood group substances), degraded ABH substances, and hydatid cyst fluid. Four of five anti-i resembled each other, but the fifth differed in its reaction with hydatid cyst fluid and milk.

Burnie [18] and Cooper et al. [21] have shown that normal plasma can be shown to contain I and i substances in small quantities.

Rosse and Lauf, [106] using *n*-butanol, extracted the antigens ("I") reacting with cold autoagglutinins from human red cells. A fascinating observation was made that although the antigen and antibody were not able to react at 37° C when the antigen was present in the intact red cell, after solubilization antigen and antibody reacted equally well at 37° C and 0° C. In addition, the amount of "I" antigen extracted from the red cells of adults and newborns appeared to be about the same! In a previous study, [107] it had been suggested that the effect of temperature changes was not upon the antibody but was rather upon the antigen or the red cell membrane. This conclusion was based upon the fact that the change in affinity of antibody for red cells of newborn infants (i_{cord}) or of i_{adult} red cells was much greater than for red cells of normal adults. Since any effect on the antibody of change of temperature would have been the same in both situations, they concluded that a change in configuration of the antigen or the red cell surface must be responsible for the characteristic cold reactivity of the antigen-antibody interaction. They further concluded that their later experiments indicated that the reactivity of cold agglutinins only in the cold was due to an effect of cold upon the red cell membrane, since the antigen-antibody reaction occurred as well at 37° C as at 0° C when the antigen was removed from the membrane. They suggested that at 37° C the antigen on the intact membrane may be "hidden," whereas at 0° C the antigen may become available for reaction with the antibody. Their studies led them to believe that the difference between "I" and "i" is largely a difference between the number of I antigenic sites. When the "affinity" of the antigen and antibody were increased by enzyme-treatment of the red cells or by incubation in the cold, the total amount of antibody fixed by both types of cells became nearly equal.

Gardas and Koscielak [39] isolated an I-active substance from human red cells by *n*-butanol extraction and found it to be identical with A, B, H isolated antigens. The materials were sialic acid free and comprised about 90 percent carbohydrate, 7 to 7.5 percent of amino acids, and 2 percent of sphingosine. A, B, and H blood group activities were completely recovered in immune precipitates of appropriate water soluble antigens with anti-I precipitating serum; on the contrary, I activity could be recovered from precipitates prepared with anti-A and -B precipitating sera. Thus, the water phase left after extraction of stroma with *n*-butanol comprises a single antigenic material in which all A, B, H, and I blood group activities are located on the same molecule. This conclusion offers an explanation for the anti-I that are influenced by the ABH group of the test red cells (e.g., anti-IH, HI, IA, IB) in that the adjacent A, B, H, and I active structures may give rise to antibodies of mixed ABH and I specificity. The results obtained in this study, like those of Marcus et al. [71] and Feizi et al. [35] indicate that terminal galactopyranosyl residues are part of the I structure.

It is interesting to note that the isolated I and H blood group substances were easily absorbed onto human red cells *in vitro* and thus group Oi red cells could easily be changed to OI. One finding contrasted with the finding of Rosse and Lauf [106] described earlier; isolated preparations of I-active antigens precipitated only at 4° C, and no reactions occurred at 37° C.

Red cell glycoproteins contain two kinds of oligosaccharide chains: (1) alkali-labile chains consisting of galactose, N-acetygalactosamine and a large proportion of sialic acid; and (2) alkali-stable chains containing galactose, N-acetyglucosamine, mannose, and low amounts of sialic acid and fucose. [1,29,69,71,113,114] Alkali-stable chains are required for I activity, [49] whereas MN activity depends on alkali-labile chains. [113,114] Red cells contain one major glycoprotein (glycophorin) and a few minor ones. I activity has been reported to be associated with the minor glycoprotein by some workers [29] and glycophorin by others. [49]

Lisowska et al. [70] tested three fractions of red cell glycoproteins obtained from sepharose 4-B chromatography for I activity with 10 anti-I sera. Fraction 1 was further purified by separating ABHI-active substances from MN active sialoglycoprotein. This fraction had the greatest I activity and contained the lowest amount of alkali-labile oligosaccharide chains. The most abundant fraction (II), which was the major sialoglycoprotein of red cell membranes, showed no or only weak I activity but I-active glycopeptides could be isolated by digestion of fraction II with trypsin. The major product of digestion, sialoglycopeptide II T-2, showed I activity only after alkaline elimination of alkali-labile oligosaccharide chains. Fraction III showed weak I activity but was slightly stronger than Fraction II. Fraction III showed less MN activity than Fractions I and II.

Lisowska et al. [70] concluded that I-active receptors were present in all fractions of the erythrocyte glycoproteins they studied, but that in some fractions they were "masked" and could be exposed by enzymatic and chemical degradation of glycoproteins. The I activity appeared to be associated with alkali-stable oligosaccharide chains. Sialic acid-rich alkali-labile oligosaccharides appeared to be responsible for the steric hindrance for the reaction between anti-I and some anti-I antigens. The results were in favor of the concept that a unique I substance is not present on red cells, but that I-active receptors are located on different ABH or MN-active molecules, in a position less or more available for reaction with anti-I.

It is interesting to note that as early as 1953, Wiener et al. [130] suggested that the cold autoantibodies associated with AIHA might be directed at the "nucleus" of ABO, which is exactly what I now appears to be!

Other Autoantibody Specificities Associated With Cold Agglutinin Syndrome

Specificities other than anti-I or anti-i are rare. Of this rare group, the most common is an antibody that usually reacts with all human red cells tested (adult and cord red cells acting equally). This antibody was first popularly called, rather facetiously, anti-"not-I." (In fact, L. W. Marsh, who first used the term, tells us he is chagrined that it ever appeared in print, and in fact called it anti-Sp$_1$ when he published the first extensive serologic data on this antibody.[74])

Marsh and Jenkins [74] called the antibody anti-Sp$_1$ (species) as no human blood sample lacking the reacting antigen could be found, and no red cells from 25 other species reacted. The Sp$_1$ antigen showed a striking difference from I and i in that the Sp$_1$ antigen could be destroyed or markedly reduced by treating the red cell with proteolytic enzymes (trypsin, bromelin, papain and ficin); both I and i give enhanced reactions following enzyme treatment (Table 7-13). The antigen was found to be well developed at birth; the antibody was found to react better if the serum was at pH 6.5 or below (e.g., titer of 16 at pH 9.0 and 8000 at pH 6.2). In a series of 268 cold autoantibodies investigated, two were designated as anti-Sp$_1$. Both of these were high titer antibodies associated with AIHA; no examples of naturally occurring anti-Sp$_1$ were found in healthy individuals in the course of many thousand cold antibody investigations.

Independently, Roelcke [94] described an antibody called anti-HD ("Heidelberg"); this antibody appeared to be reacting with an antigen identical to Sp$_1$. In 1969, Roelcke published an extensive study showing heterogeneity of the HD (Sp$_1$)-receptor. HD$_1$ antigen could be demonstrated only on human red cells, in contrast to the HD$_2$ antigen, which could be demonstrated on rat and guinea pig red cells, as well as on human red cells. Neuraminidase and proteases inactivated both antigens. However, quantitative differences were observed; the HD$_2$ antigen showed more resistant to neuraminidase and proteases than HD$_1$.[102]

In 1970, Roelcke and Uhlenbruck [101] suggested replacing the terms "Sp" and "HD" with "Pr" (indicating the property of antigen inactivation by proteases). Over the next eight years, Roelcke and his co-workers published some elegant studies on the unusual characteristics of the Pr system. A complex heterogeneity has been discovered.[95] Pr$_1$ (HD$_1$) has now been subdivided into Pr$_{1h}$ and Pr$_{1d}$. Pr$_{1h}$ is found only on human red cells. Pr$_{1d}$ is present only on red cells from human and some animal species, including dogs. Pr$_2$ has a similar species distribution, but, in contrast to Pr$_{1d}$, is increased on dog red cells and not destroyed by protease treatment of dog red cells. The anti-Sp$_1$ described by Marsh and Jenkins is probably identical to anti-Pr$_{1d}$ or -Pr$_2$ since Sp$_1$ was found to be inactivated by neuraminidase and to be present on guinea pig red cells. Of 24,150 human red cells tested by Roelcke, all have so far been

Table 7-13. COMPARISON OF REACTIONS SEEN WITH ANTI-I, -i, -I+i AND ANTI-Pr

	OI	OI (enzyme-treated)	Oi	Oi (enzyme-treated)
Anti-I	1024	4096	4	16
Anti-i	4	16	1024	4096
Anti-I+i	1024	4096	1024	4096
Anti-Pr (Sp)	1024	2	1024	2

found to contain Pr_{1h} and Pr_2. In 1971, a new determinant, Pr_a, was described.[95] Two IgG cold autoagglutinins causing transient hemolytic anemia were detected in children. They reacted with all red cells tested, and the reacting determinant was inactivated by proteolytic enzyme, but in contrast to Pr_1 and Pr_2, it was not inactivated by neuraminidase.

The latest determinant in the Pr system to be described is Pr_3.[99] A monoclonal IgM (kappa) antibody, associated with cold agglutinin syndrome, occurring after rubella infection, was shown to react as anti-Pr. Pr_3 determinants are found on cat and sheep red cells that lack Pr_1 and Pr_2 determinants. By carbodiimide treatment of human red cell glycoproteins, which causes the intramolecular coupling of N-acetylneuraminic acid carboxyl group and nucleophilic centers of the glycoprotein backbone, Pr_3 antigen activity is greatly increased, while Pr_1 and Pr_2 are inactivated.

Chemistry of Pr Blood Groups

Pr antigens are associated with the red cell glycoproteins and are represented by the alkali-labile bound oligosaccharides. N-acetylneuraminic acid (NANA) is the terminal amino-sugar of the Pr_{1h}, Pr_{1d}, and Pr_2 determinants.[97] Electrostatic interactions between NANA carboxyl groups and free ϵ-amino lysine groups which are essential for the expression of MN antigenicity are not required for the expression of Pr, thus anti-Pr is not anti-"M+N." In addition, M^k and En(a−) red cells, which have an inherited NANA deficiency, have normal Pr activity.

It is interesting that only four examples of IgA high titer cold autoagglutinins have ever been reported,[41,96,97,98] and all four have been shown to be monoclonal (kappa) and have anti-Pr_1 specificity.[96] Most anti-I associated with chronic cold agglutinin syndrome are IgM monoclonal (kappa) proteins, but rare examples of IgM (lambda) cold agglutinins have been reported.[97] Three of these were reported as having anti-"Not-I" specificity, and one of these has since been identified as anti-Pr_1.[97] The restricted nature of anti-I cold agglutinins is not limited to their constant regions; their light chain variable regions are predominantly VKII subgroup, and their heavy chain variable regions are predominantly VHI subgroup.[45,97] Wang et al.[124] studied the amino acid sequence of the IgA cold agglutinin "Rob" that we had reported as having anti-Pr specificity in 1973.[41] They were able to define a new kappa chain variable region subgroup which was designated VKIV. Since the anti-Pr and anti-I cold agglutinins had variable region subgroups which clearly differed, and since these specificities correspond to chemical differences in the red cell membrane, Wang et al.[124] suggested that their study illustrated a direct correlation between antibody specificity and the structure of the light and heavy chain variable regions.

The case "Rob" that we described[41] had an interesting history. The patient was a 51-year-old white male, who first developed symptoms compatible with cold agglutinin syndrome in 1944. His major symptoms consisted of extreme sensitivity to the cold, as manifested by bluish discoloration of the extremities, ears and face. With intense exposure to cold his entire appearance was purplish and his hands and particularly his feet became extremely painful. The presence of a high titer cold agglutinin was not determined until 21 years later. At this time electrophoresis of his serum showed a monoclonal spike in the β-globulin region, which was shown by immuno-electrophoresis to be IgA. The bone marrow was hypercellular and contained approximately 10 percent mature plasma cells. A diagnosis of multiple myeloma was considered, although the patient did not develop osteolytic bone lesions or urine protein abnormalities. Physical examination revealed no lymphadenopathy, splenomegaly, or hepatomegaly. Bone marrow examinations over the next five years showed an increase in plasma cells, and the serum IgA level rose to a concentration of 1.01 gm/dl. His cold agglutinin titer was 16,000, reacting up to 35° C. The serum caused no hemolysis *in vitro* of normal or enzyme-treated red cells. The antibody, being IgA, was incapable of activating complement; thus, although the patient had clinical signs due to the powerful cold autoagglutinin (e.g., Raynaud's phenomenon), no evidence of hemolytic anemia was ever detected.

Isolated Examples of Antibodies Other Than Anti-I, -i or -Pr Associated With Cold Agglutinin Syndrome

An unusual antibody first described by Brendemoen [17] and later named anti-H_T by Jenkins and Marsh [59], has been described associated with cold agglutinin syndrome. This antibody will not react with any fresh red cells, but it will react with the same red cells if stored, heat-treated, or enzyme-treated. Other workers [4, 9, 88] have also described this phenomenon, but none have yet explained it.

In 1977, two examples of cold autoagglutinins with new specificities were described associated with cold agglutinin syndrome. The antibodies were named anti-Gd. They reacted with all red cells tested. The antigen was not destroyed by papain, but it was denatured by neuraminidase. [100]

One case of auto anti-N of high titer and thermal range was described. [15] The anti-N reacted to a titer 512 at 4° C and reacted up to 37° C. The patient suffered from a severe transient hemolytic anemia. The authors demonstrated that the anti-N possessed strong complement binding properties (which is very unusual, as MN antibodies usually do not activate complement).

Recently, a new antibody related to the Sd^a blood group has been described in a patient with acute hemolysis. The antibody has been called anti-Sd^x, as it is inhibited by fluids rich in Sd^a (e.g., guinea pig urine) but reacts with all human red cells tested so far (i.e., Sd(a+) and Sd(a−)). [75]

There are reports in the early literature of auto anti-P$_1$, -O, -M and -B, [23] but the data presented are not complete enough to be convincing.

AUTOANTIBODY SPECIFICITY ASSOCIATED WITH PAROXYSMAL COLD HEMOGLOBINURIA

In 1963, Levine et al.[68] reported that the sera from six patients with paroxysmal cold hemoglobinuria failed to react with the rare Tj(a−) red cells, but they reacted with all other red cells tested. Thus, Levine et al. suggested the specificity of the autoantibodies in PCH was anti-PP$_1$P^k(-Tj^a). Worlledge and Rousso [136] extended these findings by testing 11 patients with PCH, using the rare P^k red cells in addition to p (Tj(a−)) red cells. (Levine et al. had mentioned in an addendum to their paper that three of their sera tested did not react wth P^k red cells.) All 11 sera reacted with P$_1$ and P$_2$ red cells but not with p or P^k cells, which suggested a specificity similar to that of the anti-P naturally occurring in the rare P^k individuals. Other workers have also since reported cases of PCH with P specificity. [13, 61, 62, 93, 119]

The only other specificities that have been related to PCH have been a single case report of an anti-p by Engelfriet et al.,[32] one example of anti-I by Bell et al.,[10] and an anti-HI by Weiner.[128]

Our experiences have been similar to the reports described in references 13, 61, 62, 68, 93, 119, and 136 in that all six cases of paroxysmal cold hemoglobinuria in our series were associated with anti-P specificity.

REFERENCES

1. Adamany, A. M., and Kathan, R. H.: Isolation of a tetrasaccharide common to MM, NN, and MN antigens. Biochem. Biophys. Res. Commun., *37:*171, 1969.
2. Allen, F. H., Jr., Issitt, P. D., Degnan, T. J., et al.: Further observations on the Matuhasi-Ogata phenomenon. Vox. Sang., *16:*47, 1969.
3. Angevine, C. D., Andersen, B. R., and Barnett, E. V.: A cold agglutinin of the IgA class. J. Immunol., *96:*578, 1966.
4. Beaumont, J. L., Lorenzelli, L., Delplanque, B., et al.: A new serum lipoprotein associated erythrocyte antigen which reacts with a monoclonal IgM. Vox. Sang., *30:*36, 1976.
5. Beck, M. L., Butch, S. H., Armstrong, W. D., et al.: An autoantibody with U-specificity in a patient with myasthenia gravis. Transfusion, *12:*280, 1972.
6. Beck, M. L., Dixon, J., and Oberman, H. A.: Variation of specificity of autoantibodies in autoimmune hemolytic anemia. Am. J. Clin. Path., *56:*475, 1971.
7. Beck, M. L., Marsh, W. L., Pierce, S. R., et al.: Auto-anti-Kp^b associated with weakened antigenicity in the Kell blood group system: A second example. Transfusion, *19:*197, 1979.
8. Bell, C. A., and Zwicker, H.: Further studies on the relationship of anti-En^a and anti-Wr^b in warm autoimmune hemolytic anemia. Transfusion, *18:*572, 1978.
9. Bell, C. A., Zwicker, H., and Nevius, D. B.: Nonspecific warm hemolysins of papain-treated cells: serologic characterization and transfusion risk. Transfusion, *13:*207, 1973.
10. Bell, C. A., Zwicker, H., and Rosenbaum, D. L.: Paroxysmal cold hemoglobinuria (PCH) following mycoplasma infection: anti-I specificity of the biphasic hemolysin. Transfusion, *13:*138, 1973.
11. Bell, C. A., Zwicker, H., and Sacks, H. J.: Autoimmune hemolytic anemia: Routine serologic evaluation in a general hospital population. Amer. J. Clin. Path., *60:*903, 1973.

12. Bird, G. W. G., and Wingham, J.: Changes in specificity of erythrocyte autoagglutinins. Vox. Sang., *22:*364, 1972.
13. Bird, G. W. G., Wingham, J., Martin, A. J., et al.: Idiopathic non-syphilitic paroxysmal cold haemoglobinuria in children. J. Clin. Path., *29:*215, 1976.
14. Booth, P. B., Jenkins, W. J., and Marsh, W. L.: Anti-I^T: A new antibody of the I blood-group system occurring in certain Melanesian sera. Brit. J. Haemat., *12:*341, 1966.
15. Bowman, H. S., Marsh, W. L., Schumacher, H. R., et al.: Auto-anti-N immunohemolytic anemia in infectious mononucleosis. Am. J. Clin. Path., *61:*465, 1974.
16. Bove, J. R., Holburn, A. M., and Mollison, P. L.: Non-specific binding of IgG to antibody-coated red cells (The Matuhasi-Ogata phenomenon). Immunology, *25:*793, 1973.
17. Brendemoen, O. J.: A cold agglutinin specifically active against stored human red blood cells. Acta Path. Microbiol. Scand., *31:*574, 1952.
18. Burnie, K.: Ii antigens and antibodies. Canad. J. Med. Technol., *55:*5, 1973.
19. Celano, M. J., and Levine, P.: Anti-LW specificity in autoimmune acquired hemolytic anemia. Transfusion, *7:*265, 1967.
20. Cohen, D. W., Garratty, G., Morel, P., et al.: Autoimmune hemolytic anemia associated with IgG auto anti-N. Transfusion, *19:*329, 1979.
21. Cooper, A. G., and Brown, M. C.: Serum i antigen: A new human blood-group glycoprotein. Biochem. Biophys. Res. Commun., *55:*297, 1973.
22. Dacie, J. V.: Acquired hemolytic anemia. With special reference to the antiglobulin (Coombs') reaction. Blood, *8:*813, 1953.
23. Dacie, J. V.: The Haemolytic Anaemias. Part II: The Auto-Immune Haemolytic Anaemias. 2nd Ed. New York, Grune & Stratton Inc., 1963.
24. Dacie, J. V.: Autoimmune hemolytic anemia. Arch. Intern. Med., *135:*1293, 1975.
25. Dacie, J. V., and Cutbush, M.: Specificity of auto-antibodies in acquired haemolytic anaemia. J. Clin. Path., *7:*18, 1954.
26. Dacie, J. V., and Worlledge, S. M.: Auto-immune hemolytic anemias. Prog. Hemat., *6:*82, 1969.
27. Dausset, J., Colombani, J., Jean, R. G., et al.: Sur un cas d'anemie hemolytique aigue de l'enfant avec presence d'une hemolysine immunologique et d'un pouvoir anticomplementaire du serum. Sang., *28:*351, 1957.
28. Dube, V. E., House, R. F., Jr., Moulds, J., et al.: Hemolytic anemia caused by auto anti-N. Amer. J. Clin. Path., *63:*828, 1975.
29. Dzierzkowa-Borodej, W., Lisowska, E., and Seyfriedowa, H.: The activity of glycoproteins from erythrocytes and protein fractions of human colostrum towards anti-I antibodies. Life Sci., *9:*111, 1970.
30. Dzierzkowa-Borodej, W., Seyfried, H., and Lisowska, E.: Serological classification of anti-I sera. Vox. Sang., *28:*110, 1975.
31. Dzierzkowa-Borodej, W., Seyfried, H., Nichols, M., et al.: The recognition of water-soluble I blood group substance. Vox. Sang., *18:*222, 1970.
32. Engelfriet, C. P., Beckers, D., Borne, A. E. G. Kr. von dem, et al.: Haemolysins probably recognizing the antigen p. Vox. Sang., *23:*176, 1971.
33. Eyster, M. E., and Jenkins, D. E., Jr.: γG erythrocyte autoantibodies: comparison of in vivo complement coating and in vitro "Rh" specificity. J. Immunol., *105:*221, 1970.
34. Feizi, T., and Kabat, E. A.: Immunochemical studies on blood groups: LIV. Classification of anti-I and anti-i sera into groups based on reactivity patterns with various antigens related to the blood group A, B, H, Le^a Le^b and precursor substances. J. Exp. Med. *135:*1247, 1972.
35. Feizi, T., Kabat, E. A., Vicari, G., et al.: Immunochemical studies on blood groups. XLVII. The I antigen complex-precursors in the A, B, H, Le^a, and Le^b

blood group system—hemagglutinin-inhibition studies. J. Exp. Med., *133:*39, 1971.

36. Flückiger, P., Ricci, C., and Usteri, C.: Zur Frage der Blutgruppenspezifität von Autoantikörpern. Acta Haemat., *13:*53, 1955.
37. Freedman, J., Newlands, M., and Johnson, C. A.: Warm IgM anti-I[T] causing autoimmune haemolytic anaemia. Vox. Sang., *32:*135, 1977.
38. Fudenberg, H. H., Rosenfield, R. E., and Wasserman, L. R.: Unusual specificity of auto-antibody in auto-immune hemolytic disease. Mt. Sinai Hospital J., *25:*324, 1958.
39. Gardas, A., and Koscielak, J.: I-active antigen of human erythrocyte membrane. Vox. Sang., *26:*227, 1974.
40. Garratty, G., Haffleigh, B., Dalziel, J., et al.: An IgG anti-I[T] detected in a Caucasian American. Transfusion, *12:*325, 1972.
41. Garratty, G., Petz, L. D., Brodsky, I., et al.: An IgA high-titer cold agglutinin with an unusual blood group specificity within the Pr complex. Vox. Sang., *25:*32, 1973.
42. Garratty, G., Petz, L. D., Wallerstein, R. O., et al.: Autoimmune hemolytic anemia in Hodgkin's disease associated with anti-I[T]. Transfusion, *14:*226, 1974.
43. Garratty, G., Sattler, M. S., Petz, L.D., Flannery, E.P.: Immune hemolytic anemia associated with anti-Kell and a carrier state for chronic granulomatous disease. Blood Transfusion and Immunohematology. In Press.
44. Gerbal, A., Homberg, J. C., Rochant, H., et al.: Les auto-anticorps d'anemies hemolytiques acquises. I. Analyse de 234 observations. Nouv. Rev. Francaise. Hemat., *8:*155, 1968.
45. Gergely, J., Wang, A. C., and Fudenberg, H. H.: Chemical analyses of variable regions of heavy and light chains of cold agglutinins. Vox. Sang., *24:*432, 1973.
46. Giblett, E. R., and Crookston, M. C.: Agglutinability of red cells by anti-i in patients with thalassaemia major and other haematological disorders. Nature, *201:*1138, 1964.
47. Giblett, E. R., Klebanoff, S. J., Pincus, S. H., et al.: Kell phenotypes in chronic granulomatous disease: A potential transfusion hazard, correspondence. Lancet, *i:*1235, 1971.
48. Goldfinger, D., Zwicker, H., Belkin, G. A., et al.: An autoantibody with anti-Wr[b] specificity in a patient with warm autoimmune hemolytic anemia. Transfusion, *15:*351, 1975.
49. Hamaguchi, H., and Cleve, H.: Solubilization of human erythrocyte membrane glycoproteins and separation of the MN glycoprotein from a glycoprotein with I, S, and A activity. Biochem. Biophys. Acta, *278:*271, 1972.
50. Holländer, L.: Specificity of antibodies in acquired haemolytic anaemia. Experientia (Basel), *9:*468, 1953.
51. Ishimori, T., and Hasekura, H.: A Japanese with no detectable Rh blood group antigens due to silent Rh alleles or deleted chromosomes. Transfusion, *7:*84, 1967.
52. Issitt, P. D.: Applied Blood Group Serology. Oxnard, Spectra Biologicals, 1970.
53. Issitt, P. D.: Autoimmune hemolytic anemia and cold hemagglutinin disease: clinical disease and laboratory findings. Prog. Clin. Path., *7:*137, 1977.
54. Issitt, P. D., and Pavone, B. G.: Critical re-examination of the specificity of auto-anti-Rh antibodies in patients with a positive direct antiglobulin test. Brit. J. Haemat., *38:*63, 1978.
55. Issitt, P. D., Pavone, B. G., Goldfinger, D., et al.: An En(a−) red cell sample that types as Wr(a−b−). Transfusion, *15:*353, 1975.
56. Issitt, P. D., Pavone, B. G., Goldfinger, D., et al.: Anti-Wr[b] and other autoantibodies responsible for positive direct antiglobulin tests in 150 individuals. Brit. J. Haemat., *34:*5, 1976.
57. Issitt, P. D., Pavone, B. G., Wagstaff, W., et al.: The phenotypes En(a−),

Wr(a−b−) and En(a+), Wr(a+b−), and further studies on the Wright and En blood group systems. Transfusion, *16:*396, 1976.

58. Issitt, P. D., Zellner, D. C., Rolih, S. D., et al.: Autoantibodies mimicking alloantibodies. Transfusion, *17:*531, 1977.
59. Jenkins, W. J., and Marsh, W. L.: Autoimmune haemolytic anaemia. Three cases with antibodies specifically active against stored red cells. Lancet, *ii:*16, 1961.
60. Jenkins, W. J., Marsh, W. L., Noades, J., et al.: The I antigen and antibody. Vox. Sang., *5:*97, 1960.
61. Johnsen, H. E., Brostrphøm, K., and Madsen, M.: Paroxysmal cold haemoglobinuria in children: 3 cases encountered within a period of 7 months. Scand. J. Haemat., *20:*413, 1978.
62. Knapp, T.: The laboratory investigation of three cases of paroxysmal cold haemoglobinuria. Canad. J. Med. Tech., *26:*172, 1964.
63. Lalezari, P., and Berens, J. A.: Specificity and cross reactivity of cell-bound antibodies. *In:* Human Blood Groups, Proceedings of the 5th International Convocation of Immunology, Buffalo, N.Y., 1976, Mohn, J. F., Plunkett, R. W., Cunningham, R. K., and Lambert, R. M., Eds. New York: S. Karger, 1977, 44.
64. Lau, F. O., and Rosse, W. F.: The reactivity of red blood cell membrane glycoprotein with "cold-reacting" antibodies. Clin. Immunol. Immunopath., *4:*1, 1975.
65. Layrisse, Z., and Layrisse, M.: High incidence cold autoagglutinins of anti-I^T specificity in Yanomama Indians of Venezuela. Vox. Sang., *14:*369, 1968.
66. Leddy, J. P., Peterson, P., Yeaw, A., et al.: Patterns of serologic specificity of human γG erythrocyte autoantibodies. Correlation of antibody specificity with complement-fixing behavior. J. Immunol., *105:*677, 1970.
67. Levine, P., and Celano, M. J.: Agglutinating specificity of LW factor in guinea pig and rabbit anti-Rh serums. Science, *156:*1744, 1967.
68. Levine, P., Celano, M. J., and Falkowski, F.: The specificity of the antibody in paroxysmal cold hemoglobinuria (PCH). Transfusion, *3:*278, 1963.
69. Lisowska, E.: The degradation of M and N blood group glycoproteins and glycopeptides with alkaline borohydride. Europ. J. Biochem., *10:*574, 1969.
70. Lisowska, E., Dzierzkowa-Borodej, W., Seyfried, H., et al.: Reactions of erythrocyte glycoproteins and their degradation products with various anti-I sera. Vox. Sang., *28:*122, 1975.
71. Marcus, D. M., Kabat, E. A., and Rosenfield, R. E.: The action of enzymes from clostridium tertium on the I antigenic determinant of human erythrocytes J. Exp. Med., *118:*175, 1963.
72. Marsh, W. L.: Anti-i: A cold antibody defining the Ii relationship in human red cells. Brit. J. Haemat., *7:*200, 1961.
73. Marsh, W. L., and Jenkins, W. J.: Anti-i: A new cold antibody. Nature, *188:*753, 1960.
74. Marsh, W. L., and Jenkins, W. J.: Anti-Sp$_1$: The recognition of a new cold autoantibody. Vox. Sang., *15:*177, 1968.
75. Marsh, W. L., Johnson, C., Øyen, R., et al.: Anti-Sd^x: A "new" auto-agglutinin related to the Sd^a blood group. Transfusion, in press, 1979.
76. Marsh, W. L., Nichols, M. E., and Allen, F. H.: Inhibition of anti-I sera by human milk. Vox. Sang., *18:*149, 1970.
77. Marsh, W. L., Nichols, M. E., and Reid, M. E.: The definition of two I antigen components. Vox. Sang., *20:*209, 1971.
78. Marsh, W. L., Øyen, R., Nichols, M. E., et al.: Chronic granulomatous disease and the Kell blood groups. Brit. J. Haemat., *29:*247, 1975.
79. Marsh, W. L., Reid, M. E., and Scott, E. P.: Autoantibodies of U blood group specificity in autoimmune haemolytic anaemia. Brit. J. Haemat., *22:*625, 1972.
80. Matuhasi, T., Kumazawa, H., and Usui, M.: Question of the presence of so-called cross-reacting antibody. J. Jap. Soc. Blood. Transf., *6:*295, 1960.

81. Mino, P.: La panemoagglutinina del sangue umane. Policlinico, Sez. Prat., *31:*1355, 1924.
82. Morel, P., Garratty, G., and Willbanks, E.: Another example of anti-IB. Vox. Sang., *29:*231, 1975.
83. Morton, J. A., Pickles, M. M., and Sutton, L.: The correlation of the Bg^a blood group with the HL-A7 leucocyte group: demonstration of antigenic sites on red cells and leucocytes. Vox. Sang., *17:*536, 1969.
84. Morton, J. A., Pickles, M. M., Sutton, L., et al.: Identification of further antigens on red cells and lymphocytes. Vox. Sang., *21:*141, 1971.
85. Nugent, M. E., Colledge, K. I., and Marsh, W. L.: Auto-immune hemolytic anemia caused by anti-U. Vox. Sang., *20:*519, 1971.
86. Ogata, T., and Matuhasi, T.: Problems of specific and cross reactivity of blood group antibodies. Proceedings of the 8th Congress of the International Society for Blood Transfusion, Tokyo, 1960; Basel/New York, Karger, 1962, 208–211.
87. Ogata, T., and Matuhasi, T.: Further observations on the problems of specific and cross reactivity of blood group antibodies. Proceedings of the 9th Congress of the International Society for Blood Transfusion, Mexico City, 1962; Basel/New York, Karger, 1964, 528–531.
88. Ozer, F. L., and Chaplin, H., Jr.: Agglutination of stored erythrocytes by a human serum. Characterization of the serum factor and erythrocyte changes. J. Clin. Invest., *42:*1735, 1963.
89. Patten, E., Beck, C. E., Scholl, C., et al.: Autoimmune hemolytic anemia with anti Jk^a specificity in a patient taking aldomet. Transfusion, *17:*517, 1977.
90. Pirofsky, B., and Pratt, K.: The antigen in autoimmune hemolytic anemia. I. Reactivity of human autoantibodies and rhesus antibodies with primate and non-primate erythrocytes. Amer. J. Clin. Path., *45:*75, 1966.
91. Race, R. R., Sanger, R., and Selwyn, J. G.: Possible deletion in human Rh chromosome: A serological and genetical study. Brit. J. Exp. Path., *32:*124, 1951.
92. Rand, B. P., Olson, J. D., Garratty, G., et al.: Coombs' negative immune hemolytic anemia with anti-E occurring in the red blood cell eluate of an E-negative patient. Transfusion, *18:*174, 1978.
93. Ries, C. A., Garratty, G., Petz, L. D., et al.: Paroxysmal cold hemoglobinuria: report of a case with an exceptionally high thermal range Donath-Landsteiner antibody. Blood, *38:*491, 1971.
94. Roelcke, D.: A new serological specificity in cold antibodies of high titre: anti-HD. Vox. Sang., *16:*76, 1969.
95. Roelcke, D., Anstee, D. J., Jungfer, H., et al.: IgG-type cold agglutinins in children and corresponding antigens. Detection of a new Pr antigen: Pr$_a$. Vox. Sang., *20:*218, 1971.
96. Roelcke, D.: Specificity of IgA cold agglutinins: Anti-Pr$_1$. Eur. J. Immunol., *3:*206, 1973.
97. Roelcke, D.: Cold agglutination. Antibodies and antigens. Clin. Immunol. Immunopath., *2:*266, 1974.
98. Roelcke, D., and Dorow, W.: Besonderheiten der Reaktionswerte eines mit Plasmocytom-γA-Paraprotein identischen Kalteagglutinins. Klin. Wschr., *46:*126, 1968.
99. Roelcke, D., Ebert, W., and Geisen, H. P.: Anti-Pr$_3$: serological and immunochemical identification of a new anti-Pr subspecificity. Vox. Sang., *30:*122, 1976.
100. Roelcke, D., Riesen, W., Geisen, H. P., et al.: Serological identification of the new cold agglutinin specificity anti-Gd. Vox. Sang., *33:*304, 1977.
101. Roelcke, D., and Uhlenbruck, G.: Letter to the Editor. Vox. Sang., *18:*478, 1970.
102. Roelcke, D., Uhlenbruck, G., and Bauer, K.: A heterogeneity of the HD-receptor, demonstrable by HD-cold antibodies: HD$_1$/HD$_2$. Scand. J. Haemat., *6:*280, 1969.

103. Rosenfield, R. E.: Unpublished observations, 1974. Cited by Issitt, P. D., and Issitt, C. H., In Applied Blood Group Serology. 2nd Ed. Oxnard, Spectra Biologicals, 1975.

104. Rosenfield, R. E., Allen, F. H., Jr., Swisher, S. N., et al.: A review of Rh serology and presentation of a new terminology. Transfusion, 2:287, 1962.

105. Rosse, W. F.: Fixation of the first component of complement (C'1a) by human antibodies. J. Clin. Invest., 47:2430, 1968.

106. Rosse, W. F., and Lauf, P. K.: Reaction of cold agglutinins with I antigen solubilized from human red cells. Blood, 36:777, 1970.

107. Rosse, W. F., and Sherwood, J. B.: Cold-reacting antibodies: Differences in the reaction of anti-I antibodies with adult and cord red blood cells. Blood, 36:28, 1970.

108. Schmidt, P. J., and Vos, G. H.: Multiple phenotypic abnormalities associated with Rh_{null} (– – –/– – –). Vox. Sang., 13:18, 1967.

109. Seyfried, H., Gorska, B., Maj, S., et al.: Apparent depression of antigens of the Kell blood group system associated with autoimmune acquired haemolytic anaemia. Vox. Sang., 23:528, 1972.

110. Svardal, J. M., Yarbro, J., and Yunis, E. J.: Ogata phenomenon explaining the unusual specificity in eluates from Coombs positive cells sensitized by autogenous anti-I. Vox. Sang., 13:472, 1967.

111. Szymanski, I. O., Roberts, P. L., and Rosenfield, R. E.: Anti-A autoantibody with severe intravascular hemolysis. N. Eng. J. Med., 294:995, 1976.

112. Tegoli, J., Harris, J. P., Issitt, P. D., et al.: Anti-IB, an expected "New" antibody detecting a joint product of the I and B genes. Vox. Sang., 13:144, 1967.

113. Thomas, D. B., and Winzler, R. J.: Structural studies on human erythrocyte glycoproteins. Alkali-labile oligosaccharides. J. Biol. Chem., 244:5943, 1969.

114. Thomas, D. B., and Winzler, R. J.: Structure of glycoproteins of human erythrocytes. Alkali-stable oligosaccharides. Biochem. J., 124:55, 1971.

115. Tonthat, H., Rochant, H., Henry, A., et al.: A new case of monoclonal IgΛ Kappa cold agglutinin with anti-Pr₁d specificity in a patient with persistent HB antigen cirrhosis. Vox. Sang., 30:464, 1976.

116. Van Loghem, J. J., Peetoom, F., Van der Hart, M., et al.: Serological and immunochemical studies in haemolytic anaemia with high-titre cold agglutinins. Vox. Sang., 8:33, 1963.

117. Van Loghem, J. J., and Van der Hart, M.: Varieties of specific auto-antibodies in acquired haemolytic anaemia. Vox. Sang., 4:2, 1954.

118. Vicari, G., and Kabat, E. A.: Immunochemical studies on blood groups. XLV. Structures and activities of oligosaccharides produced by alkaline degradation of a blood group substance lacking A, B, H, Le^a and Le^b specificities. Biochem., 9:3414, 1970.

119. Vogel, J. M., Hellman, M., and Moloshok, R. E.: Paroxysmal cold hemoglobinuria of nonsyphilitic etiology in two children. J. Pediat., 81:974, 1972.

120. Vos, G. H., Vos, Dell, Kirk, R. L., and Sanger, R.: A sample of blood with no detectable Rh antigens. Lancet. i: 14, 1961.

121. Vos, G. H., Petz, L., and Fudenberg, H. H.: Specificity of acquired haemolytic anaemia autoantibodies and their serological characteristics. Brit. J. Haemat., 19:57, 1970.

122. Vos, G. H., Petz, L. D., and Fudenberg, H. H.: Specificity and immunoglobulin characteristics of autoantibodies in acquired hemolytic anemia. J. Immunol., 106:1172, 1971.

123. Vos, G. H., Petz, L. D., Garratty, G., et al.: Autoantibodies in acquired hemolytic anemia with special reference to the LW system. Blood, 42:445, 1973.

124. Wang, A. C., Fudenberg, H. H., and Wells, J. V.: A new subgroup of the Kappa chain variable region associated with anti-Pr cold agglutinins. Nature New Biol., 243:126, 1973.

125. Watkins, W. M., and Morgan, W. T. J.: Possible genetical pathways of blood group mucopolysaccharides. Vox. Sang., *4:*97, 1959.
126. Weiner, W., and Vos, G. H.: Serology of acquired hemolytic anemias. Blood, *22:*606, 1963.
127. Weiner, W., Battey, D. A., Cleghorn, T. E., et al.: Serological findings in a case of haemolytic anaemia, with some general observations on the pathogenesis of this syndrome. Brit. Med. J., *ii:*125, 1953.
128. Weiner, W., Gordon, E. G., and Rowe, D.: A Donath-Landsteiner antibody. Vox. Sang., *9:*684, 1964.
129. Wiener, A. S., and Gordon, E. B.: Quantitative test for antibody-globulin coating human blood cells and its practical applications. Amer. J. Clin. Path., *23:*429, 1953.
130. Wiener, A. S., Gordon, E. B., and Gallop, C.: Studies on autoantibodies in human sera. J. Immunol., *71:*58, 1953.
131. Wiener, A. S., Unger, L. J., Cohen, L., et al.: Type-specific cold auto-antibodies as a cause of acquired hemolytic anemia and hemolytic transfusion reactions: Biologic test with bovine red cells. Ann. Intern. Med., *44:*221, 1956.
132. Wilkinson, L. S., Petz, L. D., and Garratty, G.: Reappraisal of the role of anti-i in haemolytic anaemia in infectious mononucleosis. Brit. J. Haemat., *25:*715, 1973.
133. Wilkinson, S. L., Vaithianathan, T., and Issitt, P. D.: The high incidence of anti-HL-A antibodies in anti-D typing reagents. Illustrated by a case of Matuhasi-Ogata phenomenon mimicking a 'D with anti-D' situation. Transfusion, *14:*27, 1974.
134. Worlledge, S. M.: A classification of AIHA, based on clinical grounds and the use of antiglobulin sera for immunoglobulin class and various complement components, and its use in clinical practice. *In* Program of the 25th Annual Meeting of the American Association of Blood Banks and the 13th Congress of the International Society for Blood Transfusion, 1972, p. 43 (abstract).
135. Worlledge, S. M., and Dacie, J. V.: Haemolytic and other anaemias in infectious mononucleosis. *In* Infectious Mononucleosis. Carter, R. L., and Penman, H. G., Eds., Oxford, Blackwell Scientific Publications, 1969.
136. Worlledge, S. M., and Rousso, C.: Studies on the serology of paroxysmal cold haemoglobinuria (PCH) with special reference to its relationship with the P blood group system. Vox. Sang., *10:*293, 1965.
137. Yokoyama, M., Eith, D. T., and Bowman, M.: The first example of auto-anti Xg[a]. Vox. Sang., *12:*138, 1967.

8

Drug-induced Immune Hemolytic Anemia

The administration of drugs may lead to the development of a wide variety of hematologic abnormalities, including immunohemolytic anemia. The clinical importance of drug-induced immune hemolytic anemia is emphasized by the fact that, among patients with acquired immune hemolytic anemia, 12.4 percent of our series of 347 patients (Table 2-3) and 18 percent of 79 patients reported by Dacie and Worlledge in 1969 [18] had anemias that were caused by drugs. A knowledge of the clinical manifestations and laboratory aids to diagnosis will prevent confusion with other causes of immune hemolysis, particularly idiopathic autoimmune hemolytic anemia. In addition, immunohematologic abnormalities caused by drugs are a source of confusion in the blood transfusion laboratory, where they may interfere with compatibility procedures.

This chapter considers the immune response to drugs, the various mechanisms leading to the development of cellular sensitization by drug-related antibodies, the clinical and laboratory features of drug-induced immunohematologic abnormalities involving red cells, methods of diagnosis, compatibility testing, management, and prognosis.

IMMUNOLOGIC MECHANISMS

General Concepts Regarding Drug-Induced Immune Cytopenias

Since the fundamental work of Landsteiner, [71, 72, 73] it has generally been accepted that simple chemicals (i.e., well defined organic compounds of molecular weight under 500 to 1,000 daltons) act as haptens and can be immunogenic only after first irreversibly binding to a macromolecular carrier, such as a protein. The specificity of the conjugated antigen (hapten-protein complex) is determined mainly by the structure of the hapten, but to a lesser degree by the nature of the carrier protein and the configuration of the conjugate. [28, 29, 46, 125] These principles were incorporated into Ackroyd's classic study regarding immune thrombotopenia induced by allylisopropylcarbamide (Sedormid). [3]

Since many of the concepts regarding mechanisms of drug-induced immune hemolytic anemia were based on pioneering work concerning drug-induced thrombocytopenia, it is pertinent to review these early studies.

Hapten Mechanism. Ackroyd demonstrated a number of serologic reactions involving platelets and drugs. He demonstrated that, in the presence of the patient's serum and the drug, platelets were agglutinated and complement was fixed in the reaction; clot retraction was inhibited if the reaction took place in freshly drawn whole blood. Ackroyd proposed that a haptenlike binding of the drug to a component of the cell (platelet) formed a new "complete" immunogen. This immunogen was conceived to elicit antibody with specificity for stuctural features of both drug and cell. The resultant antibody then reacted with drug-coated platelets leading to fixation of complement and cytolysis. This mechanism of cellular sensitization is frequently referred to as the hapten mechanism.

Shortly after Ackroyd's report, similar mechanisms were described for thrombocytopenia caused by quinine [64] and quinidine. [13, 120] Steinkamp et al. [130] reported a patient who was sensitive to quinine and developed bleeding and thrombocytopenia with a platelet count of 32,000 several hours after ingesting the drug. Quinine-dependent antibodies were proven not only by *in vitro* drug-dependent agglutination tests, but also by passive transfer of the patient's plasma to a normal volunteer. The plasma of the quinine-sensitive patient caused thrombocytopenia only when the recipient ingested quinine shortly before the infusion.

Immune Complex Mechanism. Later work by Miescher and Gorstein [93] led to the proposal that the platelet-drug complex was too labile to be strongly immunogenic, and that a more likely immunogen might be a drug-plasma protein complex. Shulman studied steps in a quinidine-antibody platelet reaction. [120–123] He studied the effect of quinidine concentration on the adsorption of antibody, on complement fixation, and on agglutination. He quantitated the equilibrium concentrations of the reactants in each step and pointed out that quinidine adsorbed on blood cells is easily eluted by washing in saline. He found that the affinity of the drug for its antibody is far stronger than the affinity of the drug for the cell membrane. From this and other evidence, Shulman proposed that the mechanism of drug-induced immune cytolysis consists of the formation of an immunogenic complex of drug and plasma protein, which leads to the production of antibodies that react with the drug with high affinity. The antibody-drug complex is then adsorbed nonspecifically by one or another of the cellular elements of the blood. Indeed, the cells have been considered "innocent bystanders" in this reaction. [19] Although the adsorption of the immune complex on the cell is nonspecific, complement may be activated and react with the cell, thereby augmenting the immune cytolysis. This mechanism of cellular sensitization is called the immune complex mechanism.

Physicochemical Characteristics of Antibodies. The physicochemical characteristics (size, configuration, charge, etc.) of the antibodies that result in

cytolysis of platelets or other cellular elements of the blood are largely uniden-
tified, although in some patients the immunoglobulin class of antibody appears to be of significance. Some reports have indicated that the IgG antibodies are more likely to affect platelets, and IgM antibodies are more likely
to affect red cells. Shulman reported that in six cases of quinidine or quinine
thrombocytopenia, the antibodies were 7S globulins (presumably IgG), but in
two cases of stibophen hemolytic anemia, the antibodies were 19S (presumably IgM). [123] Two forms of quinidine antibody were found in one patient, a 7S
globulin reacting only with platelets and a 19S globulin reacting only with red
cells. [21, 123] Similarly, rifampicin-dependent antibodies that bind complement
to normal red cells have been shown to be mainly IgM. [12, 126]

However, more recent data have suggested that such immunoglobulin
class specificity for an individual cell type may not always exist. Eisner and
Korbitz [30] reported both IgG and IgM quinine-dependent anti-platelet antibodies in a patient who developed severe thrombocytopenia after ingesting
the drug. Also, antibodies that cause lysis of platelets in the presence of rifampicin have been found in both the IgM and IgG fractions. [12] Croft et al. [17]
described a patient with quinine-induced thrombocytopenia whose serum
contained an anti-quinine antibody of high molecular weight (probably IgM).
Although the direct antiglobulin test was positive, there was no anemia or
evidence of increased hemolysis. Furthermore, the immune hemolytic
anemias provoked by other drugs, for example, Pyramidon, [10] dipyrone, [74]
melphalan, [32] sulphonylurea derivatives [11, 87] and insulin [35] appear to be due to
IgG antibodies.

**Summary of Data Regarding Hapten and Immune Complex Mecha-
nisms.** Although the mechanism described by Shulman consisting of the
nonspecific adsorption of immune complexes to the cellular elements of the
blood appears well documented as a mechanism of drug-induced immune
cytopenia, subsequent data suggest that this is not the only immunologic
mechanism of cell sensitization and cytolysis. Indeed, in many instances, the
antibody-antigen-drug reaction with complement fixation does not occur *in
vitro* until platelets are added, indicating that Ackroyd's thesis cannot be entirely discounted. [92] Evidence indicates that some drug antibodies are bivalent,
reacting with drug and platelet or drug-protein complex and platelet. Indeed,
Okuma [100] described an antibody that reportedly had two specificities—one
for platelet phosphatide and the other for ovalbumin, the carrier. Levine [76]
has emphasized that anti-hapten antibodies show immunologic specificity for
the amino acid residues through which they are covalently bound to protein,
and also for structural configurations of the carrier protein presumably ad-
joining the hapten's site of attachment (i.e., "carrier specificity"). If the conjugate inducing drug hypersensitivity is derived from cell protein (for example,
platelet surface protein), then the antibodies formed would show some
specificity toward normal platelets. Young [156] described an IgG antidigitoxin
antibody in a patient's serum that reacted with tritiated digitoxin (but not with
other forms of digitalis), and he demonstrated that the complex then fixed to
platelets. This latter reaction demonstrated specificity for platelets to the ex-

tent that the drug-antibody complex failed to react with red cells, latex particles, platelets disrupted by sonication, or sodium cyanide-treated platelets.

In summary, the evidence supporting the Miescher-Shulman "innocent bystander" theory is as follows:

1. The union between most drugs and blood cells has been shown to be weak.[38] Shulman reported that the association constants of quinine, quinidine, and stibophen with the appropriate cells were quite low, and thus if the drug were capable of becoming immunogenic after this loose union, it would differ from all known haptens. Also, the amount of drug bound to the cells seemed to be too small to account for the large amount of antibody that the cells could adsorb.

2. The reaction of antibody with excess drug does not inhibit subsequent antibody adsorption by the cells.

3. Some drug antibodies combine with drug in the absence of blood cells. Although the binding affinity of drug for platelets if often weak, the binding affinity of the same drug for antibody is considerably stronger, as is the binding affinity of drug-antibody complexes for platelets.

The arguments supporting the Ackroyd hypothesis are as follow:

1. The theory explains the rarity of drug-induced immune cytopenias in that the combination of drug with cells is postulated as being so labile that antibody formation is only rarely stimulated.

2. Better than any other hypothesis, it explains the apparent specificity of the drug antibody for a given target cell (platelets, red cells, or leukocytes).

It is probable that both proposed mechanisms are valid. Indeed, recent reports suggest the likelihood that, in individual patients, either the hapten mechanism or the immune complex mechanism may result in immune cytopenias caused by drugs such as quinidine.[7, 8, 157]

Hemolytic Anemia. Although the first drug-induced immune cytopenias to be reported concerned platelets, reports of immunologically mediated hemolytic anemias soon appeared.

In 1953 Snapper studied a patient with Coombs'-positive hemolytic anemia and pancytopenia secondary to Mesantoin ingestion who recovered completely after cessation of the drug.[125] Harris[52, 53] described a patient with schistosomiasis treated for the second time with stibophen (Fuadin) in whom acute intravascular hemolysis developed. *In vitro* studies revealed that the patient's serum agglutinated his own or normal red cells or sensitized them to agglutination with antiglobulin serum only in the presence of the drug. After cessation of stibophen therapy, the patient's hemoglobin concentration returned to normal within 20 days, and the direct antiglobulin test gradually became weaker and was negative about 60 days later. Passive transfer of the plasma containing the agglutinin to a normal volunteer resulted in a positive direct antiglobulin test and hemolytic anemia only after the volunteer also received a stibophen injection. Since this early work, numerous other drugs have been described as causing a positive direct antiglobulin test and immune hemolytic anemia (Table 8-1).

Table 8-1. DRUGS THAT HAVE BEEN REPORTED TO CAUSE A POSITIVE DIRECT
ANTIGLOBULIN TEST AND HEMOLYTIC ANEMIA *

Drug	References
Stibophen (Fuadin)	24, 52, 53
Quinidine	7, 8, 37, 157
P-aminosalicylic acid (PAS)	88, 96, 139
Quinine	98
Phenacetin	11, 22, 88, 139
Penicillins	42, 61, 82, 107, 110, 132
Insecticides (chlorinated hydrocarbons)	97
Antihistamine (Antazoline, Antistin)	9, 89
Sulfonamides	41, 134
Isoniazid (INH, Rifamate, Nydrazid)	39, 41, 112
Chlorpromazine (Thorazine)	51, 83
Pyramidon (Aminopyrin)	10
Dipyrone	74
Methyldopa (Aldomet, Aldoril, Aldoclor)	6, 15, 16, 150, 154
Melphalan (Alkeran)	32
Cephalosporins	49, 50, 95
Mefenamic acid (Ponstel)	33, 111, 116
Carbromal (Carbrital, Carbropent) †	129
Sulfonylurea derivatives (Diabenese, Dymelor, Orinase, Tolinase)	11, 87
Insulin	35
Levodopa (Levodopa, Sinemet)	43, 54, 59, 84, 136
Rifampin (Rifadin, Rifamate, Rimactane)	27, 55, 70, 113, 151
Methadone †	119
Tetracycline	147
Methysergide (Sansert)	124
Intravenous contrast media ‡	65
Acetaminophen	90
Hydrochlorothiazide	45a, 140
Streptomycin	91
Procainamide (Pronestyl, Sub-Quin)	58
Ibuprofen (Motrin)	66
Hydralazine (Apresoline, Hydralazide, Unipres)	101

* Some brand names are listed, but it is impractical to list the names of all products containing each drug. For example, the American Drug Index (J.B. Lippincott Co., Philadelphia, 1979) lists 235 products containing acetaminophen.

† Carbromal and methadone have been reported to cause positive direct antiglobulin tests but not hemolytic anemia.

‡ Serum drug-related antibodies were detected by the indirect antiglobulin test and hemolysis was suspected. However, the direct antiglobulin test was negative and hemolysis was not proven.

Additional mechanisms of red cell sensitization by drug-related antibody have been described and are of particular significance since there is generally a correlation between the responsible drug, the mechanism of sensitization, clinical manifestations, and laboratory methods of diagnosis (Table 8-2).[45, 108, 109]

Mechanisms of Drug-induced Positive Direct Antiglobulin Tests and Immune Hemolysis

Immune Complex Mechanism. The proposed "immune complex" mechanisms described by Miescher, Shulman, and others regarding thrombocytopenia appear also to be responsible for erythrocyte sensitization and hemolysis in some patients (Figure 8-1).

Not only is this immunologic mechanism of red cell destruction similar to drug-induced thrombocytopenia, but it is also true that some of the drugs that have caused hemolysis (e.g., stibophen, quinidine, p-aminosalicylic acid, quinine, and sulfonamides) are known to provoke thrombocytopenia and/or leukopenia in other patients.[149] At least four compounds have induced hemolytic anemia and thrombocytopenia at the same time in the same patient, namely quinine, quinidine, paraaminosalicylic acid, and amidopyrine.[23] Further, the clinical features of these disorders are distinctly similar in that: (1) both hemolysis and thrombocytopenia may occur after the ingestion of only a small quantity of the drug in a sensitive individual, (2) the cytolysis is

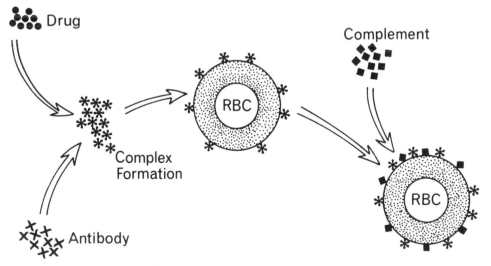

Figure 8-1. *The immune complex mechanism. Anti-drug antibody reacts with the drug to form an immune complex. The antibody-drug complex is then adsorbed onto red cells; the cell bound complex may activate complement and result in intravascular hemolysis. Red cells have been considered "innocent bystanders" in this reaction. Quinidine and phenacetin are prototype drugs.*

abrupt in onset, and (3) the cytolysis may be severe enough to be life-threatening.

The immune complex mechanism is probably responsible for the hemolytic anemias caused by most of the drugs in Table 8-1. Other immunologic mechanisms have been described regarding hemolytic anemias and/or positive direct antiglobulin tests, particularly in cases caused by methyldopa, L-dopa, mefenamic acid, penicillins, cephalosporins, carbromal, and tetracycline (described in detail later in this chapter).

The clinical and laboratory findings in patients with immune hemolytic anemia occurring as a result of the development of immune complexes are as follow.

• The patient needs to take only a small quantity of the drug if sensitized by prior exposure.

• Acute intravascular hemolysis with hemoglobinemia and hemoglobinuria is the usual clinical presentation (16 of 19 reported cases in one series).[149]

• Renal failure is frequent.[24, 74, 83, 88, 98]

• The serum anti-drug antibody may be IgG or IgM and capable of activating complement.

• The direct antiglobulin test is positive, often due to the presence of complement components on the red cell surface, usually without detectable immunoglobulins. This result may be explained by the fact that the immune complex does not bind very firmly to the red cells and it may dissociate from the cells and be free to react with other cells. This in turn may explain why such a small amount of drug complex can cause so much red cell destruction.[17] Furthermore, red cell sensitization by IgM antibodies is not readily detectable by the antiglobulin test.[44] Some reports of negative direct antiglobulin tests, particularly in the earlier literature, may result from inadequate anticomplement properties of the antiglobulin serum.[44]

• *In vitro* reactions (agglutination, lysis and/or sensitization to antiglobulin serum) are generally observed only when patient's serum, drug, and red cells are all incubated together (Table 8-2).

Drug Adsorption Mechanism. Penicillin is the prototype of drugs that cause direct antiglobulin tests and immune hemolytic anemia by the drug adsorption mechanism.

Early Reports of Penicillin-induced Immunohematologic Abnormalities

Antipenicillin antibody was first reported in 1958 by Ley et al.[82] During routine blood banking procedures the serum of a prospective transfusion recipient was found to agglutinate an entire panel of erythrocytes that had been stored with penicillin as part of the preservative; erythrocytes from the same donors, when not exposed to penicillin, were not agglutinated by this serum. Ley and his co-workers [82] and Watson, Joubert, and Bennett,[144] in tests

Table 8-2. CORRELATION BETWEEN MECHANISM OF RED CELL SENSITIZATION AND CLINICAL AND LABORATORY FEATURES IN DRUG-INDUCED IMMUNOHEMATOLOGIC ABNORMALITIES

Mechanism	Prototype Drugs	Clinical Findings	Serologic Evaluation Direct Antiglobulin Test	Antibody Identification
I. Immune complex formation (drug and anti-drug antibody)	Quinidine, phenacetin	Small doses of drug; acute intravascular hemolysis usual; renal failure common; thrombocytopenia occasionally	Usually only complement components detected, but IgG can be present	Drug + patient's serum + RBC (especially enzyme-treated) → hemolysis, agglutination or sensitization; antibody frequently IgM and capable of fixing complement; RBC eluate often non-reactive
II. Drug adsorbed onto red cell membrane; reacts with high titer serum drug antibody	Penicillins, cephalosporins	Large doses of penicillin (10 million units or more daily); other manifestations of allergy not necessarily present; usually subacute extravascular hemolysis; penicillin one of most common causes of drug-induced immune hemolysis; rare cases of immune hemolytic anemia caused by cephalosporins	Strongly positive (IgG) when hemolytic anemia present; complement sensitization also in a minority of patients	Drug-coated RBC + serum → agglutination or sensitization (rarely hemolysis); high titer antibody associated with hemolytic anemia is always IgG; RBC eluate reacts only with antibiotic-coated RBC

Table 8-2. (CONTINUED)

III. Membrane modification (nonimmunologic absorption of proteins)	Cephalosporins	No cases of cephalosporin-induced hemolytic anemia caused by nonimmunologic mechanisms	Positive with antiserums to a variety of serum proteins	Drug-coated RBC + serum → sensitization to antiglobulin serums in low titer (non-immunologic protein absorption); RBC eluate non-reactive
IV. Unknown	Methyldopa	Hemolysis in 0.8 percent of patients taking drug for at least 3 months; gradual onset of hemolytic anemia; most common cause of drug-induced immune hemolysis	Strongly positive (IgG) when hemolytic anemia present; rarely cells are sensitized with complement as well	Antibody sensitizes normal RBC without drug; antibody in serum and eluate identical to that found in warm antibody AIHA; no *in vitro* relationship to drug demonstrable

on 2,000 and 3,000 unselected sera, respectively, found this antibody only in donors who had previously received penicillin.

Between 1959 and 1965, four patients were reported who had hemolytic anemia during penicillin administration, and who also had a positive direct antiglobulin test and serum antipenicillin antibodies. However, all these patients had serious systemic infection and were also receiving other drugs.

Ley et al.[144] described a patient receiving 18,000,000 units of penicillin daily who was found to have a positive direct antiglobulin test. (No prior negative reactions had been recorded.) On the seventh day of penicillin therapy, probenecid was added to the regimen, and at that time the hematocrit level began to fall. Despite blood transfusion the fall continued. Therapy with both penicillin and probenecid was then stopped; after more transfusions, the hematocrit level remained stable. The patient subsequently died; antipenicillin antibody was demonstrated in a sample of blood drawn on the day of death.

Strumia and Raymond [131] reported a case of acute bacterial endocarditis caused by hemolytic coagulase-positive *Staphylococcus aureus*. The hemoglobin dropped from 10.9 to 6.2 gm/dl between the tenth and twenty-first days of antibiotic therapy, which included aqueous penicillin, 34,000,000 units daily. The patient's serum contained antipenicillin antibody, and an eluate from the patient's red cells was active against penicillin-sensitized cells. On the twenty-first day the reticulocyte count was 15 percent. After transfusion of 1 unit of blood on the twenty-first and twenty-fourth days of therapy, the hemoglobin "stabilized" at 10 gm/dl, and reticulocytes dropped to 11 percent, although penicillin was continued for a total of 27 days. The patient was also treated with novobiocin, probenecid, a short course of streptomycin and, because of an urticarial rash, prednisone and antihistamines. These investigators concluded that there was no direct proof of the relation between the antipenicillin antibodies, the positive direct antiglobulin test, and the hemolytic anemia, although a "strong implication" for a cause-and-effect relation existed.

Van Arsdel and Gilliland [138] described two patients who acquired "apparent hemolytic anemia" during treatment with large doses of penicillin for bacterial endocarditis and staphlococcal septicemia, respectively. One patient had a hematocrit level of 27 percent and a reticulocyte count of 3 percent even before therapy with penicillin was begun, and in the other, the degree of anemia remained unchanged more than six weeks after the administration of penicillin was discontinued. Thus, doubt remained concerning the causative role of penicillin in these cases of hemolytic anemia.

In 1966, Petz and Fudenberg [107] described a patient who developed hemolytic anemia during therapy with high doses of penicillin for suspected bacterial endocarditis (Figure 8-2). Serologic tests revealed a strongly positive direct antiglobulin test with anti-IgG antiglobulin serum but negative reactions using an "anti-non-gamma" serum. In spite of the strongly positive antiglobulin test, no abnormal antibodies could be detected in the patient's serum or eluate using standard serologic techniques (Table 8-3). However, using penicillin sensitized erythrocytes, anti-penicillin antibody was demonstrable in the serum by direct agglutination and by the indirect antiglobulin test, and in an eluate from the patient's red cells. After the cessation of all drugs except prednisone, hemolysis persisted for about three weeks and then gradually resolved. The direct antiglobulin test became progressively weaker and was negative six weeks after cessation of the drug.

Seven months later, the patient was challenged with penicillin at a time when there was no evidence of infection, to clarify the role of penicillin in production of hemolysis. All the original findings were reproduced (Figure 8-3), thereby documenting the etiologic role of penicillin.

Binding of Penicillin by Red Cells

Further observations indicated that penicillin differed from drugs that had previously been described as causing hemolytic anemia in that it was strongly bound to the red cell membrane *in vitro* in the absence of antibody. [107] Indeed, when one reacts a serum containing penicillin antibody against erythrocytes sensitized with penicillin, there is no fall in hemagglutination titer even after the red cells are washed 20 to 25 times with buffered saline solution

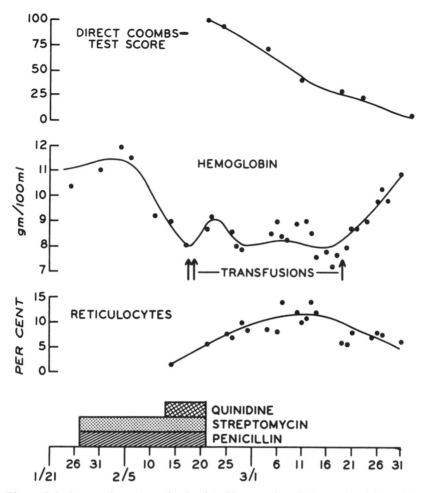

Figure 8-2. *Course of a patient who developed immune hemolytic anemia while receiving intravenous penicillin for suspected bacterial endocarditis. The direct antiglobulin (Coombs') test was known to have been negative prior to initiation of penicillin therapy. (Petz, L. D. and Fudenberg, H. H.: Coombs-positive hemolytic anemia caused by penicillin administration. New Eng. J. Med., 274:171, 1966.)*

over a one week period; studies with tritium-labeled penicillin also indicate that penicillin derivative is "firmly bound" to the erythrocytes.[137]

Penicillin can be detected on the surface of the red cells of most patients who are receiving high doses of the drug intravenously.[2, 17, 79, 92, 107, 148] Using rabbit anti-penicillin antibody, Levine and Redmond[79] demonstrated the drug on the red cells of 30 percent of the patients taking 1.2 to 2.4 million units per day, and on the RBC of all patients taking 10 million units or more daily. This coating is not by itself injurious, but some patients develop a high titer anti-penicillin antibody that reacts with cell-bound penicillin. In striking contrast to hemolytic anemia caused by the immune complex mechanism, penicillin-induced hemolytic anemia occurs only during the administration of

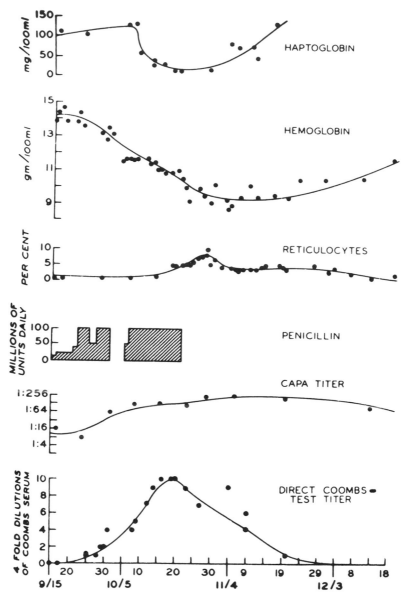

Figure 8-3. Documentation of etiologic role of penicillin in causation of immune hemolytic anemia. The patient is the same as in Figure 8-2, and a repeated administration of penicillin caused recurrence of all the original findings. (Petz, L. D., and Fudenberg, H. H.: Coombs-positive hemolytic anemia caused by penicillin adminstration. New Eng. J. Med., 274:171, 1966.)

Table 8-3. DIRECT ANTIGLOBULIN TEST TITERS IN A PATIENT WITH PENICILLIN-
INDUCED IMMUNE HEMOLYTIC ANEMIA *

| | Dilutions of Antiglobulin Serum | | | | | | |
	1:4	1:16	1:64	1:256	1:1024	1:4000	Saline
Anti-whole serum	3+	4+	4+	3+	2+	2+	0
Anti-IgG	3+	3½+	3½+	3½+	2+	1+	0
"Anti-non-gamma"	0	0	0	0	0	0	0

* Tests for abnormal erythrocyte antibodies were as follows: cold agglutinins, normal; agglutination titration at 23°C, 30°C and 37°C, using normal red cells, negative; agglutination titration at 23°C, 30°C and 37°C using pretrypsinized red cells, negative; indirect antiglobulin test, negative; lysis screening tests, negative; and tests for activity of eluate from patient's red cells, negative.

(Petz, L. D., and Fudenberg, H. H.: Coombs—positive hemolytic anemia caused by penicillin adminis-tration. N. Engl. J. Med., *274:*171, 1966.)

high doses of the drug. Large doses of the drug appear to be necessary to coat red cells sufficiently to furnish enough antigenic sites for reaction with anti-penicillin antibody. Thus, the mechanism of red cell sensitization and resul-tant hemolysis differs from the immune complex mechanism described previ-ously; it appears to result from the coating of red cells by penicillin during the administration of high doses of the drug, and the reaction of anti-penicillin antibodies with such drug-coated cells (Figure 8-4). The quantity of penicillin antibody sensitizing the red cell is related to the concentration of penicillin antigenic determinants on the cell membrane, the plasma concentration of anti-penicillin antibody, and the avidity of the antibody.[79]

We refer to this mechanism as the drug adsorption mechanism since it appears analogous to *in vitro* passive hemagglutination. Others have used the term "hapten mechanism" in reference to penicillin-induced immune hemolysis, but this term implies that the haptenlike binding of penicillin to red cells is essential for the drug to be immunogenic, as was postulated by Ackroyd. However, there is no evidence that red cell binding by penicillin is necessary for the drug to be immunogenic. Instead, the immunogenicity of penicillin may relate to its binding with serum proteins, and hemolysis may result from the reaction of anti-penicillin antibody with penicillin that has been non-specifically adsorbed to the red cell membrane.

The immunogenicity of penicillin results from its ability to react chemi-cally with proteins to form several different haptenic groups.[25, 26, 77, 78, 80, 102, 104, 117, 137] The major haptenic determinant is the benzylpenicilloyl (BPO) group. When sensitive hemagglutination techniques are used, anti-BPO an-tibodies can be demonstrated in over 90 percent of normal sera.[45] Most sera contain IgM antibodies only, but the antibodies associated with immune hemolytic anemia are of the IgG immunoglobulin class. About 3 percent of the patients who receive large doses of penicillin intravenously develop a positive direct antiglobulin test, and some of these patients develop hemolytic anemia. Complement is not usually involved in this reaction, and acute in-travascular hemolysis is rare. Instead, hemolysis is characteristically much less

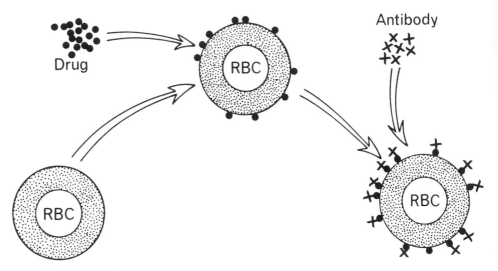

Figure 8-4. *The drug adsorption mechanism. Penicillin is the prototype drug. The essential feature is that the drug is non-specifically bound to red cells and remains firmly adherent to the cells regardless of whether the patient develops an antibody to the drug. If a patient develops a potent anti-drug antibody, it will react with the cell bound drug. Such red cells will yield a positive result in the direct antiglobulin test, and hemolytic anemia may ensue. Complement is usually not activated by anti-penicillin antibodies.*

acute in onset, with anemia developing over a week or more. Thus, both the mechanism of red cell sensitization and the clinical manifestations of hemolysis differ from those produced by drugs reacting by the immune complex mechanism.

Complement Activation

Exceptions to the typical findings already described have been reported. Kerr et al.[61] described a patient whose red cells reacted strongly with both anti-IgG and anticomplement antiglobulin sera, and they suggested that complement activation may contribute to immune hemolysis in some cases. In addition, we [110] described a patient with penicillin-induced immune hemolytic anemia who had intravascular hemolysis of life-threatening severity with hemoglobinemia and hemoglobinuria (Figure 8-5). Significant amounts of complement components C3 and C4 were detected on the patient's red cells, in addition to the usual IgG antibody to penicillin. The patient's serum caused agglutination of penicillin-coated red cells and sensitized them to agglutination by antiserum to IgG. However, it did not sensitize such cells to agglutination by antisera to C3 and C4 or cause their lysis *in vitro,* even in the presence of fresh complement.

However, complement fixation could be demonstrated by incubating the patient's serum with normal serum and then measuring residual hemolytic complement activity. Similar complement fixation could also be demonstrated

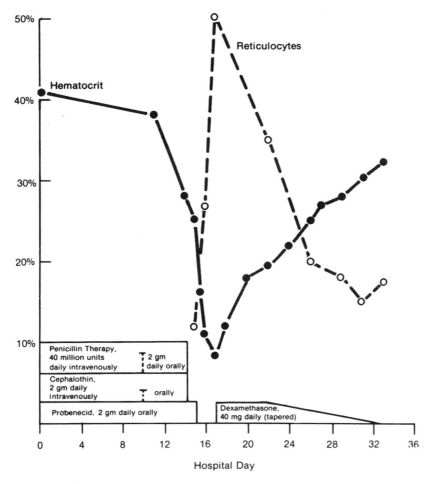

Figure 8-5. *Clinical course of a patient with penicillin-induced hemolytic anemia with intravascular hemolysis of life-threatening severity. The patient's serum contained anti-penicillin antibody to a titer of 8,000, and her red cells were sensitized with IgG, C3, and C4. She refused transfusion because of religious beliefs and was treated with oxygen, parenteral fluids, and corticosteroids.* (Ries, C. A., Rosenbaum, T. J., Garratty, G., Petz, L. D., and Fudenberg, H. H.: Penicillin-induced immune hemolytic anemia. J.A.M.A., 233:432, 1975.)

using serum from a patient with penicillin-induced serum sickness, but fixation could not be demonstrated with the serum of a patient with penicillin-induced hemolytic anemia without intravascular hemolysis, or with the sera of three people with relatively high titers of antibody to penicillin without hemolytic anemia. The presence of complement components on the patient's red cells and the finding that her serum fixed complement *in vitro* suggested that penicillin-anti-penicillin immune complexes were present in her serum. We further suggested that red cell damage mediated by immune complexes may have augmented the non-complement, IgG-mediated hemolysis that is usually seen in penicillin-induced immune hemolytic anemia. The unusual severity of hemolysis appeared to result from the high titer of antibody to penicillin (8,000) and to participation of the complement system in hemolysis.

More recently, Funicella et al.[42] reported a patient who was treated with ampicillin, oxacillin, and penicillin over an 11-day period. Hemolytic anemia ensued, and the direct antiglobulin test was positive with both anti-IgG and anti-C4/C3 antiglobulin sera. The authors demonstrated the presence of immune complexes using a radiolabelled C1q binding test, and they suggested that erythrocyte destruction occurred both by the immune complex mechanism and the drug absorption mechanism (which they referred to as the "haptene type").

Our findings in 10 patients with penicillin-induced hemolytic anemia in the present series (which includes the patient with intravascular hemolysis described above) indicate that in a majority of patients, the direct antiglobulin test is positive only with anti-IgG antiglobulin serum. However, four patients in our series and several patients reported by others [75] also had complement components on their red cells. Although these numbers are small, they suggest that hemolysis may be augmented by complement activation in a significant number of patients.

One should also appreciate that a positive direct antiglobulin test occurring during penicillin administration is not, in itself, an indication for cessation of the drug. Approximately 3 percent of the patients receiving high doses of intravenous penicillin will develop a positive direct antiglobulin test.[2, 105, 106] Hemolysis may not ensue, even with the continued administration of the drug.

Characteristic Features of Penicillin-induced Hemolytic Anemia

The usual clinical and laboratory features of penicillin-induced immune hemolytic anemia can be summarized by the following statements.

1. Hemolysis develops only in patients who are receiving large doses of penicillin intravenously (at least 10 million units daily in an adult for a week or more).

2. Hemolytic anemia is less acute in onset than that caused by the immune complex mechanism, and it usually develops over a period of 7 to 10 days. However, hemolysis may be life-threatening if the etiology is not promptly diagnosed and if penicillin administration is continued.

3. A high titer IgG penicillin antibody is present in the serum. Using the technique described later in this chapter the titer is usually 1,000 or greater.

4. The direct antiglobulin test is strongly positive due to erythrocyte sensitization with IgG. In a minority of patients, complement components are detected as well.

5. Antibody eluted from the patient's red cells will react against penicillin-treated red cells, but negative reactions will be obtained using red cells not treated with the drug.

6. Cessation of penicillin therapy is followed by complete recovery, al-

though hemolysis of decreasing severity and a "mixed-field" positive anti-globulin test may persist for several weeks.

7. Other manifestations of penicillin allergy are not necessarily present.

Other Drugs

Other drugs that bind firmly to red cells and cause positive direct anti-globulin tests by the same mechanism as penicillin are cephalothin [50, 95] and possibly carbromal. [129] Cephalothin [49] has been reported as a rare cause of immune hemolytic anemia, but carbromal, to date, has not. Using cephalothin-coated red cells and penicillin-coated red cells, [127, 128] several groups of investigators have shown that penicillin antibodies may cross-react with cephalothin-treated red cells. [2, 105, 106, 128] In addition, specific anti-cephalothin antibodies have been identified both in serum [1] and in eluates made from red cells of patients having a positive direct antiglobulin test due to cephalothin. [2, 49, 128]

Tetracycline also binds to red cells and has been the cause of immune hemolytic anemia. [135, 147] The mechanism of hemolysis is different because red cell sensitization with the drug requires the presence of a plasma factor, whereas penicillin and cephalothin-coated cells may be prepared using washed cells incubated with drug in buffer. [127] Also, acute hemolysis with severe anemia developed in a patient within two days after a repeat exposure to tetracycline. [147]

Finally, some recent reports indicate that serum antibodies in some patients with quinidine-induced hemolytic anemia react with red cells sensitized with the drug even after thorough washing of the red cells. Thus, the drug-absorption mechanism may contribute to hemolysis in some cases of quinidine-induced hemolytic anemia. [7, 8, 157]

Nonimmunologic Protein Absorption. Cephalothin is unique among drugs, in that it has been well documented as causing a positive direct anti-globulin test by three different mechanisms. The drug may combine with the red cell membrane and then react with anti-cephalothin antibody in a manner similar to that described previously for penicillin. [2, 49, 128] Alternatively, the cephalothin-coated red cell may react with cross-reacting penicillin antibodies since immunohematologic cross-reactivity between penicillin and cephalothin has been documented. [2, 48, 50, 99, 128]

Finally, cephalothin may modify the red cell membrane so that the cells adsorb proteins nonimmunologically [50, 95, 128] (Figure 8-6). When incubated in normal plasma *in vitro*, cephalothin-sensitized cells become coated with numerous plasma proteins including albumin, IgG, IgA, IgM, α_1-antitrypsin, α_2-macroglobulin, C3, C4 and fibrinogen. [108, 128]

One can generally determine whether the positive direct antiglobulin test has resulted from nonimmunologic protein adsorption or by antibody fixation (see Table 8-4). Non-immunologic adsorption of proteins will result in the direct antiglobulin test being positive with antiglobulin sera raised to a variety

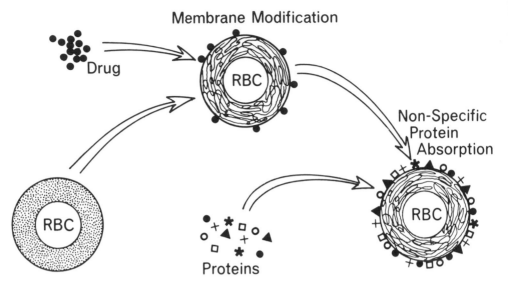

Figure 8-6. *Non-immunologic protein adsorption. One of the ways that cephalosporins cause a positive direct antiglobulin test is by modification of the red cell membrane so that plasma proteins are adsorbed nonimmunologically. Among the proteins adsorbed are β and γ globulins, and therefore the red cells will react positively in the direct antiglobulin test. Hemolytic anemia does not occur as a result of this mechanism of cellular sensitization.*

of proteins (e.g., α, β, and γ globulins, albumin and fibrinogen), the red cell eluate will be nonreactive, and the serum will contain no anti-drug antibody or antibody in low titer. In contrast, an immunologic reaction similar to that occurring with penicillin will result in the direct antiglobulin test being positive (due primarily to sensitization with IgG), the red cell eluate will be reactive against cephalothin-treated but not against untreated red cells, and the serum can be expected to contain a high titer antibody against cephalothin-treated red cells. Hemolytic anemia has not been described as a result of nonimmunologic protein adsorption.

Early reports regarding several small series of patients indicated that a high percentage of patients receiving cephalosporins developed a positive antiglobulin test.[50, 95] However, a prospective study in which more than 600 direct antiglobulin tests were performed on multiple samples from 169 patients receiving penicillin(s) intravenously (mainly penicillin G) and 124 patients receiving cephalosporin drugs (primarily cephalothin) indicated that five patients receiving penicillin and four receiving cephalosporins had positive direct antiglobulin tests, i.e., an incidence of about three percent in each instance.[2, 106, 128] Swisher's experience is in agreement with this low figure of incidence of positive direct antiglobulin tests caused by cephalosporins.[133]

Although the direct antiglobulin test has been most extensively studied with cephalothin, positive tests have also been ascribed to other cephalosporins, such as cephalexin,[67, 69, 115] cephaloridine,[34, 155] and cefazolin.[69, 94]

Table 8-4. CHARACTERISTICS OF CEPHALOSPORIN-INDUCED ABNORMALITIES

Non-immunologic
   1. Direct antiglobulin test positive with antiglobulin sera to a variety of proteins (e.g., gamma, beta, alpha globulins, albumin, and fibrinogen)
   2. Red cell eluate usually nonreactive
   3. Serum may contain low titer anticephalosporin or cross-reacting anti-penicillin antibodies
   4. Hemolytic anemia not described

Immunologic
   1. Direct antiglobulin test positive due to sensitization with IgG mainly
   2. Red cell eluate reacts with cephalosporin-treated, but not untreated red cells
   3. Serum usually contains high titer antibody against cephalosporin-treated cells
   4. Hemolytic anemia is rare

The principal clinical importance of positive direct antiglobulin tests caused by cephalosporins is that they cause apparent incompatibility in the minor "cross-match" test (which is not an essential part of compatibility testing) and may confuse the evaluation of hemolytic disorders of other etiology. [106, 108] Since penicillin is the second most common cause of drug-induced immune hemolytic anemia, and since the mechanism of red blood cell sensitization with cephalosporins is, in some cases, similar to that resulting from the administration of penicillin, Abraham et al. [2] stated in 1968 that it was "surprising" that hemolytic anemia due to the administration of cephalosporins had not been reported. Since that time several cases of cephalosporin-induced immunohemolytic anemia have been reported, [36, 49, 57, 60] but such cases are much rarer than those occurring during penicillin therapy.

Autoimmune Hemolytic Anemia Caused by Drugs. Carstairs et al. [15] and Worlledge et al. [154] first reported positive direct antiglobulin tests and autoimmune hemolytic anemia due to the antihypertensive drug, methyldopa (Aldomet). It was soon apparent from the characterization of the antibodies in the sera and red cell eluates of such patients that the mechanism by which this drug caused hemolytic anemia differed from the previously described mechanisms. The antibodies from such patients react directly with normal red cells in the absence of drug *in vitro* and, upon further characterization, are found to be indistinguishable from those found in patients with idiopathic warm antibody autoimmune hemolytic anemia. Indeed, no serologic proof of a relationship between the antibodies and the drug has ever been demonstrated, and proof that methyldopa causes autoimmune hemolytic anemia in such patients has come from clinical observations. Cessation of the drug in such patients causes a prompt remission of the hemolytic anemia, and the direct antiglobulin test slowly reverts to negative. Readministration of the drug causes the syndrome to reappear. The incidence of methyldopa-induced autoimmune hemolytic anemia exceeds the total of all other drug-induced immune hemolytic anemias both in our experience (Table 2-3, page 29) and in the experience of others.[149]

Proposed Mechanisms of Autoantibody Development Caused by Methyldopa

Several hypotheses have been proposed to explain the development of warm autoantibodies during the administration of methyldopa. One hypothesis is that the drug alters normal red cell antigens in such a way that they are no longer recognized as "self." Weigle has demonstrated loss of tolerance to antigens that have been minimally altered.[145] For example, he produced thyroiditis and antibodies to native thyroglobulin by injecting rabbits with rabbit thyroglobulin that has been picrylated or coupled with diazonium derivatives of sulfanilic acid.[146] Worlledge et al.[154] speculated that methyldopa might combine with the red cell membrane or enter the red cell and alter Rhesus antigens in such a way as to lead to the development of autoantibody by the patient's normal immune system.

Another possibility is that the drug acts as a hapten and that the resultant antibodies cross-react with normal red cell antigens. However, neither methyldopa nor several of its known metabolites or closely related substances inhibit or enhance the reaction of the antibodies with normal cells.[85, 154] The lack of chemical similarity between methyldopa and mefenamic acid, both of which result in the development of autoimmune hemolytic anemia with antibodies of similar specificity, also detracts from the probability that the antibodies develop as a result of this mechanism. Further, if the drug acts as a hapten, a secondary type of response might be expected on readministration of the drug to a patient who previously had had a positive direct antiglobulin test. This response, however, is not observed, and reappearance of immunohematologic abnormalities with readministration of the drug takes as long as with the initial administration (usually several months), and the strength of such reactions is not obviously enhanced.[14] The persistence of a positive direct antiglobulin test in some patients for seven to twenty-four months after cessation of the drug is also poorly explained by this hypothesis.

Gottlieb and Wurzel[47] have reported that immune globulin treated *in vitro* with methyldopa reacts with red cells or latex particles, and this phenomenon can be demonstrated by the antiglobulin reaction. They proposed that red cell sensitization *in vivo* during the administration of methyldopa occurs as a result of the uptake of serologically detectable altered gamma globulin on the red cell surface. As these authors point out, this hypothesis does not explain the fact that autoantibodies associated with the administration of methyldopa are commonly reported to show Rhesus specificity. Gottlieb and Wurzel were not able to confirm the presence of such specificity, perhaps because in autoimmune hemolytic anemias specificity is frequently defined on the basis of subtle differences in titer and/or cross-absorption and elution studies, especially when using rare cells of varying genotypes.[6, 45, 141, 142, 143] This finding is in contrast to the clear pattern one sees with blood group alloantibodies. Gottlieb and Wurzel[47] point out that there are abnormalities of the red cell membrane of such rare cells as Rh $_{null}$ cells, and that it might be mistaken to infer antibody specificity solely on the basis of altered reactivity with such a marred membrane.

Dameshek [20] proposed that methyldopa may produce aberrations in the proliferation of normal lymphocytes, thus yielding clones of abnormal but nevertheless immunologically competent cells. Although functional, these cells would be intolerant of normal antigens, "especially those of the ubiquitous red cell." Jandl and LoBuglio [56] have criticized this hypothesis because detailed studies of the structure of methyldopa-induced antibodies directed against the Rh locus revealed that they were composed of both κ and λ light chains and three distinct H-chain subclasses. [6] Thus, at least three different clones of immunocytes must be postulated as having lost the ability to recognize the Rh locus of the red cell as "self." Nevertheless, no other proposed mechanism is as consistent with the prolonged period of time necessary to induce such immunohematologic abnormalities in patients even on repeated challenge with the drug, or, even more significantly, for the prolonged persistence of such findings. The possibility that numerous clones of altered lymphocytes persist in producing antibody for months beyond the life span of erythrocytes is a plausible explanation for the findings of a positive direct antiglobulin test for seven to twenty-four months after cessation of the drug, and this hypothesis should therefore not be disregarded.

More recently Kirtland and co-workers have presented data in support of the possibility that altered lymphocyte function caused by methyldopa may relate to the pathogenesis of the autoimmune hemolytic anemia. [62, 63] They studied the effect of methyldopa on IgG synthesis *in vitro* and concluded that the drug exerts a direct effect on T lymphocytes, leading to a loss of suppressor function and elaboration of autoantibodies by B cells. [63] Further work to confirm such preliminary findings is necessary, but their conclusions thus far are consistent with modern hypotheses concerning the mechanism of development of autoimmune disorders. [4, 40, 68, 103]

Characteristic Features of Methyldopa-induced Immunohematologic Abnormalities

The clinical and laboratory features of methyldopa-induced abnormalities are as follow.

1. The direct antiglobulin test becomes positive after 3 to 6 months of therapy in from 10 to 36 percent of the patients receiving methyldopa.

2. The development of the positive direct antiglobulin test appears to be dose-dependent. The incidence of a positive direct antiglobulin test is 36 percent in patients taking more than 2 gm per day, 19 percent in patients taking 1 to 2 gm per day, and 11 percent in patients taking less than 1 gm daily.

3. Approximately 0.8 percent of the patients receiving methyldopa develop hemolytic anemia. [149] This is a cumulative incidence with individual reports varying from 0 to 5 percent.

4. A strongly positive direct antiglobulin test occurs in all cases, and this result is due to sensitization with IgG. In a minority of patients in our series, the direct antiglobulin test was also weakly positive with anti-C3. All positive reactions with anti-C3 antiglobulin serum were ½ to 1+ in strength (see Tables 6-3 and 6-4). Worlledge [153] reported that all patients thought to have autoimmune hemolytic anemia caused by methyldopa had a negative antiglobulin test using anti-C3 antiserum.

5. The indirect antiglobulin test is positive in all patients who have hemolytic anemia. This finding is in contrast to patients who have warm antibody AIHA not associated with the administration of methyldopa in whom the indirect antiglobulin test is positive in only 57 percent of the patients.

6. The antibodies in the serum and red cell eluate are similar to those found in idiopathic warm antibody AIHA.

7. The anemia appears to develop gradually; acute hemolytic anemia with intravascular hemolysis has not been reported.

8. After the cessation of drug therapy, the symptoms and laboratory evidence of hemolysis usually regress within a few weeks, although rare exceptions have been recorded in which 10 weeks to 6 months were required before the hemoglobin level returned to normal. [31] The autoantibodies disappear from the serum but, as emphasized above, the direct antiglobulin test may take up to two years or more to become completely negative.

Other Drugs That Cause Autoimmune Hemolytic Anemia

A few other drugs have been described as causing autoimmune hemolytic anemia in a fashion similar to methyldopa. One is a closely related drug, L-dopa, which has been reported to cause positive direct antiglobulin tests [54, 59] and hemolytic anemia. [43, 84, 136] Another drug, mefenamic acid, is chemically unrelated to methldopa and has been described as causing positive direct antiglobulin tests and autoimmune hemolytic anemia in three separate reports of five patients. [33, 111, 116] The autoantibodies provoked by L-dopa and mefenamic acid seem remarkably similar to those provoked by methyldopa. [33, 54, 86, 116] Unlike patients taking methyldopa, patients taking mefenamic acid do not frequently develop a positive antiglobulin test. The red cells of only 1 of 36 patients tested by Scott and his colleagues [116] gave a positive reaction, and this was subsequently found to be negative, although the drug was continued. However, occasional patients taking the drug are found to have a positive direct antiglobulin reaction, which becomes weaker once the drug is withdrawn. [153]

Still other drugs may cause AIHA, although for each of the following drugs, the evidence is much less definite than for methyldopa, L-dopa, and mefenamic acid. An apparent AIHA occurring in a patient who had received Mesantoin for four months was described in 1963 by Snapper and his colleagues; [125] a second patient, who had received long term diphenylhydantoin (Dilantin) was described in 1966. [114] Although both patients eventually recovered completely once the drug was withdrawn, only one recovered rapidly without immunosuppressive therapy, [125] and there are no reports in the literature of the results of tests for red cell autoantibodies in asymptomatic patients taking these drugs.

Jones et al. [58] reported that the antibody detected in the red cell eluate of their patient with procainamide-induced hemolytic anemia reacted by indirect antiglobulin test with all red cells tested including U negative and LW negative cells. Pretreatment of the red cells with procainamide or addition of the drug to the test system was not necessary in order to obtain a positive reaction. The authors cite several similar but less well documented cases.

Methysergide has been implicated in the development of an apparent AIHA in association with retroperitoneal fibrosis, mitral regurgitation, and edema. [124] The patient developed anemia with a hemoglobin of 6.8 to 9.0 gm/dl, a reticulocyte count of 15 percent, and a positive direct antiglobulin test. However, the case was also complicated by the development of renal insufficiency caused by ureteral obstruction secondary to retroperitoneal fibrosis. No red cell autoantibodies were demonstrated in the serum or eluate. After cessation of the drug, relief of ureteral obstruction and a course of corticosteroid therapy, the hemolytic anemia resolved. The patient was not challenged with the medication.

Two patients have been described with apparent AIHA and hepatitis associated with chlorpromazine treatment, in whom the autoantibodies disappeared quickly once the drug was withdrawn. [153]

METHODS OF DIAGNOSIS

History

A detailed history of drug ingestion should be obtained from any patient who has an acquired hemolytic anemia, or in whom the cause of a positive direct antiglobulin test is being sought. It is surprising how often patients attempt to make judgments concerning which drugs need to be mentioned. On initial questioning, patients frequently omit mention of medications that may be purchased without prescription such as analgesics [5] or medications that they do not take regularly. In contrast, other patients seem to feel that any medication that they have been taking for a number of months must be benign, e.g., antihypertensive drugs. Another problem concerns patients' lack of knowledge of trade names or the contents of combination drugs. For example, a patient may deny taking Aldomet and will not volunteer the fact that he is taking Aldoril or Aldoclor (all of which contain methyldopa). Similarly, acute hemolytic anemia has been reported in a patient known to be sensitive to phenacetin, but who took a proprietary medication, not realizing that it contained phenacetin. [88] Finally there are reports of positive direct antiglobulin tests caused by methadone, [119] and patients may be reluctant to admit to taking this drug.

Laboratory Tests

Methyldopa, L-Dopa, and Mefenamic Acid. Methyldopa, L-dopa and mefenamic acid all cause immune hemolytic anemia that is indistinguishable from idiopathic warm antibody AIHA. In a patient who has been taking one of these drugs in any dose for a period of at least three months, the documentation of the presence of warm antibody AIHA as described in Chapter 6 is all that can be done to make a presumptive diagnosis. Cessation of the drug with resolution of all immunohematologic abnormalities will tend to confirm the etiologic role of the drug.

Although there are no diagnostic laboratory features of AIHA caused by methyldopa, certain findings are particularly characteristic, and many patients with idiopathic warm antibody AIHA have laboratory findings that are inconsistent with a diagnosis of methyldopa-induced AIHA. (We have had less experience with L-dopa-induced immune hemolytic anemia, and no experience with mefenamic acid-induced hemolysis, so we do not know whether the following findings are applicable, other than in regard to methyldopa.)

One of the characteristic features of methyldopa-induced AIHA is a strongly positive direct antiglobulin test caused by IgG red cell sensitization. As indicated elsewhere (Chapter 6), when we used titrations of our anti-IgG antiglobulin serum, the direct antiglobulin test titer was 1,000 or greater in 100 percent of the patients and 2,000 or greater in 90 percent of the patients. Positive direct antiglobulin tests using anti-C3 antiglobulin serum occur in only a small minority of patients (17 percent), and these tests are uniformly only weakly positive. Red cells very strongly sensitized with IgG and negative or only weakly sensitized with C3 also occur in a minority of patients with idiopathic warm antibody AIHA, so such findings cannot be considered specific for Aldomet-induced hemolytic anemia. Nevertheless, it is possible to exclude the diagnosis of methyldopa-induced hemolytic anemia if the patient's red cells are negative in the antiglobulin test using anti-IgG, or are only weakly sensitized with IgG.

As indicated in Table 8-5, a positive indirect antiglobulin test has been an invariable finding in our series of 29 patients with methyldopa-induced AIHA. Dacie and Worlledge [18] reported similar findings. Therefore, the presence of a negative indirect antiglobulin test in a patient with warm antibody AIHA (which occurred in 43 percent of our patients with warm antibody AIHA not associated with methyldopa administration), essentially excludes the diagnosis of methyldopa-induced hemolytic anemia.

It is of interest that patients who have a moderately strongly positive direct antiglobulin test caused by methyldopa ingestion but who do not have evidence of hemolysis may nevertheless have a positive indirect antiglobulin test. Dacie and Worlledge [18] reported 18 patients who had 2+ to 4+ direct antiglobulin tests caused by methyldopa but who did not have hemolytic anemia; 11 of these patients had a positive indirect antiglobulin test.

As is also indicated in Table 8-5, none of the serum antibodies in our patients with methyldopa-induced hemolytic anemia caused lysis of enzyme-

Table 8-5. SERUM SCREENING TESTS IN 29 PATIENTS WITH METHYLDOPA-INDUCED WARM ANTIBODY AIHA

	Serum (% Positive Reactions)	Acidified Serum and Acidified Complement (% Positive Reactions)
20°C Untreated RBC		
Lysis	0	0
Agglutination	3.5	3.5
20°C Enzyme-Treated		
Lysis		
Agglutination		
37°C Untreated RBC		
Lysis	0	0
Agglutination	0	0
Indirect anti-globulin test	100	100
37°C Enzyme-Treated		
Lysis	0	0
Agglutination	100	100

treated red cells, even in acidified serum. This finding is in contrast to those in warm antibody AIHA not associated with methyldopa administration, in which serum autoantibody caused lysis of enzyme-treated cells at 37°C in 8.6 percent of cases without acidification of the serum and in 12.7 percent of cases using acidified serum (see Table 6-14, page 209).

An additional finding of interest reported by Lalezari is that methyldopa-induced hemolytic anemias can be distinguished from other acquired immune hemolytic anemias using the autoanalyzer (see Chapter 5, page 178).

Penicillins. All the patients that we have observed with penicillin-induced immune hemolytic anemia have strongly positive direct antiglobulin tests caused by red cell sensitization with IgG. The red cells of 4 of our 10 patients were also sensitized with C3, usually weakly (Table 6-4). However, more important than the direct antiglobulin test for diagnostic purposes is the demonstration of penicillin antibodies in the serum and eluate. Using the indirect antiglobulin test with penicillin-coated red cells made as described in the following paragraphs, we find that the titer of penicillin antibody in the serum is usually 1,000 or more. In addition, an eluate prepared from the patient's red cells is reactive against penicillin-coated red cells, but it gives negative reactions when tested against normal red cells. In the appropriate clinical settings, these findings are diagnostic of penicillin-induced immune hemolytic anemia.

A summary of typical serologic findings in patients with penicillin-induced immune hemolytic anemia is given in Table 8-6.

Table 8-6. LABORATORY RESULTS IN A TYPICAL PATIENT WITH PENICILLIN-INDUCED IMMUNE HEMOLYTIC ANEMIA

Direct Antiglobulin Test

Dilutions of Antiglobulin Serum:	64	128	256	512	1024	2048	4096
Anti-IgG	4+	3+	3+	2+	2+	1+	0

Dilutions of Antiglobulin Serum:	4	8	16	32	64	128	256
Anti-C3	0	0	0	0	0	0	0

Serum and eluate screening tests vs. normal and enzyme-treated red cells:

Direct agglutination	Negative
Indirect antiglobulin test	Negative
Lysis	Negative

Tests vs. penicillin-treated RBC:

Indirect antiglobulin test using patient's serum

Serum dilutions	64	128	256	512	1024	2048
Anti-IgG		4+	3+	2+	2+	1+	0

Reaction of undiluted eluate by indirect antiglobulin test: 4+

Direct agglutination using patient's serum:

Serum dilutions	4	8	16	32	64	128
	2+	1+	0	0	0	0

Test for lysis of penicillin-sensitized red cells by serum: negative

Agglutination reactions are graded as 1+ to 4+.

Preparation of Penicillin-Sensitized Red Cells

Penicillin-sensitized red cells may be made as described by Spath, Garratty, and Petz [127] as follows:

(a) Wash group O cells (preferably fresh) three times in saline.

(b) Add 10^6 units (approximately 600 mg) of potassium benzylpenicillin G dissolved in 15 ml of pH 9.6 barbital buffer to 1 ml of packed washed cells. In the original publication, T.M.A. buffer was used, but this has rather an obnoxious smell; barbital buffer (pH 9.6) has been found to be satisfactory for routine use. Sodium barbital, 0.1 M (20.6 g/liter), is adjusted to pH 9.6 with 0.1 N HCl (approximately 15 ml).

(c) Incubate for one hour at room temperature with gentle mixing.

(d) Wash cells three times in saline.

Slight lysis may occur during incubation, and a small "clot" may form in the red cells that can be removed with applicator sticks before washing cells. Once prepared, the cells may be kept in ACD at 4°C for up to one week, but they do deteriorate slowly during this time.

Cephalosporins. Only a few cases of cephalosporin-induced immune hemolytic anemia have been described.[36, 49, 57, 60] The direct antiglobulin test was positive, and cephalosporin antibody was demonstrable in the serum and eluate by indirect antiglobulin test against cephalosporin-sensitized red cells in cases caused by Cephalothin administration.[49, 57] A patient with hemolytic anemia associated with Cephaloridine administration had a positive antiglobulin test, but no tests for drug-related antibodies were performed.[60] The patient also had acute renal insufficiency, and the cause of the hemolytic anemia was considered uncertain. No serologic abnormalities were detected in one patient with acute intravascular hemolysis associated with Cephalexin administration except for a positive "2 stage" antiglobulin test.[36]

In performing the indirect antiglobulin test against cephalosporin-coated erythrocytes, one must remember that, because of nonspecific protein absorption, normal sera may give a positive reaction. However, the indirect antiglobulin test becomes negative at a serum dilution of about 1:20 unless an antibody is present. If a patient has a positive direct antiglobulin test that is clinically benign and is caused by nonspecific protein absorption, the serum does not contain a high titer cephalosporin antibody, and an eluate from the patient's red cells gives negative reactions (see Table 8-4).

Preparation of Cephalosporin-Coated Red Cells

Cephalosporin coated cells to be used in these tests may be made as described by Spath, Garratty and Petz as follows: [127]
  (a) Wash group O cells (preferably fresh) three times in saline.
  (b) Add 400 mg of Keflin dissolved in 10 ml of pH 9.6 barbital buffered saline (1 part barbital buffer and 9 parts saline) to 1 ml of washed packed cells.
  (c) Incubate at 37°C for 2 hours with gentle mixing.
  (d) Wash cells three times in saline.

Other Drugs. In a patient with immune hemolytic anemia whose serum and red cell eluate does not react with normal red cells, and who is receiving a drug other than those already described, antibodies reactive with red cells in the presence of the drug should be sought. The methods used vary widely, and for drugs in Table 8-1 the original method should be utilized.

In addition, the following should be done in instances in which the originally described method gives negative results or for a drug not previously shown to cause hemolytic anemia.

A trial and error approach is recommended. The patient's serum and eluate should be tested against normal untreated and enzyme-treated red cells in the presence of the drug that the patient is receiving. An approximate 1 mg/ml or a saturated solution of the drug should be made in buffered saline. If this causes lysis of normal red cells, dilutions should be made until the solution no longer causes lysis. An equal volume of this solution is added to the patient's serum, and an equal volume of buffered saline is added to another aliquot of serum as a control. The mixtures are usually incubated at 37°C for 1 to 2 hours, but one should consider extending these incubation times if negative results are obtained. A duplicate set of tubes with the addition of fresh normal serum (i.e., complement) is also recommended. The tubes are then inspected for agglutination, hemolysis, and sensitization to antiglobulin sera. If negative reactions are obtained, an attempt should be made to pretreat the red cells with the drug by incubating red cells with an isotonic solution of the drug.

COMPATIBILITY TESTING IN PATIENTS WITH DRUG-INDUCED IMMUNOHEMATOLOGIC ABNORMALITIES

Hemolytic Anemias Caused by Immune Complex Mechanism or Drug Absorption Mechanism

The major compatibility test will be compatible (unless coincidental red cell alloantibodies are present) in all instances of drug-induced immune hemolytic anemias in which the hemolysis is mediated by the immune complex mechanism or the drug absorption mechanism. This is true since the drug is necessary in the *in vitro* test system in order to demonstrate the drug-related antibody (Table 8-2). However, the transfused red cells may not survive normally if drug administration is continued, or if the serum level of drug or drug-related immune complexes remains high.

Autoimmune Hemolytic Anemia Caused by Drugs

As previously mentioned, we have found that, in patients who have autoimmune hemolytic anemia caused by methyldopa, the indirect antiglobulin test is invariably positive. In these cases, compatibility testing is similar to that described for warm antibody AIHA (see Chapter 10). Although no data are available, it is probable that donor red cells will survive as well as the patient's own red cells.

Other patients receiving methyldopa may have a positive direct antiglobulin test but no evidence of hemolysis. In many of these patients, the indirect antiglobulin test is negative, so that the major compatibility test is compatible and donor blood can be expected to survive normally.

Still other patients receiving methyldopa have a positive direct antiglobulin test and positive indirect antiglobulin test caused by autoantibody, but have no evidence of hemolytic anemia or of compensated hemolysis.[18] In performing the compatibility test, one must search for alloantibodies that may be present as described in Chapter 10. However, even if alloantibodies do not appear to be present, all compatibility tests will be incompatible, and the question then arises as to whether the autoantibody will cause shortened survival in donor red cells, even though not causing shortened survival of the patient's own red cells. Silvergleid et al. [118] studied the survival of radiolabelled donor cells in two such patients and demonstrated acceptable survival after one hour in each patient. Subsequent experience of our own and in association with Drs. Howard and Grumet at Stanford University indicates that, in such circumstances, donor units appear to survive normally, and clinical evidence of transfusion reactions does not result. That is, in 21 transfusion episodes in 19 patients who were receiving methyldopa and who had positive direct and indirect antiglobulin tests caused by autoantibody but who did not have hemolytic anemia, there were no clinical manifestations of transfusion reactions, and adequate post-transfusion increments in the hemoglobin and hematocrit resulted in each case. Although this point merits further study, it presently appears that methyldopa-induced red cell autoantibody does not cause hemolytic transfusion reactions if the patient's own red cell survival is normal.

Although no data are available concerning compatibility testing and blood transfusion in patients with drug-induced positive antiglobulin tests and autoimmune hemolytic anemia caused by drugs other than methyldopa, e.g., L-dopa and mefenamic acid, one might assume that similar principles would apply.

MANAGEMENT AND PROGNOSIS

The most common drug-induced immune hemolytic anemia is caused by methyldopa. The onset of hemolysis has been diagnosed as early as 18 weeks and as late as 4 years after the start of therapy. [152] Direct antiglobulin tests or hemoglobin or hematocrit measurements at intervals of three to four months during the first year, and semi-annually or with the development of any symptoms attributable to anemia thereafter, would seem an adequate safeguard against severe anemia since hemolysis appears to be gradual in onset.

Although other antihypertensive agents should be substituted for methyldopa in any patient with hemolytic anemia, many patients taking the drug have a positive direct antiglobulin test without hemolysis, and in this situation the drug need not be discontinued. Patients who have both a positive direct and indirect antiglobulin test but who do not have hemolytic anemia constitute a group in which continued administration of the drug may be considered optional. Our recommendation would be to discontinue the drug in this circumstance if at all possible, because the positive indirect antiglobulin test interferes with compatibility testing. Even though the autoantibody appears not to cause shortened red cell survival of donor blood if signs of hemolysis are lacking in the patient (see above), nevertheless the autoantibody may obscure the presence of alloantibody in the compatibility test, thus adding an element of risk to any required transfusion.

Corticosteroids are usually not necessary during recovery from hemolytic anemia, and their efficacy is difficult to evaluate. Nevertheless, they may be indicated for short periods of time in patients with severe anemia. Transfusion is rarely necessary, and it will be impossible to find compatible blood. In spite of *in vitro* incompatibility, transfused red cells can be expected to provide temporary benefit, and they are indicated in the face of life-threatening hemolysis. The usual indications and precautions regarding compatibility testing and transfusion in the presence of red cell autoantibodies should be kept in mind (Chapter 10).

Although rare, penicillin-induced hemolytic anemia is probably second in incidence only to that caused by methyldopa among drug-induced immune hemolytic anemias. The clinical setting is most often a life-threatening infection (especially bacterial endocarditis) in which penicillin may have distinct advantages over alternative drugs. Thus, penicillin should be discontinued only in the presence of overt hemolytic anemia; it should not be stopped merely because of the development of a positive direct antiglobulin test, since clinically significant hemolysis may not develop even in the presence of continued penicillin administration. When hemolytic anemia does occur, it usually develops over a period of weeks and may develop even in the presence of corticosteroid administration.[107] If transfusion is necessary, the major crossmatch test will be compatible, since the patient's serum antibody will not react with red cells unless they have been coated with the antibiotic. In the continued presence of the drug *in vivo*, however, transfused cells will show decreased survival, although there are no reports of acute hemolytic transfusion reactions. The substitution of a different penicillin is not likely to be of benefit because of immunologic cross-reactivity.

Since hemolytic anemia associated with cephalothin is rare, and positive direct antiglobulin tests occur in only a small percentage of patients, these immunohematologic abnormalities should not be considered an important disadvantage in the use of cephalosporins.[105, 106] Principles of management are the same as in hemolytic anemias caused by penicillins.

Other drugs cause drug immune hemolysis very rarely. However, since such cases are often characterized by the abrupt onset of severe hemolysis, an immediate cessation of the offending drug is essential. Corticosteroids and transfusions may be necessary, and adequate renal blood flow should be maintained in an effort to prevent acute renal failure.

The prognosis in patients with drug-induced hemolytic anemias is generally excellent. However, life-threatening hemolysis, hemoglobinuria, renal failure, and death have all been reported,[153] particularly in drug-induced syndromes caused by the immune complex mechanism. Such indications of acute intravascular hemolysis have been reported in patients exposed to Stibophen, para-aminosalicytic acid, quinine, phenacetin, insecticides, antistin, sulphonamides, isonicotinic acid, chlorpromazine, pyramidone, dypyrone, sulphonylurea derivatives, and rifampicin.[153]

Penicillin-induced hemolytic anemia is often not severe, but in one patient that we described, massive intravascular hemolysis did occur.[110] The patient refused blood transfusion because of religious beliefs, and the hematocrit level reached a low of 9 percent (Figure 8-5), at which time her sensorium was clouded and her respirations labored. The following day her hematocrit level had reached 12 percent, and complete recovery subsequently ensued.

Although we have no personal experience with fatalities associated with the administration of methyldopa, the hemolytic anemia may be quite severe, and mortality has been reported. Indeed, 14 deaths caused by methyldopa-induced hemolytic anemia were reported to the WHO Research Center for International Monitoring of Adverse Reactions to Drugs between 1968 and 1973.[23]

REFERENCES

1. Abraham, G. N., Petz, L. D., and Fudenberg, H. H.: Cephalothin hypersensitivity associated with anti-cephalothin antibodies. Int. Arch. Allergy, *34:*65, 1968
2. Abraham, G. N., Petz, L. D., and Fudenberg, H. H.: Immunohaematological cross-allergenicity between penicillin and cephalothin in humans. Clin. Exp. Immunol., *3:*343, 1968.
3. Ackroyd, J. F.: The pathogenesis of thrombocytopenic purpura due to hypersensitivity to Sedormid (allylisopropyl-acetylcarbamide). Clin. Sci., *7:*249, 1949.
4. Allison, A. C., Denman, A. M., and Barnes, R. D.: Cooperating and controlling functions of thymus-derived lymphocytes in relation to autoimmunity. Lancet, *i:*135, 1971.
5. Azen, E. A., Bryan, G. T., Shahidi, N. T., Rossi, E. C., and Clatanoff, D. V.: Obscure hemolytic anemia due to analgesic abuse. Amer. J. Med., *48:*724, 1970.
6. Bakemeier, R. F., and Leddy, J. P.: Erythrocyte autoantibody associated with alpha-methyldopa: Heterogeneity of structure and specificity. Blood, *32:*1, 1968.
7. Ballas, S. K., Caro, J. F., and Miguel, O.: Quinidine-induced hemolytic anemia: Immunohematologic characterization. Transfusion, *18:*215, 1978.
8. Bell, C. A., Zwicker, H., Lee, S., and Alpern, H.: Quinidine hemolytic anemia in the absence of thrombocytopenia in a patient with hemoglobin D. Transfusion, *13:*100, 1973.
9. Bengtsson, U., Ahlstedt, S., Aurell, M., and Kaijser, B.: Antazoline-induced immune hemolytic anemia, hemoglobinuria and acute renal failure. Acta Med. Scand., *198:*223, 1975.
10. Bernasconi, C., Bedarida, G., Pollini, G., and Sartori, S.: Studio dei meccanismo di emolisi in un caso di anemia emolitica acquista da piramidone. Haematologica (Pavia), *46:*697, 1961.
11. Bird, G. W. G., Eeles, G. H., Litchfield, J. A., Rahman, M., and Wingham, J.: Haemolytic anaemia with antibodies to tolbutamide and phenacetin. Brit. Med. J., *1:*728, 1972.
12. Blajchman, M. A., Lowry, R. C., Pettit, J. E., et al.: Rifampicin-induced immune thrombocytopenia. Brit. Med. J., *3:*24, 1970.
13. Bolton, F. G.: Thrombocytopenic purpura due to quinidine. II. Serologic mechanisms. Blood, *11:*547, 1956.
14. Breckenridge, A., Dollery, C. T., Worlledge, S. M., Holborrow, E. J., and Johnson, G. D.: Positive direct Coombs tests and antinuclear factor in patients treated with methyldopa. Lancet, *ii:*1265, 1967.
15. Carstairs, K. C., Breckenridge, A., Collery, C. T., and Worlledge, S. M.: Incidence of a positive direct Coombs' test in patients on α-methyldopa. Lancet, *2:*133, 1966.

16. Carstairs, K. C., Worlledge, S., Dollery, C. T., and Breckenridge, A.: Methyldopa and haemolytic anaemia. Lancet, *1:*201, 1966.

17. Croft, J. D., Swisher, S. N., Gilliland, B. C., et al.: Coombs'-test positivity induced by drugs. Mechanisms of immunologic reactions and red cell destruction. Ann. Intern. Med., *68:*176, 1968.

18. Dacie, J. V., and Worlledge, S. M.: Auto-immune hemolytic anemias. Progr. Hematol., *6:*82, 1969.

19. Dameshek, W.: Autoimmunity: Theoretical aspects. Ann. N.Y. Acad. Sci., *124:*6, 1965.

20. Dameshek, W.: Correspondence. Alpha-methyldopa red cell antibody: Cross reaction or forbidden clones? N. Engl. J. Med., *276:*1382, 1967.

21. Dausset, J., and Barge, A.: Anaemia, leucopenia, and thrombocytopenia due to drug allergy: The importance of cross-reactions. *In* Wolstenholm, G., and Porter, R., Eds. Drug Responses in Man. London, J. & A. Churchill, 1967, 91.

22. Dausset, J., and Contu, L.: A case of haemolytic anaemia due to phenacetin allergy. Vox. Sang., *9:*599, 1964.

23. de Gruchy, G. C.: Drug-Induced Blood Disorders. Oxford, Blackwell Scientific Publications, 1975.

24. De Torregrosa, M. V. V., Rosada Rodriguez, A. L., and Montilla, E.: Hemolytic anemia secondary to stibophen therapy. J.A.M.A, *186:*598, 1963.

25. De Weck, A. L.: Studies on penicillin hypersensitivity. I. The specificity of rabbit "anti-penicillin" antibodies. Int. Arch. Allergy Appl. Immunol., *21:*20, 1962.

26. De Weck, A. L.: Newer developments in penicillin immuno-chemistry. Int. Arch. Allergy Appl. Immunol., *22:*245, 1963.

27. Poole, G., Stradling, P., and Worlledge, S.: Potentially serious side effects of high-dose twice-weekly rifampicin. Brit. Med. J., *3:*343, 1971.

28. Eisen, H. N., Belman, S., and Carsten, M. E.: The reaction of 2, 4-dinitrobenzenesulfonic acid with free amino groups of proteins. J. Am. Chem. Soc., *75:*4583, 1953.

29. Eisen, H. N., Kern, M., Newton, W. T., and Helmreich, E.: A study of the distribution of 2, 4-dinitrobenzene sensitizers between isolated lymph node cells and extracellular medium in relation to induction of contact skin sensitivity. J. Exp. Med., *110:*187, 1959.

30. Eisner, E. V., and Korbitz, B. C.: Quinine-induced thrombocytopenic purpura due to an IgM and an IgG antibody. Transfusion, *12:*317, 1972.

31. Ewing, D. J., Hughes, C. J., and Wardle, D. F.: Methyldopa-induced autoimmune haemolytic anaemia—a report of two further cases. Guy's Hosp. Rep., *117:*111, 1968.

32. Eyster, M. E.: Melphalan (Alkeran) erythrocyte agglutinin and hemolytic anemia. Ann. Intern. Med., *66:*573, 1967.

33. Farid, N. R., Johnson, R. J., and Low, W. T.: Haemolytic reaction to mefenamic acid. Lancet, *2:*382, 1971.

34. Fass, R., Perkins, R., and Saslow, S.: Positive direct Coombs' tests associated with cephaloridine therapy. J.A.M.A., *213:*121, 1970.

35. Faulk, W. P., Tomsovic, E. J., and Fudenberg, H. H.: Insulin resistance in juvenile diabetes mellitus. Immunologic studies. Amer. J. Med., *49:*133, 1970.

36. Forbes, C. D., Craig, J. A., Mitchell, R., and McNicol, G. P.: Acute intravascular hemolysis associated with cephalexin therapy. Postgrad. Med. J., *48:*186, 1972.

37. Freedman, A. L., Barr, P. S., and Brody, E. A.: Hemolytic anemia due to quinidine: Observations on its mechanism. Amer. J. Med., *20:*806, 1956.

38. Freedman, A. L., Brody, E. A., and Barr, P. S.: Immunothrombocytopenic purpura due to quinidine. Report of four new cases with special observations on patch testing. J. Lab. Clin. Med., *48:*205, 1956.

39. Freedman, J., and Lim, F. C.: An immunohematologic complication of isoniazid. Vox. Sang., *35:*126, 1978.

40. Fudenberg, H. H.: Are autoimmune diseases and malignancy due to selective

T-cell deficiencies. *In* Critical Factors in Cancer Immunology. New York, Academic Press, Inc., 1975, 179.

41. Fukase, M., Nakano, H., Konda, S., Tajima, H., Takeuchi, S., Tsunematsu, T., Nishida, R., Kanagawa, K., Sugano, A., Watanabe, K., Suzuka, H., and Inagaki, M.: Two cases of drug-allergy followed by acquired autoimmune hemolytic anemia. Acta Haematol. Jap., *23:*70, 1960.

42. Funicella, T., Weinger, R. S., Moake, J. L., Spruell, M., and Rossen, R. D.: Penicillin-induced immunohemolytic anemia associated with circulating immune complexes. Amer. J. Hematol., *3:*219, 1977.

43. Gabor, E. P., and Goldberg, L. S.: Levodopa induced Coombs positive haemolytic anaemia. Scand. J. Haemat., *11:*201, 1973.

44. Garratty, G., and Petz, L. D.: An evaluation of commercial antiglobulin sera with particular reference to their anticomplement properties. Transfusion, *11:*79, 1971.

45. Garratty, G., and Petz, L. D.: Drug-induced immune hemolytic anemia. Amer. J. Med., *58:*398, 1975.

45a. Garratty, G., Petz, L. D., Houston, M., Love, J. C., and Webb, M.: Acute hemolytic anemia associated with antibodies to hydrocholorthiazide (Hydrodiuril). Transfusion, *16:*528, 1976.

46. Gell, P. G. H., and Benacerraf, B.: Studies on hypersensitivity. IV. The relationship between contact and delayed sensitivity: A study on the specificity of cellular immune reactions. J. Exp. Med., *113:*571, 1961.

47. Gottlieb, A. J., and Wurzel, H. A.: Protein-quinone interaction: In vivo induction of indirect antiglobulin reactions with methyldopa. Blood, *43:*85, 1974.

48. Gralnick, H. R., and McGinniss, M. H.: Immune cross-reactivity of penicillin and cephalothin. Nature, *215:*1026, 1967.

49. Gralnick, H. R., McGinniss, M. H., Elton, W., and McCurdy, P.: Hemolytic anemia associated with cephalothin. J.A.M.A., *217:*1193, 1971.

50. Gralnick, H. R., Wright, L. D., and McGinniss, M. H.: Coombs' positive reactions associated with sodium cephalothin therapy. J.A.M.A., *199:*725, 1967.

51. Hadnagy, C.: Coombs-positive haemolytic anaemia provoked by chlorpromazine. Lancet, *I:*423, 1976.

52. Harris, J. W.: Studies on the mechanism of a drug-induced hemolytic anemia. J. Lab. Clin. Med., *44:*809, 1954.

53. Harris, J. W.: Studies on the mechanism of a drug-induced hemolytic anemia. J. Lab. Clin. Med., *47:*760, 1956.

54. Henry, R. E., Goldberg, L. S., Sturgeon, F., and Ansel, R. D.: Serologic abnormalities associated with L-dopa therapy. Vox. Sang., *20:*306, 1971.

55. Homberg, J. C., Pujet, J. C., and Salmon, C.: A study of rifampicin antigenic site. Scand. J. Resp. Dis., *84:*36, 1973.

56. Jandl, J. H., and LoBuglio, A. F.: Alpha-methyldopa red-cell antibody crossreaction or forbidden clones? (Correspondence). N. Engl. J. Med., *276:*1382, 1967.

57. Jeannet, M., Block, A., Dayer, J. M., Farquet, J. J., Girard, J. P., and Cruchaud, A.: Cephalothin-induced immune hemolytic anemia. Acta Haematol., *55:*109, 1976.

58. Jones, G. W., George, T. L., and Bradley, R. D.: Procainamide-induced hemolytic anemia. Transfusion, *18:*224, 1978.

59. Joseph, C.: Occurrence of positive Coombs' test in patients treated with levodopa. N. Engl. J. Med., *286:*140, 1972.

60. Kaplan, K., Reisberg, B., and Weinstein, L.: Cephaloridine—studies of therapeutic activity and untoward effects. Arch. Intern. Med., *121:*17, 1968.

61. Kerr, R. O., Cardamone, J., Dalmasso, A. P., et al.: Two mechanisms of erythrocyte destruction in penicillin-induced hemolytic anemia. N. Engl. J. Med., *287:*1322, 1972.

62. Kirtland, H. H., and Mohler, D. N.: Chronic stimulation of lymphocyte cyclic

amp: A proposed etiology for methyldopa-induced autoimmunity. Blood, *50:*295, 1977.

63. Kirtland, H. H., Horwitz, D. A., and Mohler, D. N.: Inhibition of suppressor T cell function by methyldopa: A proposed cause of autoimmune hemolytic anemia. Blood, *52:*151, 1978.

64. Kissmeyer-Nielsen, F.: Thrombocytopenic purpura following quinine medication. Immunological study. Acta Med. Scand., *154:*289, 1956.

65. Kleinknecht, D., Deloux, J., and Homberg, J. C.: Acute renal failure after intravenous urography: Detection of antibodies against contrast media. Clinical Nephrology, *2:*116, 1974.

66. Korsager, S.: Haemolysis complicating ibuprofen treatment. Brit. Med. J., *1:*79, 1978.

67. Kosakai, N., and Miyakawa, G.: Fundamental studies on the positive Coombs' tests due to cephalosporins. Postgrad. Med. J., *46:*107, 1970.

68. Krüger, J., Rahman, A., Mogk, K. U., and Mueller-Eckhardt, C.: T cell deficiency in patients with autoimmune hemolytic anemia ('warm type'). Vox. Sang., *31:*1, 1976.

69. Kuwahara, S., Mine, Y., and Nishida, M.: Immunogenicity of Cefazolin. Antimicrob. Agents Chemother., *10:*374, 1970.

70. Lakshminarayan, S., Sahn, S. A., and Hudson, L. D.: Massive haemolysis caused by rifampicin. Br. Med., J., *2:*282, 1973.

71. Landsteiner, K.: The Specificity of Serologic Reactions. Cambridge, Harvard University Press, 1947.

72. Landsteiner, K., and Jacobs, J.: Studies on the sensitization of animals with simple chemical compounds. J. Exp. Med., *64:*625, 1936.

73. Landsteiner, K., and Van Der Scheer, J.: On cross reactions of immune sera to azoproteins. J. Exp. Med., *63:*325, 1936.

74. Lay, W. H.: Drug-induced haemolytic reaction due to antibodies against the erythrocyte/dipyrone complex. Vox. Sang., *11:*601, 1966.

75. Leddy, J. P., and Swisher, S. N.: Acquired immune hemolytic disorders (including drug-induced immune hemolytic anemia). *In* Immunological Diseases. 3rd Ed. Samter, M., Ed. Boston, Little, Brown, 1978, Vol. 1, 1187.

76. Levine, B. B.: Induction of immune response and the role of antibody specificity in drug hypersensitivity-type hemolytic anemias and thrombocytopenias. Seminars Hematol., *2:*338, 1965.

77. Levine, B. B., and Ovary, Z.: Studies on the mechanism of the formation of the penicillin antigen. III. The N- (D-alpha-benzylpenicilloyl) group as an antigenic determinant responsible for hypersensitivity to penicillin G. J. Exp. Med., *114:*875, 1961.

78. Levine, B. B., and Price, V. H.: Studies on the immunological mechanisms of penicillin allergy. II. Antigenic specificities of allergic wheal-and-flare skin responses in patients with histories of penicillin allergy. Immunology, *7:*542, 1964.

79. Levine, B. B., and Redmond, A.: Immunochemical mechanisms of penicillin induced Coombs positivity and hemolytic anemia in man. Int. Arch. Allergy Appl. Immunol., *31:*594, 1967.

80. Levine, B. B., and Redmond, A. P.: Minor haptenic determinant-specific reagents of penicillin hypersensitivity in man. Int. Arch. Allergy Appl. Immunol., *35:*445, 1969.

81. Ley, A. B., Cahan, A., and Mayer, K.: Circulating antibody directed against penicillin. Bibl. Haemat., *10:*539, 1959.

82. Ley, A. B., Harris, J. P., Brinkley, M., Liles, B., Jack, J. A., and Cahan, A.: Circulating antibodies directed against penicillin. Science, *127:*1118, 1958.

83. Lindberg, L. G., and Norden, A.: Severe hemolytic reaction to chlorpromazine. Acta Med. Scand., *170:*195, 1961.

84. Lindström, F. D., Lieden, G., and Engström, M. S.: Dose-related levodopa-induced haemolytic anaemia. Ann. Intern. Med., *86:*298, 1977.

85. LoBuglio, A. F., and Jandl, J. H.: The nature of the alpha-methyl-dopa red-cell antibody. N. Engl. J. Med., *276:*658, 1967.
86. LoBuglio, A. F., Masouredis, S. P., Pisciotta, A. V., et al.: Characteristics of red cell autoantibodies induced by L-dopa. Clin. Res., *17:*333, 1969.
87. Logue, G. L., Boyd, A. E., and Rosse, W. F.: Chlorpropamide-induced immune hemolytic anemia. N. Engl. J. Med., *283:*900, 1970.
88. MacGibbon, B. H., Loughridge, L. W., Hourihane, D. B., and Boyd, D. W.: Autoimmune haemolytic anaemia with acute renal failure due to phenacetin and p-aminosalicylic acid. Lancet, *1:*7, 1960.
89. Malassenet, R., Dreyfus, B., and Antoine, B.: Anemia hemolytique immunologique due a l'antistine. Proceedings of the 7th Congress International Society of Haematology, Rome, 1958. New York, Grune & Stratton, 1960, Vol. 2, 614.
90. Manor, E., Marmor, A., Kaufman, S., and Leiba, H.: Massive hemolysis caused by acetaminophen. J.A.M.A., *236:*2777, 1976.
91. Martinez, L., Letona, J., Barbolla, L., Frieyro, E., Bouza, E., Gilsanz, F., and Fernandez, M. N.: Immune haemolytic anaemia and renal failure induced by streptomycin. Brit. J. Haemat., *35:*561, 1977.
92. McVie, J. G.: Drug induced thrombocytopenia. *In* Blood Disorders Due to Drugs and Other Agents. Girdwood, R. H., Ed. Amsterdam, Excerpta Medica, 1973, 187.
93. Miescher, P. A., and Gorstein, F.: Mechanisms of immunogenic platelet damage. *In* Blood Platelets. Johnson, S. A., Monto, R. W., Rebuck, J. W., and Horn, R. C., Eds. London, J. & A. Churchill, 1961, 671.
94. Mine, Y., and Nishida, M.: Studies on direct Coombs reaction by cefazolin in vitro. J. Antibiot., *23:*575, 1970.
95. Molthan, L., Reidenberg, M. M., and Eichman, M. F.: Positive direct Coombs' tests due to cephalothin. N. Engl. J. Med., *277:*123, 1967.
96. Mueller-Eckhardt, C., Kretschmer, V., and Coburg, K. H.: Allergic, immunohemolytic anemia due to para-aminosalicylic acid (PAS). Immunohematologic studies of three cases. Dtsch. Med. Wochenschr., *97:*234, 1972.
97. Muirhead, E. E., Groves, M., Guy, R., Halden, E. R., and Bass, R. K.: Acquired hemolytic anemia, exposures to insecticides and positive Coombs' test dependent on insecticide preparations. Vox. Sang., *4:*277, 1959.
98. Muirhead, E. E., Halden, E. R., and Groves, M.: Drug-dependent Coombs' (antiglobulin) test and anemia. Arch. Intern. Med., *101:*87, 1958.
99. Nesmith, L. W., and Davis, J. W.: Hemolytic anemia caused by penicillin. Report of a case in which antipenicillin antibodies cross-reacted with cephalothin sodium. J.A.M.A., *203:*27, 1968.
100. Okuma, M.: Studies on experimental immune thrombocytopenia. III. Serological studies of rabbits sensitized with platelet phosphatides mixed with foreign protein. Acta Haematol. Jap., *30:*354, 1967.
101. Orenstein, A. A., Yakulis, V., Eipe, J., and Costea, N.: Immune hemolysis due to hydralazine (letter). Ann. Intern. Med., *86:*450, 1977.
102. Parker, C. W., Shapiro, J., Kern, M., et al.: Hypersensitivity to penicillenic acid derivatives in human beings with penicillin allergy. J. Exp. Med., *115:*821, 1962.
103. Parker, A. C., Stuart, A. E., and Dewar, A. E.: Activated T-cells in autoimmune haemolytic anaemia. Brit. J. Haematol., *36:*337, 1977.
104. Parker, C. W., De Weck, A. L., Kern, M., et al.: The preparation and some properties of penicillenic acid derivatives relevant to penicillin hypersensitivity. J. Exp. Med., *115:*803, 1962.
105. Petz, L. D.: Immunologic reactions of humans to cephalosporins. Postgrad. Med. J., *47:* suppl., 64, 1971.
106. Petz, L. D.: Immunologic cross-reactivity between penicillins and cephalosporins: A review. J. Infect. Dis., *137:*S74, 1978.

107. Petz, L. D., and Fudenberg, H. H.: Coombs-positive hemolytic anemia caused by penicillin administration. N. Engl. J. Med., *274:* 171, 1966.
108. Petz, L. D., and Fudenberg, H. H.: Immunologic mechanisms in drug-induced cytopenias. *In* Progress in Hematology. Vol. IX. Brown, E. B., Ed. New York, Grune & Stratton, 1975, 185.
109. Petz, L. D., and Garratty, G.: Drug-induced haemolytic anaemia. Clinics in Haematology, *4:*181, 1975.
110. Ries, C. A., Rosenbaum, T. J., Garratty, G., Petz, L. D., and Fudenberg, H. H.: Penicillin-induced immune hemolytic anemia. J.A.M.A., *233:*432, 1975.
111. Robertson, J. H., Kennedy, C. C., and Hill, C. M.: Haemolytic anaemia associated with mefenamic acid. Ir. J. Med. Sci., *140:*226, 1971.
112. Robinson, M. G., and Foadi, M.: Hemolytic anemia with positive Coombs' test. Association with isoniazid therapy. J.A.M.A., *208:*656, 1969.
113. Schubothe, H., and Weber, S.: Rifampicin-dependent reactions against erythrocytes in the sera of patients receiving rifampicin therapy. Scand. J. Res. Dis., *84:*53, 1973.
114. Schwartz, R. S., and Costea, N.: Autoimmune hemolytic anemia: Clinical correlations and biological implications. Semin. Hemat., *3:*2, 1966.
115. Schwarz, S., Gabl, R., Huber, H., and Spath, P.: Positive direct antiglobulin (Coombs') test caused by cephalexin administration in humans. Vox. Sang., *29:*59, 1975.
116. Scott, G. L., Myles, A. B., and Bacon, P. A.: Autoimmune haemolytic anaemia and mefenamic acid therapy. Brit. Med. J., *3:*534, 1968.
117. Siegel, B. B., and Levine, B. B.: Antigenic specificities of skin-sensitizing antibodies in sera from patients with immediate systemic allergic reactions to penicillin. J. Allergy, *35:*488, 1964.
118. Silvergleid, A. J., Wells, R. P., Hafleigh, E. B., Korn, G., et al.: Compatibility test using ^{51}chromium-labeled red blood cells in crossmatch positive patients. Transfusion, *18:*8, 1978.
119. Sivamurthy, S., Frankfurt, E., and Levine, M. E.: Positive antiglobulin tests in patients maintained on methadone. Transfusion, *13:*418, 1973.
120. Shulman, N. R.: Immunoreactions involving platelets. IV. Studies on the pathogenesis of thrombocytopenia in drug purpura using test doses of quinidine in sensitized individuals; their implications in idiopathic thrombocytopenic purpura. J. Exp. Med., *107:*711, 1958.
121. Shulman, N. R., Marden, V. J., Aledort, L. M., and Hiller, M. C.: Complement-fixing isoantibodies against antigens common to platelets and leukocytes. Trans. Assoc. Am. Physicians, *75:*89, 1962.
122. Shulman, N. R.: Mechanism of blood cell destruction in individuals sensitized to foreign antigens. Trans. Assoc. Am. Physicians, *76:*72, 1963.
123. Shulman, N. R.: A mechanism of cell destruction in individuals sensitized to foreign antigens and its implications in autoimmunity. Combined clinical staff conference at the National Institutes of Health. Ann. Intern. Med., *60:*506, 1964.
124. Slugg, P. H., and Kunkel, R. S.: Complications of methysergide therapy. J.A.M.A., *213:*297, 1970.
125. Snapper, I., Marks, D., Schwartz, L., and Hollander, L.: Hemolytic anemia secondary to Mesantoin. Ann. Intern. Med., *39:*619, 1953.
126. Sors, C., Sarrazin, A., and Homberg, J. C.: Accidents hemolytiques recidivants d'origine immuno-allergique au cours d'un traitement intermittent par la rifampicine. Rev. Tuberc. (Paris), *36:*405, 1972.
127. Spath, P., Garratty, G., and Petz, L. D.: Studies on the immune response to penicillin and cephalothin in humans. I. Optimal conditions for titration of hemagglutinating penicillin and cephalothin antibodies. J. Immunol., *107:*854, 1971.
128. Spath, P., Garratty, G., and Petz, L. D.: Studies on the immune response to

penicillin and cephalothin in humans. II. Immunohematologic reactions to cephalothin administration. J. Immunol., *107:*860, 1971.

129. Stefanini, M., and Johnson, N. L.: Positive antihuman globulin test in patients receiving carbromal. Am. J. Med. Sci., *259:*49, 1970.
130. Steinkamp, R., Moore, C. V., and Doubek, W. G.: Thrombocytopenic purpura caused by hypersensitivity to quinine. J. Lab. Clin. Med., *45:*18, 1955.
131. Strumia, P. V., and Raymond, F. D.: Acquired hemolytic anemia and antipenicillin antibody: Case report and review of literature. Arch. Int. Med., *109:*603, 1962.
132. Swanson, M. A., Chanmougan, D., and Schwartz, R. S.: Immunohemolytic anemia due to antipenicillin antibodies. N. Engl. J. Med., *274:*178, 1966.
133. Swisher, S. N.: Antibiotics and red blood cells. *In* Drugs and Hematologic Reactions. Dimitrov, N. V., and Nodine, J. H., Eds. New York, Grune & Stratton, 1974, 123.
134. Tajima, H.: Clinical studies on hemolytic anemia. I. Autoimmune hemolytic anemia. Acta Haematol. Jap., *23:*188, 1960.
135. Takahashi, R., Tsukada, T., and Hasegawa, M.: Tetracycline-induced hemolytic anemia. Keio. J. Med., *12:*161, 1963.
136. Territo, M. C., Peters, R. W., and Tanaka, K.: Autoimmune hemolytic anemia due to levodopa therapy. J.A.M.A., *226:*1347, 1973.
137. Thiel, J. A., Mitchell, S., and Parker, C. W.: Specificity of hemagglutination reactions in human and experimental penicillin hypersensitivity. J. Allergy, *35:*399, 1964.
138. VanArsdel, P. P., and Gilliland, B. C.: Anemia secondary to penicillin treatment: Studies on two patients with "non-allergic" serum hemagglutinins. J. Lab. Clin. Med., *65:*277, 1965.
139. Van Loghem, J. J.: Autoimmune haemolytic anaemia with renal failure due to phenacetin and PAS. Lancet, *1:*434, 1960.
140. Vila, J. M., Blum, L., and Dosik, H.: Thiazide-induced immune hemolytic anemia. J.A.M.A., *236:*1723, 1976.
141. Vos, G. H., Petz, L., and Fudenberg, H. H.: Specificity of acquired haemolytic anaemia autoantibodies and their serological characteristics. Brit. J. Haematol., *19:*57, 1970.
142. Vos, G. H., Petz, L. D., and Fudenberg, H. H.: Specificity and immunoglobulin characteristics of autoantibodies in acquired hemolytic anemia. J. Immunol., *106:*1172, 1971.
143. Vos, G. H., Petz, L. D., Garratty, G., and Fudenberg, H. H.: Autoantibodies in acquired hemolytic anemia with special reference to the LW system. Blood, *42:*445, 1973.
144. Watson, K. C., Joubert, S. M., and Bennett, M. A. E.: Occurrence of haemagglutinating antibody to penicillin. Immunology, *3:*1, 1960.
145. Weigle, W. O.: The antibody response in rabbits to previously tolerated antigens. Ann. N.Y. Acad. Sci., *124:*133–142, 1965.
146. Weigle, W. O.: The induction of autoimmunity in rabbits following injection of heterologous or altered homologous thyroglobulin. J. Exp. Med., *121:*289, 1965.
147. Wenz, B., Klein, R. L., and Lalezari, P.: Tetracycline-induced immune hemolytic anemia. Transfusion, *14:*265, 1974.
148. White, J. M., Brown, D. L., Hepner, G. W., and Worlledge, S. M.: Penicillin-induced haemolytic anaemia. Brit. Med. J., *3:*26, 1968.
149. Worlledge, S. M.: Immune drug-induced haemolytic anemias. Semin. Hematol., *6:*181, 1969.
150. Worlledge, S. M.: Autoantibody formation associated with methyldopa (Aldomet) therapy. Brit. J. Haematol., *16:*5, 1969.
151. Worlledge, S. M.: The detection of rifampicin-dependent antibodies. Scand. J. Resp. Dis., *84:*60, 1973.

152. Worlledge, S. M.: Immune drug-induced haemolytic anaemias. *In* Blood Disorders Due to Drugs and Other Agents. Girdwood, R. H., Ed., Amsterdam, Excerpta Medica, 1973, 11.
153. Worlledge, S. M.: Immune drug-induced hemolytic anemias. Seminars in Hematol., *10:*327, 1973.
154. Worlledge, S. M., Carstairs, K. C., and Dacie, J. V.: Autoimmune haemolytic anaemia associated with methyldopa therapy. Lancet, *2:*135, 1966.
155. York, P., Landes, R., and Seay, L.: Coombs' positive reactions associated with cephaloridine therapy. J.A.M.A., *206:*1086, 1968.
156. Young, R. C., Nachman, R. L., and Horowitz, H. I.: Thrombocytopenia due to digitoxin. Demonstration of antibody and mechanisms of action. Amer. J. Med., *41:*605, 1966.
157. Zeigler, Z., Shadduck, R. K., Winkelstein, A., and Stroupe, T. K.: Immune hemolytic anemia and thrombocytopenia secondary to quinidine: In vitro studies of the quinidine-dependent red cell and platelet antibodies. Blood, *53:*396, 1979.

9

Unusual Problems Regarding Autoimmune Hemolytic Anemias

CONTENTS OF CHAPTER

A. Autoimmune Hemolytic Anemia with a Negative Direct Antiglobulin Test
B. Autoimmune Hemolytic Anemia during Pregnancy
C. Differentiation between a Delayed Hemolytic Transfusion Reaction and Autoimmune Hemolytic Anemia
D. The Development of Autoimmune Hemolytic Anemia following Blood Transfusion
E. Serum Complement in Autoimmune Hemolytic Anemia
F. Chronic Paroxysmal Cold Hemoglobinuria
G. Warm Antibody Autoimmune Hemolytic Anemia Associated with Abnormal Cold Agglutinins
H. Warm Antibody Autoimmune Hemolytic Anemia in Patients whose Direct Antiglobulin Test is Positive Only with Anti-IgA Antiserum
I. Autoimmune Hemolytic Anemia in Infancy and Childhood

A. AUTOIMMUNE HEMOLYTIC ANEMIA ASSOCIATED WITH A NEGATIVE DIRECT ANTIGLOBULIN TEST

Patients with acquired hemolytic anemia whose red cells are not agglutinated by antiglobulin serum have been reported by numerous investigators. In some instances, the hemolysis is clearly not antibody-induced as, for example, hemolytic anemia caused by oxidant drugs in patients with glucose 6-phosphate dehydrogenase deficiency, mechanical hemolytic anemias, paroxysmal nocturnal hemoglobinuria, etc. However, in other patients, extensive evaluation fails to reveal a non-immunologic etiology, and clinical findings are suggestive of autoimmune hemolytic anemia. That is, these patients destroy transfused normal compatible red cells at a rate approximating destruction of their own, thus indicating an extrinsic mechanism for red cell destruction. In addition, they usually respond to steroid therapy and/or splenectomy as do patients with more typical serologic findings of autoimmune hemolytic anemia.[54] In many such patients, evidence supporting the hypothesis that these are, indeed, autoimmune hemolytic anemias can be obtained by utilizing techniques more sensitive than standard serologic procedures.

Incidence: The exact incidence of autoimmune hemolytic anemia with a negative direct antiglobulin test is not known. Evans and Weiser [39] described four patients with negative antiglobulin tests who were clinically similar to 37 other patients with serologic abnormalities indicative of autoimmune hemolytic anemia. Dacie also noted persistently negative antiglobulin tests in some patients who otherwise appeared to have autoimmune hemolytic anemia. [33] Worlledge and Blajchman [143] reported 10 similar cases in their series of 333 cases consisting of all types of autoimmune hemolytic anemia. In eight of these cases, survival of ^{51}Cr-tagged compatible normal red cells was shortened. Chaplin [19] reported that 2 to 4 percent of the patients with autoimmune hemolytic anemia have a negative antiglobulin test.

Relationship of Antibody Concentration to Rate of Hemolysis: The inability to demonstrate autoantibodies on red cells of some patients with immune hemolytic anemia results from the concentration of antibody being too low for detection by the usual antiglobulin test. That such small concentrations of IgG autoantibody are capable of producing red cell destruction is supported by observations with alloantibodies. Mollison and Hughes-Jones [91] studied the clearance of Rh-positive red cells by low concentrations of Rh antibody. They injected anti-Rh$_o$(D) into an Rh negative person, and followed the injection by ^{51}Cr-tagged Rh$_o$(D) positive red cells; they demonstrated that when red cells were coated with about 10 molecules of antibody per cell, their survival (halftime) was approximately 100 hours. They also demonstrated that the lowest concentration of antibody capable of bringing about red cell destruction *in vivo* was about $^1/_{50}$ of the lowest concentration detectable by the indirect antiglobulin test *in vitro*. This finding must not be taken to mean, however, that all antibodies have the same degree of potency in regard to their ability to cause red cell destruction *in vivo*. Indeed, there are ample data indicating that the ability of autoantibodies to produce red cell destruction varies among patients. Although hemolytic anemia occurs in some patients who have low concentrations of antibody on their red cells, other patients have mild or no red cell destruction with a strongly positive antiglobulin test. Constantoulakis et al. [25] demonstrated that the rate of hemolysis depends more on the characteristics of the individual antibody than on the antibody concentration. Although wide variations of antibody concentration per red cell and hemolytic activity are observed among patients, in the individual patient with autoimmune hemolytic anemia the rate of red cell destruction usually is related to the concentration of red cell-bound antibody. [68, 92, 116] (Also see Chapter 6, page 204.)

Sensitivity of the Direct Antiglobulin Test: The concentration of IgG antibody on the red cell required for a positive antiglobulin test is quite variable. Also of importance are the characteristics of the red cell, the red cell antibody, and the antiglobulin serum.[54] Gilliland reported that red cells of some patients were agglutinated by antiglobulin serum with 150 molecules of IgG per cell, while red cells from other patients were not agglutinated although they were sensitized with 475 molecules per cell.[55] With manually performed antiglobulin tests, Dupuy et al.[37] observed weak agglutination of red cells coated with 100 molecules of anti-Rh$_o$(D) per cell by some antiglobulin sera; however, with other antiglobulin sera, 10 to 20 times more cell-bound antibody was required for agglutination. Other observers, using red cells coated with either IgG anti-A or anti-Rh$_o$(D), have observed minimally detectable agglutination by antiglobulin serum with antibody concentrations ranging from 100 to 500 molecules per cell.[14, 65, 115]

Results carried out in our laboratory with an anti-Rh$_o$(D) antibody are indicated in Table 9-1. Negative results were obtained in the antiglobulin test with red cells coated with fewer than 120 molecules per cell. Progressively stronger reactions occurred with higher concentrations of IgG. The concentration of IgG on the red cells was determined using the complement-fixing antibody consumption test (described later in this chapter).

Table 9-1. THE STRENGTH OF THE ANTIGLOBULIN TEST USING RED CELLS COATED WITH VARYING CONCENTRATIONS OF IgG AS DETERMINED BY THE COMPLEMENT FIXING ANTIBODY CONSUMPTION TEST. (A SINGLE ANTI-IgG ANTIGLOBULIN SERUM WAS USED AT OPTIONAL DILUTION.)

RBC sensitized *in vitro* with anti-Rh$_o$(D)	
Antiglobulin Test	IgG Molecules per RBC
negative	<25–120
±	120
1+	200
2+	300–500
3+, 4+	>500

Measurement of Small Amounts of Red Cell-Bound Antibodies: Small amounts of red cell antibodies can be measured by techniques not available in most laboratories. A sensitive method is the detection of agglutination augmented by polyvinylpyrrolidone (PVP)[14] performed on the Auto-Analyzer (Technicon Corp.) This method has been shown to detect as few as eight molecules of anti-Rh$_o$(D) per red cell. Radioimmunoassay, utilizing a radiolabelled anti-IgG, has also been used to measure red cell antibodies. In the past this technique has tended to suffer from nonspecific binding of the radiolabelled anti-IgG to the red cell. In a more recently described technique, nonspecific binding was reduced by using white-cell-free blood cells and non-radioactive protein diluent.[69]

A complement-fixing antibody consumption test has been described by Gilliland for the quantitation of IgG on human red cells.[55, 56] A known number of thoroughly washed patient's red cells are incubated with a pre-determined amount of rabbit anti-human IgG. The amount of IgG after absorption is measured by a quantitative complement fixation test, which by reference to a standard curve can then be expressed as a quantity of cell-bound IgG or molecules of IgG per red cell. The latter calculations can be considered valid only by accepting the assumption that the binding ratio of anti-IgG to cell-bound IgG is the same with antibodies used to develop the standard curve as with other IgG antibodies.[69]

Laboratory Investigation of Patients with Acquired Hemolytic Anemia with a Negative Direct Antiglobulin Test: In the original study of Gilliland et al.,[55] the red cells of five of six patients with acquired hemolytic anemia with a negative direct antiglobulin test were found to have abnormal quantities of IgG, as measured by the complement-fixing antibody consumption test. The amount of IgG per red cell ranged from 70 to 434 molecules, as compared with 35 molecules or less of IgG per cell found on the red cells of normal persons. Red cells of patients with other varieties of hemolytic anemia had less than 35 molecules per cell. These included red cells of two patients with chronic hemolytic anemia due to cold agglutinins, two patients with paroxysmal nocturnal hemoglobinuria, two with hereditary spherocytosis and one with burr cells related to chronic liver disease.

In patients who had abnormal concentrations of IgG on their red cells, eluates prepared from 50 to 200 ml of blood and concentrated to a final volume of 1 ml contained IgG as demonstrated by the indirect antiglobulin test. Eluates prepared from red cells of normal subjects or from subjects with other types of hemolytic anemia gave negative reactions. Further evidence that the IgG in the red cell eluates had antibody characteristics was shown by their specificities. Three of the eluates reacted with red cells of common Rh phenotypes but did not react with Rh_{null} red cells, thus reflecting the diversity of specificity seen in patients with acquired hemolytic anemia and positive antiglobulin tests.

One of the six patients with acquired hemolytic anemia had a normal concentration of IgG on her red cells as measured by the complement-fixing antibody consumption test and no IgG, IgA, or IgM red cell antibodies could be identified in a concentrated eluate prepared from 200 ml of blood. Further, no free antibody was detected in her serum. However, survival of transfused normal compatible red cells was greatly shortened. The authors speculated that part of the population of IgG molecules found on her red cells, which was in the quantitative range found on cells from normal persons, might represent antibody.

More recently, Gilliland extended these findings by reporting an additional nine patients.[54] The amount of IgG per red cell in these patients ranged from 76 to 350 molecules. Six of the nine responded to corticosteroid therapy, one did not improve, one died of chronic lymphocytic leukemia before results of therapy could be assessed, and one patient was lost to follow-up. The patient who showed no improvement had the same quantity of IgG on his red cells three weeks later. Follow-up quantitative red cell antibody data were obtained in some of the patients that responded to therapy, and these data revealed a decrease in the amount of antibody per red cell.

Rosse [117] used a similar technique to demonstrate small quantities of IgG on red cells of patients with the clinical picture of immune hemolytic anemia. He detected 50 to 450 molecules of IgG per cell in certain patients with autoimmune hemolytic anemia. Prednisone or splenectomy resulted in clinical remission and a reduction in the amount of antibody detectable on the red cells.

Parker et al.[98] used an erythrophagocytosis test to study one patient with acquired hemolytic anemia who had a persistently negative direct antiglobulin test. *In vitro* erythrophagocytosis by mouse macrophages was graded as 3+ (greater than 25 percent phagocytosis) when the patient's serum and red cells were used, 2+ (20 to 25 percent phagocytosis) when the patient's serum was used with normal red cells, but negative if normal serum was used with the patient's red cells or with normal red cells. The patient responded to corticosteroid therapy on two occasions and had a permanent remission after splenectomy. The erythrophagocytosis test revealed little change soon after initiation of corticosteriod therapy but there was a marked reduction in phagocytosis (5 to 10 percent) just prior to splenectomy.

Idelson et al.[66] have reported on the use of an aggregate-hemagglutination test for the diagnosis of autoimmune hemolytic anemia with a negative direct antiglobulin test. Two procedures have been developed, both based on the agglutination of the patient's red cells upon the addition of test erythrocytes coated with aggregated proteins from antiglobulin serum.

In procedure I ("antiglobulin variant") the red blood cells examined are mixed with test erythrocytes sensitized with aggregated rabbit anti-human globulins. In procedure II ("antiantiglobulin variant") the test consists of two stages. It begins with a preliminary incubation of the red cells under examination with rabbit anti-human globulin (monovalent or polyvalent) serum. After that the red cells are separated from the unbound proteins by washing with saline. Then they are mixed with test erythrocytes sensitized with aggregated sheep and donkey antiglobulin serum against rabbit γG. In both procedures positive results are recorded in 10 minutes.

In these authors' series of 303 patients with an assumed diagnosis of autoimmune hemolytic anemia, an exceptionally high percentage had a negative direct antiglobulin test, i.e., 43.9 percent. They detected antibodies in 33 of these patients using their procedure I and in additional 88 patients using their procedure II. In 12 patients both tests were negative. Both tests were negative in 720 normal donors and in 155 patients with anemias including non-immune hemolytic anemias.

The Value of Standard Serologic Tests in Diagnosis: One facet of the laboratory investigation of a patient with acquired hemolytic anemia with a negative direct antiglobulin test that has generally been ignored or under-emphasized is that relatively sensitive serologic tests that can readily be performed by blood bank technologists in a community hospital without special resources often demonstrate the presence of red cell autoantibodies. [102] We have previously reported [43, 52] a series of six patients with acquired hemolytic anemia in whom the direct antiglobulin test was repeatedly negative with polyspecific antiglobulin serum as well as with monospecific antisera against IgG, IgM, IgA, C3, and C4. Antiglobulin tests were also negative when done at 4°C. Further, there was no agglutination after centrifugation of the patients' cells with proteolytic enzymes or albumin. However, three patients had autoantibodies in their sera detectable using enzyme-treated red cells, and in one of these patients an unconcentrated ether eluate was strongly reactive. Our further experience has confirmed these findings and, in particular, tests using a red cell eluate made from just 3 to 5 ml of red cells may be positive, especially if the eluate is concentrated by a factor of 2 to 5 times before testing. This is easily accomplished using Minicon filters (Amicon Corporation, Lexington, Massachusetts).

Although Gilliland did not use enzyme-treated red cells for the detection of autoantibodies, he did report that eluates from red cells of patients showing greater than 70 molecules of IgG per cell have always contained red cell antibody activity. [54] However, Gilliland has used large volumes of blood (50 to 200 ml) for preparing the eluates, and they were also highly concentrated (to a final volume of 1 ml). We have not found such extraordinary measures for preparation of the eluates to be necessary routinely.

On the basis of the previously described studies, we recommend that patients with an acquired hemolytic anemia with a negative direct antiglobulin test (in whom non-immunologic causes for the hemolysis are not evident) be evaluated with the sensitive serologic screening tests described in Chapters 5 and 6. Emphasis should be placed on the results of screening tests with enzyme treated red cells and with an eluate which has preferably been concentrated 2 to 5 times. If these tests yield negative results, a complement-fixing antibody consumption test may yield a positive result (described later), although most laboratories will find it impractical to perform the test.

The Use of the Complement-fixing Antibody Consumption Test in Patients with Suspected Immune Hemolytic Anemia Who Have a Negative Direct Antiglobulin Test: We have performed 82 complement-fixing antibody consumption tests on 59 subjects who were normal or who had disorders other than idiopathic acquired hemolytic anemia. In addition, we have studied 27 patients who were referred to our laboratory with a diagnosis of acquired hemolytic anemia with a negative direct antiglobulin test.

Results in the former group of patients are summarized in Table 9-2. Of 54 studies on 31 normal subjects, only one was positive, that is, indicated greater than 25 molecules of IgG/red blood cell. Of 11 patients with heredi-

Table 9-2. COMPLEMENT FIXING ANTIBODY CON-
SUMPTION TEST IN NORMAL SUBJECTS AND IN PA-
TIENTS WITH DISORDERS OTHER THAN IDIOPATHIC
ACQUIRED HEMOLYTIC ANEMIA.

Diagnosis	Number of Studies	Number with >25 Molecules of IgG/RBC
Normal persons	54	1
Hereditary spherocytosis	11	1 *
Pyruvate kinase deficiency	1	0
Gilbert's syndrome	2	0
Post-splenectomy	3	0
Mechanical hemolytic anemia (prosthetic heart valves)	11	1

* Patient also had Hodgkin's disease.

tary spherocytes, one was positive in a patient who also had Hodgkin's disease.
Tests in one patient with pyruvate kinase deficiency and two with Gilbert's
syndrome with a mild reticulocytosis were negative, as were tests in three
patients who had had splenectomy for a myeloproliferative disorder. Only
one of 11 patients with mild hemolysis associated with the presence of a
prosthetic heart valve produced a positive reaction to the test.

Our experience with 27 patients who were referred to our laboratory with
a diagnosis of acquired hemolytic anemia with a negative direct antiglobulin
test are summarized in Table 9-3. Although the direct antiglobulin test was
negative in all cases in the referral laboratory, we were able to detect complement sensitization of the patient's red cells in 11 instances using a potent
anti-C3 antiglobulin serum containing anti-C3d that was prepared in our
laboratory. In most of these instances the antiglobulin test was only weakly
positive. Also, in one instance, we obtained a weakly positive reaction using
our anti-IgG antiglobulin serum.

Autoantibodies were detected in the serum or eluate in 11 patients. Most
often, the autoantibody was detected in the serum using enzyme-treated red
cells. Less often, eluates prepared from several ml of red cells and concentrated 2 to 5 times resulted in a positive reaction. Only in one instance was
antibody detected solely by the indirect antiglobulin test.

The complement-fixing antibody consumption test revealed greater than
25 molecules of IgG per red cell in all patients and between 100 and 300
molecules of IgG per red blood cell in 15 of the 27 cases. In five instances,
greater than 400 molecules of IgG per red blood cell were detected, including
one extraordinary case in which 1400 molecules of IgG were found in spite of
a negative direct antiglobulin test in a patient with recurrent episodes of brisk
hemolysis (see case report 9-1).

Information concerning response to therapy was available in 17 patients
and, among these, follow-up complement-fixing antibody consumption tests

Table 9-3. WARM ANTIBODY AUTOIMMUNE HEMOLYTIC ANEMIC WITH A NEGATIVE DIRECT ANTIGLOBULIN TEST

| | DAT in Referral Laboratory | DAT in Authors' Laboratory | | Test for Autoantibody | | | CFAC Test: IgG Molecules per RBC (Normal = <25) | Therapy | Course | Associated Disease |
| | | | | Serum | | Eluate | | | | |
		IgG	C3d	IAT	Enzyme Treated RBC	IAT				
1	Neg	Neg	1½+	Neg	Neg	Neg	144	None	Improved	History of ITP
2	Neg	Neg	2+	Neg	Neg	Neg	>400		Improved	Wiskott-Aldrich
3	Neg	Neg	Neg	Neg	Neg	NT	126			
4	Neg	Neg	1+	Neg	3½+	Neg	251	Steroids	Improved	
5	Neg	Neg	Neg	Neg	Neg	Neg	93			
6	Neg	Neg	Neg	Neg	Neg	NT	59	Steroids	Improved	
7	Neg	Neg	1+	Neg	1½+	Neg	234			
8	Neg	½+	½+	½+	3½+	Neg	126			
9	Neg	Neg	Neg	Neg	Neg	Neg	>400	Steroids	Improved	
10	Neg	Neg	Neg	Neg	½+	Neg	166			
11	Neg	Neg	½+	2+	3½+	½+	173	Steroids	Improved	
12	Neg	Neg	1+	Neg	Neg	NT	339			
13	Neg	Neg	Neg	Neg	3+	Neg	243	Steroids	Persistent hemolysis; expired	Chronic persistent hepatitis
14	Neg	Neg	Neg	Neg	Neg	Neg	54	Steroids	Unchanged	Metastatic carcinoma; microangiopathic hemolytic anemia

No.							Count	Treatment	Response	Diagnosis
15	Neg	Neg	Neg	1+	Neg	NT	128	Steroids	Improved	
16	Neg	Neg	Neg	Neg	Neg	2+	185	Steroids	Improved	
17	Neg	Neg	Neg	Neg	Neg	Neg	70	Steroids	Unchanged	TTP
18	Neg	Neg	Neg	Neg	Neg	NT	>400	Steroids	Improved	
19	Neg	Neg	Neg	Neg	Neg	1/2+	95	Steroids	Improved	
20	Neg	1+	Neg	Neg	Neg	NT	122			Carcinoma of ovary
21	Neg	Neg	Neg	Neg	Neg	Neg	127			
22	Neg	Neg	1/2+	Neg	Neg	Neg	290	Steroids	Improved	
23	Neg	Neg	Neg	NT	NT	NT	59			
24	Neg	3+	Neg	2+	2+	1+	1400	Splenectomy	Long term remission	
25	Neg	2½+	Neg	Neg	Lysis	1½+	138	Splenic irradiation	Marked temporary improvement	
26	Neg	½+	Neg	Neg	Neg	Neg	180	Prednisone and splenectomy	Unchanged	
27	Neg	Neg	Neg	Neg	Neg	Neg	640	Steroids	Rapid improvement	

DAT = Direct antiglobulin test
IAT = Indirect antiglobulin test
CFAC = Complement fixing antibody consumption
NT = Not tested
ITP = Idiopathic thrombocytopenic purpura
TTP = Thrombotic thrombocytopenic purpura

were performed in seven. Six of these patients revealed marked clinical improvement in response to steroids or splenectomy. The subsequent complement-fixing antibody consumption test revealed less than 25 molecules of IgG per red cell in five patients, but in one patient 228 molecules of IgG were present after therapy (compared with 173 prior to therapy) in spite of clinical improvement. One patient who did not improve as a result of treatment with steroids and splenectomy had 180 molecules of IgG per red blood cell before therapy and 607 when re-tested two years later.

Twenty-two of the patients had no associated disorder and were diagnosed as having idiopathic autoimmune hemolytic anemia, although one of these had a history of having had idiopathic thrombocytopenic purpura. Five patients had active associated disease.

Although not indicated in the table, spherocytes were noted on the peripheral blood film in seven patients. This finding suggests that the interaction of antibody coated red cells with the cells of the reticuloendothelial system (as described in Chapter 4) occurred in spite of the small numbers of IgG molecules present on the red cells.

While accumulating this experience, we have also observed five patients who were referred with a diagnosis of idiopathic acquired hemolytic anemia with a negative direct antiglobulin test and in whom the complement-fixing antibody consumption test indicated that the patients' red cells were coated with fewer than 25 molecules of IgG per cell (the lower limit of sensitivity of the test in our laboratory). In four of these patients, C3d was detectable on the patients' cells by the direct antiglobulin test, but in none were autoantibodies detectable in the serum or eluate. Whether these patients' hemolytic anemia is also immunologically mediated is conjectural.

Therapy and Course: Patients with acquired hemolytic anemia who have a negative direct antiglobulin test and who do not have evidence for a non-immune cause of the hemolysis, but who have abnormal numbers of IgG molecules on their red cells, should be treated similarly to patients who have more characteristic findings of warm antibody autoimmune hemolytic anemia (see Chapter 11). The variable responses to therapy indicated in Table 9-3 and described previously are similar to these observed in patients who present with a positve direct antiglobulin test and typical serologic findings of warm antibody autoimmune hemolytic anemia. Gilliland [54] has also demonstrated that, in many patients, a reduction of cell-bound IgG antibody can be documented after remission induced by corticosteroids or splenectomy. However, other patients develop a well-compensated hemolytic anemia with little change in the abnormal quantity of IgG per cell. He further indicated that some patients who originally presented with autoimmune hemolytic anemia with a positive antiglobulin test have shown a reduction of cell-bound IgG antibody with corticosteroid therapy to levels that are still elevated, but below detection by routine antiglobulin testing. The quantity of IgG antibody in some of these patients has remained at these low levels for several years, while in others the quantity of IgG per cell has increased, and hemolytic anemia has recurred after therapy with steroids was decreased or stopped. In still other patients, the quantity of IgG per red cell has fallen to the range observed on normal red cells, and therapy has been discontinued without an increase of cell-bound antibody or exacerbation of hemolytic disease.

The following case reports illustrate the value of sensitive serologic tests and the complement-fixing antibody consumption test in evaluating patients with acquired hemolytic anemia with a negative direct antiglobulin test.

Case 9-1: A twelve-year history of episodic acquired hemolytic anemia with a negative direct antiglobulin test. (Referred by Neil W. Culp, M.D.)

J.T., a 49-year-old man, had a history of recurrent episodes of hemolytic anemia for 12 years. In June 1963 he developed malaise, fatigue, gastrointestinal symptoms, jaundice, and dark urine. An acute hemolytic anemia was diagnosed, and there were no evident precipitating events. The hemolysis resolved spontaneously without therapy and, over the next two years the patient had recurrent episodes at approximately 60 to 90 day intervals. The episodes gradually decreased in severity and he was free of symptoms from 1965 until November 1971 when the pattern was re-established.

He then developed recurrent attacks consisting of progressive weakness, darkening of the urine, malaise, pallor, and, by the fourth or fifth day, jaundice and symptoms of anemia. The nadir of hemoglobin depression was generally in the range of 5 to 7 gm/dl and occurred 7 to 10 days after the onset of symptoms. Reticulocytopenia (1 percent or less) was present during the period of progressive fall in hemoglobin, and usually for about 72 hours after reaching the nadir. Leukopenia and thrombocytopenia also occurred, with the white cell count dropping to about $2000/\mu l$ with a normal differential, and the platelets falling to about $80,000/\mu l$. Then followed a progressive reticulocytosis to a value of about 20 percent over the succeeding 7 to 10 days and complete recovery at the end of approximately three weeks. At this time the patient's hemoglobin was in the range of 14 gm/dl, and the reticulocyte count, white cell count, and platelet count were normal. These episodes continued to recur at 60 to 90 day intervals for the next four years, during which time numerous studies were undertaken.

The patient was repeatedly questioned about any environmental factor relating to occupation or hobbies that might be of significance in precipitating attacks, but none could be identified. There was no history of drug ingestion. Physical examination was remarkable for the presence of mild tachycardia and icterus during periods of marked anemia. In addition, he had persistent splenomegaly, the edge of the spleen usually palpable 4 cm below the left costal margin.

Laboratory data revealed characteristic findings of hemolysis during periods of progressive anemia. In a typical episode the total bilirubin was 1.6 mg/dl with 0.3 mg direct reacting, haptoglobin absent, LDH 390, and urine hemosiderin weakly positive. The red cell morphology was essentially normal, although an occasional target cell and rare spherocyte were present. A bone marrow aspirate performed at a point of maximum anemia revealed intense erythroid hyperplasia with some "megaloblastoid" features. A repeat bone marrow study performed during a phase of remission revealed some residual erythroid hyperplasia that was normoblastic. A red cell survival study using ^{51}Cr labelled red cells was begun near the onset of an episode of hemolysis. The curve initially began with a steady exponential fall revealing a halftime of 17 days (normal = 25 to 35 days). Suddenly on the eleventh day of the study, the chromium disappearance became markedly accelerated with a halftime of three days. Excessive splenic sequestration was noted. Another red cell survival study was begun when the patient's hematocrit was 12.5 percent. During the study his hematocrit level rose to 24 percent on the tenth day and 38 percent on the seventeenth day. The disappearance curve of the radioactive chromium was within normal limits.

Extensive diagnostic studies to determine the cause of the hemolysis were negative. Tests performed included the direct antiglobulin test, Ham's acid serum test, the sucrose hemolysis test, osmotic fragility before and after incubation at 37°C for 24 hours, hemoglobin electrophoresis, quantitation of hemoglobins A_2 and F, isopropanol and heat tests for unstable hemoglobins, and biochemical measurement of red cell G-6PD, 6-phosphogluconic dehydrogenase, hexokinase, pyruvate kinase, aldolase, catalase, pyruvate, and lactate.

One type of therapy that was tried included prednisone at a dose of 80 mg per day given at the onset of symptoms. This regimen had no significant effect on the progression of the hemolytic episode. The patient was also treated with folic acid without effect. Transfusions were given during his first episode in 1963, but thereafter the patient learned to tolerate symptoms in spite of striking drops in hemoglobin. However, when his disease became progressively more severe in 1975, he was given two units of red cells during each of two successive hemolytic episodes after his hemoglobin had dropped to 3.5 gm/dl.

When referred for immunohematologic evaluation in December 1975, his direct antiglobulin test was negative with anti-IgG antiglobulin serum but moderately strongly positive with anti-C3 antiserum. His serum contained an antibody that reacted equally with all enzyme-treated red cells of a panel. An alloantibody (anti-Wr[a]) was also detectable by indirect antiglobulin test. An eluate prepared from the patient's red cells contained a weak antibody without evident specificity.

In spite of the negative direct antiglobulin test using anti-IgG antiserum, the complement fixing antibody consumption test revealed a surprising value of 1400 molecules of IgG per red cell at a time when the patient's hemoglobin was 5.9 gm/dl. A repeat test in January 1979, when the hemoglobin was 13.6 gm/dl, revealed 396 molecules of IgG per red blood cell.

On January 27, 1976, splenectomy was performed. The spleen weighed 1164 gm and revealed congestion of the red pulp, follicular center hyperplasia, and abundant iron.

Subsequently, the patient has been asymptomatic and has had no further hemolytic episodes during a three-year follow-up period. His hemoglobin is 17.2 gm/dl, hematocrit level 51.4 percent, white cell count 11,200/μl, platelets 329,000/μl, and reticulocytes 1.7 percent. A repeat complement-fixing antibody consumption test performed in July 1976 revealed <25 molecules of IgG per red blood cell. In March, 1979, the complement-fixing antibody consumption test revealed 240 molecules of IgG per red blood cell; his direct antiglobulin test was negative with anti-IgG and anti-C3 reagents, and no antibody was detected in his serum or in a red cell eluate.

Comment: This patient had a long history of recurrent attacks of hemolysis without evident cause. Attacks occurred every 60 to 90 days, and his hemoglobin fell to as low as 3.5 gm/dl. Immunohematologic evaluation including the use of the complement-fixing antibody consumption test revealed evidences of warm antibody autoimmune hemolytic anemia. The patient responded to splenectomy with complete cessation of episodes of hemolysis and follow-up immunohematologic evaluations revealed significant improvement.

Case 9-2: Acquired hemolytic anemia with a negative direct antiglobulin test with anti-E occurring in the red blood cell eluate of an E-negative patient.

We have previously described [112] a patient who presented with two unusual phenomena. Not only did he have an acquired hemolytic anemia with a negative direct antiglobulin test, but he also had an apparently specific Rhesus antibody in his red cell eluate that appeared to be directed against an antigen not present on his own red cells. Although the occurrence of either of these phenomena is not unique, this was the first report in which both findings were present in the same patient.

A previously untransfused 20-year-old man presented with a seven-day history of malaise, fatigue, jaundice, dark urine, and splenomegaly. Hemolytic anemia was indicated by a hemoglobin of 8.7 gm/dl, reticulocyte count 8 percent, lactic dehydrogenase 389 iu/L, bilirubin 4.3 mg/dl (direct 0.1 mg/dl), and undetectable haptoglobins. Tests for nonimmunologic causes of hemolytic anemia were negative. The direct antiglobulin test was repeatedly negative with polyspecific, anti-IgG, -IgA, -IgM, and anti-C3 antisera. The patient's serum contained a weak anti-I, anti-E strongly reactive by indirect antiglobulin test, and an antibody reactive against all cells tested. The latter antibody reacted weakly by the indirect antiglobulin test but strongly against enzyme-treated cells (titer 160). Eluates from the patient's red blood cells only reacted with E+ red blood cells. The patient was E negative. He was treated for warm antibody autoimmune hemolytic anemia with high doses of prednisone. By the twelfth day his response allowed the medication to be tapered and by one month from the onset of treatment laboratory studies had returned to normal. The direct antiglobulin test remained negative; however, following recovery, anti-E could not be eluted from the red blood cells. Anti-E remained in his serum and the titer of the enzyme reactive antibody had decreased to 16. It was suggested that the anti-"E-like" antibody may represent auto anti-Hr preferentially reacting with E+ red blood cells.

Our experience has indicated that when IgG antibody is present in an eluate prepared from red blood cells, the complement-fixing antibody consumption test is always abnormal. Thus, we performed the assay only on red cells obtained five months following remission at which time the eluate gave negative results. The antibody-fixing complement consumption test revealed normal findings (<25 molecules IgG/RBC).

Case 9-3: Warm antibody autoimmune hemolytic anemia erroneously diagnosed as cold agglutinin syndrome.

D.P., a 17-year-old boy, was admitted to the hospital for evaluation of severe hemolytic anemia. Physical examination revealed an icteric young man in no acute distress. The spleen was palpable 2 cm below the left costal margin. The hemoglobin was 7.6 gm/dl, reticulocytes 10.8 percent, white cell count 7,600/μl, serum bilirubin 7.2 mg/dl (0.8 direct reacting), the urine hemoglobin was 4+, and the mono spot test negative. The peripheral blood film revealed anisocytosis, polychromasia, and numerous spherocytes. The patient required transfusion of 10 units of blood in a 10-day period to maintain a hematocrit level of about 25 percent. The direct antiglobulin test was negative. The only free antibody detectable in his serum was a cold agglutinin with anti-I specificity that had a maximum titer of 512 at 4°C and demonstrated weak reactivity up to 22°C. The Donath-Landsteiner test was negative. A diagnosis of atypical cold agglutinin syndrome was made, and the patient was treated by keeping the temperature of his room at 37°C. However, brisk hemolysis continued. He received 16 additional units of red cells during the next month without his hematocrit level rising above 30 percent.

Studies on blood referred to our laboratory revealed that the direct antiglobulin test was negative using antisera against IgG, IgA, IgM, and C3. No warm autoantibodies were detected in the serum by indirect antiglobulin test or by agglutination of enzyme-treated red cells. A cold agglutinin was present to a titer of 8 at 4°C in saline; it did not cause agglutination in saline or albumin at 25°C. The complement-fixing antibody consumption test revealed greater than 400 molecules of IgG per red cell. The patient was subsequently treated with therapy appropriate for warm antibody autoimmune hemolytic anemia, had a partial response to steroids, but subsequently required splenectomy before achieving remission.

Case 9-4: Relapsing hemolytic anemia of pregnancy with a negative direct antiglobulin test.

It is important to diagnose autoimmune hemolytic anemia when present during pregnancy because hemolysis frequently worsens as pregnancy progresses and the disorder may become life-threatening. A case in which the complement-fixing antibody consumption test was very helpful in diagnosing autoimmune hemolytic anemia in a patient with recurrent hemolytic anemia of pregnancy is described in section B, "Autoimmune Hemolytic Anemia during Pregnancy."

The Complement-Fixing Antibody Consumption Test in Patients with Sickle Cell Anemia and other Hemoglobinopathies: In extending our studies to include a representative sample of other non-immune hemolytic anemias, we have studied patients with a variety of congenital hemolytic anemias.[141] Rather surprisingly, we have found that 27 of 36 patients (75 percent) who were homozygous for hemoglobin S had between 25 and 890 molecules of IgG per red cell; the median value was 156 and the mean was 203.

The patients ranged in age from 11 months to 30 years, the hemoglobin from 6.0 to 11.1 gm/dl and the reticulocytes from 0.8 to 20 percent. There were no differences that we could discern between the patients with or without IgG on their red cells.

Eluates were made from the red cells of 21 of the 27 patients with sickle cell disease who had increased numbers of IgG molecules per red cell. Although only small volumes of red cells were generally available for preparing eluates, six of the 21 eluates demonstrated antibody activity against normal red cells by the indirect antiglobulin test. In each case specificity tests revealed no definite specificity, thus suggesting autoantibody.

The relationship of the red cell sensitization in patients with sickle cell anemia to blood transfusion was considered. Many of the patients had a history of blood transfusions but none included in the study had received blood products in the preceding three months. One patient's case history illustrates the possible significance of these studies.

The patient was a 24-year-old woman with sickle cell anemia who had received multiple transfusions during childhood, although in the past four years she had received only three units of packed red cells, which were administered six months previously. Her hematocrit level was 18 percent and the reticulocyte count 18.1 percent. She was admitted to the hospital for an elective cholecystectomy and it was elected to transfuse her until her hematocrit level was about 36 percent in an attempt to reduce her anesthetic risk. Her direct antiglobulin test was negative, but a complement-fixing antibody consumption test done at the onset of the transfusions revealed 533 molecules of IgG per red cell, and a red cell eluate was weakly reactive with no definable specificity. She was known to have had anti-M and anti-C antibodies in the past, as well as multiple leukocyte antibodies, and she was therefore transfused with leukocyte-poor red cells lacking these red cell antigens, even though these antibodies were not detectable at this time.

After transfusion of eight units of leukocyte-poor packed red cells over a four-day period, her hematocrit level reached 36.8 percent. Two days later she began to have shaking chills, abdominal pain and fever, and she experienced a life-threatening hemolytic reaction with a hematocrit level dropping to 13 percent in 48 hours and ultimately reaching a low of 7.4 percent. The serum hemoglobin reached 283 mg/dl, and she had hemoglobinuria and hemosiderinuria. She also suffered a hyporegenerative crisis with a reticulocyte count of 0.

A direct antiglobulin test was negative. Repeat screening of her serum for alloantibodies revealed negative results except for very weak reactions with enzyme-treated cells with no antibody specificity detectable. She was treated with high doses of corticosteroids and two additional units of leukocyte-poor packed red cells, and she gradually improved to a hematocrit level of 19.8 percent.

This patient's course was consistent with that of a delayed transfusion reaction, although there were no detectable alloantibodies. Our data offer a possible alternative explanation in that autoimmunization may have played a key role.

Autoimmunization was suggested by the presence of 533 molecules of IgG on the patient's red cells at the onset of transfusions, by a red cell eluate that was weakly reactive by the indirect antiglobulin test, and by the response to corticosteroids. It is possible that the transfusions stimulated the further production of autoantibodies, which also reacted with the donor cells, causing a transient autoimmune hemolytic anemia. The lack of strongly reactive serologic abnormalities usually found in autoimmune hemolytic anemia may be analogous to the cases of immune hemolytic anemia with a negative direct antiglobulin test previously described.

The suggestion that an augmentation of autoantibody production could be of significance in this clinical setting is strengthened by reports of numerous investigators concerning the production of autoantibodies after immunization with red cells, as is reviewed in detail in Section D. In addition, Constantoulakis et al.[25] have indicated that above a certain level ("hemolytic threshold"), minute increases of red cell-bound antibody induce pronounced effects on red cell survival. These authors emphasized that an acute, explosive hemolytic crisis in a patient with an otherwise chronic, compensated autoimmune hemolytic anemia could result from a relatively small increment in antibody production, and that this increase in antibody production would not be detected by conventional serologic tests. The patient's hyporegenerative crisis may also be immunologically mediated since there is ample precedent for reticulocytopenia as a part of an acute autoimmune hemolytic anemia (see Chapter 2).

Thus, this unusual type of hyperhemolytic "sickle cell crisis" associated with severe anemia and marked reticulocytopenia may be immunologically mediated and related to transient augmentation of autoantibody production.

Other investigators have also described hyperhemolytic crises in patients with sickle cell anemia that occurred after transfusion and that were associated with destruction of donor red cells, but in the absence of detectable alloantibodies. Chaplin and Cassell's detailed account [20] describes numerous serologic studies and 17 measurements of *in vivo* red cell survival carried out over a two-year period in one patient. They also mention an identical clinical pattern observed in a second patient with sickle cell anemia.

Similarly, Issitt* has observed patients with sickle cell anemia who have no serologically demonstrable autoantibodies or alloantibodies, yet in whom red cells are destroyed following transfusion. Their declining levels of hemoglobin appear too rapid to be explained by marrow shutdown of sickle cell production.

Although our initial studies have concerned patients with sickle cell anemia, hemolytic transfusion reactions without detectable alloantibodies have been reported by numerous investigators, [90] and the use of sensitive means of detecting red cell antibodies may assist in understanding their pathogenesis whether caused by autoantibody, alloantibody, or both.

Further Studies in Patients with Hemoglobinopathies: We have extended our studies in patients with hemoglobinopathies and have now tested 98 samples from 56 patients with sickle cell anemia, 69 samples from 59 patients with sickle cell trait, 16 samples from 11 patients with hemoglobin S-C disease, and 13 samples on 9 patients with thalassemia syndromes including heterozygous β-thalassemia, homozygous β-thalassemia, and patients doubly heterozygous for sickle cell homoglobin and β-thalassemia.

Our results indicated that 34 of the 56 patients with sickle cell anemia (61 percent) had increased numbers of IgG molecules on their red cells (>25 molecules of IgG/red blood cell) on at least one occasion. Twenty-two patients had more than 250 molecules of IgG/red blood cell. In most patients, follow-up examinations revealed a relatively consistent pattern; i.e., those patients without abnormal red cell sensitization with IgG had normal values when re-tested, and those subjects with abnormal red cell sensitization on initial testing continued to have abnormal results on follow-up examination.

Ten patients with sickle cell trait yielded abnormal results (17 percent). Six patients had more than 250 molecules of IgG/red blood cell on at least one occasion. Of the five patients in whom repeat samples were obtained, only one patient was found to have consistently abnormal results. Six of the 11 patients

* Issitt, P.: Personal communication, 1978.

with S-C disease had increased numbers of IgG/red blood cell as did six of the nine patients with thalassemia syndromes.

We have not observed additional examples of hyperhemolytic crises in sickle cell anemia and, to date, we have not detected a significant correlation between the number of molecules of IgG per red cell and the severity of anemia, painful sickle cell crises, reticulocyte count, or the history of blood transfusions.

B. AUTOIMMUNE HEMOLYTIC ANEMIA DURING PREGNANCY

Since hemolytic anemia commonly occurs in young women, it is surprising that the medical literature concerning autoimmune hemolytic anemia during pregnancy is scanty. Indeed, Chaplin et al.,[21] in an excellent review in 1973, were able to find only 19 reports of pregnancy in patients with presumed autoimmune hemolytic anemia. All patients had unequivocal evidence for acquired hemolysis, but evidence for an autoimmune basis of hemolysis was often incomplete, especially in the pre-antiglobulin test era. Among the 19 cases reviewed, the direct antiglobulin test on maternal cells was positive in 7, negative in 5, and not performed in 7. Four of the 5 mothers with a negative direct antiglobulin test were treated with corticosteroids and all improved.

Maternal Hazards: The hazard to maternal survival was often extremely serious. In 9 patients the hemoglobin fell below 5 gm/dl, and in another 8 instances the hemoglobin values were in the range of 5 to 8 gm/dl. Leukopenia was present in 4 pregnancies and thrombocytopenia in 3 pregnancies. Vigorous transfusion therapy, high doses of corticosteroids, and/or early induction of labor were employed as life-saving measures in critically ill patients.

Particularly significant is the observation that hemolysis worsened as the pregnancy progressed in 18 of the 19 patients. Following delivery, complete or partial remissions of hemolysis occurred in 16 patients within 3 months of delivery. The two patients who did not improve were subsequently diagnosed as having systemic lupus erythematosus.

Fetal Hazards: Four of the 19 pregnancies resulted in the delivery of a stillborn premature infant, and a fifth premature infant died at 48 hours of bronchopneumonia. No hematologic data were reported on these 5 infants, and none were described as having pallor, jaundice, or hydrops. However, all were born to mothers with severe anemia (hemoglobin less than 5 gm/dl), which suggests that fetal death was related more to the critical maternal state than to autoantibody-induced hemolytic disease of the newborn. Indeed, 11 other infants were considered normal despite the fact that they were born to mothers who had evidence of brisk hemolysis during the latter months of pregnancy.

However, severe hemolytic disease of the newborn did occur in three infants. In one infant, two exchange transfusions were required; the mother and infant were both group A, Rh-positive, and there was no evidence of maternal alloimmunization.[15] A second infant became severely anemic and jaundiced in the fourth week of life and seemed to respond to therapy with corticosteroids.[127] The third infant was severely anemic (hemoglobin 2.5 gm/dl; reticulocytes 22 percent) and leukopenic (WBC 1800/μl) at 2 months of age, and required multiple transfusions.[125] The mother, who had systemic lupus erythematosus, also had leukopenia during pregnancy. Although the anemia in these infants was attributed to placentally transferred IgG autoantibody, two of the infants had a negative direct antiglobulin test and the reaction was equivocal in the other.

Case Reports: On the basis of the preceding data that indicate that pregnancy in association with autoimmune hemolytic anemia may provoke life-threatening anemia in 40 to 50 percent of mothers and stillbirth or severe postpartum hemolytic anemia in 35 to 40 percent of their infants, Chaplin et al.[21] recommend frequent antepartum maternal hemotologic evaluation (every two weeks until the eighth month, and weekly thereafter until delivery) with frequent adjustment of corticosteroid dosage in an effort to maintain a hemoglobin level above 10 gm/dl. These investigators meticulously followed this regimen in a patient who had brisk hemolysis (hemoglobin 10 gm/dl; reticulocytes 32 percent) when she presented in the third month of her first pregnancy. The direct antiglobulin test was strongly positive using anti-IgG and anti-C3d and a warm reactive IgG autoantibody was present in her serum and red cell eluate. The antibody reacted with all cells of a panel including Rh$_{null}$, U-negative, and Tj^a-negative cells. She also developed a cold agglutinin with a titer of 256. No significant change in titers of the autoantibodies was documented during pregnancy. Amniocentesis was performed at the beginning of the eighth and ninth months of pregnancy and amniotic fluid pigment analysis was consistent with either a normal fetus or one afflicted with mild hemolytic disease.

The mother's hemolytic anemia subsided following delivery and therapy with corticosteroids was tapered and then discontinued. Six months postpartum the hemoglobin and the reticulocyte count were normal, although serologic findings showed no significant change compared with results obtained during pregnancy.

The infant exhibited a mild hemolytic syndrome associated with a weakly positive direct antiglobulin test and autoantibody demonstrable in the cord serum and in an eluate from the cord cells. However, no tranfusions or steroid therapy were required.

Other recent case reports have generally emphasized similar findings. Baumann and Rubin [7] described a patient who was well until the 36th week of her second pregnancy, at which time she experienced the onset of rapidly progressive symptoms of severe anemia. One week later she was admitted to hospital with a hemoglobin of 3 gm/dl, a hematocrit of 6.2 percent, and 58 percent reticulocytes. The direct antiglobulin test was strongly positive with anti-IgG antiglobulin serum, and an antibody was detected in both the serum and eluate which revealed no specificity when tested against a red cell panel including Rh$_{null}$ cells. The patient was treated with 100 mg of prednisone daily and was transfused with 4 units of packed red cells. Four days after admission she delivered a female infant weighing 2350 g. The mother's hemolysis gradually subsided, and therapy with prednisone was reduced. Five months later her hemoglobin level was 11.9 gm/dl, and her reticulocyte count was normal, although the direct antiglobulin test remained weakly positive. The baby had a positive direct antiglobulin test, and her bilirubin level peaked at 13.2 mg/dl on the third day of life. The infant's direct antiglobulin test became negative at the age of one month; the hemoglobin level decreased to a low of 9.7 gm/dl at 6 weeks of age and then gradually improved. The authors cite an additional case reported in the French literature in which antiglobulin positive hemolytic anemia occurred in the fifth month of pregnancy, resulting in death of the mother and of the premature infant.[58]

Blajchman and Gordon [12] reported a patient who had been treated for Hodgkin's disease for 6 years and then became pregnant. The patient, who was group O with probable rhesus genotype of R_2R_2, developed warm antibody autoimmune hemolytic anemia during pregnancy and also had an alloantibody of anti-e specificity. Before therapy with prednisone, the patient's hemoglobin level was 5.9 gm/dl, and the reticulocytes were 24.4 percent. The alloantibody titer was 512 and the autoantibody titer was 16 by indirect antiglobulin test. After the therapy and before delivery the hemoglobin level was 12 gm/dl, the reticulocytes 7 percent, the anti-e titer was 32, and the autoantibody titer was 1. A healthy boy was delivered weighing 3280 g; the cord hemoglobin was 18.2 gm/dl and the direct antiglobulin reaction was positive. The titer of autoantibody and alloantibody in the cord serum was the same as their titer in the maternal serum. The phenotype of the infant's red blood cells was 0 ccDEe (probable genotype R_2r) and the antibodies eluted from the baby's red blood cells showed both the autoantibody and the alloantibody. The baby's bilirubin rose to a peak of 11 mg/dl on day 5. The mother's prednisone therapy was gradually decreased, her hemoglobin improved, and 5 months later her hemoglobin and reticulocyte count were normal. Autoantibody was no longer demonstrable by indirect antiglobulin test, but it was present to a titer of 8 using enzyme-treated erythrocytes. The authors emphasized that the alloantibody titer also continued to decrease after delivery, and five months later the titer was only 8 by indirect antiglobulin test; the researchers suggested that the corticosteroid therapy may have affected both the alloantibody and the autoantibody.

Pirofsky [108] also reported two patients who first manifested signs of autoimmune hemolytic anemia during pregnancy, but he comments that two other patients became pregnant during remission and did not have an exacerbation of their disease. He concluded that his series was too small to draw definite conclusions concerning the influence of pregnancy on autoimmune hemolytic anemia.

Relapsing Hemolytic Anemia in Pregnancy: Since hemolysis so frequently worsens during pregnancy and improves spontaneously after delivery, it is not unexpected that cases of relapsing hemolytic anemia of pregnancy have been described. Swisher [132] described an interesting patient with idiopathic autoimmune hemolytic anemia, whose degree of hemolysis increased with each of three pregnancies and remitted with each parturition.

More recently, Eldor et al. [38] and Hershko et al. [61] described four patients who had relapsing hemolytic anemia of pregnancy with a negative antiglobulin reaction. Seven episodes of hemolytic anemia associated with pregnancy were observed during a follow-up period of two to 16 years. Normal hemoglobin levels were found both before and after pregnancy. Hemolysis became progressively more severe during pregnancy and remitted promptly after delivery. An autoimmune mechanism was suggested in spite of negative serologic findings because of rapid destruction of transfused blood, a favorable response to corticosteroids, and the development of transient hemolytic anemia in three of the infants.

Yam, Wilkinson, Petz, and Garratty [144] studied a patient with hemolytic anemia of pregnancy with a negative direct antiglobulin test and applied the complement-fixing antibody consumption test in order to document support for an immune pathogenesis. The patient was a 34-year-old woman who had had seven previous pregnancies. She had a single blood count during her seventh pregnancy; the hematocrit level was 29 percent and reticulocytes were 6.7 percent; a single hematocrit level of 39 percent was available from her records in the non-gravid state. On referral, during the second trimester of her second pregnancy, her hemoglobin level was 9.6 gm/dl, the hematocrit level 28 percent and the reticulocyte count 10.3 percent. The white blood cell count, differential count, and platelet count were normal. The blood film showed a moderate number of spherocytes. No abnormalities were detected by the following tests: red cell glucose 6-phosphate dehydrogenase, hemoglobin electrophoresis, lactic dehydrogenase, bilirubin, VDRL, HBs-antigen, and liver function tests.

She had a hemolytic anemia as manifested by persistent anemia (hematocrit 24 to 27 percent) and reticulocytosis (6.3 to 10.3 percent) (Figure 9-1). The direct antiglobulin test was negative throughout her pregnancy using polyspecific antiglobulin serum and multiple dilutions of monospecific anti-IgG, anti-C3, and anti-C4 antisera. No antibody was detected in her serum or in an eluate from her red cells. Hereditary spherocytosis was suspected but six of her seven children were examined and none showed evidence of spherocytosis. The peripheral blood films, hematocrits and reticulocyte counts were normal in all, thus making hereditary spherocytosis very unlikely.

A complement-fixing antibody consumption test performed on the patient's blood revealed 212 IgG molecules per red cell. The patient was treated with 50 mg of prednisone daily throughout the remainder of her pregnancy.

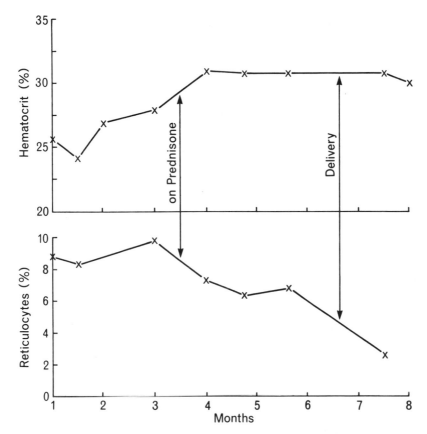

Figure 9-1. *The clinical course of a patient with relapsing hemolytic anemia of pregnancy with a negative direct antiblobulin test. Hemolytic anemia was evident prior to the initiation of therapy with prednisone as manifested by anemia with reticulocytosis. The anemia resolved, but reticulocytosis persisted during prednisone therapy until the delivery of the patient's baby. Thereafter the reticulocytosis subsided and prednisone therapy was gradually withdrawn (see text).*

Three weeks after initiation of therapy with prednisone her hematocrit level rose to 31 percent with a reticulocyte count of about 7.5 percent. The reticulocytosis persisted until delivery. Therafter the reticulocyte count decreased to a level that was persistently less than 1 percent. Prednisone was gradually decreased and then discontinued. Postnatal serologic findings remained negative. The complement-fixing antibody consumption test performed two weeks postpartum revealed a significant reduction in red cell sensitization. At this time only 53 molecules of IgG per red cell were present. The baby was anemic at birth, with a hemoglobin of 12.2 gm/dl. The complement-fixing antibody consumption test on a cord blood sample revealed 250 molecules of IgG per red blood cell. The infant did not require therapy, and 14 days later only 25 molecules of IgG per red blood cell were detectable (Table 9-4).

Table 9-4. COMPLEMENT FIXING ANTIGLOBULIN CONSUMP-
TION TEST IN A PATIENT WITH RELAPSING HEMOLYTIC
ANEMIA OF PREGNANCY AND A NEGATIVE DIRECT ANTI-
GLOBULIN TEST.

	Molecules of IgG/RBC	
	Pre Partum	Post Partum
Mother	212	53
Newborn	–	250 (cord blood)
		<25 (14 days post partum)

This case represents the first instance in which evidence has been presented supporting the hypothesis that the hemolysis in a case of relapsing
hemolytic anemia of pregnancy is immunologically mediated.

In two other cases described by Yam et al.,[144] the maternal hemolytic
anemia persisted after delivery. Since future pregnancies were possible, and
since life-threatening exacerbations of hemolysis occur so frequently during
pregnancy, an elective splenectomy was performed in the postpartum period
in each case at a time when only mild to moderate hemolytic disease was
present. In both patients hemolysis subsided and continued therapy with
corticosteriods was unnecessary.

The Cause of Hemolytic Anemia in Pregnancy: The cause of exacerbation of hemolysis or the recurrent development of hemolytic anemia during
pregnancy remains speculative, particularly since pregnancy is not invariably
associated with worsening of several disease states commonly thought of as
autoimmune. Exacerbations of systemic lupus erythematosus during the third
trimester of pregnancy are uncommon and, moreover, about 50 percent of
the patients are improved during pregnancy, as are a majority of patients with
rheumatoid arthritis. Thus, immune aberrations associated with pregnancy
cannot adequately explain the extremely frequent worsening of autoimmune
hemolytic anemia during pregnancy. Others have postulated [21, 61] that fetal-
maternal transplacental hemorrhage leads to stimulation of maternal au-
tosensitized immunocompetent cells, increasing their autoantibody production as pregnancy progresses. This hypothesis may offer at least a partial
explanation in those patients in whom evidence of increased antibody production during pregnancy can be documented. However, changes in the intensity
of hemolysis are not necessarily correlated with changes in strength of
the direct antiglobulin test or in titers of autoantibodies present in the
serum.[21]

Changes in function of elements of the cellular immune system during
pregnancy resulting in an increased rate of red cell destruction of antibody
coated cells perhaps contribute to the exacerbation of hemolysis that so regu-

larly occurs during pregnancy. Studies of macrophage activity during pregnancy would certainly be of interest in this regard.

Alternatively, non-immunologic factors related to pregnancy may be responsible for some cases, as has recently been suggested by Goodall et al.[57]

Management: Although the cause of exacerbation of hemolysis in pregnancy is not well defined, the potential seriousness of pregnancy in autoimmune hemolytic anemia justifies very close observation of the patient. Antenatal hematologic evaluation appears indicated every two weeks until the 8th month of pregnancy and weekly therafter until delivery. Such evaluations should include as a minimum a blood count and reticulocyte count. Determining the titer of the serum autoantibody may offer additional information, although there is as yet little data on correlation of autoantibody titers and the severity of autoantibody-induced hemolytic disease of the newborn. Corticosteroid therapy should be given in doses adequate to suppress hemolysis in an effort to maintain a hemoglobin level above 10 gm/dl. Amniocentesis appears indicated in the presence of brisk hemolysis which is mediated by an IgG autoantibody.[21, 144] If steroids are not effective in controlling hemolysis and/or if amniocentesis indicates high fetal risk, splenectomy may be indicated, although we are not aware of its having been performed for this indication during pregnancy. In some instances, early induction of labor has been employed in critically ill patients.[21] Since exacerbation of autoimmune hemolytic anemia so frequently occurs during pregnancy, an elective splenectomy appears warranted in the postpartum period, particularly if evidence of hemolysis persists.[144] However, the effectiveness of splenectomy in preventing hemolytic anemia in subsequent pregnancies has not yet been demonstrated.

C. THE DIFFERENTIATION BETWEEN A DELAYED HEMOLYTIC TRANSFUSION REACTION AND AUTOIMMUNE HEMOLYTIC ANEMIA

Delayed hemolytic transfusion reactions are a recognized risk of blood transfusion. The reaction is caused by the reappearance of an antibody, presumably first stimulated by pregnancy or a previous transfusion. Unlike immediate transfusion reactions, which are usually caused by human error,[106] delayed reactions are usually not avoidable. Since hemolysis is delayed in onset (typically 3 to 14 days after transfusion) the relationship of hemolytic anemia to prior transfusion may not be suspected, and a diagnosis of autoimmune hemolytic anemia may seem more appropriate.

As in any patient with the acute onset of hemolysis, findings may include fever, pallor, jaundice, hemoglobinemia, hemoglobinuria and, rarely, disseminated intravascular coagulation or renal failure.[30] Further, laboratory tests are likely to reveal the presence of positive direct and indirect antiglobulin tests, spherocytosis, and reticulocytosis. If multiple alloantibodies or an alloantibody against a high incidence antigen are formed, the findings may be difficult to differentiate from autoimmune hemolytic anemia. The diagnostic problem is compounded by the fact that, in some cases, autoimmune hemolytic anemia may actually develop as a consequence of blood transfusion (described later in this chapter). Indeed, therapy with corticosteroids for suspected autoimmune hemolytic anemia has been instituted [31, 134] or contemplated [63, 118] in some reported cases of delayed hemolytic transfusion reactions before the correct diagnosis was made.

A characteristic example of a patient who had a delayed hemolytic transfusion reaction simulating autoimmune hemolytic anemia was reported by Croucher, Crookston, and Crookston.[31] They described a patient with vaginal bleeding who was transfused with 10 units of blood over a period of 8 days. Despite the arrest of hemorrhage her hemoglobin level continued to fall. The patient was found to be pale and jaundiced; her urine was dark and contained "urobilin" but did not contain hemoglobin or bile. The spleen was just palpable. Her hemoglobin, which had been 8.5 gm/dl at a time that hemorrhage ceased, dropped to about 6 gm/dl. At this time her reticulocyte count was 13 percent and it subsequently rose to a peak of 24 percent. The blood film showed small agglutinates, many spherocytes, and some myelocytes and normoblasts. The serum bilirubin was 4.5 mg/dl and serum haptoglobin [42] was absent. The direct antiglobulin test was strongly positive. The patient's serum reacted with her own cells and with samples from more than 30 donors, and thus appeared to have a "non-specific" autoantibody.

However, careful serologic studies documented the presence of anti-Fy[a], anti-Ce and anti-e alloantibodies, and the patient's hemolytic anemia resolved without therapy. The direct antiglobulin test rapidly weakened and became negative 10 days after the last transfusion, but the indirect antiglobulin test remained strongly positive throughout hospitalization.

Diagnostic Aids: As mentioned in Chapters 5 and 6, a presumptive diagnosis of warm antibody autoimmune hemolytic anemia may be entertained in a patient who has not been transfused during the previous 4 months, has an acquired hemolytic anemia with a positive direct antiglobulin test, does not have a cold agglutinin of high thermal amplitude, has not been taking drugs, and has a warm antibody with broad reactivity in the serum or red cell eluate. This diagnosis tends to be correct because, if donor red cells no longer remain in the patient's circulation, alloantibodies cannot be causing either the acquired hemolytic anemia or the positive direct antiglobulin test. Even in this setting, we recommend further tests to characterize the patient's red cell antibody(ies) in order to avoid diagnostic error, and to have results of specificity tests available should transfusion be necessary. If a patient has been transfused within recent weeks, such additional testing is mandatory to distinguish between a delayed hemolytic transfusion reaction and autoimmune hemolytic anemia. Some simple measures may afford important clues.

"Mixed Field" Direct Antiglobulin Test: Since donor red cells as well as the patient's own red cells are circulating, the direct antiglobulin test may be positive with a "mixed field" type of reaction. The alloantibody that has been stimulated by transfusion of donor red cells will not react with the patient's own cells, and therefore only a portion of the circulating red cells will be agglutinated by antiglobulin serum. However, if the patient has been transfused with large volumes of red cells, and if he has an alloantibody or a mixture of alloantibodies having a broad range of reactivity, the "mixed field" reaction may be difficult to detect.

Comparison of Direct and Indirect Antiglobulin Tests: Another simple observation that may yield valuable information is the comparison of the strength of the direct and indirect antiglobulin tests. As is stressed in Chapter 10, the direct antiglobulin test is almost always stronger than the indirect antiglobulin test in warm antibody autoimmune hemolytic anemia. It appears that autoantibody is largely adsorbed onto the patient's red cells, and only when the cells are heavily coated does one find a large amount of antibody in the serum. In contrast, strongly reactive alloantibodies may be present in a patient's serum, but this finding cannot result in a strongly positive direct antiglobulin test unless large numbers of transfused cells of appropriate antigenic type are present. Thus the presence of a weakly positive direct antiglobulin test in association with a strongly positive indirect antiglobulin test is strong evidence for the presence of an alloantibody. These findings may be present in a delayed hemolytic transfusion reaction, particularly if only a relatively small volume of red cells of appropriate antigenic type have been transfused or if many of the transfused red cells have already been destroyed. Further, even if the direct antiglobulin test is strongly positive at the time of initial evaluation, it may soon become weaker in subsequent tests as a result of the destruction of the transfused red cells as was true in the case of Croucher et al. that was previously described. In contrast, a rapid diminution in the strength of the direct antiglobulin test would not be expected in autoimmune hemolytic anemia except as a result of treatment (as with corticosteroids or splenectomy).

Antibody Specificity: An important means of differentiating autoimmune hemolytic anemia from a delayed hemolytic transfusion reaction relates to the specificity of the antibody(ies) present in the serum and in a red cell eluate. Some antibodies that commonly cause delayed hemolytic transfusion reactions have not been found or have been reported only rarely as autoantibodies in autoimmune hemolytic anemia. The outstanding example is anti-Jk^a, which is the antibody that has been most commonly incriminated in published cases of delayed hemolytic transfusion reactions.[30, 107] Similarly, the finding of anti-Jk^b, -Fy^a, or Kell antibodies would be strong evidence for alloimmunization.

Many autoantibodies in warm antibody autoimmune hemolytic anemia demonstrate specificity within the Rh system but, even here, a distinction between autoantibodies and alloantibodies with Rh specificity is often possible. Whereas alloantibodies demonstrate truly specific reactions and give clearly negative reactions with cells lacking the appropriate antigen, autoantibodies almost always demonstrate "relative specificity." That is, autoantibodies that are described as having specificity within the Rh system react more strongly or to a higher titer against red cells bearing a particular Rh antigen, but they will nevertheless react with red cells lacking the antigen. Thus a truly specific Rh antibody strongly suggests that it is an alloantibody, whereas an antibody demonstrating "relative specificity" is characteristic of autoantibody. However, a mixture of an Rh alloantibody and an autoantibody reacting equally but less strongly with all normal red cells will appear similar to an autoantibody. A differentiation of these two possibilities would be difficult, except by using the patient's pre-transfusion red cells for cell typing or for the warm autoabsorption test, or by utilizing the differential absorption test (see Chapter 10).

A further clue to the differentiation of autoantibodies and alloantibodies having Rh specificity is the specificity itself. That is, anti-e has only once been incriminated in a delayed hemolytic transfusion reaction,[30] but it is the most frequently described autoantibody against common Rh antigens (i.e., C, c, D, E, e). In contrast, anti-E is the most common Rh alloantibody responsible for delayed hemolytic transfusion reactions,[30, 107] but it is a relatively unusual autoantibody. Again, if pre-transfusion red cells are still available, it will be possible to use them to distinguish alloantibody from autoantibody with certainty.

Separating Donor and Recipient's Red Cells: Another method that has been described as beneficial [31] in distinguishing alloantibodies from autoantibodies is based on the fact that reticulocytes can be separated from older red cells by centrifugation.[24, 113] This method is particularly practical if the reticulocyte count is 10 percent or more. In this case it may be possible to incriminate an alloantibody by finding that the reticulocytes, which are the patient's own cells, have a negative direct antiglobulin test, while the older cells that contain the transfused cells have a positive direct antiglobulin test. It may also be possible to do cell typing on the reticulocyte rich and reticulocyte poor portions of blood.[31]

Additional Approaches: If the recipient's direct antiglobulin test was known to be negative prior to transfusion, or if the recipient's red cells are still available for the performance of the direct antiglobulin test and it is demonstrated to be negative, this can be valuable information. An abrupt change in the antiglobulin test from negative to positive is strong evidence that the patient has a hemolytic transfusion reaction rather than autoimmune hemolytic anemia.

If it is possible to test the donor units of blood, this procedure may be of significance if an antibody having specificity that could be either an alloantibody or autoantibody is detected, such as, for example, anti-E. If by chance, none of the donor units contained the E antigen, autoimmune hemolytic anemia or an alloantibody-induced hemolytic transfusion reaction caused by an undetected antibody must be considered.

Thus, with careful serologic testing, it is possible to distinguish a delayed hemolytic transfusion reaction from autoimmune hemolytic anemia in almost all cases. However, if pre-transfusion red cells are not available (as, unfortunately, is usually the case), and if the patient has an alloantibody or mixture of alloantibodies with a broad range of reactivity, and if a large volume of donor cells have been transfused, the distinction may be difficult.

D. THE DEVELOPMENT OF AUTOIMMUNE HEMOLYTIC ANEMIA FOLLOWING BLOOD TRANSFUSION

Our interest in the role of blood transfusion as a possible cause of autoimmune hemolytic anemia was stimulated by the observation that one of our patients who developed two red cell alloantibodies also developed a positive direct antiglobulin test and autoimmune hemolytic anemia after receiving blood transfusions. Patient J.O. was a type O Rh-negative elderly man with gastrointestinal bleeding of undetermined origin; he received 2 units of group O Rh-positive blood. The direct and indirect antiglobulin tests were negative at this time. Eight weeks later anti-Rh$_o$(D) was present in his serum, but the direct antiglobulin test remained negative. Two units of group O, Rh-negative blood were transfused, and subsequently no further transfusions were required. Two months later anti-Rh$_o$(D) (titer of 1024), anti-rh″(E) (titer of 8) and anti-rh′(c) (titer of 8) were detected in his serum, as was a weak IgG "nonspecific" antibody that reacted with all red cells of a panel. The direct antiglobulin test was positive, and IgG antibody eluted from the red cells showed no evident blood group specificity. Three weeks later the direct antiglobulin test remained positive, the "nonspecific" autoantibody in the serum had increased in titer, and the patient developed mild signs of hemolytic anemia. The direct antiglobulin test was performed biweekly for the next four months and remained positive without any diminution in the strength of the reaction. Signs of hemolysis gradually subsided spontaneously, and performance of the direct antiglobulin test monthly indicated a gradual weakening of the reaction during the subsequent six months. The patient was next evaluated two years later, at which time the direct antiglobulin test was negative.

Previous Reports of the Development of Autoantibodies Following Transfusion of Foreign Red Cells: Although the development of autoantibodies after blood transfusion is not frequently recognized, there are a significant number of recorded observations relating to this phenomenon.

Dameshek and Levine in 1943 [35] first suggested that multiple transfusions could lead to alloimmunization and a resulting hemolytic crisis. They reported a case in which successive transfusions resulted in extreme, almost fatal, hemolysis. They suggested that an irreversible autohemolytic process had been established by the multiple transfusions, and that this was then intensified by a severe hemolytic transfusion reaction. Allen, in discussing a paper presented at the Eighth Congress of the International Society of Blood Transfusion, stated that he had seen acute acquired hemolytic anemia complicating hemolytic transfusion reactions.[1]

Polesky and Bove [109] described a fatal hemolytic transfusion reaction in a woman with marrow hypoplasia associated with acute leukemia. Radioactive chromium studies, which were in progress at the time, made it possible to demonstrate that a severe autohemolytic crisis was part of the reaction. The authors postulated the presence of autoantibodies but could not demonstrate their presence.

Zmijewski [145] immunized chimpanzees with human blood. As expected, a circulating antibody against human red cells was produced. In addition autoantibodies were produced that reacted against the chimpanzees' own cells. The chimpanzee cells were shown to be sensitized with IgG and complement. The antibody eluted from the chimpanzee cells showed some allospecificity when tested against other chimpanzee cells, and it also reacted with human cells. Zmijewski postulated that the autoantibody was produced as a result of a breakdown in immunologic tolerance after the administration of closely related antigens, as previously described by Weigle.[140]

Ovary and Spiegelman [96] employed a rabbit test system. They documented the formation of allo- and auto-panhemagglutinins directed against both the donor and recipient erythrocytes when a rabbit was immunized with donor erythrocytes. The alloantibodies produced were a mixture of IgG and IgM antibodies; the auto-panhemagglutinin was an IgM antibody reactive only at 4°C.

Liu and Evans [79] described the occurrence of a positive direct antiglobulin test in three of 12 rabbits, following intraperitoneal injections of homologous blood. These experiments were performed to simulate the observation of a transient positive direct antiglobulin test in a patient with anemia secondary to intraperitoneal bleeding from a ruptured ectopic pregnancy. It was suggested that relatively bland treatment of red cells may result in modification of surface structure sufficient to produce antibody formation.

Fudenberg, Rosenfield, and Wasserman [51] described two patients who produced alloantibodies as a result of transfusion and then deliberate immunization. Both patients developed strongly positive direct antiglobulin tests, with autoantibodies as well as alloantibodies present in the serum. The authors suggested that an explanation of this finding is the lack of control over antibody production that is always taking place. Thus it might be assumed that all individuals are subject to autoerythrocytic antibody production, but that hemolytic anemia results only when this "horror autotoxicus" outruns normal curbs. Another possible explanation is that of immunization to an Rh structure common to all Rh antigens, yielding results suggestive of complete nonspecificity. Such immunization could arise either *de novo* as the initial sensitization or as a result of initial immunization to a blood factor in the Rh system, with subsequent widening of the "spectrum of specificity" as further stimulation occurred.

Chown et al. [22] described two Rh-negative women who produced anti-Rh during pregnancy and later developed positive direct antiglobulin tests. Beard et al.[8] described an Rh-negative patient who was transfused with 400 ml of Rh-positive blood. The foreign cells were eliminated from the circulation over a period of 5 days by large doses of anti-D immunoglobulin assisted by a rapid immune response. Six months later the patient developed a positive direct antiglobulin test that persisted for 3 months.

Lalezari et al.[75] described a 40-year-old black woman who had the rare Rh phenotype $Rh^d(D)$, Category III, which lacks a component of Rh antigenic material. She had been transfused with several units of $Rh_o(D)$ positive blood, and 10 years later received three additional units. She developed a high titer anti-$Rh_o(D)$ and this anamnestic response was associated with the development of an autoantibody. The direct antiglobulin test, which was negative prior to transfusion, became positive and remained so for 6 months. A red cell eluate revealed a strong anti-$Rh_o(D)$ and a weak "panagglutinin" by the Polybrene technique.

Cook[26] immunized 34 Rh negative male volunteers with Rh positive blood. In addition to the development of the expected anti-$Rh_o(D)$ in 68 percent of the volunteers, 11 men developed an antibody that reacted with Rh negative enzyme-treated red cells; two developed a positive direct antiglobulin test (inhibited by pure IgG) that persisted for about 4 months. No evidence of hemolytic anemia was present, although red cell survival studies were not performed.

Cox and Keast[27, 28] produced erythrocyte autoantibodies in mice immunized with rat erythrocytes. They suggested that immunologic tolerance can be terminated temporarily by immunization with antigens cross-reacting with self.

Worlledge[142] has stated that persistent alloimmunization may lead eventually to autoimmunization, and that one certainly sees patients who have had repeated transfusions and who have developed multiple alloantibodies, in whom a positive antiglobulin test appears even though compatible red cells have been given. The antibody eluted from the red cells in this situation often seems to react with all cells except Rh_{null} cells.

Evidence that Autoantibodies in the Recipient are Produced by the Immune Apparatus of the Donor: Viable lymphocytes, capable of responding to phytohemagglutinin have been demonstrated in blood stored in A.C.D. solution for up to one month.[81, 100, 135] Further, graft-versus-host reactions have been described following blood transfusion in immunologically deficient individuals.[60, 64] Immunohemolytic anemia is an outstanding feature of graft-versus-host reactions. In chickens,[23] mice,[95] and rabbits[110] the syndrome is typical, with positive antiglobulin tests, reticulocytosis, and shortening of red cell survival time. Shapiro[126] described a case of autoimmune hemolytic anemia with the clinical features of runt disease in a three-month-old child. He suggested that maternal blood may have gained access to the baby's circulation, and that maternal lymphoid cells had survived and set up a graft-versus-host reaction. It was further suggested that the immunologic activity of the graft was triggered by an infection. Similar cases have been described in adults with acquired hypogammaglobulinemia [50, 62] and in children with dys-gammaglobulinemia. [121]

Delayed hypersensitivity can be transferred by blood transfusion in humans. Mohr et al. [89] demonstrated a passive transfer of delayed skin hypersensitivity to purified protein derivative of tuberlin (tuberculin PPD) in 5 recipients who previously had negative reactions to tuberculin, after receiving transfusions of whole blood from donors with known positive reactions. The reactivity persisted for at least 8 months.

Lawrence [76] has shown that the delayed sensitivity acquired in individuals injected with viable circulating leukocytes or leukocyte extracts (e.g., transfer factor) can be effective in man for several years.

Fishman and Adler,[45] and Mitsuhashi et al.[86] have shown that "immune-RNA" prepared from culture filtrates of macrophages or extracted from the spleens of immunized animals could induce antibody formation *in vitro,* when added to cells of non-immunized animals. Kawakami et al. [72] showed that spleen cells from individual mice produced autoantibody against their own red cells when the spleen cells were treated *in vitro* with RNA preparations obtained from the spleen of an allogeneic mouse immunized with red cells from that individual. Watanabe and Mitsuhashi [139] have shown that the injection into animals of "immune-RNA" obtained from the culture filtrate of peritoneal macrophages, derived from immunized animals, would induce proliferation of antibody-forming cells *in vivo.* "Memory" cells capable of responding to a secondary stimulus with an antigen to produce a high titer serum antibody were shown to be present. Bell and Dray[9-11] have shown that RNA extracts obtained from peritoneal exudate cells or lymph node cells of rabbits immunized with a single injection of sheep cells would convert spleen cells from nonimmunized animals to antibody-forming cells. They were able to produce IgG and IgM antibodies showing light- and heavy-chain allotypic specificity of the RNA donor, which were foreign to the allotype of the animal from which the antibody-producing cells were obtained. The active synthesis of IgM and IgG antibody with foreign allotype by "RNA-converted" cells was explained by attributing a messenger role for the RNA.

Schechter et al. [122] noted a fivefold or greater rise in atypical lymphocytes or *in vitro* ^{3}H-thymidine incorporation by blood leukocytes (or both) occurring one week after blood transfusion. These values declined to pretransfusion levels by the third week. The results were significantly greater than in patients undergoing surgery without transfusion, autotransfused patients, or patients receiving frozen-thawed leukocyte-poor blood. Lymphocytotoxic reactivity was also detected in 6 of 12 patients. It was suggested that the frequency and timing of this cellular activation and its absence after the administration of leukocyte-depleted red cells favored an immunologic response to HLA antigens on the transfused leukocytes and platelets.

A later report by Schechter et al,[123] described cytogenetic studies that were performed on the peripheral blood leukocytes of 10 adult patients who received fresh blood from donors of the opposite sex. Nine of the 10 patients had spontaneously dividing mononuclear cells of the recipient or host karyotype circulating during the latter part of the first week after transfusion. In two patients, the spontaneously dividing cells were of donor as well as of host origin. The authors suggested that these data indicated the counterpart of the *in vitro* mixed leukocyte reaction, and that dividing donor cells may represent a subclinical graft-versus-host reaction.

Production of Autoantibodies by Transfusion of Alloantibodies: Mohn et al.[87, 88] performed a unique set of experiments that led to the production of autoantibodies in humans but did not involve transfusion of donor cells. These investigators transfused volunteers with potent incompatible Rhesus (anti-CD) antibodies. Approximately 240 ml of antibody-containing plasmas were transfused into three recipients of cDE/cDE, CDe/cDE and cde/cde genotypes. Acute hemolytic anemia ensued in the D positive recipients. Direct antiglobulin tests on the red cells were positive immediately, remaining so for 168 and 202 days respectively for the cDE/cDE and CDe/CDe recipients. Eluates from the red cells of the cDE/cDE recipient revealed activity for his pretransfusion cells and cDe/cde cells to the end of the study. A surprising finding was the presence of a specific anti-E in the red cell eluate. This antibody appeared on the 70th day post-transfusion and persisted at a high level through the 229-day observation period. The authors concluded that the anti-E could represent only new autoantibody formation by the recipient himself. They hypothesized that the autoantibodies were produced in response to alterations brought about at the Rh sites on the erythrocyte membrane by the antigen-antibody reactions between the D antigen receptors on the recipient's red cells and the transfused anti-CD alloantibodies, involving the E antigen receptors in the autoimmunization process by reason of their proximity.

The Possible Role of Genetic Factors and T-cell Responsiveness in the Development of Autoimmune Hemolytic Anemia: Additional factors that may be of significance in the development of idiopathic autoimmune hemolytic anemia may play a role in those cases in which autoantibodies appear to develop as a result of blood transfusion. In this regard, a significant body of data has been developed implicating genetic factors and T-cell responsiveness.

Recent evidence has suggested that susceptibility to certain autoimmune disease, as well as other pathologic states, is determined by specific immune response genes.[3, 82] This concept was fostered by the observations that specific immune responsiveness to a variety of antigens appeared to be determined by genes linked to the species major histocompatability locus.[83] Indeed, there are now numerous reports of association of particular major histocompatability locus specificities and specific disease states.[85, 120] Susceptibility to immunologic disorders, which may be multigenic in nature, could in part be determined by specific immune response genes governing responsiveness to certain exogenous and endogenous antigens.

Warner has reported [138] that two genes, one dominant and one recessive, are carried by NZB mice and are associated with the spontaneous production of anti-red cell autoantibody in that strain, and that NZC mice carry only the recessive gene. In attempts to induce expression of this gene in NZC mice, groups of mice of various inbred strains were immunized with syngeneic or allogeneic mouse erythrocytes emulsified in complete Freunds adjuvant. At various intervals, the mice were then tested for the development of a positive antiglobulin test. Whereas mice of most strains immunized with allogeneic red cells failed to show positive direct antiglobulin tests, most of the NZC mice developed positive reactions. Two injections of allogeneic red cells in adjuvant were necessary for the induction of this autoantibody production; injection of either allogeneic red cells without adjuvant, or syngeneic red cells with adjuvant were ineffective. Thus, the data indicated that red cells constitute an effective stimulus to the development of anti-red cell autoantibodies, and that there is a genetic control of the production of both spontaneous and induced examples of these autoantibodies.

Another body of evidence has suggested that T-cells play an important role in the homeostatic control of antibody production. Baker and Stashak found that treatment of BALB/c mice with anti-lymphocyte serum prior to immunization with pneumococcal polysaccharide type III resulted in enhanced anti-Pn III antibody production.[4] Moreover, administration of syngeneic thymocytes to these animals resulted in dimunution in antibody titer.[5] Other evidence has been provided by the model of Jacobson et al. of allotype suppression [67] and Okumura's demonstration of control of homocytrophic antibody production of T-cells.[94]

That this regulatory function encompasses autoantibody production as well has been suggested by numerous investigators.[2,47,48] Fudenburg[48] has suggested that the T suppressor cells, presumably coming from the appendix and Peyer patches of normal man, affect the level of autoimmune cells in lymph nodes, spleen and other organs to modulate the levels of both autoantibodies and cellular autoimmunity to various body organs and tissue. In T-cell immune deficiency, T suppressor cells may be disporportionately diminished either in number or in function, so that the autoimmune clones increase and cause disease.

In a series of reports by Dewar, Parker, Stuart, et al.[36,97,99] measurements were made of homologous and autologous rosetting cells in the peripheral blood of patients with autoimmune hemolytic anemia. In 12 of 14 patients, high levels of rosetting cells were present. In 10 of these patients, who were observed over a period of two years, the levels bore a direct relationship to the activity of the disease.[99] Ultrastructural studies[97] indicated that the predominant homologous rosette-forming cell was lymphocytic and the evidence favored the conclusion that they were nonimmune in nature. Forty-four percent of the total lymphocytic rosette-forming cells had features consistent with activated T cells, and the remainder had no features that allowed their identification as T or B cells.

Krüger et al. also studied patients with warm antibody autoimmune hemolytic anemia for abnormalities of cellular immune reactions.[74] In contrast to the data of Parker et al.,[99] evidence was obtained for a reduction of rosette-forming cells in 36 of 41 determinations in 19 patients. The authors interpreted their results as evidence that a reduction of T-cells may be operative in autoimmune hemolytic anemia, leading to an imbalance between reduced T-cells and an increased but uncontrolled humoral immune response toward red cell autoantigens. Both Krüger et al.[74] and Parker et al.[99] suggested that further studies were indicated employing methods for discrimination of T-cell subpopulations.[2, 16, 119, 137]

Further evidence that disordered T-cell regulatory function is important in autoimmune disorders is derived from the following observations: I. occurrence of autoantibodies in chickens and rabbits neonatally thymectomized;[84, 131] II. the increased propensity of neonatal obese strain chickens to develop autoimmune thyroiditis following neonatal bursectomy;[49] III. demonstration of impaired T-cell function in NZB mice [17, 78, 130] and the results of lymphoid cell transfers in this strain;[2] IV. thymocyte transfer studies in aging A strain mice.[133]

Thus it is possible that some autoimmune states are characterized by a genetically determined aberrant responsiveness to specific exogenous antigens, and that impaired responsiveness of modulating T-cells could eventuate in the unbridled production of autoantibody.

Summary: There is ample clinical and experimental evidence to suggest that transfusion may lead to the development of autoantibodies. This phenomenon may result from a graft-versus-host type of reaction due to prolonged survival of donor mononuclear leukocytes. However, autoantibodies have also been produced merely by transfusions of plasma-containing alloantibodies, thus suggesting that in at least some instances, the host immune system is the source of the autoantibodies.

Mounting evidence suggests that genetic factors and alterations of T-cell responsiveness are of significance in the pathogenesis of autoimmune hemolytic anemia.

E. SERUM COMPLEMENT IN AUTOIMMUNE HEMOLYTIC ANEMIA

The significance of complement in red cell destruction in autoimmune hemolytic anemia has been reviewed in detail in Chapters 3 and 4, and, in addition, we have previously reviewed selected aspects of the role of complement in immunohematology.[43, 101, 103–105] The serum concentration of complement in autoimmune hemolytic anemia has been studied by several investigators and has been found to be low in some patients with autoimmune hemolytic anemia associated with warm or cold antibodies.

Studies reported in the older medical literature utilized hemolytic assays for "total complement." Raeder [111] found subnormal levels in 7 out of 15 patients suffering from miscellaneous types of hemolytic anemia. Van Loghem et al.[136] reported low complement levels in 20 percent of patients with incomplete warm antibodies and in 50 percent of those forming cold agglutinins. Dacie [32] reported subnormal serum complement concentrations in 5 of 8 patients with warm antibody autoimmune hemolytic anemia and in 9 of 9 patients with cold agglutinin syndrome. In 3 of the patients with cold agglutinin syndrome, a normal concentration of serum complement was recorded at other times during their disease. In paroxysmal cold hemoglobinuria, serum complement is frequently low during an acute attack. Jordan [71] reported low complement levels in 3 of 4 patients, and van Loghem et al. [136] reported low levels in all of 17 patients. The possibility of a low complement level must be considered in performing the Donath-Landsteiner test (see page 175).

More recently, Kretschmer and Mueller-Eckhardt [73] reported results of direct antiglobulin tests and serum C3 and C4 levels as determined by radial immunodiffusion in 69 patients with warm antibody autoimmune hemolytic anemia. They found that serum C3 was normal in all 17 patients who had IgG but not complement demonstrable on their red cells as indicated by the direct antiglobulin test. Low serum C3 levels were found in 9 of 33 (27 percent) patients who had both IgG and complement on their red cells and in 4 of 19 (21 percent) patients whose cells were coated with complement but not IgG. Similarly, serum C4 was normal in 17 patients who had only IgG on their red cells, and was low in 14 of 19 (74 percent) patients with IgG and complement on their red cells, and in 9 of 19 (47 percent) patients whose red cells were sensitized with complement but not with IgG. The authors reported that there was an inverse correlation between serum C3 and serum C4 and the degree of hemolysis. Further, in 23 patients who were repeatedly investigated during the course of the disease, a significant correlation was found between improvement of hemolysis and the rise of serum C3 and C4.

The concentrations of serum C3 and C4 as measured by radial immunodiffusion in 55 patients with warm antibody autoimmune hemolytic anemia studied in our laboratory are indicated in Figure 9-2. Of 13 patients whose red cells were sensitized only with IgG, 2 patients had a low serum C3 and 2 had low serum C4 values. Among 37 patients with IgG and C3 on their red cells, 12 had low levels of C3, and 16 had low levels of C4. There were 5 patients whose red cells were sensitized only with complement, and 3 of these had a low serum C3 and 4 had a low serum C4.

Among 16 patients with cold agglutinin syndrome (Figure 9-3), 6 had low C3 levels and 10 had low C4.

Not indicated are the serum concentrations of C3 and C4 in 8 patients who had warm antibody autoimmune hemolytic anemia associated with the use of methyldopa. In 6 of the 8 patients, both C3 and C4 were normal, but in 2 patients the C3 value was minimally reduced (85 mg/dl).

Our previous studies of the metabolism of radiolabelled C3 in patients with warm antibody autoimmune hemolytic anemia [105] indicated that the *in vivo* catabolism was increased in the patients that we studied whose red cells were sensitized at least in part by C3. In some patients, a moderate increase in catabolic rate is balanced by an increased rate of synthesis, thus maintaining a normal serum concentration. Thus a normal concentration of serum C3 can-

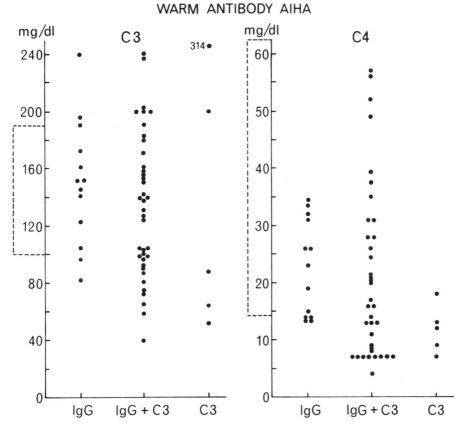

WARM ANTIBODY AIHA

Figure 9-2. Serum C3 and C4 levels as measured by radial immundiffusion in 55 patients with warm antibody AIHA. The patients are divided into three categories on the basis of results of the direct antiglobulin test using monospecific IgG and C3 antisera. The normal ranges are indicated by the dotted lines.

not be taken to indicate that complement is playing no role in the mechanism of red cell destruction.

Occasionally, the use of washed red cells [40] or frozen-thawed red cells for transfusion is suggested with the rationale that supplying complement in the donor plasma may augment a patient's hemolysis. Indeed, Evans et al. [40, 41] studied red cell survival and serum complement levels in 4 patients with cold agglutinin syndrome. All patients studied had reduced levels of serum hemolytic complement with values of 34, 35, 40, and 70 CH_{50} units/ml (normal = 85–125 CH_{50} units/ml). Their data indicated that a small volume of radiolabelled normal red cells were removed with a half-time of less than 24 hours when infused into a patient, yet transfusion of 500 ml of red cells was given without reaction, and the half-time of these cells as measured by the Ashby technique was 19 days or roughly one third of normal. This finding suggested that the mechanism for hemolysis of normal red cells by cold agglutinin was limited, perhaps by depletion of complement. In experiments

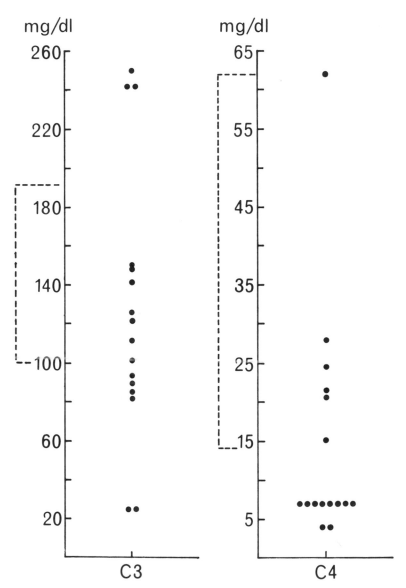

Figure 9-3. *Serum C3 and C4 levels as measured by radial immunodiffusion in 16 patients with cold agglutinin syndrome. In all cases the direct antiglobulin test was positive with anti-C3 and negative with anti-IgG. The normal ranges are indicated by the dotted lines.*

in two other patients they measured red cell survival of ^{51}Cr labelled cells before and after transfusion of about 2 units of red cells and found improved survival in the period following transfusion. They further determined that a drop in serum complement followed the infusion of the large volumes of red cells, presumably due to the utilization of complement during complement sensitization and lysis of the transfused red cells. They suggested that the fall in serum complement levels that followed the introduction of large volumes of red cells was the most obvious explanation for the improved red cell survival found after transfusion. On the basis of these findings, the authors transfused red cells that were washed in order to avoid the infusion of complement that might augment the hemolysis of the transfused red cells. It appears that no additional experiments of this type have been reported.

However, as indicated in Figures 9-2 and 9-3, C3 and C4 are frequently normal, and are only strikingly reduced in a minority of patients with autoimmune hemolytic anemia. Even in patients with reduced levels of complement, evidence that such reductions in complement components are a rate limiting factor in causing hemolysis is inconclusive. Thus, further data are needed to assess the significance of complement that is transfused in association with red cells in patients with autoimmune hemolytic anemia. This topic is discussed further in Chapter 10.

F. CHRONIC IDIOPATHIC PAROXYSMAL COLD HEMOGLOBINURIA

One of the rarest forms of autoimmune hemolytic anemia is chronic idiopathic paroxysmal cold hemoglobinuria. We have observed one such patient, whose early course has previously been reported in detail by Ries, Garratty, Petz, et al.[114] The serologic features were unique because of the presence of a Donath-Landsteiner antibody of exceptionally high thermal range. Further, she had a remarkable response to splenectomy, which has only rarely been utilized as therapy for this disorder.

Case 9-5: L.Z., a 60-year-old widow of Portuguese-Irish heritage, who resided in northern California, had been well except for mild labile hypertension and "hypothyroidism" until late July 1970, when she first had intermittent fevers, chills, and night sweats, followed by progressive weakness, fatigue, and malaise. Subsequently, gross hemoglobinuria was also observed, occurring daily in urine voided at about 11 a.m. No exposure to cold could be identified, and the patient experienced no prodromal symptoms except mild, vague back discomfort which occurred 30 minutes before the hemoglobinuria.

The patient's past medical history and review of systems were unremarkable except for mild labile hypertension, intermittently treated with reserpine and thiazides, and "hypothyroidism" treated with thyroglobuin (Proloid). There was no past history of syphilis, and no symptoms suggestive of Raynaud's phenomenon or other vasomotor abnormality.

On physical examination, the patient was moderately obese and pale, but otherwise appeared relatively healthy. She was in no distress. Her temperature was 38.0°C, pulse was 100, respirations were 20 and blood pressure was 140/80. Examination was otherwise within normal limits; there were no lymphadenopathy or hepatosplenomegaly.

Laboratory Data: Blood tests revealed a hematocrit level of 25 percent, hemoglobin of 8.1 gm/dl, and reticulocytes of 15.8 percent; the white cell count was 10,600/μl (78 percent neutrophils, 18 percent lymphocytes and 4 percent monocytes), and the platelet count was 312,000/μl. The peripheral blood film showed moderate anisocytosis and polychromatophilia. The urine was dark reddish-brown and contained free hemoglobin and hemosiderin. Stool specimens contained no occult blood. Total serum bilirubin was 4.1 mg/dl (3.0 mg/dl indirect), lactic dehydrogenase was 1411 international units (IU)/liter, serum glutamic oxaloacetic transaminase was 41 IU/liter, serum glutamic pyruvic transaminase was 49 IU/liter, alkaline phosphatase was 154 IU/liter, creatinine phosphokinase was 49 IU/liter, uric acid was 7.2 mg/dl and fasting blood glucose was 123 mg/dl. Serum electrolytes, calcium, phosphorus, and creatinine were normal. Serum total hemolytic complement and complement component C3 were normal; serum protein electrophoresis and immunoelectrophoresis appeared normal. Haptoglobins were absent. Tests for antinuclear antibody, thyroid antibody, rheumatoid factor, and heterophile antibody, and serologic tests for syphilis were all negative. Serum iron, total iron-binding capacity, and vitamin B_{12} and folate levels were normal. Red-cell glucose-6-phosphate dehydrogenase activity and osmotic fragility were normal. Thyroid function tests were normal. Routine direct antiglobulin test using commercial polyspecific antiserum was weakly positive; indirect antiglobulin test was negative. The cold hemagglutinin titer was 1:64; Ham's test was negative.

Chest and abdominal radiographic studies and the electrocardiogram were normal. Cultures of blood, urine, sputum, and stool grew no pathogens, and PPD and fungal skin-sensitivity tests were negative. Bone marrow showed marked erythroid hyperplasia and diminished iron stores. Imaging of liver, spleen and bone marrow with ^{99}Tc-sulfur colloid showed a normal-sized liver and spleen, and peripheral extension of the active bone marrow.

Serologic Studies: The direct antiglobulin test was strongly positive (titer 128). Testing with specific antisera showed that this result was due to the presence of complement component C3 on the red cells; no IgG, IgA, IgM, or C4 was detected. The results of initial testing of the patient's serum at 0, 20, and 37°C are shown in Table 9-5. The Donath-Landsteiner test was strongly positive to a titer of 64. Cold hemagglutination titer was 64 at 0°C.

Table 9-5. RESULTS OF INITIAL TESTING OF PATIENT'S SERUM FOR ANTIBODY ACTIVITY

	0°C				20°C				37°C			
	S	AS	S+C	AS+AC	S	AS	S+C	AS+AC	S	AS	S+C	AS+AC
Untreated red cells												
Agglutination	4+	4+	4+	4+	2+	2+	2+	2+	0	0	0	0
Lysis	0	0	0	0	2+	2+	3+	3+	0	0	0	0
Indirect antiglobulin test *												
Antiserum to IgG					1+	1+	1+	1+	0	0	0	0
Antiserum to C3					4+	4+	4+	4+	0	0	0	0
Papain-treated red cells												
Agglutination	4+	4+	4+	4+	4+	4+	4+	4+	0	0	0	0
Lysis	0	0	0	0	3+	3+	4+	4+	0	0	0	0

S, Untreated patient's serum; AS, patient's serum + 1/10 vol N/5 HCl (final pH 6.5); C, fresh compatible serum (complement); AC, fresh compatible serum + 1/10 vol N/5 HCl (final pH 6.5).
* The indirect antiglobulin test could not be interpreted at 0°C because of strong cold agglutination.
(From Ries, C. A., Garratty, G., Petz, L. D., and Fudenberg, H. H.: Paroxysmal cold hemoglobinuria: Report of a case with an exceptionally high thermal range Donath-Landsteiner antibody. Blood, *36:*491, 1971.)

Maximum lysis occurred in the Donath-Landsteiner test when the cold phase of incubation was at 0°C and decreasing titers were noted as initial incubation temperatures were increased, as is typical of paroxysmal cold hemoglobinuria (Figure 9-4). Antibody activity is ordinarily not detected above 10 to 12°C [80] although exceptional cases in which antibody binding could be detected at temperatures of 20 to 25°C have been reported.[33, 124] Antibodies with these higher thermal ranges would be expected to produce some degree of monophasic hemolysis, since complement would be active within the thermal range of antibody binding. Our patient's Donath-Landsteiner antibody was unique in being capable of binding to red cells at temperatures as high as 32°C, thereby producing vigorous monophasic hemolysis.

Further studies revealed that the antibody had anti-P specificity with both agglutination and hemolysis mediated by the same antibody. When the patient's serum proteins were separated by starch-block electrophoresis and gel filtration, the hemolytic and agglutinating activity was found to reside in the fraction identified as IgG by immunoelectrophoresis and ultracentrifugation. No antibody activity against red cells could be identified in the IgM fraction.[114]

The patient's treatment was directed toward keeping her as warm as possible,

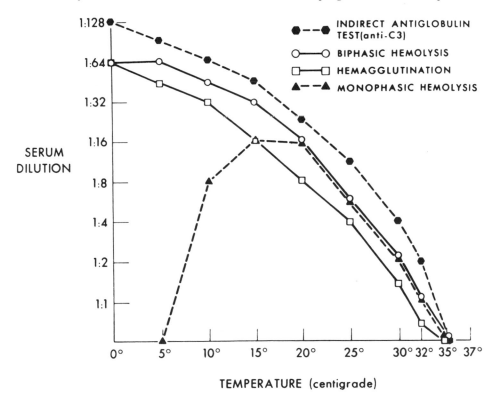

Figure 9-4. *Thermal characteristics of the patient's Donath-Lansteiner antibody as demonstrated by hemagglutination, by monophasic and biphasic hemolysis, and by the indirect antiglobulin test (antiserum to C3) after biphasic incubation. (From Ries, C. A., Garratty, G., Petz, L. D., and Fudenberg, H. H.: Paroxysmal cold hemoglobinuria: Report of a case with an exceptionally high thermal range. Donath-Landsteiner antibody. Blood, 36:491,1971.)*

with strict avoidance of even minimal exposure to cold. She was also treated with varying doses of prednisone and was somewhat improved, but she continued to have chronic symptomatic hemolytic anemia. There were no changes in the direct antiglobulin test or in the thermal amplitude, titer, or score of her Donath-Landsteiner antibody.

Splenectomy was performed in March of 1972 and thereafter the patient evinced marked clinical improvement. Her hematocrit level has remained in the range of 38 to 40 percent with a reticulocyte count of about 1 percent. There was a marked decrease in the strength of her direct antiglobulin test and a significant change in the thermal amplitude, titer, and score of her Donath-Landsteiner antibody (Table 9-6).

We know of only one other reported instance in which splenectomy has been performed for chronic paroxysmal cold hemoglobinuria.[6] That patient, who had serologic evidence for syphilis, also had striking benefit from the procedure (see Chapter 11, page 427).

Table 9-6. REPEATED DETERMINATIONS OF THE DIRECT ANTIGLOBULIN TEST AND DONATH-LANDSTEINER TEST. (THE PATIENT WAS TREATED WITH CORTICOSTEROIDS FROM AUGUST 1970 TO MARCH 1972, AT WHICH TIME SPLENECTOMY WAS PERFORMED.)

Direct Antiglobulin Test	12/27/70 Titer	Score	5/4/71 Titer	Score	7/25/72 Titer	Score	12/10/73 Titer	Score
Anti-IgG	0	0	0	0	0	0	0	0
Anti-C3	128	38	128	39	32	22	0	0

Donath-Landsteiner Test	Titer	Score	Titer	Score	Titer	Score	Titer	Score
4°→37°	64	26	64	25	32	19	32	19
10°→37°	32	20	32	19	16	12	16	12
20°→37°	4	8	4	7	0	0	0	0
37°→37°	0	0	0	0	0	0	0	0

G. WARM ANTIBODY AUTOIMMUNE HEMOLYTIC ANEMIA ASSOCIATED WITH ABNORMAL COLD AGGLUTININS

Characteristic laboratory findings of warm antibody autoimmune hemolytic anemia, cold agglutinin syndrome, and paroxysmal cold hemoglobinuria were described in Chapter 6, and a majority of hemolytic anemias can be readily diagnosed as one of these three types. However, unusual serologic findings may be a source of confusion.

One of the more commonly encountered problems is the interpretation of abnormal cold agglutinins. Cold agglutinins are normally present to a titer of less than 64 at 4°C [32] and, although no extensive studies have been carried out regarding the thermal amplitude of normal cold agglutinins, experience indicates that they are not reactive at room temperature (about 20°C). Not infrequently, abnormal cold agglutinins are encountered that react to a titer greater than 64 at 4°C and/or react up to a temperature of 20°C or above. As with all red cell antibodies, a precise correlation between *in vitro* serologic characteristics and *in vitro* pathogenetic significance does not exist. Thus, it is impossible to state precise criteria that allow one to determine whether a cold agglutinin in a given patient is responsible for a short red cell survival time.

We have approached this problem by performing a detailed serologic characterization of cold agglutinins in patients who have hemolytic anemia with typical features of cold agglutinin syndrome and comparing such antibodies with cold agglutinins found in patients who have no evidence of hemolytic anemia [53] (see Chapter 6, page 214). Our data indicated that the thermal amplitude of the antibody was the most important serologic characteristic and this finding is in agreement with statements of other investigators.[34, 77, 108] In particular, cold agglutinins that reacted up to 30°C in albumin were associated with hemolytic anemia. On this basis we developed criteria for the diagnosis of cold agglutinin syndrome (page 217).

Warm Antibody Autoimmune Hemolytic Anemia with Clinically Insignificant Abnormal Cold Agglutinins: Of particular interest are those patients with acquired hemolytic anemia who have serologic findings characteristic of warm antibody autoimmune hemolytic anemia but who also have abnormal cold agglutinins. Indeed, in our series of 244 patients with warm antibody autoimmune hemolytic anemia, 34.8 percent of patients had antibodies that caused agglutination of normal red cells (i.e., not enzyme-treated) at 20°C (Table 6-14, page 209). The specificity of the cold agglutinin, when determined, was anti-I, and the titer at 4°C was usually normal in spite of the abnormal thermal amplitude. Although reactive at room temperature, the antibodies did not react up to 30°C in albumin and therefore did not seem likely to be a contributing factor in causing shortened red cell survival. Thus, we believe that these patients have warm antibody autoimmune hemolytic anemia with a clinically insignificant albeit abnormal cold agglutinin.

As is also indicated in Table 6-14, the sera of 4.9 percent of the patients with warm antibody autoimmune hemolytic anemia also agglutinated normal red cells at 37°C. However, in these cases the specificity of the agglutinin was not anti-I but was the same as that of the warm autoantibody as determined by indirect antiglobulin test or agglutination of enzyme treated-red cells.

Warm Antibody Autoimmune Hemolytic Anemia with Concomitant Serologic Findings of Cold Agglutinin Syndrome: Rarely, a patient will be found who has serologic findings characteristic of warm antibody autoimmune hemolytic anemia while also having a cold agglutinin of high titer and thermal amplitude, thus satisfying the criteria for both warm antibody autoimmune hemolytic anemia and cold agglutinin syndrome. Such a case was described by Crookston [29] who reported findings in a 70-year-old man with a lymphoproliferative disorder who developed a hemolytic anemia.

The patient's hemoglobin level was 4.7 gm/dl, reticulocytes 5 percent, white blood cell count 6,500/μl with a normal differential count, and platelets 130,000/μl. The blood film showed moderate autoagglutination and marked spherocytosis. A bone marrow biopsy showed a very hypercellular specimen almost completely replaced by small lymphocytic lymphosarcoma cells. Serum bilirubin was 2.8 mg/dl (direct-reacting, 0.5 mg/dl), serum C3 105 mg/dl, and a sharp "M" spike was present in the γ-globulin region. The paraprotein was identified as an IgM protein containing only λ-light chains.

The direct antiglobulin test was strongly positive with anti-IgG and anti-C3 antiglobulin reagents. The patient's serum contained anti-E and anti-K alloantibodies but a warm IgG autoantibody was also identified in his serum and eluate. The autoantibody reacted at 37°C with all red cells tested except Rh$_{null}$ cells. The patient also had a cold agglutinin of anti-i specificity that reacted to a titer of 1024 at 4°C with cord cells and reacted with his own red cells up to a temperature of 33°C. Fractionation of the patient's serum showed that the anti-i activity was confined to the IgM fraction. Therapy with prednisone caused his warm autoantibody to become weaker, but his hemoglobin level rose only slightly, and there was a progressive rise in his anti-i titer. He was therefore treated with cyclophosphamide with marked improvement, which was maintained with the daily administration of prednisone, chlorambucil, and fluoxymesterone.

We have observed 4 patients with autoimmune hemolytic anemia who had serologic findings characteristic of both warm antibody autoimmune hemolytic anemia and cold agglutinin syndrome. The findings in these patients are summarized in Table 9-7. In all patients, the red cells were coated with IgG and C3; a cold agglutinin was present in high titer at 4°C and reacted up to 37°C. In 3 patients in whom the cold agglutinin specificity was identified, the specificity was anti-i. All patients had a warm autoantibody readily demonstrable by indirect antiglobulin test using serum and/or eluate and, in tests against a routine panel of red cells, no specificity was evident. Three of the 4 patients were diagnosed as having an associated lymphoproliferative disorder, but in each instance this diagnosis was based only on the finding of excessive numbers of lymphocytic cells and plasmacytoid lymphocytes in the bone marrow. None of the patients had other manifestations of lymphoma such as lymphadenopathy and, in particular, laparotomy and splenectomy in 2 patients failed to reveal evidence of lymphoma. All patients responded to therapy during the period of follow-up which ranged from 2 weeks to 2 years.

Additional Cases of Autoimmune Hemolytic Anemia with Both IgM and IgG Autoantibodies: Further cases have been described in which both IgM and IgG autoantibodies have been detected in patients with autoimmune hemolytic anemia, but in these cases both autoantibodies were cold antibodies.

Moore and Chaplin [93] described a patient with autoimmune hemolytic anemia who had a direct antiglobulin test that was strongly positive with anti-IgG and anti-C3 antisera. The patient's serum contained an IgM cold agglutinin reactive to a titer of 256 at 4°C, and also an IgG cold autoantibody.

Table 9-7. SUMMARY OF FINDINGS OF FOUR PATIENTS WITH AIHA WHO HAD SEROLOGIC FINDINGS CHARACTERISTIC OF BOTH WARM ANTIBODY AIHA AND COLD AGGLUTININ SYNDROME.

Patient	Age/Sex	Hb (gm/dl)	Reticulocytes (%)	DAT*: Titer/Score				IgG Warm IAT* at 37°C with anti-IgG	Autoantibody Specificity (routine panel by IAT)
				Anti-IgG	Anti-IgA	Anti-IgM	Anti-C3		
M.P.	43/F	5.0	21	4096/47	0	0	16/15	positive	"non-specific"
R.M.	52/M	10.0	2.1	1024/35	0	0	32/26	positive	"non-specific"
C.S.	80/F	8.7	7.0	32,000/61	80/11	0	256/36	positive	"non-specific"
A.M.	28/F	4.5	12	512/28	20/6	40/16	32/30	positive	"non-specific"

Patient	Cold Agglutinin 4°C: Titer/Score	Thermal range	Specificity	Serum IgM (N=45−200)	Serum IgG (N=664−825)	Serum IgA (N=59−311)	Miscellaneous
M.P.	4096/110	37°C	anti-i	NT	NT	NT	R.M.: Biclonal "M" spikes on serum electrophoresis; cryoglobulin present.
R.M.	1024/94	37°C	anti-i	600	1166	83	
C.S.	2048/102	37°C	unidentified	650	600	84	C.S.: Further testing revealed anti-dl and anti-En[a] warm autoantibodies.
A.M.	128/59	37°C	anti-i	NT	NT	NT	

Patient	Associated Diagnosis	Therapy	Response
M.P.	Lymphoproliferative disease	Prednisone, cytotoxic drugs	Hb improved to 9-10 gm/dl; Stable on therapy for two years.
R.M.	Lymphoma	Chlorambucil	Hb improved to 13.2 gm/dl during 5 month follow-up.
C.S.	Lymphoproliferative disorder	Prednisone, cytotoxic drugs, splenectomy	Improved during short period of follow-up. Hb 9.8 gm/dl; Retics 2.4%
A.M.	None	Prednisone, splenectomy	Gradual resolution of hemolysis. 2 years later RBC were weakly coated with C3 only; IgG antibody no longer detected; IgM antibody reactive only at 4°C

* DAT=Direct Antiglobulin Test; IAT=Indirect Antiglobulin Test; NT=Not tested

The IgM antibody demonstrated anti-I specificity, but no blood group specificity of the IgG antibody could be defined. The titer of the serum IgG autoantibody was 64 at 4°C, 16 at 32°C, and 4 at 37°C. In contrast, IgG autoantibodies from 4 patients with warm antibody autoimmune hemolytic anemia reacted to a higher titer at 37°C than at 4°C. The IgG cold autoantibody caused complement-mediated lysis of enzyme treated red cells at 37°C. Unfortunately, the thermal amplitude of the IgM antibody was not determined. The patient did not respond well to therapy with corticosteroids, but splenectomy caused significant improvement, and the patient maintained a hemoglobin level of 10.5 to 12.0 gm/dl without therapy.

Freedman and Newlands[46] described 2 patients with autoimmune hemolytic anemia who had positive direct antiglobulin tests with anti-IgG anti-C3 antisera. Both patients had an IgM anti-I autoantibody that was maximally reactive at 4°C, but that also caused agglutination of red cells up to 37°C (although in one of the patients, only papainized red cells were agglutinated at that temperature). The IgG antibody present in each case was an incomplete autoantibody of wide thermal range and also had anti-I specificity. Both patients had a prompt and marked response to therapy with corticosteroids.

H. WARM ANTIBODY AUTOIMMUNE HEMOLYTIC ANEMIA IN PATIENTS WHOSE DIRECT ANTIGLOBULIN TEST IS POSITIVE ONLY WITH ANTI-IgA ANTISERUM

There have been several reports of patients with warm antibody autoimmune hemolytic anemia in whom the direct antiglobulin test was positive only with anti-IgA antiglobulin serum. Worlledge and Blajchman[143] and Dacie[34] reported 3 such patients among a series of 121 patients of warm antibody autoimmune hemolytic anemia (2.4 percent). The authors indicated that the autoantibody in the eluate from these patients' red cells demonstrated Rh specificity in 2 of the 3 cases. Stratton et al.[128] and Sturgeon et al.[129] have also reported instances in which warm antibody AIHA was associated with an IgA autoantibody demonstrating Rh specificity.

Our own results after performing the direct antiglobulin test with antisera to IgG, IgM, IgA, and C3 in 104 patients with warm antibody autoimmune hemolytic anemia are indicated in Table 6-6. The direct antiglobulin test was positive only with anti-IgA in 2 patients (1.9 percent). One of these patients is of particular significance in that, although IgG, IgM, and complement components could not be detected by the antiglobulin test, it was possible to demonstrate IgG on the patient's red cells by the complement-fixing antibody consumption test.

Case Report 9-6 (Warm antibody autoimmune hemolytic anemia with only IgA detectable by the direct antiglobulin test and with IgG detectable by the complement-fixing antibody consumption test): C.P., a 54-year-old man, was admitted to hospital because of arthralgias involving the knees and hips, weight loss of about 20 pounds, and anorexia. Physical examination revealed matted masses of lymph nodes bilaterally in axillae and in the inguinal and femoral areas. No cervical lymphadenopathy, hepatomegaly or splenomegaly were noted.

Laboratory data revealed the hemoglobin level to be 7.6 gm/dl, hematocrit level 23 percent, and reticulocytes 24 percent; the white cell count was 30,930 / μl with a normal differential. Platelets were 344,000/μl. The direct and indirect antiglobulin tests were negative using licensed polyspecific antiglobulin reagents. In spite of the fact that the direct antiglobulin test was negative, numerous spherocytes were present in the peripheral blood film, a finding leading to a suspicion of autoimmune hemolytic anemia. The total bilirubin was 2.1 mg and the direct reacting bilirubin was 0.55 mg/dl. Stools were negative for occult blood. A lymph node biopsy revealed nodular poorly differentiated lymphocytic lymphoma, and a bone marrow biopsy revealed lymphoid nodules compatible with bone marrow involvement.

Serologic findings revealed that the direct antiglobulin test was negative using multiple dilutions of monospecific antisera to IgG, IgM and C3. However, using anti-IgA, a 3+ reaction was obtained and positive reactions were obtained to a titer of 640. No autoantibodies were detected in the patient's serum, but an eluate caused a 3+ indirect antiglobulin test with anti-IgA antiserum.

A complement-fixing antibody consumption test was performed on two separate samples of blood and revealed 211 and 140 molecules of IgG per red cell, respectively. The patient was treated with high doses of prednisone (80 mg daily) and with combination drug chemotherapy. His hemolytic anemia resolved and his lymphoma went into partial remission.

Comment: It is, of course, not possible to determine whether the small concentration of IgG on the patient's red cells, the more readily detectable IgA, or both the IgG and IgA were responsible for the hemolytic anemia. Careful exclusion of the presence of IgG by techniques more sensitive than the direct antiglobulin test is advisable before ascribing pathogenetic significance to the IgA autoantibody.

I. AUTOIMMUNE HEMOLYTIC ANEMIA IN INFANCY AND CHILDHOOD

Although autoimmune hemolytic anemia in infancy and childhood is similar in many ways to autoimmune hemolytic anemia in adults, some distinctive findings have been emphasized. Zuelzer, et al.[146, 147] reported a series of cases of autoimmune hemolytic anemia in children and, more recently, several reviews have been published.[13, 18, 59, 70, 148]

Most authors indicate that a higher percentage of children have an acute self-limited disease than is found in adults. This tendency was particularly striking in the series reported by Buchanan et al.,[13] in which this course was recorded in 17 of 22 children (77 percent). The authors commented that, in this respect, autoimmune hemolytic anemia in childhood resembles idiopathic thrombocytopenic purpura, which is also usually acute and transient in childhood but chronic in adults.

Zuelzer[147] divided his patients into three groups: Group I was characterized by a fairly short uncomplicated course, usually ending in recovery,

Group II by a similarly uncomplicated but very prolonged course with persistent or recurrent hemolysis, and Group III by extreme chronicity, high intercurrent morbidity, poor response to therapy, and a high mortality. The authors suggested that a patient's ultimate course is determined by his immunologic adequacy. Cytomegalovirus infection was incriminated in 10 of 17 suitably studied cases, and the authors speculated that the infection might somehow be involved in the genesis of the hemolytic state. This etiology was suggested by a parallelism in several children between hemolytic episodes and massive recurrent cytomegalovirus lymphadenitis; they indicated that other occult viruses may also be involved. Autoantibodies correlated poorly with hemolysis. Zuelzer et al. believed that their observations supported the hypothesis that the basic disturbance in autoimmune hemolytic anemia is an immunologic handicap predisposing to occult viral infections, which in an undetermined manner cause hemolysis and may induce autoantibody formation.

Habibi et al.[59] published an excellent review of 80 children with autoimmune hemolytic anemia who were followed in the same department for from 4 months to 14 years with an average follow-up of 3 years. They pointed out clinical and immunologic features that tended to distinguish transient cases (duration less than 3 months) from chronic cases (Table 9-8). Steroid therapy seemed to be effective frequently, but it was often difficult to exclude the possibility of a spontaneous remission, especially in acute cases. Splenectomy was performed in 16 patients who showed corticosteroid resistance or dependence with severe side effects. Eight patients were fully cured of hemolysis, although positive serologic findings remained in 3; moderate improvement occurred in 4 patients, and 4 others were not evaluable. A close correlation was found between the degree of splenic sequestration of ^{51}Cr-labelled erythrocytes and the diminution of the anemia following splenectomy. The efficacy of immunosuppressive agents was estimated in 7 patients who had been given regular and sufficient doses for a period of longer than 4 months. Four patients were judged to have benefited with development of compensated hemolysis and reduced corticosteroid dosage. Blood transfusions were judged as ineffective in 16 of 23 patients in that there was no rise in the hemoglobin level the day after transfusion. The mortality in chronic cases was 11.2 percent and these patients generally had associated disorders and inherent complications at the time of death: thrombocytopenia and cerebral hemorrhage, malignant varicella, septicemia, cytomegalovirus infection, marrow aplasia, and immunologic deficiency disease.

Carapella de Luca et al.[18] also divided their patients into categories of transient or chronic, depending on whether the initial episode of increased hemolysis was either shorter or longer than 3 months. If a relapse occurred, the autoimmune hemolytic anemia was considered to be chronic. Fifteen patients had transient autoimmune hemolytic anemia and 14 had the chronic form of the disease. The authors noted that 4 cases that had been considered chronic ultimately recovered completely from the autoimmune hemolytic anemia.

Johnson and Abildgaard[70] reviewed the literature regarding immuno-

Table 9-8. COMPARISON OF CLINICAL FEATURES IN CHILDREN WITH TRAN-
SIENT OR CHRONIC AUTOIMMUNE HEMOLYTIC ANEMIA.[59]

	Transient Cases	Chronic Cases
Onset in first 4 years of life	Frequent (80%)	Moderate incidence (44%)
Clinical presentation	Invariably acute or hypera-cute	Acute in only 34% of cases
Hemoglobinuria	45%	4%
Prodromal acute infection	70%	4%
Underlying disorders	5.8%	58%
Effectiveness of corticos-teroid therapy	Rapid and constant	Variable
Clinical course	Full recovery in less than 3 months	Intermittent or permanent course for months or years
Direct antiglobulin test	Only complement detected on RBC in 67.6% of cases	IgG or IgG with complement in 84.7% of cases
Mortality	None	11.2%

suppressive therapy in children and reported that about 60 percent of the
children (9 of 15) were improved. The authors believed that these results
warranted additional clinical trials.

REFERENCES

1. Allen, F. H.: Proceedings of 8th Congress of the International Society of Blood Transfusion. 1960, 359.
2. Allison, A. C., Denman, A. M., and Barnes, R. D.: Cooperating and controlling functions of thymus-derived lymphocytes in relation to autoimmunity. Lancet, 2:135, 1971.
3. Bach, F. H.: Disease and the HL-A histocompatability system. Ann. Intern. Med., 75:962, 1971.
4. Baker, P. J., and Stashak, P. W.: Quantitative and qualitative studies on the primary antibody response to pneumococcal polysaccharides at the cellular level. J. Immunol., 103:1342, 1969.
5. Baker, P. J., Stashak, P. W., Amsbaugh, D. F., Prescott, B., and Barth, R. F.: Evidence for the existence of two functionally distinct types of cells which regulate the antibody response to type III pneumococcal polysaccharide. J. Immunol., 105:1581, 1970.
6. Banov, C. H.: Paroxysmal cold hemoglobinuria: Apparent remission after splenectomy. J.A.M.A., 174:1974, 1960.
7. Baumann, R., and Rubin, H.: Autoimmune hemolytic anemia during pregnancy with hemolytic disease in the newborn. Blood, 41:293, 1973.

8. Beard, M. E. J., Pemberton, J., Blagdon, J., and Jenkins, W. J.: Rh immunization following incompatible blood transfusion and a possible long-term complication of anti-D immunoglobulin therapy. J. Med. Genet., 8:317, 1971.
9. Bell, C., and Dray, S.: Conversion of non-immune spleen cells by ribonucleic acid of lymphoid cells from an immunized rabbit to produce γM antibody of foreign light chain allotype. J. Immunol., 103:1196, 1969.
10. Bell, C., and Dray, S.: Conversion of non-immune rabbit spleen cells by ribonucleic acid of lymphoid cells from an immunized rabbit to produce IgG antibody of foreign light-chain allotype. J. Immunol., 105:541, 1970.
11. Bell, C., and Dray, S.: Conversion of non-immune rabbit spleen cells by ribonucleic acid of lymphoid cells from an immunized rabbit to produce IgM and IgG antibody of foreign heavy-chain allotype. J. Immunol., 107:83, 1971.
12. Blajchman, M. A., and Gordon, H.: Successful pregnancy in a patient with Hodgkin's disease complicated by warm autoimmune hemolytic anemia and anti-e alloimmunization. Transfusion, 12:276, 1972.
13. Buchanan, G. R., Boxer, L. A., and Nathan, D. G.: The acute and transient nature of idiopathic immune hemolytic anemia in childhood. J. Pediat., 88:780, 1976.
14. Burkart, D., Rosenfield, R. E., Hsu, T. C. S., et al.: Instrumented PVP-augmented antiglobulin test. 1. Detection of allogenic antibodies coating otherwise normal erythrocytes. Vox. Sang., 26:289, 1974.
15. Burt, R. L., and Prichard, R. W.: Acquired hemolytic anemia in pregnancy: Report of a case. Obstet. Gynecol., 90:444, 1957.
16. Cantor, H., and Boyse, E. A.: Development and function of subclasses of T-cells, J. Reticuloendothel. Soc., 17:115, 1975.
17. Cantor, H., Asofsky, R., and Talal, N.: Synergy among lymphoid cells mediating the graft-versus-host response. J. Exp. Med., 131:223, 1970.
18. Carapella de Luca, E., Casadei, A. M., di Piero, G, et al.: Auto-immune haemolytic anaemia in childhood. Vox. Sang., 36:13, 1979.
19. Chaplin, H., Jr.: Clinical usefulness of specific antiglobulin reagents in autoimmune hemolytic anemias. Prog. Hematol., 7:25, 1973.
20. Chaplin, H., Jr., and Cassell, M.: The occasional fallibility of in vitro compatibility tests. Transfusion, 6:375, 1962.
21. Chaplin, H. R., Cohen, R., Bloomberg, B., et al.: Pregnancy and idiopathic autoimmune hemolytic anemia: A prospective study during 6 months gestation and 3 months postpartum. Br. J. Haematol., 24:219, 1973.
22. Chown, B., Daita, H., Lowen, B., and Lewis, M.: Transient production of anti-LW by LW-positive people. Transfusion, 11:220, 1971.
23. Cock, A. G., and Simonsen, M.: Immunological attack on newborn chickens by injected adult cells. Immunology, 1:103, 1958.
24. Constantoulakis, M., and Kay, H. E. M.: Observations on the centrifugal segregation of young erythrocytes. A possible method of genotyping the transfused patient. J. Clin. Path., 12:312, 1959.
25. Constantoulakis, M., Costea, N., Schwartz, R. S., et al.: Quantitative studies of the effect of red-blood-cell sensitization on in vivo hemolysis. J. Clin. Invest., 42:1790, 1963.
26. Cook, I. A.: Primary rhesus immunization of male volunteers. Brit. J. Haemat., 20:369, 1971.
27. Cox, K. O., and Keast, D.: Erythrocyte autoantibodies induced in mice immunized with rat erythrocytes. Immunology, 25:531, 1973.
28. Cox, K. O., and Keast, D.: Autoimmune haemolytic anaemia induced in mice immunized with rat erythrocytes. Clin. Exp. Immunol., 17:319, 1974.
29. Crookston, J. H.: Hemolytic anemia with IgG and IgM autoantibodies and alloantibodies. Arch. Intern. Med., 135:1314, 1975.
30. Croucher, B. E. E.: Differential diagnosis of delayed transfusion reaction. In: Laboratory Management of Hemolysis. Washington, American Association of Blood Banks (Publisher), 1979.
31. Croucher, B. E. E., Crookston, M. C., and Crookston, J. H.: Delayed haemolytic transfusion reactions simulating auto-immune haemolytic anaemia. Vox. Sang., 12:32, 1967.
32. Dacie, J. V.: The Hemolytic Anaemias. Part II. Auto-immune hemolytic anaemias. 2nd Ed. London, J. & A. Churchill, 1962, 460.

33. Dacie, J. V.: The Haemolytic Anaemias: Congenital and Acquired. Part II. The auto-immune haemolytic anaemias. Ed. 2. New York, Grune and Stratton, 1962, 416.
34. Dacie, J. V.: Autoimmune hemolytic anemia. Arch. Intern. Med., *135:*1293, 1975.
35. Dameshek, W., and Levine, P.: Isoimmunization with Rh factor in acquired hemolytic anemia. New Eng. J. Med., *228:*641, 1943.
36. Dewar, A. E., Stuart, A. E., Parker, A. C., and Wilson, C.: Rosetting cells in autoimmune haemolytic anaemia. Lancet, *2:*519, 1974.
37. Dupuy, M. E., Elliot, M., and Masouredis, S. P.: Relationship between red cell bound antibody and agglutination in the antiglobulin reaction. Vox. Sang., *9:*40, 1964.
38. Eldor, A., Yatziv, S., and Hershko, C.: Relapsing Coombs-negative haemolytic anaemia in pregnancy with haemolytic disease in the newborn. Brit. Med. J., *4:*625, 1975.
39. Evans, R. S., and Weiser, R. S.: The serology of autoimmune hemolytic disease: Observations on forty-one patients. Arch. Intern. Med., *100:*371, 1957.
40. Evans, R. S., Bingham, M., and Turner, E.: Autoimmune hemolytic disease: Observations of serological reactions and disease activity. Ann. N.Y. Acad. Sci., *124:*422, 1965.
41. Evans, R. S., Turner, E., Binghan, M., and Woods, R.: Chronic hemolytic anemia due to cold agglutinins. II. The role of C' in red cell destruction. J. Clin. Invest., *47:*691, 1968.
42. Fink, D. J., Petz, L. D., and Black, M. B.: Serum haptoglobin. A valuable diagnostic aid in suspected hemolytic transfusion reactions. J.A.M.A., *199:*615, 1967.
43. Fischer, J., Petz, L. D., and Garratty, G.: Characterization of immune hemolytic anemias with negative direct antiglobulin (Coombs') tests. Clin. Res., *21:*265, 1973.
44. Fischer, J. T., Petz, L. D., Garratty, G., and Cooper, N. R.: Correlations between quantitative assay of red cell-bound C3, serologic reactions, and hemolytic anemia. Blood, *44:*359, 1974.
45. Fishman, M., and Adler, F. L.: Role of macrophage-RNA in immune response. Cold Spring Harbor Symp., Quart. Biol., *32:*343, 1967.
46. Freedman, J., and Newlands, M.: Autoimmune haemolytic anaemia with the unusual combination of both IgM and IgG autoantibodies. Vox. Sang., *32:*61, 1977.
47. Fudenberg, H. H.: Genetically determined immune deficiency as the predisposing cause of "autoimmunity" and lymphoid neoplasia. Amer. J. Med., *51:*295, 1971.
48. Fudenberg, H. H.: Are autoimmune diseases and malignancy due to selective T-cell deficiencies? *IN:* Critical Factors in Cancer Immunology. Schultz, J., and Leif, R. C., Eds. New York, Academic Press, 1975, 179.
49. Fudenberg, H. H., and Holman, H. R.: Autoimmune diseases: Genetics, mechanisms and diagnostic approaches. *IN:* Progress in Immunology. Amos, B., Ed. New York, Academic Press, 1971, 1319.
50. Fudenberg, H. H., and Solomon, A.: "Acquired agammaglobulinemia" with autoimmune hemolytic disease: Graft-versus-host reaction? Vox. Sang., *6:*68, 1961.
51. Fudenberg, H. H., Rosenfield, R. E., and Wasserman, L. R.. Unusual specificity of autoantibody in autoimmune hemolytic anemia. J. Mt. Sinai Hosp., *25:*324, 1958.
52. Garratty, G., and Petz, L. D.: Acquired hemolytic anemia associated with negative direct antiglobulin tests but enzyme reactive autoantibodies in the serum. Presented at the American Association of Blood Banks, 24th Annual Meeting, Chicago, 1971.
53. Garratty, G., Petz, L. D., and Hoops, J. K.: The correlation of cold agglutinin titrations in saline and albumin with haemolytic anaemia. Brit. J. Haemat., *35:*587, 1977.
54. Gilliland, B. C.: Coombs-negative immune hemolytic anemia. Seminars in Hematol., *13:*267, 1976.
55. Gilliland, B. C., Baxter, E., and Evans, R. S.: Red-cell antibodies in acquired hemolytic anemia with negative antiglobulin serum tests. N. Engl. J. Med., *285:*252, 1971.

56. Gilliland, B. C., Leddy, J. P., and Vaughan, J. H.: The detection of cell-bound antibody on complement-coated human red cells. J. Clin. Invest., *49:*898, 1970.
57. Goodall, H. B., Ho-Yen, D. O., Clark, D. M., et al.: Haemolytic anaemia of pregnancy. Scand. J. Haematol., *22:*185, 1979.
58. Grislain, J. R., Mainard, R., and de Berranger, P.: Ictère hémolytique néonatale par anticorps froids d'origine maternelle. Arch. Fr. Pediatr., *20:*853, 1963.
59. Habibi, B., Homberg, J. C., Schaison, G., and Salmon, C.: Autoimmune hemolytic anemia in children: A review of 80 cases. Amer. J. Med., *56:*61, 1974.
60. Hathaway, W. F., Githens, J. H., Blackburn, V., Fulginiti, and Kempe, C. H.: Aplastic anemia, histiocytosis and erythrodermia in immunologically deficient children. Probable human runt disease. New Eng. J. Med., *273:*953, 1965.
61. Hershko, C., Berrebi, A., Resnitzky, P., and Eldor, A.: Relapsing haemolytic anaemia of pregnancy with negative antiglobulin reaction. Scand. J. Haematol., *16:*135, 1976.
62. Hobbs, J. R., Russell, A., and Worlledge, S. M.: Dysgammaglobulinemia. Type IV C. Clin. Exp. Immunol., *2:*589, 1967.
63. Holland, P. V., and Wallerstein, R. O.: Delayed hemolytic transfusion reaction with acute renal failure. J.A.M.A., *204:*1007, 1968.
64. Hong, R., Gatti, R. A., and Good, R. A.: Hazards and potential benefits of blood transfusion in immunological deficiency. Lancet, *2:*388, 1968.
65. Hughes-Jones, N. C., Polley, M. J., Telford, R., et al.: Optimal conditions for detecting blood group antibodies by the antiglobulin test. Vox. Sang., *9:*385, 1964.
66. Idelson, L. L., Koyfman, M. M., Gorina, L. G., and Olovnikov, A. M.: Application of a high sensitivity aggregate-haemagglutination test for the diagnosis of autoimmune haemolytic anaemia with a negative direct antiglobulin test. Vox. Sang., *31:*401, 1976.
67. Jacobson, E. B., Herzenberg, Lenore A., Riblet, R., and Herzenberg, L. A.: Active suppression of immunoglobulin allotype synthesis. II. Transfer of suppressing factor with spleen cells. J. Exp. Med., *135:*1163, 1972.
68. Jandl, J. H., and Kaplan, M. E.: The destruction of red cells by antibodies in man. III. Quantitative factors influencing the patterns of hemolysis in vivo. J. Clin. Invest., *39:*1145, 1960.
69. Jenkins, D. E. Jr., Moore, W. H., and Hawiger, A.: A method for radioactive antiglobulin testing with ^{125}I labeled anti-IgG. Transfusion, *17:*16, 1977.
70. Johnson, C. A., and Abildgaard, C. F.: Case report: Treatment of idiopathic autoimmune hemolytic anemia in children. Review and report of two fatal cases in infancy. Acta Paediatr. Scand., *65:*375, 1976.
71. Jordan, F. L. F.: The role of complement in immunohemolytic disease. Proceedings of the 6th Congress of the International Society for Hematology, Boston, 1956, 825.
72. Kawakami, M., Kitamura, K., Mikami, H., and Mitsuhashi, S.: Transfer agent of immunity. III. Autoantibody formation by mouse spleen cells treated with immune ribonuleic acid preparation. Jap. J. Microbiol., *13:*247, 1969.
73. Kretschmer, V., and Mueller-Eckhardt: Significance of complement activation in autoimmune haemolytic anaemia of "warm type." Blut, *35:*447, 1977.
74. Krüger, J., Rhaman, A., Mogk, K. U., and Mueller-Eckhardt, C.: T cell deficiency in patients with autoimmune hemolytic anemia ("warm type"). Vox. Sang., *31:*1, 1976.
75. Lalezari, P., Talleyrand, N. P., Wenze, B., Schoenfeld, M. E., and Tippett, P.: Development of direct antiglobulin reaction accompanying alloimmunization in a patient with Rh[d] (D, Category III) phenotype, Vox. Sang., *28:*19, 1975.
76. Lawrence, H. S.: Transfer factor. Adv. Immunol., *11:*195, 1965.
77. Leddy, J. P., and Swisher, S. N.: Acquired immune hemolytic disorders (including drug-induced immune hemolytic anemia). *In:* Immunological Diseases. Samter, M., 3rd Ed. Boston, Little Brown, 1978, 1187.
78. Leventhal, B. G., and Talal, N.: Response of NZB and NZB/NZW spleen cells to mitogenic agents. J. Immunol., *104:*918, 1970.
79. Liu, C. K., and Evans, R. S.: Production of positive antiglobulin serum test in rabbits by intraperitoneal injection of homologous blood. Proc. Soc. Exp. Biol. Med., *79:*194, 1952.

80. Mackenzie, G. M.: Paroxysmal hemoglobinuria; Review Medicine (Balt.), *8:*159, 1929.
81. McCullough, J., Benson, S. J., Yunis, E. J., et al.: Effect of blood-bank storage on leukocyte function. Lancet, *2:*1333, 1969.
82. McDevitt, H. O., and Bodmer, W. F.: Histocompatibility antigens, immune responsiveness and susceptibility to disease. Amer. J. Med., *52:*1, 1972.
83. McDevitt, H. O., Bechtol, K. B., Grumet, F. C., Mitchell, G. F., and Wegmann, T. G.: Genetic control of the immune response to branched synthetic polypeptide antigens in inbred mice. *In:* Progress in Immunology. Amos, B., Ed. New York, Academic Press, 1971, 495.
84. Miller, J. F. A. P., and Howard, J. G.: The use of reticuloendothelial function for studying graft-versus-host reaction in the presence of potential host-versus-graft reaction. J. Reticuloendothelial. Soc., *1:*29, 1964.
85. Miller, W. V.: The human histocompatibility complex: A review for the hematologist. Prog. Hematol., *10:*173, 1977.
86. Mitsuhashi, S., Kurashige, S., Kawakami, M., and Nojima, T.: Transfer agent of immunity. I. Immune ribonucleic acid which induces antibody formation to Salmonella flagella. Jap. J. Microbiol., *12:*261, 1968.
87. Mohn, J. F., Lambert, R. M., Bowman, H. S., and Brason, F. W.. The formation of Rh specific autoantibodies in experimental isoimmune hemolytic anemia in man. Communications of the 10th Congress of the International Society for Blood Transfusions, Stockholm, 1964.
88. Mohn, J. F., Lambert, R. M., Bowman, H. S., and Brason, R. W.: Experimental production in man of autoantibodies with Rh specificity. Ann. N. Y. Acad. Sci., *124:*477, 1965.
89. Mohr, J. A., Killebrew, L., Muchmore, H. G., Felton, F. G., and Rhoades, E. R.: Transfer of delayed hypersensitivity. J.A.M.A., *297:*517, 1969.
90. Mollison, P. L.: Blood Transfusion in Clinical Medicine. 6th Ed. Oxford, Blackwell Scientific Publications, 1979, 537.
91. Mollison, P. L., and Hughes-Jones, N. C.: Clearance of Rh-positive red cells by low concentrations of Rh antibody. Immunology, *12:*63, 1967.
92. Mollison, P. L., Crome, P., Hughes-Jones, N. C., et al.: Rate of removal from the circulation of red cells sensitized with different amounts of antibody. Br. J. Haematol., *11:*461, 1965.
93. Moore, J. A., and Chaplin, H., Jr.: Autoimmune hemolytic anemia associated with an IgG cold incomplete antibody. Vox. Sang., *24:*236, 1973.
94. Okumura, K.: Regulation of hemocytotropic antibody formation in the rat. VI. Inhibitory effect of thymocytes on the hemocytotropic antibody response. J. Immunol., *107:*1682, 1971.
95. Oliner, H., Schwartz, R., and Dameshek, W.: Studies in experimental autoimmune disorders. I. Clinical laboratory features of autoimmunization (runt disease) in the mouse. Blood, *17:*20, 1961.
96. Ovary, Z., and Speigelman, J.: The production of "cold autoagglutinins" in the rabbit as a consequence of immunization with isologous erythrocytes. Ann. N.Y. Acad. Sci., *124:*147, 1965.
97. Parker, A. C., and Stuart, A. E.: Ultrastructural studies of leucocytes which form rosettes with homologous erythrocytes in human autoimmune haemolytic anaemia. Scand. J. Haematol., *20:*129, 1978.
98. Parker, A. C., Habeshaw, J., and Cleland, J. F.: The demonstration of a 'plasmatic factor' in a case of Coombs' negative haemolytic anemia. Scand. J. Haemat., *9:*318, 1972.
99. Parker, A. C., Stuart, A. E., and Dewar, A. E.: Activated T-cells in autoimmune haemolytic anaemia. Brit. J. Haemat., *36:*337,1977.
100. Petrakis, N. L., and Politis, G.: Prolonged survival of viable, mitotically competent mononuclear leukocytes in stored whole blood. New Eng. J. Med.,*267:*286, 1962.
101. Petz, L. D.: The role of complement in immune hemolysis in vitro and in vivo.*In:* Protides of the Biological Fluids. Oxford and New York, Pergamon Press, 1975, 535.
102. Petz, L. D.: Autoimmune and drug-induced immune hemolytic anemias. *In:* Manual of Clinical Immunology. Rose, N. R., and Friedman, H., Eds. American Society for Microbiology (Publisher). 2nd Ed in press.

103. Petz, L. D., and Garratty, G.: Complement in immunohematology. Prog. Clin. Immunol., *2:*175,1974.
104. Petz, L. D., and Garratty, G.: Antiglobulin sera—past, present and future. Transfusion, *18:*257, 1978.
105. Petz, L. D., Fink, D. J., Letsky, E. A., Fudenberg, H. H., and Müller-Eberhard, H. J.: In vivo metabolism of complement. I. Metabolism of the third component (C′3) in acquired hemolytic anemia. J. Clin. Invest., *47:*2469, 1968.
106. Pineda, A. A., Brzica, S. M., Jr., and Taswell, H. F.: Hemolytic transfusion reaction: Recent experience in a large blood bank. Mayo Clin. Proc., *53:*378, 1978.
107. Pineda, A. A., Taswell, H. F., and Brzica, S. M., Jr.: Delayed hemolytic transfusion reaction. Transfusion, *18:*1, 1978.
108. Pirofsky, B.: Autoimmunization and the Autoimmune Hemolytic Anemias. Baltimore, Williams and Wilkins, 1969, 25.
109. Polesky, H. F., and Bove, J. R.: A fatal hemolytic transfusion reaction with acute autohemolysis. Transfusion, *4:*285, 1964.
110. Porter, K. A.: Immune Hemolysis: A feature of secondary disease and runt disease in the rabbit. Ann. N.Y. Acad. Sci., *87:*391, 1960.
111. Raeder, R.: Complement in acquired haemolytic anemia. Aust. Ann. Med., *4:*279, 1955.
112. Rand, B. P., Olson, J. D., Garratty, G., and Petz, L. D.: Coombs' negative immune hemolytic anemia with anti-E occurring in the red blood cell eluate of an E-negative patient. Transfusion, *18:*174, 1978.
113. Renton, P. H., and Hancock, J. A.: A simple method of separating erythrocytes of different ages. Vox. Sang., *9:*183, 1964.
114. Ries, C. A., Garratty, G., Petz, L. D., and Fudenberg, H. H.: Paroxysmal cold hemoglobinuria: Report of a case with an exceptionally high thermal range Donath-Landsteiner antibody. Blood, *38:*491, 1971.
115. Romano, E. L., Hughes-Jones, N. C., and Mollison, P. L.: Direct antiglobulin reaction in ABO-haemolytic disease of the newborn. Br. Med. J., *1:*524, 1973.
116. Rosse, W. F.: Quantitative immunology of immune hemolytic anemia. II. The relationship of cell-bound antibody to hemolysis and the effect of treatment. J. Clin. Invest., *50:*734, 1971.
117. Rosse, W. F.: The detection of small amounts of antibody on the red cell in autoimmune hemolytic anemia. Series Haematol., *7:*358, 1974.
118. Rothamn, I. K., Alter, H. J., and Strewler, G. J.: Delayed overt hemolytic transfusion reaction due to anti-U antibody. Transfusion, *16:*357, 1976.
119. Sampson, D., Gotelueschen, C., and Kauffman, H. M., Jr.: The human splenic suppressor cell. Transplantation, *20:*362, 1975.
120. Sasazuki, T., and McDevitt, H. O.: The association between genes in the major histocompatibility complex and disease susceptibility. Ann. Rev. Med., *28:*425, 1977.
121. Schaller, J., Ching, Yi-chuan, Williams, C. P. S., et al.: Hypergammaglobulinemia, antibody deficiency, autoimmune hemolytic anemia and nephritis in infant with familial lymphopenic immune defect. Lancet, *2:*825, 1966.
122. Schechter, G. P., Soehnlen, F., and McFarland, W.: Lymphocyte response to blood transfusion in man. N. Eng. J. Med., *287:*1169, 1972.
123. Schechter, G. P., Whang-Peng, J., and McFarland, W.: Circulation of donor lymphocytes after blood transfusion in man. Blood, *49:*651, 1977.
124. Schubothe, H.: Serology and clinical significance of autoantibodies to red blood cells (in German). Bibl. Haemat., *8:*1, 1958.
125. Seip, M.: Systemic Lupus Erythematosus in pregnancy with haemolytic anaemia, leucopenia and thrombocytopenia in the mother and her newborn infant. Arch Dis. Childh., *35:*364, 1960.
126. Shapiro, M.: Familial autohemolytic anemia and runting syndrome with Rh_0-specificity antibody. Transfusion, *7:*281, 1967.
127. Söderhjelm, L.: Non-spherocytic haemolytic anaemia in mother and newborn infant. Acta Paediat., *48*(Suppl. 117):34, 1959.
128. Stratton, F., Rawlison, V. I., Chapman, S. A., Pengelly, C. D. R., and Jennings, R. C.: Acquired hemolytic anemia associated with IgA anti-e. Transfusion, *12:*157, 1974.
129. Sturgeon, P., Smith, L. E., Chun, H. M. T., Hurvitz, C. H., Garratty, G., and

Goldfinger, D.: Autoimmune hemolytic anemia associated exclusively with IgA of Rh specificity. Transfusion, *19:*324, 1979.

130. Stutman, O., Yunis, E. J., and Good, R. A.. Deficient immunologic functions of NZB mice. Proc. Soc. Exp. Biol. Med., *127:*1204, 1968.

131. Sutherland, D. E. R., Archer, O. K., Peterson, R. D. A., Elkert, E., and Good, R. A.: Development of "autoimmune processes" in rabbits after neonatal removal of central lymphoid tissue. Lancet, *1:*130, 1965.

132. Swisher, S. N.: Acquired hemolytic disease. Postgrad. Med., *40:*378, 1966.

133. Teague, P. O., and Friou, G. J.: Antinuclear antibodies in mice. II. Transmission with spleen cells; inhibition or prevention with thymus or spleen cells. Immunology, *17:*665, 1969.

134. Thomson, S., and Johnstone, M.: Delayed haemolytic transfusion reaction due to anti-Jk[a] and anti-M. Can. J. Med. Tech., *34:*159, 1972.

135. Turner, J. H., Hutchinson, D. L., and Petricciani, J.: Cytogenic and growth characteristics of human lymphocytes derived from stored donor blood packs. Scand. J. Haemat., *8:*169, 1971.

136. van Loghem, J. J., van der Hart, M., and Dorfmeier, H.: Serologic studies in acquired hemolytic anemia. Proceedings of the 6th Congress of the International Society for Hematology, Boston, 1956, 858.

137. Waldman, T. A., Broder, S., Blaese, R. M., Durm, M., Blackmann, M., and Strober, W.: Role of suppressor T-cells in pathogenesis of common variable hypogammaglobulinaemia. Lancet, *2:*609, 1974.

138. Warner, N. L.: Genetic control of spontaneous and induced antierythrocyte autoantibody production in mice. Clin. Immunol. Immunopath., *1:*353, 1973.

139. Watanabe, K., and Mitsuhashi, S.: The role of transfer agent in immunity. Tohoku J. Exp. Med., *103:*1, 1971.

140. Weigle, W. O.: Natural and Acquired Immunologic Unresponsiveness. Cleveland, World Publishing Company, 1967.

141. Wilkinson, L., Yam, P., Petz, L. D., and Garratty, G.: Erythrocyte autoantibodies in sickle cell disease. Tranfusion, *15:*512, 1975.

142. Worlledge, S. M.: The interpretation of a positive direct antiglobulin test. Brit. J. Haemat., *39:*157, 1978.

143. Worlledge, S. M., and Blajchman, M. A.: The autoimmune haemolytic anaemias. Br. J. Haemat., *23:*(Suppl) 61, 1972.

144. Yam, P., Wilkinson, L., Petz, L. D., and Garratty, G.: Studies on hemolytic anemia in pregnancy with evidence for autoimmunization in a patient with a negative direct antiglobulin (Coombs') test. Amer. J. Hematol., *8:*23, 1980.

145. Zmijewski, C. M.: The production of erythrocyte autoantibodies in chimpanzees. J. Exp. Med., *121:*657, 1965.

146. Zuelzer, W. W., Stulberg, C. S., Page, R. H., Teruya, J., and Brough, A. J.: Etiology and pathogenesis of acquired hemolytic anemia. Transfusion, *6:*438, 1966.

147. Zuelzer, W. W., Mastrangelo, R., Stulberg, C. S., Poulik, M. D., Page, R. H., and Thompson, R. I.: Autoimmune hemolytic anemia. Natural history and viral immunologic interactions in childhood. Amer. J. Med., *49:*80, 1969.

148. Zupanska, B., Lawkowicz, W., Gôrska, B., et al.: Autoimmune haemolytic anaemia in children. Br. J. Haemat, *34:*511, 1976.

10

Blood Transfusion in Autoimmune Hemolytic Anemias

Patients with autoimmune hemolytic anemia frequently present with anemia of sufficient severity to suggest the possible need for blood transfusion. Indeed, when anemia of such severity is discovered, physicians frequently refer a sample of blood to the blood transfusion laboratory while simultaneously initiating diagnostic studies to determine the cause of the anemia. A diagnosis of autoimmune hemolytic anemia is often first made by the blood transfusion service when autoantibodies are detected during the performance of the compatibility ("crossmatch") test.

Nowhere in the management of patients with immune hemolytic anemias is the communication between clinician and laboratory personnel more important than in regard to blood transfusion. As with all clinical decisions concerning therapy, the possible benefits must be weighed in relationship to potential risks. The advisability of blood transfusion is related to the severity of the anemia, whether the anemia is rapidly progressive, and especially to the associated clinical findings. However, a clinical decision based on such facts must be tempered by the knowledge that blood transfusion has a greater than usual risk in patients with autoimmune hemolytic anemia.

In this chapter, we first discuss the indications (and lack of indications) for blood transfusion in specific clinical settings, and we apply such principles to patients with AIHA. We then describe, from the point of view of practicing clinicians, the nature and clinical significance of the unique risks encountered when transfusion is necessary in a patient with AIHA. In essence, the risks relate to two factors. The autoantibody often complicates the compatibility test and may make it difficult to detect co-existing alloantibodies or to exclude their presence with confidence, thereby increasing the risk of an alloantibody-induced hemolytic transfusion reaction; secondly, the autoantibody itself may cause marked shortening of the survival of donor red cells. In spite of these added risks, we emphasize that blood should never be denied a patient with a justifiable need (e.g., a progressively severe, life-threatening anemia) even though the compatibility test may be strongly incompatible. On the other hand, in discussing the difficulties faced by laboratory personnel, and adverse reactions to blood transfusion that are unique to patients with acquired hemolytic anemia, we hope to justify the view that frequently the course of lesser risk is to withhold blood transfusions in some settings in which the initial clinical judgment would suggest their need.

We next review the principles and give technical details of the methods that should be utilized for the optimal selection of blood for patients with autoimmune hemolytic anemias of various types. Finally, we discuss the optimal volume of blood to be transfused (which may be of critical importance in safely treating patients with severe hemolytic anemia), we consider the use of warm blood for patients with cold antibody AIHA, and we discuss the use of washed red cells.

GENERAL PRINCIPLES CONCERNING INDICATIONS FOR TRANSFUSION

It is useful to compare the indications for blood transfusion in autoimmune hemolytic anemias with those in several more common causes of anemia that vary in abruptness of onset and in the need for transfusion such as acute blood loss, severe megaloblastic anemia, and chronic refractory anemias. In these instances, the requirement for blood transfusion is analogous to that in AIHA in that the most critical aspects of the clinical evaluation are the symptoms and signs resulting from the anemia and evidence of probable progression of its severity. The hemoglobin and hematocrit values are of significance, but they are too often overemphasized as criteria for transfusion.

The following familiar clinical settings illustrate fundamental principles. A patient with hematemesis, melena, a hemoglobin level of 9 gm/dl, a blood pressure of 100/60 mm Hg, and a pulse of 128/minute, should, of course, be transfused. Such anemia is producing life-threatening signs because of hypovolemia; the manifestations of hypovolemia (hypotension and tachycardia) indicate that the anemia is acute in onset because compensatory increases in plasma volume will occur in slowly developing anemias, thus keeping total blood volume near normal.[33(a)] Further, the hematemesis and melena indicate that the anemia and hypovolemia are likely to become progressively and acutely more severe.

The severity of reduction in blood volume must be estimated and managed according to its effect on the cardiovascular system. The evaluation takes place at the bedside, with the assessments of volume loss, transfusion requirements, and response to therapy being made from the signs and symptoms of volume depletion.[19] Normally, the blood volume in an adult male is 69 ml per kg (30 ml RBC per kg and 39 ml plasma per kg) and in females is 65 ml per kg (25 ml RBC per kg and 40 ml plasma per kg).[54] Most patients can withstand an acute loss of up to 20 percent of their blood volume (about 1000 ml in an adult of average size) without signs of vascular insufficiency. When the loss exceeds 1000 ml, rising to the range of 20 to 30 percent of blood volume, signs of cardiovascular distress appear. At first, these signs are limited to tachycardia at rest and postural hypotension.[19] The pulse rate is an unreliable guide to hypovolemia, but a persistent rate of 100 or more per minute without other evident explanation (e.g., fever) may be caused by hypovolemia and suggests that the blood volume is less than 80 percent of normal.[26] A 70 kg patient may compensate for an acute loss of blood volume of up to about 1,500 ml by vasoconstriction and may appear normal if lying flat.[30] However, such a patient is in latent shock and may faint when placed in the upright position. If the systolic blood pressure is below 100 mm Hg as a result of acute blood loss, the blood volume is probably less than 70 percent of normal.[2] Loss of 40 percent of intravascular volume produces overt shock in most patients. Other clinical manifestations of hypovolemia include pallor, sweating, thirst, light-headedness, air-hunger, and restlessness.

In contrast to the preceding example of a patient with acute blood loss, a patient with megaloblastic anemia with a hemoglobin level of 8 gm/dl who has normal vital signs, no signs of hypovolemia, and whose symptoms are weakness, lethargy and palpitations should not be transfused.[33(b)] The symptoms and signs do not warrant blood transfusion, and effective and safer therapy is available. The stable vital signs with this level of hemoglobin indicate that the anemia cannot have been acute in onset. Unless there is concomitant evidence of blood loss, there are no indications that the anemia will rapidly become more severe.

A third familiar clinical example is that of a patient with a chronic anemia that may be quite severe but is stable and is not correctable by specific therapy (e.g., anemia associated with renal insufficiency, liver disease, carcinoma, chronic rheumatoid arthritis, and "refractory" anemias such as hypoplastic anemia and sideroblastic anemia). Such a patient should not be transfused unless it is required to correct associated symptoms of marked severity. Transfusions will temporarily improve the anemia and the patient's symptoms, but if the underlying disease is not improved, anemia of similar severity will recur within weeks. For example, a 70 kg male has a red cell volume of about 2,100 ml (30 ml/kg). If, for convenience, we use a figure of 100 days as the normal red cell life span, he must produce 21 ml of red cells per day. To maintain a hemoglobin of 10 gm/dl (about 2/3 of normal) requires 14 ml/day. Freshly obtained donor red cells are of all ages and therefore will have an average life expectancy of $\frac{100}{2}$ or 50 days. Thus, the daily requirement of transfused red cells to maintain a hemoglobin level of 10 gm/dl in a 70 kg male who is making no red cells is 14×2 or 28 ml per day or 196 ml/week. A unit of red cells contains about 200 ml, so that an average of one unit per week will need to be transfused. Thus, after transfusion of 3 units of red cells, the hemoglobin will return to the pre-transfusion value in 3 weeks. Since transfusion does suppress erythropoiesis,[33(b)] such estimates often turn out to be clinical realities. The return of the patient's hemoglobin level to pre-transfusion levels within weeks is often misinterpreted as an indication of poor survival of transfused red cells and as an indication that the hemoglobin will continue to decline. However, the marrow may be able to maintain a stable hemoglobin at a relatively low level and optimal management may be the education of the patient to tolerate this degree of anemia rather than to repeatedly transfuse. Chronic transfusion therapy exposes the patient to all the acute dangers of transfusion and may also result in iron overload and immunologic reactions that make subsequent transfusions more difficult. In some patients multiple red cell alloantibodies may develop, thus making transfusion therapy much more difficult at a later time of urgent need.

Physicians should also consider that improvement in symptoms may be related to the strong placebo effect of blood transfusion, and its benefit may be exaggerated by the patient or by the physician himself. Patients with chronic anemia have compensatory increases in plasma volume, cardiovascular compensatory mechanisms, and increased red cell 2,3-diphosphoglycerate (2,3-DPG), which results in improved oxygen delivery to tissues, so that they usually manage quite well. For example, the results of controlled studies have indicated that patients with iron deficiency anemia with hemoglobin levels of 8 gm per dl had no change in symptoms as a result of iron therapy and improvement in hemoglobin.[10-12, 36] Indeed, large studies have failed to demonstrate any evidence of an association between hemoglobin levels above 8 gm per dl and the severity of symptoms.[12, 56]

Nevertheless, it is certainly true that some patients with chronic severe anemia must be transfused in order for them to sustain a reasonable level of activity. Although it is impossible to give strict criteria for transfusion of such patients, some guidelines should be considered.

If the hemoglobin level is above 10 gm/dl, transfusion therapy for a chronic stable anemia is almost never indicated. If the patient's hemoglobin is stable at a level of 8 to 10 gm/dl, transfusion is rarely necessary or desirable. Such patients may have mild symptoms such as some decrease in exercise tolerance, but will do better ultimately if a program of chronic transfusions is not undertaken. For anemias of greater severity (hemoglobin level of 5 to 8 gm/dl), symptoms of anemia such as fatigue, a more marked decrease in exercise tolerance, and palpitations will usually be present and may prove intolerable to some patients. It is in this group of patients that clinical judgment is most critical. Many, but by no means all, such patients can make an adequate adjustment to their decreased exercise tolerance and thus avoid the problems associated with a program of chronic transfusion. At a level of hemoglobin below 5 gm/dl, most patients will require repeated transfusions but, even here, such a program must be embarked upon reluctantly and is not always necessary. Indeed, patients with chronic renal failure undergoing dialysis regularly sustain normal organ function in the presence of hemoglobin levels of 3 or 4 gm per dl.[31]

These rather fundamental examples are cited as a basis for the following discussion which emphasizes that, although physicians may be somewhat ill at ease in the rather unfamiliar setting of AIHA, similar principles should be utilized in formulating a clinical decision concerning the advisability of blood transfusion. Thus, the clinician should assess the patient's symptoms and signs caused by the anemia, the acuteness of the hemolysis, the rapidity of progression of the anemia, and the probable effectiveness of therapy other than transfusion.

The clinical decision should be tempered by an assessment of the increased risk of transfusion, which varies depending on the type and severity of the hemolytic anemia, the difficulties imposed on the laboratory by the patient's autoantibodies, and the patient's history of prior transfusions and pregnancies.

ASSESSING THE NEED FOR TRANSFUSION IN PATIENTS WITH AUTOIMMUNE HEMOLYTIC ANEMIA

Assessing the Acuteness of Onset and Rapidity of Progression of Autoimmune Hemolytic Anemia

When a patient presents with autoimmune hemolytic anemia and a moderately severe anemia, it is not possible to predict with certainty whether or not the anemia will rapidly become more severe. Thus, serial determinations of the hemoglobin and hematocrit should be performed at intervals determined by the results of the evaluation of the severity of the illness. In particular, the physician should note whether the patient appears acutely ill with symptoms attributable to acute hemolysis such as fever, malaise, and pain in the back, abdomen, and legs.[48] The presence or absence of hemoglobinuria and hemoglobinemia should be noted. These findings are usually manifestations of severe hemolysis.

If a patient is acutely ill, has a history of an abrupt onset of the illness, or has grossly evident hemoglobinuria, the hematocrit level should be determined every 2 to 4 hours initially, whereas in less acutely ill patients, initial testing may be at 12 to 24 hour intervals. The frequency of testing may soon be decreased if the severity of the anemia proves to be essentially constant. In some cases of fulminant hemolysis, a significant fall in the hematocrit may occur within hours, whereas in a majority of patients with autoimmune hemolytic anemia, the anemia is essentially stable or only slowly progressive over a period of days.

The Appropriate Use of Blood in Various Clinical Settings in Patients with Autoimmune Hemolytic Anemia

Severe but Stable Anemia During Initial Evaluation. Patients with an anemia that is essentially stable during the initial period of evaluation generally should not be transfused at this point, even though they may have such symptoms as a marked decrease in exercise tolerance and palpitations with exertion. Even severe anemia found in patients with AIHA is generally well tolerated, even in the elderly, if bed rest is employed.[41] Furthermore, the response to therapy or spontaneous improvement may be rapid. For example, 50 percent of the patients with warm antibody autoimmune hemolytic anemia will respond to adequate doses of corticosteriods during the first week of therapy (Chapter 11), and acute paroxysmal cold hemoglobinuria seldom lasts longer than 7 to 10 days.[43]

Progressively Severe Anemia. Some patients do, however, have an anemia that is steadily progressive in severity, thus leading to the development of symptoms of hypoxemia. There usually is no evidence of vascular collapse because blood volume remains near normal, but progressively more severe angina and cardiac decompensation may occur. Extremely anemic patients (hematocrit level of 12 percent or hemoglobin level of 4 gm/dl) may develop neurologic signs beginning as marked lethargy and weakness, and progressing to somnolence, mental confusion, obtundation, and death. In patients with anemia of such severity (or in those patients whose rate of progression of anemia indicates that this point will probably be reached) red cells are urgently needed and nothing can substitute for their use, although oxygen should also be administered. In the management of these acutely ill patients who have not yet had time to respond to therapy, the use of packed red cells sufficient to maintain a modest increase in hematocrit until therapy of the AIHA becomes effective is probably optimal (see page 384).

In some patients, in spite of adequate therapy, hemolysis proceeds chronically at a rate greater than that of their red cell production, resulting in a relentlessly progressive anemia. In this situation, chronic transfusion is necessary to sustain life, and the attendant risks, cost, and inconvenience must be accepted.

Chronic Stable Anemia. Many patients (especially those with cold agglutinin disease) are able to partially compensate for their shortened red cell survival and maintain a relatively stable albeit occasionally quite severe degree of anemia. In such patients, in whom transfusion may be considered as a means of relieving symptoms, the advantages and disadvantages of such management are similar to those with other "refractory anemias" and must be very carefully weighed (for example, see Case Report: Patient V. W.; Chapter 6, page 218).

As in any patient with chronic anemia, transfusions should be given as packed red cells, although a leukocyte poor red cell preparation may ultimately be required to prevent febrile reactions.

Transfusions will at least partially suppress erythropoiesis, and the frequency of transfusions will need to be determined arbitrarily and will depend on the rate of hemolysis. It is usually convenient to give 2 to 4 units of packed red cells at a time when necessary. It is not advisable to completely correct the anemia, and transfusion to a level of hemoglobin of 8 to 11 gm/dl is perhaps optimal.

Fulminant Hemolytic Anemia. Least common among the indications for transfusion in immune hemolytic anemia is rapidly progressive anemia caused by acute massive hemolysis. Nevertheless, such fulminant hemolysis does occur and such patients may even be hypotensive. Signs of shock should be sought in patients with acute hemolytic anemia in a manner similar to that described regarding acute blood loss.

Patients who have AIHA of such severity can be expected to have gross evidences of hemolysis, particularly hemoglobinuria and hemoglobinemia. Diagnoses such as *Clostridium perfringens (welchii)* septicemia and drug-induced immune hemolytic anemia caused by drug-antibody immune complexes (Chapter 8) should also be quickly investigated. The onset may be so acute that a reticulocytosis may not be present, since the bone marrow may not have had time to compensate. Indeed, an increase in the reticulocyte count in response to a sudden decrease in red cell mass requires 7 to 10 days.[19]

Although such patients are uncommon, transfusion is urgent. If manifestations of shock are present, the immediate aim of transfusion is improvement in vital signs, which may be temporarily restored by the use of electrolyte or colloid solutions. Simultaneously the physician should communicate a sense of urgency to the blood transfusion laboratory (a maneuver rarely omitted*) to find optimal red cells for transfusion. Rarely will these red cells be "compatible" in the crossmatch, but, nevertheless, their use is mandatory in this acute life-threatening setting.

THE RISKS OF TRANSFUSION IN PATIENTS WITH AUTOIMMUNE HEMOLYTIC ANEMIA

AN OVERVIEW OF THE PROBLEM

In autoimmune hemolytic anemia, the risks of blood transfusion beyond the usual risks relate to the presence of the patient's red cell autoantibody. Autoantibodies usually react with all normal red cells so that any transfused cells may have a shorter than normal life span. This reaction cannot be avoided, assuming that optimal therapeutic measures are being utilized to treat the AIHA. The red cell autoantibody may react strongly *in vitro* (e.g., 2+ to 4+ by indirect antiglobulin test) with all available donor red cells to be transfused, thus making it impossible to obtain compatible blood for transfusion. Nevertheless, acute symptomatic transfusion reactions occur only infrequently. Subsequent survival is about as good as the patient's own red cells, and the net result is that transfusion generally causes temporary benefit. Thus, the reactivity *in vivo* of the autoantibody causes shortened survival of transfused red cells but usually does not contribute greatly to the acute risk of transfusion.

Although this finding is generally true, if the patient has very severe hemolysis, the autoantibody may cause striking destruction of transfused red blood cells, resulting in no benefit [18] or in dangerous degrees of hemolysis with hemoglobinemia, hemoglobinuria,[7] renal failure,[1] and clinical deteriora-

---

* Personal communication from technologists and blood bank directors too numerous to name.

tion.[24, 7] This observation is probably particularly true if relatively large volumes of blood are given (see *Optimal Volume of Blood to Be Transfused,* page 384).

In some patients, the autoantibody demonstrates clinically significant "relative specificity" in that it reacts more strongly with red cells bearing certain common Rh antigens than with red cells lacking these antigens. Tests for determining autoantibody "relative specificity" should be performed, since red cells lacking the more strongly reactive antigen may survive significantly better than cells containing the more reactive antigen.

Further, when the patient's serum reacts with all red cells in routine compatibility and antibody identification tests, the blood transfusion laboratory must utilize additional techniques in an attempt to demonstrate red cell antibodies other than the autoantibody. This is a critical aspect of selection of donor blood because, if the patient has previously been transfused or has been pregnant, and has developed red cell alloantibodies (e.g., anti-Rh, anti-Kell, anti-Kidd), donor red cells lacking such antigens must be selected for transfusion or a severe alloantibody-induced hemolytic transfusion reaction may ensue.

THE SELECTION OF DONOR BLOOD FOR TRANSFUSION IN SPECIFIC KINDS OF AUTOIMMUNE HEMOLYTIC ANEMIA

Warm Antibody Autoimmune Hemolytic Anemia

The selection of blood for transfusion to patients with warm antibody AIHA is one of the most difficult tasks faced by a blood transfusion laboratory. Also, laboratories vary in their resources, so methods that are readily available in reference laboratories may not be feasible in many hospital blood banks. Thus, absorption of aliquots of a patient's serum with red cells of various types (e.g., Jk^a negative, Fy^a negtive, and Kell negative) may present no problem for reference laboratories, but it may be very impractical for hospital blood banks to obtain adequate supplies of the appropriate cells.

In addition, the problems presented by individual patients with warm antibody AIHA vary greatly. For example, if a patient has not been recently transfused, determination of the patient's Rh phenotype and the use of autoabsorption techniques are practical and are of significant value. However, some patients may be transferred to referral centers after first being transfused, in which case determining the Rh phenotype of the patient and the use of autoabsorption techniques may be unreliable.

In any case, a significant commitment of time is required both in understanding the problems presented and in actually performing the tasks necessary for their resolution. We have divided the discussion of these problems into a consideration of ABO and Rh typing, the detection of alloantibodies, and the significance of autoantibody specificity.

ABO and Rh Cell Typing. ABO and Rh cell typing in AIHA are discussed in Chapter 5. For all patients with warm antibody AIHA who require transfusion, we strongly recommend determining the Rh phenotype of the patient prior to the initial transfusion. The reason for this recommendation is made evident in the following paragraphs.

Detection of Alloantibodies. If the patient's autoantibody reacts with all normal red cells, several techniques should be performed in order to detect alloantibodies that may also be present. These procedures are quite practical, not excessively time-consuming, and should be performed in all cases except when extreme urgency precludes adequate pre-transfusion evaluation.

Comparison of Direct and Indirect Antiglobulin Tests. A comparison of the strength of reactivity of the direct and indirect antiglobulin tests sometimes affords extremely valuable information.

In patients with warm antibody AIHA, the indirect antiglobulin test caused by autoantibody is generally weaker than the direct antiglobulin test. Apparently, most of the antibody is absorbed to the patient's red cells *in vivo.* A co-existing alloantibody will not, of course, be absorbed by the patient's red cells, and may result in a strongly positive indirect antiglobulin test. Thus, if the indirect antiglobulin test is significantly stronger than the direct antiglobulin test, the presence of an alloantibody is strongly suspected.

If the direct antiglobulin test is 4+, or if it is equal to or stronger than the indirect antiglobulin test, no conclusion can be reached concerning the presence or absence of alloantibodies.

Testing of Patient's Serum Against a Red Cell Panel. If the screening tests for serum antibody reveal an antibody reactive at 37°C, the serum should be tested against a panel of phenotyped cells as is routine in any blood bank determining specificities of alloantibodies. If a weakly reactive autoantibody and a strongly reactive alloantibody are present, the differences in the strength of reaction of various cells of the panel will make this evident. For example, Table 10-1 shows a strong anti-Kell together with a weak autoantibody.

However, one has no assurance that a patient's alloantibody will react more strongly than the autoantibody, so additional tests to detect alloantibody are necessary.

Warm Autoabsorption Technique. In our experience, the best technique for determining whether alloantibodies are present in addition to autoantibodies is to absorb the autoantibody from the patient's serum at 37°C using the patient's own red blood cells after first eluting some of the autoantibody. The earliest description of this technique that we are aware of is in a laboratory reference manual;[21a] it was subsequently also mentioned by Dorner, Parker, and Chaplin[9] and seemed to us to be a logical approach.[40] The technique may be modified by enzyme treatment of the patient's red cells after the elution procedure.[35] After absorption of the autoantibodies, the serum can then be tested for other red cell antibodies, since alloantibodies will not be

Table 10-1. REACTIONS OBTAINED WITH A SERUM CONTAINING ALLO ANTI-K AND AN UNDEFINED AUTOANTIBODY WHEN REACTED WITH A PANEL OF RED CELLS

Donor No.	Rh Phenotype	Rh								Kell						Duffy		Kidd		Lewis		MNS				P_1	Lutheran		Sex Linked	Results		
		C	D	E	c	e	f	C^w	V	K	k	Kp^a	Kp^b	Js^a	Js^b	Fy^a	Fy^b	Jk^a	Jk^b	Le^a	Le^b	M	N	S	s	P1	Lu^a	Lu^b	Xg^a	IC	37	IAT
1	rr	0	0	0	+	+	+	0	0	0	+	0	+	0	+	+	0	+	+	+	0	+	0	+	0	0	0	+	+	0	0	1+
2	rr	0	0	0	+	+	+	0	0	+	0	0	+	0	+	0	+	+	0	0	+	+	0	+	0	+	0	+	+	0	0	3+
3	rr	0	0	0	+	+	+	0	0	+	+	0	+	0	+	+	+	+	0	+	0	0	+	0	+	+	+	+	+	0	0	3+
4	r'r	+	0	0	+	+	+	0	0	0	+	0	+	0	+	0	+	+	+	0	+	0	+	0	+	+	0	+	+	0	0	1+
5	r'r	0	0	+	+	+W	+	0	0	0	+	0	+	0	+	+	+	0	+	0	+	+	+	+	+	+	0	+	+	0	0	1+
6	$R_1^wR_1$	+	+	0	0	+	0	+	0	0	+	0	+	0	+	+	0	0	+	0	+	+	+	0	+	+	0	+	+	0	0	3+
7	R_1R_1	+	+	0	0	+	0	0	0	0	+	+	+	+	+	0	0	+	0	0	+	+	+	+	+	+	0	+	0	0	0	1+
8	R_o	0	+	0	+	+	+	0	0	0	+	0	+	0	+	+	0	+	+	0	0	+	0	+	+	+	0	+	0	0	0	1+
9	R_2R_2	0	+	+	+	0	0	0	0	0	+	0	+	0	+	+	0	+	+	0	0	+	+	+	+	+	0	+	0	0	0	1+
10	R_2R_2	0	+	+	+	0	0	0	0	0	+	0	+	+	+	0	+	0	+	+	0	0	+	+	0	+	0	+	0	0	0	1+

IC=Immediate Centrifugation; 37=Agglutination at 37°C; IAT=Indirect Antiglobulin Test
Note that 3+ reactions are obtained with K positive red cells; all other cells yield 1+ reactions.

adsorbed onto the patient's own red blood cells. Details of the technique are listed in Table 10-2 and in Figure 10-1.

It has been our experience that most autoantibodies have indirect antiglobulin test titers less than 16, and two autoabsorptions will remove all autoantibody, leaving any alloantibody present in the serum. If the autoantibody titer is higher than 16 by the indirect antiglobulin test, more autoabsorptions may be necessary to remove all autoantibody. If the autoantibody titer is not high, enzyme treatment of the eluted red cells is not necessary. Indeed, since the ratio of cells and serum is different in the *in vitro* absorption procedure than it is *in vivo* in a patient anemic enough to require transfusion, autoabsorption without prior elution of the autoantibody (with or without enzyme treatment of the red cells) may suffice.

Following the autoabsorptions, the absorbed serum is retested. If a negative reaction is obtained, it is assumed that all the serum reactions were due to autoantibody. If a positive reaction still occurs, the absorbed serum should be tested against a panel of red cells to determine whether alloantibody is present or whether autoantibody is still present, thus requiring further warm autoabsorptions.

At the 1976 American Association of Blood Banks meeting, Morel and co-workers [35] presented data on 20 patients who had 3+ or 4+ direct antiglobulin tests, and indirect antiglobulin tests of 1+ to 4+. Twelve patients had autoantibodies that could be completely removed by two autoabsorptions. Eight other patients were shown to have alloantibodies present in addition to autoantibodies. The specificities involved were anti-E (3 patients), anti-V^w (1 patient), anti-c + E (2 patients), anti-C^W(1 patient), and anti-E + K (1 patient).

Table 10.2. WARM AUTOABSORPTION TECHNIQUE

a. Wash patient's red cells 4 times.

b. To packed washed cells add saline or 6% albumin (e.g., equal volume).

c. Incubate at 56°C for 5 minutes.*

d. Remove supernatant (eluate) after centrifugation. (Heat eluate can be discarded or used for specificity studies.)

e. Wash red cells three times

f. Enzyme treated red cells.† (We routinely use papain, but ficin works well.)

g. Add enzyme-treated cells to patient's serum (equal volume).

h. Incubate at 37°C for approximately 30 minutes.

i. Centrifuge. Remove serum.

j. Usually steps g–i must be repeated at least once more. ‡

k. Test autoabsorbed serum for activity.

    If negative: Antibody was autoantibody.

    If still positive: Antibody may be alloantibody, or serum needs further autoabsorptions.

---

* Some workers prefer 3 minutes.

† It does not matter if red blood cells are "overtreated."

‡ Most autoantibodies do not have titers higher than 8; in these cases 2 autoabsorptions are usually sufficient. It has been our experience that if the titer is higher than 16, three or more autoabsorptions may be necessary.

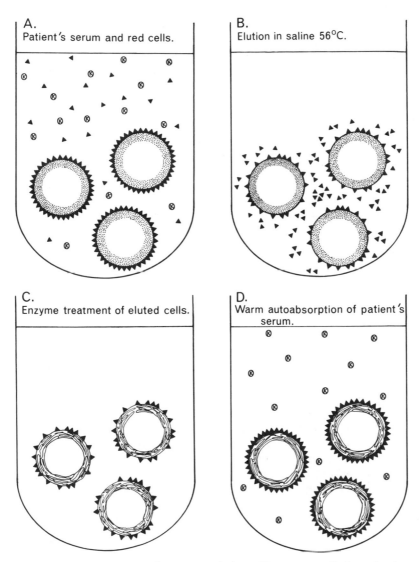

Figure 10-1. *The warm autoabsorption technique. Warm autoantibody molecules are illustrated by solid triangles, and anti-Kell allantibody molecules are indicated by the symbol K.* **Figure 10-1A** *indicates a Kell negative patient with warm antibody autoimmune hemolytic anemia who has formed anti-Kell as a result of previous transfusions. Autoantibody is present on the patient's red cells, and the serum contains both autoantibody and anti-Kell alloantibody.* **Figure 10-1B** *indicates the first step of the warm autoabsorption technique. An aliquot of the patient's red cells is washed and incubated in saline at 56°C for 5 minutes to elute some autoantibody.* **Figure 10-1C** *illustrates alteration of the red cell membrane by proteolytic enzymes such as papain or ficin. This augments the ability of the red cells to absorb antibody. These red cells are then used to absorb the patient's serum at 37°C. As indicated in* **Figure 10-1D,** *the autoantibody is removed from the serum, leaving only the alloantibody, which can then be identified by routine specificity testing against a panel of red cells.*

Since the warm autoabsorption technique is so useful, we recommend storing some of the patient's red cells obtained before the first transfusion episode so that they may be used in future autoabsorptions should continued transfusions be required. The red cells are best stored in ACD, CPD, or in the frozen state if facilities are available.

The Matuhasi-Ogata phenomenon may theoretically limit the usefulness of the warm autoabsorption technique or the differential absorption technique (described later). Matuhasi and Ogata suggested that antibodies of one specificity may adhere to antigen-antibody complexes of a different specificity.[3, 27, 37, 38] Thus, one could envision the absorption of alloantibody onto red cells that are used to absorb autoantibody from the patient's serum. Our personal experience, however, indicates that alloantibodies are indeed detectable after absorption of autoantibodies, so the extent of absorption of the alloantibody, if any, is not sufficient to nullify the usefulness of absorption techniques. Further, methods other than absorption techniques for detecting alloantibodies in the presence of autoantibodies are generally unreliable.

The preceding procedures ordinarily suffice to adequately assure detection of alloantibodies in the presence of autoantibodies, and further tests are superfluous. However, if a patient has been transfused in recent weeks, the warm autoabsorption test may not be absolutely reliable because it would seem possible that donor red cells that are still circulating could absorb alloantibody as well as autoantibody from the patient's serum *in vitro*. However, even if a patient has been recently transfused, we recommend performing the warm autoabsorption technique (although the differential absorption test is an adequate alternative when feasible—described later) because alloantibody may nevertheless be detected. Indeed, if alloantibody is not absorbed onto the circulating donor red cells *in vivo*, it seems likely that it will not be absorbed *in vitro* either. However, *in vitro* conditions may not exactly mimic *in vivo* conditions (e.g., the ratio of cells and serum are different and enzyme-treated red cells are usually recommended for *in vitro* autoabsorption), so that failure to detect alloantibodies by the warm autoabsorption technique in a recently transfused patient cannot be taken as absolutely definitive evidence of their absence. In this case, it would seem logical to omit the enzyme treatment of the red cells used for the warm autoabsorption in order to more closely mimic *in vivo* conditions. Also, the following additional tests are recommended.

Dilution Technique. Dilutions of the patient's serum are tested against a pool of two screening cells containing most common red cell antigens. A dilution is selected that reacts approximately 1+, and that dilution is then tested against a panel of red cells. This technique is efficient when the alloantibody is of higher titer than the autoantibody, but it cannot be used to confidently exclude the presence of alloantibody. Table 10-3 illustrates the results obtained in a case where the alloantibody of anti-c specificity had a titer of 64 and the autoantibody a titer of only 16. When the undiluted serum was tested, all cells reacted 3+, but a 1:64 dilution of the patient's serum reacted only with c positive red cells.

Table 10-3. RESULTS OF DILUTION TECHNIQUE TO DETERMINE PRESENCE OF ALLOANTIBODY

Dilutions of Patient's Serum:	2	4	8	16	32	64	128	256	512	1024
Indirect antiglobulin test on screening cells (pooled)	3+	3+	3+	2+	2+	1+	0	0	0	0

	Panel of Group O Cells							
	rr	rr	r'r	R₁R₁	R₁R₁	R₂R₂	R₂R₂	r"r"
Undiluted serum	3+	3+	3+	3+	3+	3+	3+	3+
Serum diluted 1:64	1+	1+	1+	0	0	1+	1+	1+

Agglutination reactions are graded as 1+ to 4+

Differential Absorption Technique. An approach that may be used instead of the warm autoabsorption method is the differential absorption technique, that is, the absorption of the autoantibody from the patient's serum using red cells of varying phenotypes. For example, performing an absorption using a Jkᵃ negative cell, of a serum containing a warm autoantibody and an anti-Jkᵃ alloantibody, will remove the autoantibody but not the anti-Jkᵃ. As with the warm autoabsorption technique, enzyme treatment of the red cells used for absorption will facilitate the removal of the autoantibody, but it is not absolutely necessary. The only practical limitation to the utilization of the differential absorption technique is obtaining an adequate supply of red cells of appropriate types for the absorption (that is, several ml of packed red cells of each type are needed).

Although this technique may seem hopelessly complicated since hundreds of red cell alloantibodies have been identified, alloantibodies of only a few specificities are responsible for a large majority of hemolytic transfusion reactions. That is, almost all hemolytic transfusion reactions are caused by ABO, Rh, Kell, Jkᵃ and Fyᵃ antibodies.[16]

ABO antibodies will present no problem, providing proper cell typing is performed as described in Chapter 5. Further, if the Rh phenotype of the patient is known, hemolytic transfusion reactions caused by Rh alloantibodies can be avoided by using blood of the same Rh phenotype as the patient. (Rh typing in AIHA is also discussed in Chapter 5.)

Thus, one may detect almost all potentially hemolytic alloantibodies by absorbing with only three cells, that is, Kell negative, Jkᵃ negative and Fyᵃ negative. As a modification of this approach one could, for example, omit the absorption with Kell-negative red cells and, instead, select Kell-negative donor red cells for transfusion to assure lack of a Kell-related transfusion reaction. Although this principle could theoretically be extended to the other blood groups as well, it is obviously unrealistic to attempt to secure donor blood that is, for example, Kell-negative, Jkᵃ-negative, Fyᵃ-negative and of the appropriate ABO and Rh type. If the cells used for absorbing are enzyme-treated and the autoantibody titer less than 16 by indirect antiglobulin test, two absorptions will most likely remove all autoantibody.

In summary, then, one need only absorb the autoantibody from the patient's serum with (enzyme-treated) Jk^a-negative and Fy^a-negative red cells to exclude the presence of these alloantibodies. If no alloantibodies are detected in the absorbed aliquots of the patient's serum, one may then transfuse with donor red cells that are Kell-negative and of the same Rh phenotype as the patient. Although the possible presence of alloantibodies of numerous specificities is ignored, the probability of an alloantibody-induced hemolytic transfusion reaction is minimal.

The differential absorption technique has another advantage in that it can be utilized even if the patient has recently been transfused. However, if the patient's Rh phenotype was not determined prior to transfusion, the strategy must be altered since Rh phenotyping is unreliable in the recently transfused patient. In this situation there is no way to avoid a rather significant degree of extra work to assure the absence of the most common and clinically important alloantibodies. In addition to absorbing with Jk^a-negative and Fy^a-negative red cells, the detection of Rh alloantibodies will require the absorption of three aliquots of the patient's serum using R_1R_1, R_2R_2 and rr red cells, respectively. Although cumbersome, this is the most reliable method to detect alloantibodies in the presence of autoantibodies in those most trying of times when a patient with warm antibody autoimmune hemolytic anemia has been recently transfused, has not had Rh phenotyping performed, and no pre-transfusion red cells are available for use in the warm autoabsorption technique.

Finally, as a note of reassurance, it should be emphasized that the probability of an alloantibody-induced hemolytic transfusion reaction is, in most instances, quite low. This finding is true since the incidence of alloantibodies capable of causing a hemolytic transfusion reaction in patients receiving blood of the same ABO and Rh types is a little over 1 percent.[16] The incidence of alloantibodies is lowest in patients who have never been pregnant or transfused, and increases with the number of exposures to blood.

Significance of Autoantibody Specificity. Techniques for demonstrating autoantibody specificity are described in Chapter 5. Ordinarily a titration technique for determining Rh specificity is the only method required regarding selection of blood for transfusion. In essence, one need only titer the patient's serum or eluate against R_1R_1, R_2R_2, and rr red cells.

Autoantibodies with Rh Specificity or "Relative Specificity." Serologists are frequently vague regarding the criteria used when reporting an autoantibody as having Rh specificity. Most warm autoantibodies react with all red cells of common Rh genotypes, but they may fail to react with gene deletion cells such as Rh$_{null}$ cells. Other autoantibodies will react with all red cells tested, but react to a higher titer or score against red cells bearing a particular Rh antigen. In either case the autoantibody is usually said to have Rh specificity without distinguishing such reactions from each other or from the clear-cut specificity of Rh alloantibodies, wherein cells lacking the appropriate antigen give strictly negative reactions. We will refer to antibodies that react with all normal red cells bearing common Rh antigens but that consistently react to a higher titer or score against red cells containing one or another Rh antigen as having "relative specificity."

Table 10-4 shows results of an eluate that would be interpreted as showing "relative specificity" against the e antigen. Such reactions should be confirmed by testing against several examples of red cells with and without the appropriate antigen before clinical decisions that are based on the "relative specificity" of the autoantibody are made.

Several investigators have studied the *in vivo* survival of red cells of varying Rh phenotypes in patients who have warm autoantibodies that were said to have Rh specificity. In most instances, detailed serologic data are not given, and the autoantibodies are likely to have demonstrated "relative specificity."

Mollison has described a case in which survival of the patient's own e-positive red cells was markedly shortened, whereas transfused e-negative red cells survived almost normally. The patient's serum contained an autoantibody with anti-e specificity.[32]

Salmon[45] described two patients who had anti-e and anti-nl autoantibodies. In the first case, the half time of ^{51}Cr-labeled red cells was 23 days for -D-/-D- red cells (e-, nl-), 24 days for cDE/cDE red cells (e-, nl+), and 12.5 days for cde/cde red cells (e+, nl+). In the second case, the half time was 14 days for cDE/cDE red cells but only 4 days for CDe/cde red cells.

Von dem Borne et al.[50] reported a patient who had auto-anti-e and anti-nl antibodies. The ^{51}Cr half time of CDe/CDe red cells was 1.9 days, and that of cDE/cDE red cells was 4.0 days.

In Holländer's patient,[21] the autoantibodies had anti-D specificity; while cde/cde blood survived for at least 31 days, CDe/cde blood survived for only 3 days. In Crowley and Bouroncle's patient,[6] two autoantibodies, anti-D and anti-E, were present, and cde/cde cells survived normally. In the patient of Wiener, Gordon, and Russow[53] the autoantibody reacted to highest titers with cells containing the rh' (C) factor; when transfused with blood lacking this factor, the patient made a complete and lasting recovery. Previously she had been treated with randomly selected Rh-positive donors and had failed to improve. Ley, Mayer, and Harris's patient was group O cde/cde. cDE/cDE

TAble 10-4. ELUATE SHOWING ANTI-e "RELATIVE SPECIFICITY"

	Dilutions of Eluate							
	2	4	8	16	32	64	128	256
rr(cde/cde)	4+	3+	3+	2+	2+	1+	0	0
R₁R₁(CDe/CDe)	4+	3+	3+	2+	2+	1+	0	0
R₂R₂(cDE/cDE)	3+	2+	1+	0	0	0	0	0

Agglutination reactions are graded as 1+ to 4+.

erythrocytes were demonstrated to survive normally (^{51}Cr half time = 25 days), but cde/cde cells survived even less well than the patient's own cells (^{51}Cr half time 5 days and 13 to 14 days, respectively).[25]

Högman, Killander and Sjölin's case was a 13-year-old child, of genotype CDe/CDe, who had formed auto-anti-e as well as an apparent "non-specific" component. The latter component did not appear to be of much importance as cDE/cDE red cells survived normally.[20]

Bell et al.[1] mention one patient with anti-e who tolerated two e-negative units with the expected rise and maintenance of hemoglobin levels. No further details are given.

Habibi et al.[18] transfused cDE/cDE red cells to 6 patients with autoantibodies of e, ce, or Ce specificities. The blood "proved normally efficient *in vivo*," but 2 of 6 homozygous ee patients developed anti-E alloantibodies.

Although the preceding data are scanty, we feel that if an autoantibody demonstrates "relative specificity" (e.g., the titer against red cells containing the e antigen is consistently two tubes higher than when tested against cells lacking the e antigen), it is preferable to avoid transfusion of blood containing the antigen in question, at least during the first few days of hospitalization, even though this may involve the deliberate administration of red cells containing Rh antigens that the patient lacks. An exception to this course is generally made if it would be necessary to give D positive blood to a D negative individual, especially in women who have not passed child-bearing age, or if repeated transfusions are necessary.

This approach is based on the fact that most patients with warm antibody AIHA respond to therapy quickly. That is, the median duration of corticosteroid therapy before discernable response was only 7 days in one large series (see Chapter 11). Thus, patients can benefit from the more prolonged survival of transfused red cells during this time when dangers of alloimmunization are as yet minimal. If transfusions are required over a more prolonged period of time, the development of alloantibodies becomes increasingly more probable. The deliberate transfusion of blood containing Rh antigens that are lacking on the patient's red cells may be continued as long as one can be confident that an alloantibody against that antigen is not present. However, a careful search for development of all clinically important red cell alloantibodies must be made at regular intervals (i.e., every 48 hours, as is required for all patients requiring frequent transfusion). When frequent transfusions are necessary, it is probably more practical, if the patient's Rh phenotype is known, to change to the transfusion of red cells of the same Rh phenotype as the patient, unless a supply of the patient's red cells obtained prior to the initial transfusion have been saved for use in the warm autoabsorption test. Without the availability of the patient's pretransfusion red cells for warm autoabsorption, the most reliable method for detecting alloantibodies requires absorption using red cells of varying antigenic types. This is cumbersome when absorptions of red cells of varying Rh types are necessary in addition to absorptions using cells of other blood groups. Further, it may not be feasible to obtain an adequate supply of the appropriate cells.

In contrast to our approach, some immunohematologists recommend ignoring the specificity of the autoantibody. This attitude is based on two considerations.

First, the evidence indicating good survival related to autoantibody "relative specificity" is not extensive. Indeed, in some reports no difference in survival *in vivo* could be demonstrated [7] and, in others the benefit was minimal.[50] In other instances, good survival of donor blood lacking the more reactive antigen was not shown to be due to the autoantibody specificity since survival of transfused cells containing the more reactive antigen was not studied.[1, 6, 18, 20]

Secondly, if one transfuses red cells that lack an antigen with which an autoantibody reacts, one may need to use red cells containing an antigen not found on the patient's own cells, thus causing the potential for alloimmunization. This does not seem to be a critical argument since typing for Rh antigens other than Rh_0 (D) is not part of routine blood transfusion practice, and we know of no data that convincingly demonstrate that patients with AIHA have an increased incidence of development of red cell alloantibodies after transfusion. However, as indicated previously, it is true that there is some advantage to be gained by ignoring Rh "relative specificity" if one instead selects blood for transfusion that is the same Rh phenotype as the patient. This will avoid Rh alloantibody-induced hemolytic transfusion reactions and is particularly significant if a patient needs multiple transfusions over a period of days or weeks.

Autoantibodies Without Demonstrated Specificity. If autoantibody specificity is not demonstrable, a seemingly logical approach is to do compatibility tests using as large a number of donor units as practical (e.g., 5 to 10 units) and then select for transfusion those units giving the weakest *in vitro* reactions. However, when such *in vitro* differences in reactivity are caused by variable reactivity of the red cell autoantibody not related to a specific Rh antigen (and not caused by the presence of alloantibody), there are no data indicating whether such comparatively weakly reactive units have better survival than more strongly reactive units. Pirofsky [41] states that the search for relatively weakly incompatible units is of no value, whereas Rosenfield and Jagathambal [44] accept that it may be of some value.

Autoimmune Hemolytic Anemia Without Serum Autoantibody. In contrast to the previously described problems frequently encountered in patients with AIHA, it should also be pointed out that in some patients with autoimmune hemolytic anemia, the autoantibody does not interfere with compatibility testing. This is true because the autoantibody may be undetectable in the patient's serum (apparently because it is entirely absorbed onto the patient's red cells) or detectable only by techniques more sensitive than are used in routine saline and albumin compatibility tests. Even though the donor blood is apparently compatible, the transfused red cells cannot be expected to survive normally because the autoantibody, although detectable only with very sensitive techniques *in vitro*, will react with donor cells *in vivo* as it has with the patient's own cells.[24] Thus, precautions concerning transfusion in patients with warm antibody AIHA apply equally even though the routine compatibility test would tend to falsely assure normal donor red cell survival.

When autoantibody is not detectable in the patient's serum by routine compatibility tests, the use of more sensitive serologic techniques may be utilized (i.e., the use of enzyme-treated red cells). In addition, autoantibody is often readily detected in an eluate prepared from the patient's red cells and, in this case, tests for specificity against common Rh antigens may be performed by titrations against R_1R_1, R_2R_2, and rr cells as described above.

In summary, in regard to selection of blood for transfusion to patients with warm antibody AIHA, we feel that it is most important to determine the Rh phenotype of the patient, save some of the patient's red cells for future warm autoabsorption tests, compare the strength of the direct and indirect antiglobulin tests, test for antibody specificity using a routine red cell panel, and perform the warm autoabsorption test. It is also important to test for autoantibody Rh "relative specificity" by performing a titration against R_1R_1, R_2R_2, and rr red cells. These tests are usually all that are necessary, but alternative approaches are acceptable and, at times, additional testing is required. Table 10-5 summarizes our recommendations.

Cold Agglutinin Syndrome

Performing Compatibility Test at 37°C in Saline. There are several approaches to compatibility testing in patients with cold agglutinin syndrome. One method is to perform the compatibility test strictly at 37°C and to use only normal saline media (i.e., without using albumin). Cold agglutinins from only 7 percent of patients with cold agglutinin syndrome react at 37°C in saline, although positive reactions will be obtained about 30 percent of the time in albumin media.[15] If positive reactions occur at 37°C in saline, one must first suspect faulty technique. If cells and serum are not prewarmed before mixing, if centrifugation is performed at a temperature less than 37°C, or if the initial washes of the cells after incubation do not utilize saline at 37°C, reactions may occur within seconds. Even if direct agglutination is not evident, complement may be bound by the antibody reactivity and result in a positive indirect antiglobulin test (one molecule of IgM antibody may bind several hundred molecules of complement).

The advantages of this method are that time-consuming autoabsorptions of the patient's serum are not necessary, and that the method can be utilized even if the patient has been recently transfused (the reliability of autoabsorption in the latter case is not certain; see page 370).

Several disadvantages are also apparent. First, it is obvious that red cell alloantibodies reacting at temperatures less than 37°C will not be detected. This finding is of little consequence since antibodies that do not react *in vitro* at temperatures less than 37°C are rarely, if ever, clinically significant. Giblett is

Table 10-5. SUMMARY OF METHODS USED IN SELECTION OF BLOOD FOR TRANSFUSION TO PATIENTS WITH WARM ANTIBODY AUTOIMMUNE HEMOLYTIC ANEMIA

I. Alloantibody Detection
   A. Patient not recently transfused
      1. Determine patient's Rh phenotype.
      2. Save as many red cells as practical in ACD, CPD, or in frozen state for use in warm autoabsorption technique should repeat transfusion be necessary in subsequent days to weeks.
      3. Compare strength of direct antiglobulin test and indirect antiglobulin test. If the indirect antiglobulin test is stronger, the presence of an alloantibody is highly suspected.
      4. Test patient's serum against a red cell panel. If an alloantibody causes stronger reactions than the autoantibody, the alloantibody specificity may be evident.
      5. Perform the warm autoabsorption test.
      6. The differential absorption test may be used instead of the warm autoabsorption test if adequate volumes of red cells of appropriate types are available.
   B. Patient recently transfused
      1. Pre-transfusion red cells available for warm autoabsorption technique.
      Follow steps 3–5 of A or use differential absorption method.
      2. Pre-transfusion red cells not available for warm autoabsorption technique.
         a) Rh phenotype of patient determined prior to first transfusion. The differential absorption technique is probably preferable for alloantibody detection. If impractical because of an inability to obtain adequate volumes of red cells for absorption, the warm autoabsorption test (using non-enzyme–treated red cells) is best compromise. Since the patient's Rh phenotype is known, reactions caused by alloantibodies of Rh specificity may be avoided by giving blood of the same Rh phenotype as the patient. For patients requiring repeated transfusions, this approach would appear safer than selecting blood on the basis of Rh "relative specificity" of the autoantibody because the dangers of undetected Rh alloimmunization outweigh the possible advantage of better cell survival related to autoantibody "relative specificity."
         b) Rh phenotype of patient not determined prior to first transfusion. If Rh phenotype was not determined prior to transfusion, it is best to use additional cells for differential absorption (i.e., R_1R_1, R_2R_2 and rr) or, if not feasible, rely on warm autoabsorption technique and the dilution technique for alloantibody detection. If the autoantibody does not demonstrate any specificity against common Rh antigens, blood of any Rh phenotype may be given—*but* D positive red cells should not be given to a D negative patient.
II. Autoantibody Specificity
   A. First transfusion episode
      Titer autoantibody in eluate or serum against R_1R_1, R_2R_2 and rr red cells. If significant "relative specificity" exists as shown by difference of titer of at least two tubes in doubling dilutions, select donor red cells lacking the more reactive antigen. An exception to this course is generally made if it would be necessary to give D positive blood to a D negative individual.

(cont. on p. 378)

Table 10-5. (CONTINUED)

B. Repeat transfusions

    1. Pre-transfusion red cells available for warm autoabsorption technique. If autoanti-body "relative specificity" is present and if repeated transfusions are necessary, one may continue to transfuse red cells lacking the more reactive antigen, providing that one can be confident that alloantibodies are not present. This is practical if pre-transfusion red cells are available for use in warm autoabsorption technique (or if it is feasible to perform differential absorption technique).

    2. Pre-transfusion red cells not available for warm autoabsorption technique.

        a) Rh phenotype of patient determined prior to first transfusion. Conditions are the same as described in section I,B,2,a.

        b) Rh phenotype of patient not determined prior to first transfusion.
        Conditions same as described in section I,B,2,b—but if autoantibody demonstrates Rh "relative specificity" one may as well continue to transfuse with red cells lacking the more reactive antigen, providing one does not transfuse D positive blood to a D negative recipient.

emphatic about this point, stating that alloantibodies that do not react at 37°C are of no concern since she has observed no *in vivo* hemolysis associated with a cold-reacting alloantibody (such as anti-A$_1$, -P$_1$, -M, -N, -Lu^a, etc.) during a 20 year period, when over one million units of blood were transfused.[16] Mollison is somewhat more cautious in his conclusions, but he does state that, in view of the small amount of destruction caused by cold agglutinins that are weakly reactive at 37°C, it seems clear that those cold agglutinins that are active only at some lower temperature than 37°C can safely be ignored.[34]

It is also true that antibodies reactive only in albumin media will be missed, but here, again, the risk is minimal because such antibodies are quite unusual.[47] Since compatibility testing at 37°C is quicker than other methods, it can be utilized even if the patient has recently been transfused, and it results in a low risk of missing clinically significant alloantibodies, we believe it is the method of choice. However, certain technical details are crucial in order to be certain that one is truly working strictly at 37°C.

A heated centrifuge or a centrifuge in a 37°C warm room may be used, a centrifuge may be placed in an incubator (Figure 10-2), or the tubes may be placed in centrifuge cups containing warm water. Samples transferred from a 37°C water bath and centrifuged immediately in a Serofuge at room temperature drop approximately 7 to 8°C after only 1 minute of centrifugation. It is necessary to keep a Serofuge in an incubator at about 45°C, to insure that the samples spin at 37°C. Similarly, saline at 40 to 45°C may be used, since it drops a few degrees when it enters a test tube and a few more degrees when centrifuging is in progress. A few simple experiments with each laboratory's equipment are all that is required to determine the conditions required to be able to carry out all procedures strictly at 37°C.

Cold Autoabsorption. An alternative approach is to absorb the cold autoantibody from the patient's serum before performing the compatibility test. This method works well for low titer cold agglutinins. However, it is very time-consuming when high titer antibodies causing cold agglutinin syndrome are present, requiring multiple absorptions even when using enzyme-treated red cells. This approach is therefore not optimal if blood is needed urgently.[40] However, the technique may be necessary in the small percentage of patients whose antibody is reactive at 37°C, even in saline. When positive reactions are obtained at 37°C, one or two autoabsorptions, followed by compatibility testing at 37°C, are useful. Table 10-6 shows the results of autoabsorbing a serum with a cold agglutinin titer of 2048 (saline) and 8096 (albumin). After three absorptions for one half hour each at 4°C using the patient's papainized red cells, the serum still reacted strongly (4+ with undiluted serum) at room temperature (25°C), but no longer reacted at 37°C.

Cold Autoabsorption Method.
a. Obtain two specimens of blood. Allow one to clot at 4°C; the other specimen should be anticoagulated and placed in a 37°C water bath for about 15 minutes.
b. Separate the serum while cold, preferably by centrifuging in ice-filled cups or in a refrigerated centrifuge.
c. Remove plasma from the 37°C incubated cells. Wash the cells 3 times in a large volume of warm (37°C) saline.
d. To one volume * of washed, packed autologous red blood cells, add one volume of enzyme solution. Any of the commonly used enzymes may be used (we usually use papain or ficin).
e. Mix and incubate at 37°C for 15 to 30 minutes. It is not important if cells are "overtreated."
f. Wash cells several times to remove enzyme solution.
g. To one volume of washed, packed, enzyme-treated cells, add one volume of patient's serum.
h. Mix and incubate in ice bath for 15 to 60 minutes, mix frequently for maximum absorption.
i. Centrifuge, preferably at 4°C, and separate serum as quickly as possible.
j. Test patient's absorbed serum against autologous cells to determine if the cold autoagglutinin has been completely removed. If not, repeat absorption with fresh enzyme-treated cells.

Other Methods. Still another approach to compatibility testing in cold agglutinin syndrome is to inactivate the IgM cold agglutinin with 2-mercaptoethanol [8, 17] or dithiothreitol (DTT).[42]

Pirofsky and Rosner [42] described the use of dithiothreitol at a concentration of 0.01M in a rapid 15 minute, 37°C incubation test system. Dialysis was not required. They reported that this procedure caused at least a fourfold or greater decrease in IgM antibody titers, without affecting the activity of IgG antibodies.

---

* Because several autoabsorptions are going to be necessary, it is wise to prepare enough enzyme-treated cells for multiple absorptions.

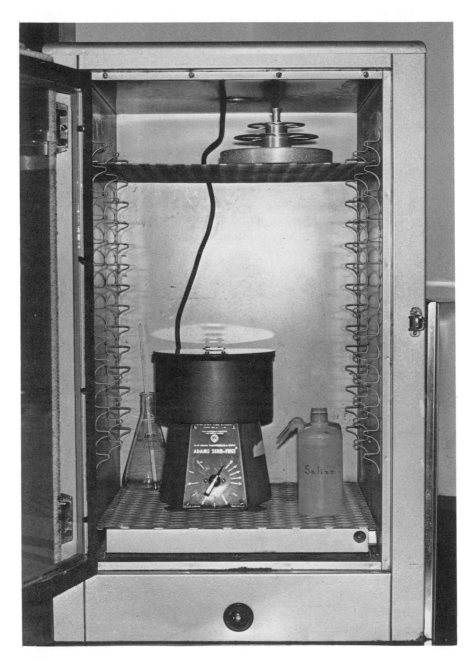

Figure 10-2. *A serologic centrifuge may by placed in an incubator to maintain the temperature at 37°C during centrifugation. The incubator must be maintained at a temperature of about 45°C so that the temperature in the tubes being centrifuged will be at least 37°C.*

Table 10-6. ABSORPTION OF COLD AGGLUTININ BY
PATIENT'S OWN CELLS AT 4°C

| | Titer against Adult OI Cells | | | | | |
| | 4°C | | 25°C | | 37°C | |
	Saline	Albumin	Saline	Albumin	Saline	Albumin
Unabsorbed	2048	8096	1024	8096	0	32
Absorbed × 1	1024	2048	256	1024	0	16
Absorbed × 2	256	256	128	256	0	8
Absorbed × 3	128	128	16	64	0	0

Olsen et al [38a] used dithiothreital in a concentration of 0.01M, added equal volumes to test sera, and incubated for 30 minutes at 37°C. Thirty sera that contained red cell antibodies reactive by the indirect antiglobulin test showed virtually no alteration in activity after dithiothreital treatment, while 20 sera containing cold-reactive red cell antibodies showed almost total elimination of activity. However, none of the cold-reactive antibodies tested were pathologic high titer cold agglutinins from patients with cold agglutinin syndrome.

Freedman et al.[14] reviewed the optimal conditions for the use of sulphydryl compounds in dissociating red cell antibodies. They noted that incubation at 37°C with 0.2M 2-mercaptoethanol provided the best conditions for inactivating IgM antibodies. However, it still failed to inactivate completely the extremely potent auto-anti-I (titer of 1,024,000) that was used. False positive reactions in the indirect antiglobulin test using anti-IgG or anti-complement antiglobulin serum were consistently obtained when sera which had been treated with 2-mercaptoethanol were not subsequently dialyzed. Although in many cases dialysis for as short as 30 minutes was sufficient, in others dialysis overnight was found to be necessary. Incubation of serum with DTT produced a slower effect than did 2-mercaptoethanol, and incubation for 2½ hours was necessary to reduce the anti-I titer from 1,024,000 to 1,024.

Using either reagent, IgM alloantibodies will, of course, be inactivated in addition to the cold agglutinins, and blood bank technologists are usually less confident with the use of such reagents than the use of 37°C apparatus or autoabsorptions.

Some investigators have suggested that adult-i red cells be used for transfusion of patients with cold agglutinin syndrome who have anti-I autoantibodies. Van Loghem et al.[49] studied the survival of I and i red cells labeled with ⁵¹Cr in one patient with chronic cold agglutinin syndrome. They demonstrated normal survival for the i donor cells with greatly shortened survival of both the patient's I cells and donor I cells. Woll et al.[55] reported one patient with transient cold agglutinin syndrome who responded to transfusion of warmed, freeze-thawed adult-i red blood cells. However, they did not test the survival of adult I red cells. Bell et al.[1] reported unfavorable experiences transfusing two patients with cold agglutinin syndrome with adult i red cells. Two adult i units given a patient with strong anti-I survived for approximately the same period of time (i.e., 3 to 4 days) as several adult I units given subsequently. In a second patient with anti-I, no elevation of hematocrit was noted after transfusion of 2 units of adult i blood. These authors suggested that the minimal I antigen present on adult i erythrocytes seemed sufficient to render them biologically incompatible.

Our own experience indicates that transfusion of adult I red cells to patients with chronic cold agglutinin syndrome usually results in an appropriate rise in hemoglobin. Unusual patients may fail to respond to transfusion of adult I red cells, but a majority of available data indicate that the use of adult i cells is not a solution to the problem. In patients with chronic cold agglutinin syndrome, the repeated use of i cells is certainly not feasible because of their extreme rarity.

Paroxysmal Cold Hemoglobinuria

Transfusion of compatible blood may be possible if the rare p or P^k cells are available through a rare donor file. Although the routine crossmatch test will appear to be compatible with other red cells since the antibody reacts only in the cold (usually <15°C), there is evidence indicating that p or P^k red cells will survive better.[43] Patients may require transfusion before such cells are available, and transfusion of red blood cells of common P types should not be withheld if transfusion is urgently needed. Although there are some reports of Donath-Landsteiner antibodies having other specificities, these are extraordinarily rare.

IN VIVO COMPATIBILITY TESTING

"*In vivo* compatibility testing" has been advocated by some and is, in general, based on testing the survival of an aliquot of red cells. Such studies should never be considered a substitute for a meticulous serologic evaluation of the patient with AIHA as described above. Red cell survival may be measured crudely by means of changes in serum bilirubin [51] or plasma hemoglobin,[19] or more precisely by utilizing ^{51}Cr-tagged cells.[22, 28, 33(c), 46] When radiolabeled cells are used, 0.5 to 1 ml of cells from a donor unit may be labeled with ^{51}Cr and injected,[22] or cells from each of two potential donors may be mixed prior to labeling.[33(c)] If the amount of radioactivity in the plasma, both at 10 and 60 minutes, does not exceed 5 percent of the radioactivity injected, and if red cell survival at 60 minutes is not less than 70 percent, some investigators feel that donor red cells may be transfused with minimum hazard.[22, 33d]

However, we feel that the significance of *in vivo* survival studies has been overemphasized regarding patients with AIHA and life-threatening anemia. If a careful serologic study has been done using the techniques and principles already described to select the best possible blood, and an *in vivo* test nevertheless demonstrates a very short cell survival, there is no logical way to select a different unit of blood for transfusion. If the patient is seriously ill and is not yet responding to appropriate therapy such as high doses of corticosteroids, such incompatible blood must still be given in the hope of obtaining temporary benefit.

In a detailed study of ^{51}Cr-labeled red cells in crossmatch positive patients, 10 ml of donor red cells were labeled, and a one hour survival of 85 percent was considered adequate.[46] In all patients the post-transfusion hematocrit level rise was appropriate for the number of units transfused, and no patient exhibited acute symptoms attributable to a hemolytic transfusion reaction. However, one patient with warm antibody autoimmune hemolytic anemia had a one hour red cell survival of 87 percent, a pre-transfusion hematocrit level of 10.5 percent, a post-transfusion hematocrit level of 20.6 percent, but a hematocrit level of only 10 percent just 16 hours post-transfusion. Another patient, with paroxysmal cold hemoglobinuria, had a one hour survival of Tj (a+) red cells of 87 percent, but only 53 percent of the radiolabeled cells survived to 48 hours. Still another patient with an alloantibody (anti-Jk^{b}) had 94 percent survival of tagged cells at one hour but only 10 percent survival at 24 hours. That a one hour red cell survival study does not accurately predict survival in subsequent hours is further indicated by an additional case report of a patient with anti-Lu^{b}; survival of radiolabeled Lu^{b} positive red cells was 84.4 percent at 1 hour but only 48 percent at 5 hours and 8.5 percent at 24 hours.[39]

It has been proposed [22,33(d)] that if at least 70 percent of a small volume of radiolabeled red cells are present in the circulation at the end of 1 hour, transfusion of a large volume of cells from the same donor will result in red cell survival better than that of the small volume. The rationale underlying this recommendation is that when survival of a small volume of red cells is at least 70 percent at 1 hour, it may be concluded that the concentration of antibody is low, and therefore there will be a big difference between the survival of small and large amounts of red cells. Mollison [33(d)] states that if a patient's serum contains potent Rh antibody, a small dose of red cells (1 ml) may be cleared with a half time of about 20 minutes, but a large dose (e.g., 400 ml) with a half time of 20 hours. More recently, data obtained in one patient with anti-A$_1$ that was weakly reactive at 37°C indicated progressively better red cell survival when volumes of ^{51}Cr labeled cells of 0.55 ml, 18.9 ml, and 178 ml were utilized.[34] Chaplin has reported similar findings in a patient with hypogammaglobulinemia who had anti-B that was barely detectable.[4]

However, Mollison also points out that with a potent hemolytic antibody both the rate and extent of destruction may be almost as great with a large as with a small amount of incompatible red cells.[33(d)] Further, the data previously cited concerning the patient with warm antibody AIHA whose hematocrit level dropped from 20.5 percent to 10 percent in 16 hours post-transfusion indicate that marked hemolysis may follow transfusion in AIHA even after adequate one hour survival of an aliquot of radiolabeled red cells.

Survival studies may be of some significance in that available data indicate that a good one-hour *in vivo* compatibility test seems to preclude the possibility of an immediate symptomatic hemolytic reaction when cells from the labeled unit are subsequently transfused.[22, 28, 33(d), 46] However, even if further data confirm the lack of an immediate symptomatic reaction, the destruction of large volumes of blood in the 16 to 24 hours after transfusion may result in significant morbidity or even mortality (see below).

Thus, *in vivo* survival studies yield disappointing results when applied to the problem of transfusing patients with AIHA. An acceptable survival of tagged cells for 1 hour may impart a false sense of security, since only a small percentage of cells may survive during the subsequent 16 to 24 hours.

Equally crucial is the realization that a patient should never be denied a needed transfusion because laboratory data (compatibility test or red cell survival study) suggest that the transfused blood will not survive well. Indeed, Mayer has reported [29] that 11 patients with AIHA who had an *in vivo* survival of ^{51}Cr tagged donor red blood cells of less than 70 percent in 1 hour nevertheless required transfusion. Only one of these patients had a complication directly attributable to the transfusion.[29] Also, Mollison [33a] states that when survival of a test sample of radiolabeled red cells at 60 minutes is subnormal, it by no means follows that there will be clinically significant red cell destruction if a unit or more of blood from the donor or donors is transfused.

When hemolysis is of life-threatening severity, the only alternatives are to allow the patient to die without transfusion or to transfuse blood that may be quite rapidly destroyed, perhaps with ensuing hemoglobinemia and hemoglobinuria, while producing only transient benefit. The obvious choice is to transfuse while simultaneously initiating appropriate therapy of the AIHA. Measures to decrease the likelihood of morbidity resulting from transfusion of patients with AIHA are discussed in the following section.

OPTIMAL VOLUME OF BLOOD TO BE TRANSFUSED

The optimal volume of blood to be transfused to patients with AIHA varies with the clinical setting. In patients who have severe hemolysis but may require transfusion only temporarily until therapy becomes effective, the transfusion of modest volumes of red cells just sufficient to maintain a tolerable hematocrit level appears advisable. Indeed, Rosenfield and Jagathambal point out that the salutary effect of just 100 ml of packed red cells may be quite remarkable when given to a patient with cardiopulmonary embarrassment from anemia.[44] They suggest that 100 ml may be given as needed (perhaps twice daily, depending on the severity of hemolysis), and that there is no need to increase the hemoglobin even to a level of 8 gm/dl. The aim of such transfusions is to supply just enough red cells to prevent hypoxemia while avoiding dangerous reactions resulting from over-transfusion.

The dangers of over-transfusion in patients with AIHA are several.

If the anemia is very severe (hematocrit 10 to 15 percent; hemoglobin 3.5 to 5.0 gm/dl), and especially if the patient is elderly or if cardiac reserve may be reduced, transfusion may easily overload the circulation and precipitate cardiac failure. In such patients red cells should be administered slowly, not exceeding 1 ml/kg/hr.[33(e)] One must look for evidence of congestive heart failure during and following the transfusion, particularly elevated venous pressure and the presence of rales on auscultation of the chest. Cardiac failure after the administration of as little as 200 ml of red cells may develop up to 6 to 12 hours later and may be fatal.[33(e)] Although diuretics are of value and probably should be given to patients with diminished cardiac reserve, responses will vary, and their administration must not replace close clinical observation of the patient.

Some physicians recommend partial exchange transfusion that can be conveniently carried out by starting a venesection in one arm and infusing red cells in the other, and by keeping the rates of blood administration and removal nearly equal. Since the hematocrit level in the blood removed is much lower than that in the blood administered, one may rapidly increase the patient's hematocrit level without changing blood volume. This can also be accomplished with cell separation by exchanging plasma for red cells. However, such measures to acutely increase the patient's red cell mass are probably contraindicated in this clinical setting for the following reasons.

An additional danger in patients with AIHA relates to the fact that the kinetics of red cell destruction always describe an exponential curve of decay, indicating that the number of cells removed in a unit of time is a percentage of the number of cells present at the start of this time interval.[44] Thus, the more cells present at zero time, the more cells in absolute number will be destroyed in the unit time span. Indeed, Chaplin indicates that the most common cause of post-transfusion hemoglobinuria in AIHA may not be alloantibody-induced hemolysis but instead may be the quantitative effect of transfusion in increasing the red cell mass subjected to on-going autoantibody mediated destruction.[5] Such marked post-transfusion hemoglobinemia and hemoglobinuria has the potential for a significant degree of associated morbidity and possibly mortality. Patients undergoing severe post-transfusion intravascular hemolysis may develop disseminated intravascular coagulation, possibly as a result of procoagulant substances present in red cell lysates.[33(b)] Further, there is evidence that complement activation may also trigger coagulation. Such coagulation abnormalities may be fatal, again emphasizing the need for restraint in transfusion of patients with AIHA.[33(b)]

The following two case summaries illustrate these points and were supplied by Chaplin.*

R.S., a 34 year old white gravida-1, para-1, with relapsing primary autoimmune hemolytic anemia for 4 months, was admitted to hospital with a hemoglobin level of 5.0 gm/dl; reticulocytes of 16 percent; direct antiglobulin test strongly positive for C3d, moderately positive for IgM, negative for IgG; and all crossmatches "incompatible." Despite high-dose therapy with corticosteroids, she required 1 to 2 units of packed red cells daily to maintain her hemoglobin level at 4.5 to 6.0 gm/dl. She experienced increasingly severe hemoglobinemia and hemoglobinuria associated with transfusions, clearing within a few hours. No alloantibodies were

* Chaplin, H., Jr.: Personal Communication, 1979.

demonstrable. On the 10th hospital day a splenectomy was performed without benefit. On the 12th hospital day, several hours following a transfusion, she developed acute respiratory distress, followed by cardiopulmonary arrest which did not respond to resuscitative measures. Autopsy revealed a single large para-aortic lymph node diagnosed as "plasmacytoid malignant lymphoma;" death was attributed to multiple fresh small pulmonary emboli.

L.F., a 56 year old white woman, never previously pregnant or transfused, was semistuporous at time of admission to the hospital. She had a hemoglobin level of 1.6 gm/dl; hematocrit level 6.2 percent; reticulocytes 19 percent; direct antiglobulin test strongly positive for C3d, moderately positive for IgG, weakly positive for IgM; and all crossmatches "incompatible." She was given corticosteroids and 3 units of packed group O D-negative red cells, developed fever and striking hemoglobinemia and hemoglobinuria which improved over the ensuing 3 hours. Her state of consciousness improved, and the hemoglobin level rose transiently to 5.7 gm/dl but was rapidly declining when she developed severe respiratory distress, followed by cardiopulmonary arrest which did not respond to resuscitation. At autopsy, no underlying cause for the autoimmune hemolytic anemia was found; death was attributed to multiple fresh small pulmonary emboli.

Transfusion of comparatively small volumes of blood as suggested by Rosenfield [44] may be the optimal means of minimizing the danger of transfusion-induced intravascular hemolysis. If post-transfusion hemoglobinuria occurs nevertheless, the use of heparin should be considered, although there is no well-documented evidence to support its prophylactic value in the prevention of disseminated intravascular coagulation.

Patients who have a chronic anemia that is unresponsive to therapy will, for practical purposes, require the transfusion of volumes of blood larger than 100 ml of RBC per transfusion. Patients with anemia causing signs and symptoms severe enough to require transfusion chronically may have only moderate degrees of hemolysis associated with a relatively poor marrow response, e.g., hemoglobin level of 5 gm/dl with less than 10 percent reticulocytes. Such patients can usually be managed as outlined on page 363 for patients with chronic anemia, i.e., with several units of red cells per transfusion as required.

Patients with chronic AIHA whose rate of hemolysis is significantly more severe and who require chronic transfusions are in greater danger of post-transfusion hemoglobinuria for reasons previously indicated. Transfusion therapy must be individualized, with an attempt being made to compromise between the impracticality of repeated use of small volumes of red cells, and the dangers inherent in transfusion of large volumes. Patients with marked shortening of red cell life span who require repeated frequent transfusions have a precarious outlook, at least in part because of the acute and chronic dangers of blood transfusions. Vigorous therapeutic measures for the AIHA are indicated (Chapter 11), and every attempt should be made to wean the patient off transfusion if a stable, albeit low, hematocrit level can be maintained.

THE USE OF WARM BLOOD FOR PATIENTS WITH COLD AGGLUTININ SYNDROME AND PAROXYSMAL COLD HEMOGLOBINURIA

Eminent authorities offer sharply differing opinions concerning the need for warm blood when transfusing patients with cold agglutinin syndrome. Dacie states that properly crossmatched blood can probably be transfused with safety if run in at a slow drip rate, in which case there is probably no need to attempt to warm it above room temperature.[7] In contrast, Rosenfield states that patients with cold agglutinin disease must receive warmed blood.[44] Mollison, in his comprehensive text,[33(g)] states that blood should be warmed before transfusion only in a few special circumstances, but he does not list cold antibody autoimmune hemolytic anemia among these indications. He does recommend that the patient be kept warm.[33(h)] Wallace comments that hemolytic reactions are unlikely, provided that the donor blood is warmed to body temperature and the recipient is kept warm.[52] Apparently the problem has not been studied in much depth, and no red cell survival studies are available comparing survival of blood transfused at various temperatures.

In regard to paroxysmal cold hemoglobinuria, Rausen does report that even compatible Tj (a−) blood needs to be warmed to 37°C before transfusion.[43] Wallace, however, states that transfusion of red cells of the common P groups (either P_1 positive or negative) is unlikely to precipitate an acute hemolytic transfusion reaction in paroxysmal cold hemoglobinuria provided the donations are warmed to 37°C and the patient is maintained at a warm temperature.[52] Johnsen et al.[23] reported the results of transfusion of 150 ml of prewarmed packed red cells (P positive) to an 18 month old boy with paroxysmal cold hemoglobinuria. The transfusion was followed by a temperature rise and passage of red-colored urine. However, the hemoglobin improved from 4.7 gm per dl to 12.4 gm per dl and remained at that level.

In the absence of extensive data, logic must prevail. Our experience in cold agglutinin syndrome has been consistent with Dacie's view, although in some instances we have empirically used an in-line blood warmer for seriously ill patients. The use of an in-line blood warmer would appear indicated if the patient has either severe paroxysmal cold hemoglobinuria or florid cold agglutinin disease. It is also logical to keep the patient warm, even if the efficacy of such a maneuver has not been proven.

If blood is to be warmed, it must be done properly. Unmonitored or uncontrolled heating of blood is extremely dangerous and should not be attempted. Red cells heated too much are rapidly destroyed *in vivo* and can be lethal to the patient.[44] In the past, blood units were pre-warmed by microwave units or by immersing in warm water. Neither practice is acceptable today. Instead, very efficient in-line blood warmers are available that are simple, efficient, and safe to use.[44]

USE OF WASHED RED BLOOD CELLS

Evans et al.[13] reported their experience in transfusing one patient with cold agglutinin syndrome. The cold antibody agglutinated red cells to a titer of 500,000 at 4°C and caused lysis of normal red cells both at room temperature and at 37°C (maximal at room temperature). A transfusion of 2 units of packed red cells was given without subjective reaction, although hemoglobinuria occurred following completion of the transfusion. A subsequent transfusion of 3 units of washed red cells was given without rise in plasma hemoglobin. The patient's serum complement was "always low." Although the data are far from conclusive, the authors speculated that the small amount of plasma present in the first transfusion of red cells provided the necessary complement for the hemolysis that followed. As indicated in Chapter 9, Section E, serum complement is often not reduced in patients with warm or cold antibody AIHA, and we would not recommend the use of washed red cells for this rationale on the basis of the limited information available.

Some investigators recommend using washed red cells for patients with AIHA to avoid febrile reactions caused by factors other than red cell antibodies. The interpretation of a febrile reaction in a seriously ill patient with AIHA is difficult and could lead to unnecessary cessation or delay of transfusion. These reactions may largely be prevented by the use of leukocyte poor red cells, and it is true that one method of preparation of these cells is by mechanical washing. The only justification for their use in AIHA beyond that applicable to other acutely ill patients is that the compatibility test procedures may be much more time consuming in AIHA. Thus, unnecessary cessation of the transfusion is more costly because of the additional technical procedures, and there may be a longer delay in selecting an alternative unit.

REFERENCES

1. Bell, C. A., Zwicker, H., and Sacks, H. J.: Autoimmune hemolytic anemia: Routine serologic evaluation in a general hospital population. Amer. J. Clin. Path., *60:*903, 1973.
2. Blackburn, E. K.: Indications for blood transfusion. Practitioner, *195:*174, 1965.
3. Bove, J. R., Holburn, A. M., and Mollison, P. L.: Non-specific binding of IgG to antibody-coated red cells (the Matuhasi-Ogata phenomenon). Immunology, *25:*793, 1973.
4. Chaplin, H., Jr.: Studies on the survival of inompatible cells in patients with hypo-gamma-globulinaemia. Blood, *14:*24, 1959.
5. Chaplin, H., Jr.: Special problems in transfusion management of patients with autoimmune hemolytic anemia. *In:* A seminar on laboratory management of hemolysis. Bell, C. A., Ed. Amer. Assoc. of Blood Banks, Wash., D.C., 1979.
6. Crowley, L. V., and Bouroncle, B. A.: Studies on the specificity of autoantibodies in acquired hemolytic anemia. Blood, *11:*700, 1956.
7. Dacie, J. V.: The Haemolytic Anemias. 2nd Ed. London, J. & A. Churchhill, Ltd, 1962, 673–676.

8. Deutsch, H. F., and Morton, J. I.: Dissociation of human serum macroglobulins. Science, *125:*600, 1957.
9. Dorner, I. M., Parker, C. W., and Chaplin, H.: Autoagglutination developing in a patient with acute renal failure. Brit. J. Haematol., *14:*383, 1968.
10. Elwood, P. C., and Hughes, D.: A clinical trial of iron therapy on psychomotor function in anaemic women. Brit. Med. J., *3:*254, 1970.
11. Elwood, P. C., and Wood, M. M.: Effect of oral iron therapy on the symptoms of anaemia. Brit. J. Preventive Social Med., *20:*172, 1966.
12. Elwood, P. C., Waters, W. E., Greene, W. J., Sweetnam, P., and Wood, M. M.: Symptoms and circulating haemoglobin level. J. Chronic Dis., *21:*615, 1969.
13. Evans, R. S., Bingham, M., and Turner, E.: Autoimmune hemolytic disease: Observations of serological reactions and disease activity. Ann. N. Y. Acad. Sci., *124:*422, 1965.
14. Freedman, J., Masters, C. A., Newlands, M., and Mollison, P. L.: Optimal conditions for the use of sulphydryl compounds of dissociating red cell antibodies. Vox. Sang., *30:*231, 1976.
15. Garratty, G., Petz, L. D., and Hoops, J. K.: The correlation of cold agglutinin titrations in saline and albumin with haemolytic anemia. Brit. J. Haematol., *35:*587, 1977.
16. Giblett, E. R.: Blood group alloantibodies: An assessment of some laboratory practices. Transfusion, *17:*299, 1977.
17. Grubb, R., and Swahn, B.: Destruction of some agglutinins but not of others by two sulfhydryl compounds. Acta Path. Microbiol. Scand., *43:*305, 1958.
18. Habibi, B.: Autoimmune hemolytic anemia in children. Am. J. Med., *56:*61, 1974.
19. Hillman, R. S.: Blood loss anemia. Postgrad. Med., *64:*88, 1978.
20. Högman, C., Killander, J., and Sjölin, S.: A case of idiopathic auto-immune haemolytic anaemia due to anti-e. Acta Paediat. (Uppsala), *49:*270, 1960.
21. Holländer, L.: Study of the erythrocyte survival time in a case of acquired haemolytic anaemia. Vox. Sang., *4:*164, 1954.
21a. Hyland Reference Manual of Immunohematology. 4th Ed. Los Angeles, Hyland Labs, 1966, 76.
22. International Committee for Standardization in Hematology: Recommended methods for radioisotope red cell survival studies. Blood, *38:*378, 1971.
23. Johnsen, H. E., Brostrom, K., and Madsen, M.: Paroxysmal cold haemoglobinuria in children: 3 cases encountered within a period of 7 months. Scand. J. Haematol., *20:*413, 1978.
24. Leddy, J. P., and Swisher, S. N.: Acquired immune hemolytic disorders (including drug-induced immune hemolytic anemia). *In* Immunological Diseases. 3rd Ed. Samter, M., Ed. Boston, Little, Brown, Vol. 1, 1978, 1187.
25. Ley, A. M., Mayer, K., and Harris, J. P.: Observations on a "specific autoantibody." Proc. 6th Congr. Int. Soc. Blood Trans., Boston, 1958, 148.
26. Masouredis, S. P.: Clinical use of blood and blood products in hematology. *In* Hematology. Williams, W. J., Beutler, E., Erslev, A. J., and Rundles, R. W., Eds. 2nd Ed. New York, McGraw-Hill, 1972, 1530–1546.
27. Matuhasi, T.: Plasma protein and antibody fractions observed from the serological point of view. Proceedings of the 15th General Assembly Japanese Medical Congress, Tokyo. *4:*80, 1959.
28. Mayer, K., Bettigole, R. E., Harris, J. P., et al.: Test in vivo to determine donor compatibility. Transfusion, *8:*28, 1968.
29. Mayer, K., Chin, B., Magnes, J., Harris, J. P., and Tegoli, J.: Further experiences with the in vivo crossmatch and transfusion of Coombs incompatible red cells. *In* XVII Congress of International Society of Hematology and XV Congress of International Society of Blood Transfusion Book of Abstracts, July 23–29, 1978, 49.
30. Metheny, D.: Clinical estimation of acute blood loss by the tilt test. Amer. Surg., *33:*573, 1967.

31. Milinan, N.: Blood transfusion requirements before and after bilateral nephrectomy in patients undergoing chronic haemodialysis. Acta Med. Scand., 195:479, 1974.
32. Mollison, P. L.: Measurement of survival and destruction of red cells in hemolytic syndromes. Brit. Med. Bull., 15:59, 1959.
33. Mollison, P. L.: Blood Transfusion in Clinical Medicine. 5th Ed. Oxford, Blackwell Scientific Publications, 1972, (a) 133, (b) 36, (c) 477, (d) 510, (e) 46–48, (f) 550–552, (g) 581, (h) 446.
33a. Mollison, P. L.: Blood Transfusion in Clinical Medicine. 6th Ed. Oxford, Blackwell, 1979, 532.
34. Mollison, P. L., Johnson, C. A., and Prior, D. M.: Dose-dependent destruction of A_1 cells by anti-A_1. Vox. Sang., 35:149, 1978.
35. Morel, P. A., Bergren, M. O., and Frank, B. A.: A simple method for the detection of alloantibody in the presence of warm autoantibody. Transfusion, 18:388, 1978 (abstract).
36. Morrow, J. J., Dagg, J. H., and Goldberg, A.: A controlled trial of iron therapy in sideropenia. Scot. J. Med., 13:78, 1968.
37. Ogata, T., and Matuhasi, T.: Problems of specific and cross reactivity of blood group antibodies. Proc. 8th Congr. Int. Soc. Blood Transf., Tokyo. Karger, Basel/New York, 1960, 208.
38. Ogata, T., and Matuhasi, T.: Further observations on the problem of specific and cross reactivity of blood group antibodies. In Proc. 9th Congr. Int. Soc. Blood Transf., Mexico. Karger, Basel/New York, 1962, 528.
38a. Olson, P. R., Weiblen, B. J., O'Leary, J. J., Moscowitz, A. J., and McCullough, J.: A simple technique for the inactivation of IgM antibodies using dithiothreitol. Vox Sang. 30:149, 1976.
39. Peters, B., Reid, M. E., Ellisor, S. S., and Avoy, D. R.: Red cell survival studies of Lu[b] incompatible blood in a patient with anti-Lu[b]. (Abstract.) Transfusion, 18:623, 1978.
40. Petz, L. D., and Garratty, G.: Laboratory correlations in immune hemolytic anemias. In Vyas, G. N., Stites, D. P., and Brecher, G., Eds. Laboratory Diagnosis of Immunologic Disorders. Grune & Stratton, 1975, 139.
41. Pirofsky, B.: Immune haemolytic disease: The autoimmune haemolytic anaemias. Clinics Haematol., 4:167, 1975.
42. Pirofsky, B., and Rosner, E. R.: DTT test: A new method to differentiate IgM and IgG erythrocyte antibodies. Vox. Sang., 27:480, 1974.
43. Rausen, A. R., LeVine, R., Hsu, T. C. S., and Rosenfield, R. E.: Compatible transfusion therapy for paroxysmal cold hemoglobinuria. Pediatrics, 55:275, 1975.
44. Rosenfield, R. E., and Jagathambal: Transfusion therapy for autoimmune hemolytic anemia. Seminars Hematol., 13:311, 1976.
45. Salmon, C.: Autoimmune hemolytic anemia. In Immunology. Bach, J., Swenson, R. S., and Schwartz, R. S., Eds. New York, John Wiley & Sons, 1978, 675.
46. Silvergleid, A. J., Wells, R. P., Hafleigh, E. B., Korn, G., et al.: Compatibility test using [51]chromium-labeled red blood cells in crossmatch positive patients. Transfusion, 18:8, 1978.
47. Stroup, M., and MacIlroy, M.: Evaluation of the albumin antiglobulin technic in antibody detection. Transfusion, 5:184, 1965.
48. Todd, D.: Diagnosis of haemolytic states. Clin. Haematol., 4:63, 1975.
49. Van Loghem, J. J., Peetom, F., Van der Hart, M., et al.: Serological and immunochemical studies in hemolytic anemia with high-titer cold agglutinins. Vox. Sang., 8:33, 1963.
50. Von Dem Borne, A. E. G., Engelfriet, C. P., Beckers, D. O., et al.: Autoimmune anaemias. Biochemical studies of red cells from patients with autoimmune

haemolytic anaemia with incomplete warm antibodies. Clin. Exper. Immunol., *8:*377, 1971.

51. Walford, R. I., and Taylor, P.: An in vivo crossmatching procedure for selected problem cases in blood banking. Transfusion, *4:*372, 1964.
52. Wallace, J.: Blood Transfusion for Clinicians. New York, Churchill Livingstone, 1977, 154–155.
53. Wiener, A. S., Gordon, E. B., and Russow, E.: Observations on the nature of the auto-antibodies in a case of acquired hemolytic anemia. Ann. Intern. Med., *47:*1, 1957.
54. Williams, W. J., Beutler, E., Erslev, A. J., and Rundles, r. W., Eds. Hematology. 2nd Ed., New York, McGraw-Hill, 1972, 239.
55. Woll, J. E., Smith, C. M., and Nusbacher, J.: Treatment of acute cold agglutinin hemolytic anemia with transfusion of adult i RBCs. J.A.M.A., *229:*1779, 1974.
56. Wood, M. M., and Elwood, P. C.: Symptoms of iron deficiency anaemia. A community survey. Brit. J. Preventive Social Med., *20:*117, 1968.

11

Management of Autoimmune Hemolytic Anemias

This chapter summarizes the information available on therapy of autoimmune hemolytic anemias and indicates a reasonable approach to therapeutic management, recognizing a lack of controlled clinical trials to clarify specific details. Most information available in the literature consists of anecdotal experiences of investigators or institutions, and there is considerable variation in dosage regimens, criteria of response, and indications for alternative therapeutic modalities. Indeed, we cannot offer results of randomized trials, since many of our patients were referred for diagnostic evaluation and were managed by their referring physicians so that therapeutic regimens varied widely.

WARM ANTIBODY AUTOIMMUNE HEMOLYTIC ANEMIA

Corticosteroid Therapy

Initial Management. Corticosteroids should be the initial therapeutic tool in treating patients with autoimmune hemolytic anemia of warm antibody type. Although detailed studies are not available concerning the efficacy of individual corticosteroids, there appears to be no selective benefit of any agent over prednisone. No advantages have been documented for parenteral administration or for the use of ACTH.

Initial dosage should be 60 to 80 mg per day in an adult. Experienced clinicians have emphasized that significantly larger doses (i.e., greater than about 1.5 mg per kg per day) will not have a greater effect.[20, 84, 114] Initial response is usually excellent, with about 80 percent of patients having a prompt and dramatic reduction in red cell destruction (Table 11-1).

The onset of the response is usually rapid. Significant hematologic improvement is often evident within a few days, and the median duration of therapy before discernable response was only seven days in one large series.[114] Only 6 of 86 patients (7 percent) responded after 2 weeks of therapy. Although therapeutic effects were occasionally noted after 3 weeks of therapy, the responses were generally poor, and high doses of prednisone were required for prolonged periods. Therefore, a lack of therapeutic response after three weeks of therapy should be considered a therapeutic failure.[114]

Table 11-1. INITIAL CORTICOSTEROID RESPONSE RATE IN IDIOPATHIC
WARM ANTIBODY AIHA

Authors (year)	Total Patients	Number of Responders	Percent Responders	Reference Number
Pirofsky (1969)	33	25	76	114
Allgood, Chaplin (1967)	44	37	84	4
Eyster, Jenkins (1969)	13	10	77	47
Dameshek, Komninos (1956)	21	20	95	32
Dacie (1962)	23	17	74	28
Horster (1961)	167	139	83	66
TOTAL	301	248	82	

Improvement of symptoms frequently occurs before a hematologic response is apparent. The patient may experience less fatigue, an improvement in strength, decreased malaise, disappearance of fever, and a sense of well being. These findings, however, are not always associated with hematologic improvement.

A transient but often substantial rise in the reticulocyte count may be discernable as the first objective evidence of a therapeutic response.[28, 114, 115] The degree of reticulocytosis attained reflects in part the pretherapeutic reticulocyte level. The elevation is less striking when the initial reticulocyte counts are high. The cause of the reticulocytosis is uncertain; some investigators have suggested that it results from temporary marrow stimulation, while others indicate that premature marrow release or a delay in maturation of the reticulocyte appears more likely.[28]

In other patients, hematologic improvement is first indicated by stabilization or improvement in the hematocrit level. Serum bilirubin values are of less significance and decrease slowly after the hematocrit and reticulocyte counts indicate improvement. Surprisingly little information is available on the use of LDH and haptoglobin values to monitor improvement.

Remission Maintenance. Sudden cessation of therapy often results in prompt relapse, and continued high dose corticosteroid therapy may lead to significant detrimental side effects. Thus, it is important to develop a general strategy for reduction of dosage, and criteria for institution of other modes of therapy.[112]

The following recommendations are influenced by the variety of approaches that have been proposed by experienced clinicians.[4, 84, 101, 115, 124] The initial dose of prednisone should be continued for three weeks unless the patient demonstrates an adequate response sooner (i.e., hematocrit level greater than 30 percent). For patients who have responded, a progressive but slow reduction of dosage is indicated. The following schedule is recommended: a weekly reduction of the daily dose of prednisone by 10 or 15 mg until a dose of 30 mg per day is reached. Thereafter, a reduction of 5 mg of the daily dose is made every week or two until a dose of 15 mg per day is reached. Subsequently, a reduction of 2.5 mg every two weeks should be employed. Although one may be tempted to discontinue steroids more rapidly, Leddy and Swisher [84] state that recurrences seem more likely unless patients are treated for a minimum of three or four months with low doses of corticosteroids following subsistence of an acute episode of hemolysis.

If a relapse occurs, one should return to the last previous dose. If small doses are adequate for maintenance therapy, it may be preferable to give alternate day therapy. In some patients remission may be maintained by relatively small doses of prednisone (5 to 10 mg per day), and occasionally what would seem to be a "ridiculously low dose" will suffice. [124] Indeed, Rosse and Logue described two patients whose hematologic remission was maintained with 5 mg of prednisone every third day; these patients relapsed if the steroid was withdrawn. [124]

If more than 15 mg per day of prednisone is required to keep the hematocrit level above 30 percent, the response should be considered inadequate and splenectomy performed or immunosuppressive drugs administered. Some have recommended that 10 mg of prednisone should be the maximum dosage acceptable for chronic therapy, [104] and Pirofsky has emphasized that long term side effects of corticosteroids are often "disastrous." [114]

The recurrence of hemolysis after corticosteroid-induced remission is usually gradual when the recommended schedule is used for tapering the dose. A majority of patients will relapse, however. Dacie [28] reported that only 3 of 23 patients (13 percent) were apparently "cured," and Allgood and Chaplin [4] indicated that 7 of 44 patients (16 percent) achieved a complete and permanent remission lasting from 9 months to 11 years following a single course of corticosteroid therapy. Dameshek and Komninos [32] reported that remission was maintained after discontinuing corticosteroids in 8 of 40 patients (18.6 percent). Some of those patients who relapse may be maintained on acceptably low doses of prednisone (10–15 mg per day or less), but about 50 percent of the patients will require other forms of therapy, such as splenectomy. [4]

Mechanisms of Corticosteroid Response. Several mechanisms have been documented as being responsible for the remissions induced by corticosteroids. The relative role of each mechanism is difficult to quantitate and probably varies from patient to patient. None of the described mechanisms offers an adequate explanation for the minority of patients who develop complete and permanent remissions, and it is more likely that such "cures" represent spontaneous remissions occurring during suppression of the disease manifestations by corticosteroids. At present the only well documented cause of transient cases of warm antibody autoimmune hemolytic anemia is the administration of certain drugs, particularly methyldopa. Other suspected causes are viral diseases or viral-like syndromes, especially in children.

Reduction of antibody synthesis: Reduction of antibody synthesis certainly plays a role in the development of remission in most patients treated for warm antibody autoimmune hemolytic anemia. Glucocorticoids are known to reduce antibody production. Rosse [123] used the C1 fixation and transfer test to study the quantative immunology of immune hemolytic anemia and demonstrated that, when patients achieved remission as a result of corticosteroid therapy, concentration of serum antibody fell to low levels. Numerous other investigators have documented similar findings by serologic studies. That is, if a patient derives substantial benefit from corticosteroid therapy, this will usually be reflected in an improvement in the serologic findings. [28] The direct antiglobulin test will become less strong and may eventually become negative, and free antibody, if originally present, most often is no longer discernable. For example, Evans reported that therapy resulted in serum antibody disappearing in 3 of 7 patients. The direct antiglobulin test became weaker in 6 patients and negative in 1. Dameshek and Komninos reported improvement in the direct antiglobulin test titer in 19 of 24 patients, although in only 1 patient did it become negative permanently. However, in 5 patients the strength of the reaction was apparently unaltered despite clinical and hematologic improvement. Serum antibody became weaker in all 19 patients in whom antibody was originally found, and became undetectable in 8.

Such serologic improvement is frequently underestimated if only the direct antiglobulin test is monitored, and particularly if only a single dilution of an antiglobulin serum is used. As emphasized elsewhere (page 204), changes in serologic findings are much more obvious if direct antiglobulin test titrations are performed and the titer of the serum antibody determined. Chaplin [19,20] illustrated a case in which apparent descrepancy between clinical improvement and lack of change in the antiglobulin test was resolved by antiglobulin test titrations. The direct antiglobulin test at an optimal dilution of antiglobulin serum was 4+ at the time corticosteroids were begun, and it remained so after 40 days of therapy. During this time, the ^{51}Cr red cell half-life improved from 7 days on initial measurement to near normal levels. However, reactions at other dilutions of the antiglobulin serum were clearly and progressively weaker when measured 14 and 40 days after the onset of therapy. Table 11-2 illustrates these findings.

The favorable effect on the direct antiglobulin test or a diminution or disappearance of free antibody in the serum of a successfully treated patient occurs relatively slowly, and it may not be discernable within the first week of treatment; thereafter the response, if it occurs, is usually relatively rapid and may be well marked by the end of the second week. [28] Thus, to the extent that serologic reactions accurately reflect concentrations of serum and cell bound antibody, it appears that the suppression of antibody synthesis is not likely to be the explanation for the very rapid improvement noted in many patients.

Table 11-2. CHANGES IN DIRECT ANTIGLOBULIN TEST REACTIVITY DURING RESPONSE TO THERAPY

	^{51}Cr-RBC Half-life, days	Reciprocal of Dilutions of Antiglobulin Reagent									
		2	4	8	16	32	64	128	256	512	1024
Before treatment	7	3+	4+	4+	4+	4+	4+	4+	4+	4+	3+
After 14 days of treatment	12	3+	3+	4+	4+	4+	4+	4+	3+	1+	2+
After 40days of treatment	20	2+	3+	3+	4+	4+	3+	2+	1+	1+	0

Agglutination reactions are graded as 1+ to 4+.

More likely, it is at least a contributing factor in long term control of autoimmune hemolytic anemia.

Altered antibody avidity: A second mechanism for therapeutic effect may be an alteration of antibody avidity for antigen on the red cell surface. Rosse [123] reported a decrease in the number of antibodies bound to the red cell and a concomitant increase in concentration of antibody in the serum within 48 hours of administration of corticosteroids in man. This finding may be the most immediate effect reported following the administration of corticosteroids in patients with autoimmune hemolytic anemia. However, *in vitro* studies with hydrocortisone have been unable to demonstrate alteration in the binding of antibody to red cells, and this effect has not been observed *in vivo* in an animal model. [5]

Altered clearance of antibody-coated red cells: A third effect of corticosteroids may be to alter the rate of clearance of antibody-coated cells by the reticuloendothelial system. Frank, Schreiber, and Atkinson [51] have shown that corticosteroid treatment caused a decrease in clearance of cells sensitized with both IgM and IgG antibody. The decrease in clearance was more marked in the case of IgG-coated red cells and was dose-dependent. The activity of the corticosteroids was first manifest after 4 to 5 days of treatment, and it became maximal after 8 days. The authors advanced the hypothesis that one of the *in vivo* effects of corticosteroids was to decrease the number and/or avidity of macrophage receptors for IgG and C3. These experiments correlate with clinical experience indicating much greater effectiveness of corticosteroids in warm antibody AIHA than in hemolytic anemia caused by IgM cold antibodies.

Kay and Douglas [80] also studied monocyte recognition of immunoprotein-coated erythrocytes *in vitro* in 21 patients with immune hemolytic anemia. They found that a majority of patients exhibited enhanced interaction between their monocytes and autologous immunoprotein-coated erythrocytes, as compared to normal monocytes exposed to the same immunoprotein-coated erythrocytes. In an animal model, 3 to 5 days of corticosteroid therapy resulted in a decreased ability to remove IgG sensitized red cells and/or complement sensitized cells from their circulation. Both splenic and hepatic receptor activity were inhibited. Macrophage activation had the opposite effect. Five days after the intravenous administration of Bacille Calmette Guerin (BCG), guinea pigs had a markedly increased rate and magnitude of clearance of IgG sensitized red cells and IgG and C3b sensitized cells.

Splenectomy

Clinical Response. The beneficial effect of splenectomy in acquired hemolytic anemia seems to have been reported for the first time by Micheli in 1911.[28] Other favorable accounts soon followed, and by 1940 Dameshek and Schwartz [33] were able to collect reports of 23 patients with acute hemolytic anemia (including 4 patients of their own), 20 of whom responded favorably to splenectomy. Later, Dameshek reported good results in 10 of 18 personally studied patients.[31]

In the last several decades, numerous reports concerning the effectiveness of splenectomy have appeared, many of which are summarized in Table 11-3.

Table 11-3. RESULTS OF SPLENECTOMY IN IDIOPATHIC WARM ANTIBODY AUTOIMMUNE HEMOLYTIC ANEMIA

Authors	Year	Number of Cases	Number Improved	Percent Improved	Reference
Stickney and Heck	1948	22	13	59	146
Robson	1949	9	7	78	119
Welch and Dameshek	1950	34	17	50	159
Dreyfus et al.	1951	5	2	40	40
Learmonth	1951	15	7	47	83
Chertkow and Dacie	1956	21	12	57	21
Young et al.	1957	18	12	67	166
Crosby and Rappaport	1957	27	17	63	26
Dausset and Colombani	1959	31	8	26	35
Dacie	1962	26	15	58	28
Goldberg	1966	13	11	85	55
Kinlough et al.	1966	9	8	89	82
Allgood and Chaplin	1967	25	18	72	4
Mapes and Fischer	1969	12	3	25	92
Schwartz et al.	1970	7	6	86	142
Devlin et al.	1970	5	4	80	37
Ahuja et al.	1972	4	4	100	3
Christensen	1973	13	12	92	22
Habibi et al.*	1974	16	12	75	58
Ikkala et al.	1974	4	3	75	69
TOTALS		316	191	60	

* Children

On the basis of this information, it is evident that splenectomy appears to offer considerable benefit in about 60 percent of patients.

Remissions are not always permanent, however. For example, Allgood and Chaplin [4] reported that 10 patients had a complete and permanent hematologic remission during a period of follow-up of from 1 to 10 years, but 6 other patients relapsed from 4 months to 8 years after splenectomy. (Two other patients benefited from splenectomy and could be maintained without corticosteroid therapy.)

If an incomplete remission develops or a relapse occurs following splenectomy, much lower doses of corticosteroids may prove effective in controlling the disease activity. [20] Indeed, Christensen reported that the requirement for prednisone decreased in 12 of 13 patients submitted to splenectomy. [22]

Mechanisms of Response to Splenectomy. As with corticosteroids, splenectomy probably produces benefit by more than one mechanism. One mechanism is decreased production of antibody. Although it may appear illogical that the removal of a small portion of the reticuloendothelial system should result in the disappearance of red cell autoantibodies, this is indeed the case in a significant number of patients. Dacie [28] emphasizes that in patients who improve, the serologic signs of the disease will become less marked. If antibody had been detected in the serum before splenectomy, it will probably disappear and the intensity of the direct antiglobulin test will lessen. Indeed, the direct antiglobulin test may become completely negative in patients with complete hematologic remission, although it often remains positive for years as the only sign of autoimmunization. Dacie reported that the direct antiglobulin test became negative in five of seven patients who had clinical cures of warm antibody AIHA by splenectomy. [28] Allgood and Chaplin did follow-up antiglobulin tests in 8 patients who had a complete remission, and the results were negative in 4. [4] Habibi [58] described 8 patients who were cured of hemolysis after splenectomy, and the serologic that results became negative in 5 of these patients.

The diminution in antibody production in patients with AIHA after splenectomy is consistent with the report of Karpatkin et al., [79] who studied the effect of splenectomy in a similar syndrome, idiopathic autoimmune thrombocytopenic purpura. They demonstrated a significant decline in serum antiplatelet antibody titer following splenectomy in 7 out of 8 patients. McMillan et al. [97] also reported that the spleen is an important site of antiplatelet antibody production.

A splenectomy also results in the removal of a potent site of red cell damage. Thus, the same degree of red cell sensitization may result in less shortening of red cell survival time. Indeed, Rosse [123] estimated that when the spleen is removed, up to 10 times as much antibody must be present on the red cell to affect the degree of lysis present prior to splenectomy. As emphasized in recent reviews of the role of the spleen in hemolytic disorders, [13, 14] factors of significance include the characteristics of particulate flow through the microvasculature, the environmental characteristics specific to the spleen, the deformability and plasticity of the red cell, and the highly specific cell-to-cell interactions between red cells and tissue cells. The latter are discussed in detail in Chapter 4.

The Value of Radiolabelled Red Cell Studies in the Selection of Patients for Splenectomy. The introduction of ^{51}Cr as a red cell label was followed shortly by the suggestion that surface detection of the radioactivity related to specific organs could be used to determine the predominant sites of red cell destruction.[67,73,74] Numerous subsequent studies have applied this technique to hemolytic anemias.[3,10,22,55,85,95,102,109,135,149,156,162]

Technical difficulties have been emphasized and related to collination of the apparatus, the marking of the surface sites for counting, and the analysis of the data.[14,149] In addition, the contribution of the red cell pool to the surface detectable radioactivity has produced a complication that has seldom been explicitly addressed in the analysis of results.[14] Clinical studies have led to various degrees of enthusiasm for the technique.

Three major deterrents exist that prevent ready acceptance of the thesis that splenic sequestration studies with ^{51}Cr labelled red cells should have a prominent role in deciding whether to perform splenectomy in patients with AIHA. First, Nightingale et al.[103] point out that many predictions of the value of splenic sequestration studies in hemolytic anemia have been largely based on, and extended from, the findings in hereditary spherocytosis in which splenectomy is always successful. Second, the concept that measurement of splenic sequestration of radiolabelled red cells can predict the outcome of splenectomy ignores the fact that the decreased production of antibody as a result of splenectomy is a major mechansim by which the operation produces clinical benefit.[4]

Third, Allgood and Chaplin[4] emphasize that few patients have been reported who have undergone splenectomy when external organ scanning failed to indicate splenic sequestration. For example. Ahuja et al.[3] selected patients for operation mainly on the basis of surface counting. No patients who showed evidence of red cell destruction in the liver alone or in whom there was no excess accumulation in either liver or spleen underwent the operation. Similarly, Kinlough et al.[82] concluded that studies with ^{51}Cr labelled red cells may lend valuable assistance in the selection of patients for operations, but all patients in their series had a "splenic uptake" sequestration pattern. Goldberg[55] selected 13 patients for splenectomy on the basis of an elevated spleen:liver ratio and concluded that results are better than in randomly selected patients reported in the literature.

Indeed, a significant number of patients with warm antibody AIHA have had a favorable response to splenectomy in spite of the fact that a ^{51}Cr sequestration study predicted a therapeutic failure. For example, Allgood and Chaplin[4] reported a good response to splenectomy in 4 of 7 patients who failed to show evidence for splenic sequestration. Parker et al.[109] studied 12 patients and found that 3 of 7 patients with spleen:liver ratios of less than 2.5 had a good result from splenectomy, and 2 of 5 patients with ratios greater than 2.5 had a poor response. They concluded that surface counting measurements are not reliable indicators of the outcome of splenectomy. Ben-Bassat et al.[10] reported that in 3 out of 5 patients the response to splenectomy was contrary to that expected from sequestration studies. Discrepant results have also been reported by other investigators,[3, 55, 156] and Crosby succinctly concludes that the test gives false-positive and false-negative results, thus vitiating its value.[25]

Therefore, clinical findings rather than ^{51}Cr sequestration studies should indicate the advisability of performing splenectomy.[4, 13, 25, 30, 114, 115] The operation need not be considered if satisfactory remission results from corticosteroid administration. If corticosteroids yield unsatisfactory results, the options are few and, in essence, include splenectomy, immunosuppressive drugs, and a variety of miscellaneous therapies that are reviewed below and that are still experimental and incompletely evaluated. The favorable results of splenectomy as listed in Table 11-3 are more impressive than any of the alternatives and, although a splenic sequestration study may predict a higher probability of response than would be true in a randomly selected patient, a good clinical response will frequently occur in spite of prediction of failure by the isotope study. In cases in which the indications for splenectomy are not compelling (e.g., an incomplete remission maintained on less than 15 mg of prednisone per day, or patients with relative contraindications to splenectomy), the sequestration study may be of some value in arriving at a decision. However, among those who require 10–15 mg per day or more of prednisone for adequate control of hemolysis, no patient should be denied the possible beneficial results of splenectomy of the basis of a ^{51}Cr splenic sequestration study.

Adverse Effects of Splenectomy. *Surgical morbidity and mortality:* The mortality and morbidity associated with splenectomy vary greatly, depending largely on the underlying disease for which the operation is performed. Thus, Schwartz et al. reported a series of 200 splenectomies for hematologic disorders [141, 142] in which a 7 percent mortality occurred during the immediate hospitalization (Table 11-4). However, all deaths were in patients with idiopathic thrombocytopenic purpura, thrombotic thrombocytopenic purpura, or in patients with lymphomas or leukemias. The immediate cause of death was usually cerebral hemorrhage caused by severe thrombocytopenia. In good risk patients who underwent elective splenectomy, no deaths occurred. Similar experience with almost identical mortality rates has been reported in other large series.[38, 131, 133]

Postoperative morbidity occurred in 18 percent of the patients reported by Schwartz et al.[142] The most frequent complication is that of left lower lobe atelectasis. Wound complications, septicemia, and development of subphrenic hematoma and abscess occurred almost exclusively in patients with myeloid metaplasia or hematologic malignancies with significant bleeding from the splenic bed.

Table 11-4. MORTALITY IN 200 PATIENTS UNDERGOING SPLENECTOMY
FOR HEMATOLOGIC DISORDERS

Disease	Number of Patients	Number of Post-operative Deaths	Percent Mortality
Idiopathic throm-bocytopenic purpura	63	7 *	11
Hereditary spherocytosis	40	0	0
Lymphomas and leukemia	26	5	19
Primary hypersplenism	12	0	0
Myeloid metaplasia	12	0	0
Thalassemia	10	0	0
Thrombotic throm-bocytopenic purpura	7	2	29
Acquired hemolytic anemia	7	0	0
Secondary hypersplenism	7	0	0
Miscellaneous	13	0	0
Splenic rupture (spon-taneous)	3	0	0
TOTALS	200	14	7

* All in-hospital postoperative deaths in idiopathic thrombocytopenic purpura occurred in patients
undergoing emergency splenectomy for uncontrollable hemorrhage or intracranial bleeding.

Fulminant bacteremia: In recent years, an appreciation has gradually developed of the risk of fulminant bacteremia as part of the hyposplenic
state. [12, 43] This risk is greatest in young children, especially for the first two
years after surgery and when the disorder for which the splenectomy was
required was a disease such as thalassemia major, histiocytosis X, or the
Wiscott-Aldrich syndrome. [43] Children subjected to splenectomy during stag-
ing laparotomy for Hodgkin's disease are also at high risk. [43] Fulminant septicemia seems rare after splenectomy for hereditary spherocytosis. [134]
Nevertheless, there is a low but significant risk even in normal subjects who
have incidental splenectomy. [56] In recent years, approximately 50 cases of
serious and often fatal post-splenectomy septicemia have been reported in
adults, many of whom underwent splenectomy for trauma. [43] In the typical
syndrome, a prevoiusly healthy normal adult develops a high fever, usually
after a brief mild upper respiratory tract infection, and within hours experiences shock and disseminated intravascular coagulation, which often proves
fatal. [12, 56, 68] The organism most commonly responsible for the infection is the
pneumococcus (*Streptococcus pneumoniae*). These patients have no obvious sites
of pneumococcal infection, and it may be that a synergistic viral infection is

needed to convert an asymptomatic carrier state into a fulminant pneumococ-cemia.[68] Blood levels of pneumococci reach extraordinary concentrations, seen only in patients with hyposplenism, and the capsular polysaccharides of these organisms trigger shock and disseminated intravascular coagula-tion.[24, 129] Although the pneumococcus has accounted for most cases, there have been reports, especially in children, of fatal septicemia caused by the meningococcus or by *H. influenzae*.

The management of hyposplenic patients includes the use of bacterial vaccines. A commercial pneumococcal vaccine is presently available, and others are being developed for meningococci and *H. influenzae*. Prophylactic adminstration of penicillin should be considered, especially for the first two years after splenectomy, and especially in children. However, the value of prophylactic regimens has not been proven, except in mice.[39] Patients should be alerted to the fact that the development of a fever without an obvious site of infection may constitute a medical emergency, and physicians should be prepared to obtain cultures and treat the patient for pneumococcemia with intravenous penicillin.[43]

Thrombocytosis: An additional potential complication is the development of postsplenectomy thrombocytosis and thromboembolism. Splenectomy is usually followed by a mild symptomless thrombocytosis that reaches a peak at about the end of the second week and gradually subsides within three months. Occasionally, however, postsplenectomy thrombocytosis persists. Hirsh and Dacie [64] studied the postsplenectomy platelet count in patients suffering from various types of anemia and in hematologically normal persons. Persistent postsplenectomy thrombocytosis was noted in all patients with continuing anemia after splenectomy, and the height of the persistent thrombocytosis was closely related to the severity of the anemia ($p < 0.001$). No such relation-ship existed between the platelet count and hemoglobin level in a comparable group of patients who had not been subjected to splenectomy. Hirsh and Dacie suggested that, in the presence of active hemopoiesis, anemia stimulates thrombopoiesis as well as erythropoiesis, but the increased thrombopoiesis does not result in persistent thrombocytosis unless the spleen is removed. They indicated that the persistence of thrombocytosis after splenectomy can usually be predicted; this happens when anemia continues after splenectomy in association with active hemopoiesis. Hirsh and Dacie also pointed out that postsplenectomy thromboembolism in association with postsplenectomy thrombocytosis has been reported after splenectomy, and they reported 5 patients in whom this complication occurred out of 80 patients who had undergone splenectomy for hematologic disease. Four of the 5 patients had congenital hemolytic anemias, but none of the patients in their series had an acquired immune hemolytic anemia. The authors were careful to point out that many other patients in their series had comparable increases in the post-splenectomy platelet count, which had been maintained for many years with-out development of thromboembolism.

Coon et al.[23] studied 86 patients who were undergoing elective splenectomy, and they detected deep vein thrombosis in five patients by using labeled fibrinogen and dye phlebography. However, in none of these 5 patients did an elevation in platelet count to 600,000/μl develop before or at the time of development of the thrombosis. None of 21 other patients who did have a rise in platelet count to greater than 1,000,000/μl had evidence of venous thrombosis. Coon et al. concluded that there was no need for the routine administration of prophylactic antithrombotic therapy in patients in whom postsplenectomy thrombocytosis develops.

Bensinger et al.[11] reported 4 patients (none of who had AIHA) who developed hemorrhagic complications associated with "spectacular" thrombocytosis postsplenectomy. Therapy with melphalan (L-phenylalanine mustard) effectively controlled the abnormal thrombocytosis and the clinical evidence of disease.

Thus, patients who have undergone splenectomy for AIHA may develop thrombocytosis if anemia persists, but there are no clear indications for treatment unless hemorrhagic or thromboembolic phenomena occur.

Immunosuppressive Drugs

Effectiveness. Although there has been less experience with the use of immunosuppressive drug therapy in AIHA than with corticosteroids or splenectomy, current evidence suggests that these drugs now have a definite role in the therapy of these patients.

In contrast to corticosteroids, which were demonstrated to have efficacy in AIHA prior to any rationale for their use, cytotoxic drugs have been selected for therapeutic trial because of demonstrated effects on the immune system. In 1957, Sterzl and Holub [147] suggested that 6-mercaptopurine might interfere with antibody synthesis. This theory was further studied by Schwartz et al.,[138,140] who demonstrated that this agent would suppress antibody formation in rabbits immunized with purified proteins. Most comparative pharmacologic studies have been accomplished in animals, but sufficient studies have been done in man to suggest similar modes of action. Drugs with the most potential for immunosuppressive therapy are cyclophosphamide, 6-mercaptopurine, methotrexate, cytosine arabinoside, and procarbazine, because they exert greater immunosuppression that myelosuppression. These agents, with the exception of cyclophosphamide, exert their principal immunosuppressive effect when administered prior to antigen, i.e., on the induction phase. Cyclophosphamide, however, effectively suppressed both the induction and the proliferative phases of the immune response.[50]

In 1960, a preliminary report concerning the use of antimetabolites in humans with AIHA was published,[34] and two years later Schwartz and Dameshek[139] reported results in 14 patients. This series includes 6 idiopathic cases, 2 associated with lupus erythematosus, and single cases associated with myxedema, hepatitis, chronic lymphocytic leukemia, Dilantin ingestion, virus infection, and rheumatoid arthritis. Two patients were exclusively treated with immunosuppressive drugs. Nine of the 14 patients experienced a beneficial effect of therapy with either 6-mercaptopurine or thioguanine at a dosage of 2.5 mg per kg. Of 9 patients who were prior steroid failures, 4 had good responses and 1 a partial response to cytotoxic therapy.

Taylor [152] reported a patient with autoimmune hemolytic anemia and possible Hodgkin's disease who failed to respond to corticosteroids and splenectomy. Over the next 6 years remissions of the hemolytic state were induced with triethylene melamine, chlorambucil, and cyclophosphamide.

Hitzig and Massimo [65] treated 3 children with AIHA with azathioprine at a dosage of 2.5 mg per kg in combination with steroid therapy. In 1 patient there was a complete response, and in 2 a partial response that permitted the reduction of steroid dosage.

Habibi et al. [58] treated 7 children with AIHA with azathioprine, and 4 obtained good responses.

Worlledge [164] reported that 6 of 14 patients treated with 75–200 mg of azathioprine daily had a good response, and 1 patient had a partial response. The duration of treatment ranged from 4 months to 6 years.

There have been several reviews of the use of immunosuppressive drugs in AIHA. Skinner and Schwartz [144] selected 42 cases of warm antibody AIHA from the literature. [65, 106, 107, 128, 130, 151, 152, 165] Most of the patients were treated with a combination of azathioprine and corticosteroids, and in many cases splenectomy was done before the azathioprine had been instituted. All patients seemed to have failed to respond to corticosteroid treatment. Twenty of the 42 patients (48 percent) were said to have improved with immunosuppressive therapy. Unfortunately, no objective criteria for improvement were listed in many cases, and the response was often merely described as "beneficial."

A similar analysis of the literature by Mueller-Eckhardt and Kretschmer [100] reported a 45 percent incidence of "good" response in 66 patients with AIHA treated with cytotoxic drugs.

Johnson and Abildgaard [75] reviewed the literature relating to pediatric patients [16, 58, 63, 65, 106, 139, 157] and described 2 additional cases. In all, 9 of 17 patients (53 percent) showed improvement. Eight of the 9 children who improved received azathioprine as one of their immunosuppressive agents, but at least 4 children who failed to improve had also received this drug.

Indications and Therapeutic Regimens. On the basis of the preceding reports, immunosuppressive drugs are indicated in some patients with warm antibody AIHA. Most clinicians suggest their use after both corticosteroids and splenectomy have failed to produce an adequate remission and if it is further demonstrated that an adequate remission is not possible using small doses of prednisone postsplenectomy. However, immunosuppressive drugs may be used instead of splenectomy if contraindications to surgery exist.

In contrast, Pirofsky [115] recommends beginning therapy with immunosuppressive drugs one week after starting prednisone if a discernable response is not evident by that time. The rationale for this approach is based on the fact that only 6 of his 62 patients who responded to corticosteroids did so after 2 weeks of therapy, and that 10 to 14 days of therapy with immunosuppressive drugs are necessary before a response is evident. Thus, if no response is evident after four weeks of drug therapy, one can proceed immediately to splenectomy or to higher doses of immunosuppressive drugs. In this case, prednisone should be reduced and eventually discontinued. For patients who do respond during the third and fourth week of therapy, immunosuppressive drugs are continued and prednisone gradually discontinued. Although this approach represents a minority viewpoint, it has the distinct advantage of allowing one to reach conclusions relatively quickly.

Several regimens for the administration of immunosuppressive drugs in patients with AIHA have been recommended.[101, 112, 115, 124] These regimens have been arbitrarily designed and are quite similar. Azathioprine in a dose of 2 to 2.5 mg per kg per day or cyclophosphamide, 1.5 to 2.0 mg per kg per day, may be used to initiate cytotoxic drug therapy. If corticosteroids have been responsible for an incomplete remission prior to the initiation of therapy with immunosuppressive drugs, they should be continued until signs of hematologic improvement occur, at which time they should be reduced in dosage as indicated on page 394, and discontinued if possible. Murphy and Lo Buglio[101] recommend continuing immunosuppressive drug therapy at the initial dosage for 6 months in those who respond, although this is evidently an empiric recommendation and a shorter period of time may be chosen. It is possible that maintenance doses of 25 mg every other day or even twice weekly may suffice.

In patients who do not respond after 4 weeks of therapy, the alternative drug may be substituted, or the dose of the initially used drug may be increased by increments of 25 mg per day every 2 weeks until a response or limiting side effects occur.[112] Particularly important adverse effects are gastrointestinal intolerance and evidence of marrow depression as manifested by leukopenia, thrombocytopenia, or increasing anemia with reticulocytopenia. Additional adverse effects of cyclophosphamide are hemorrhagic cystitis, alopecia, and adverse effects on the reproductive system.[101] Blood counts should be obtained weekly during the first month of therapy and for a similar period of time after each dose increase. Thereafter blood counts should be performed bi-weekly for several months and, if they become stable, monthly thereafter.

If a therapeutic response occurs while the patient is being maintained at full dosage, but hemolysis reappears during decrease of the cytotoxic agent, full doses should be reinstituted for several additional months. If the relapse occurs after the patient has been in remission for some time after all drugs had been withdrawn, a trial of corticosteroids alone has a chance of success and may be considered before proceeding to additional cytotoxic therapy.[101]

Adverse Effects. Although some adverse effects of immunosuppressive drug therapy have already been mentioned, a more complete discussion of possible complications is warranted. These complications are reviewed in detail by Steinberg et al.[145] and Miescher, Gerebtzoff, and Lambert.[99] In particular, several recent articles have reviewed cases in which malignancies have developed after cytotoxic agent therapy. [18a, 50a, 57a, 117a]

Infection: There is little doubt that the major immediate complication of cytotoxic drug therapy is infection. Most human data come from extremely complex clinical situations in which uremia, adrenal corticoid administration, prophylactic antibiotics, frequent hospitalizations, and many other factors are pertinent to whether or not an infection develops. In some diseases such as systemic lupus erythematosus, increased prevalence of infection is apparently a feature of the disease itself. With all this recognized, there is still an untoward incidence of infection, an apparent reduction in the ability to localize it, and a greater likelihood of an unfavorable outcome when a patient is on cytotoxic drugs.

It is also noteworthy that most patients, at the dose levels recommended in the preceding paragraphs, seem to do well over extended periods without apparent trouble from exogenous organisms. Specifically, pyogenic organisms do not seem to cause an unexpected amount of disease in these patients provided that the granulocyte count is maintained at adequate levels. Granulocytopenia of less than 1,000 polymorphonuclear leukocytes/μl is much more likely to result in disseminated pyogenic infection that is unresponsive to antibiotics.

Even without leukopenia, there are several classes of agents that can give trouble. Herpes zoster is very common but usually heals uneventfully. Dissemination of herpes zoster virus has been recognized, with death from this organism; also deaths from chickenpox pneumonia and systemic measles have been reported. Cytomegalovirus dissemination is commonly observed at autopsy, but the role of the organism in causing disease is often problematic. Rarer viral agents apparently also produce major illnesses in the immunosuppressed patient.

Pneumocystis carinii pneumonia is a potential problem, and its recognition is of the utmost importance since several specific therapeutic methods are available, notably pentamidine isethionate.

Other organisms that cause "intracellular infections" are organisms to which cellular immunity appears to be of more importance to the host's defenses than is circulating antibody. Mycotic and mycobacterial infections are in this group.

Virtually all the fungi have been seen to disseminate under cytotoxic therapy, usually with a fatal outcome. Infections with fungi that are ordinarily not of great pathogenetic significance for man, such as *Nocardia* or *Aspergillus* have been shown to be a hazard for the cytotoxic-treated patient. The same is true of a number of bacterial organisms—*Listeria, Herellea, Serratia*, and the like.

To summarize, the most important immediate problem for patients taking cytostatic drugs is infection from a great variety of organisms, some common and some exotic.

Sterilization: An important risk of some of these medications is that of sterilization. In treating non-malignant disease of various types, there are substantial chances for long term remission, periods when procreation may be of the utmost concern to the patient. This side effect is a serious problem, which must be dealt with in discussing the use of the medications, especially with youthful patients. That alkylating agents can damage animal germinal epithelium has long been apparent; the question is what can be expected in humans given ordinary doses of the drugs. Several reports have described ovarian suppression or premature menopause in roughly 10 percent of the patients given cyclophosphamide or chlorambucil.[145] Autopsy examination of the ovaries of a 13-year-old girl with juvenile rheumatoid arthritis who had received cyclophosphamide for 2½ years showed no oogonia and no follicles, only swirling masses of fibroblast-like cells.

Studies of 15 men in remission from Hodgkin's disease, months or years after treatment with six monthly cycles of four drugs in combination, revealed that two thirds of the men showed azoospermia, an absence of all germinal elements on testicular biopsy, and elevated circulating levels of follicle-stimulating hormone. The latter finding represented the loss of feedback control to the pituitary and permits the assumption that feedback was derived from the germinal epithelium in some ways.[145]

Effects on spermatogenesis may not be reflected by similar changes in oogenesis because of the great difference in turnover time of the germinal epithelium. Nevertheless, the clinical problem is clearly present in both men and women. Much more information in needed on these effects of various drugs; the results of further studies may well have a bearing on the selection of the "best" drug for an individual situation.[145]

Teratogenic Side Reactions: All drugs affecting nucleic acid and protein metabolism exhibit teratogenicity in animals. The doses necessary to trigger this effect vary greatly from compound to compound, as well as with the same compound from species to species, which makes it difficult to draw conclusions from animal to man. However, immunosuppressive therapy should be avoided in pregnant women whenever possible.

Teratogenicity may also be mediated by the father.[99] A few children exhibiting deformities have been born whose fathers were undergoing azathioprine therapy at the time of the child's conception. However, at least 38 normal children have been born to mothers married to a man receiving immunosuppressive therapy. In two instances an abortion occurred in the first trimester. Although children of fathers undergoing immunosuppressive treatment at the time of conception, or of mothers under immunosuppressive treatment during pregnancy, appear usually in good health, chromosomal changes have been observed at birth. These changes disappear during the following months.

In view of the potential teratogenicity of immunosuppressive therapy, patients must be informed accordingly. Contraception is indicated whether the husband or the wife undergoes immunosuppressive therapy. In the exceptional case of a mother who desperately wants a child, even after being informed of the potential danger, she should be assisted by proper manipulation of therapy, if possible without immunosuppressive agents during the first trimester. Since most information is available with regard to 6-mercaptopurine and azathioprine, preference should be given to these drugs.

Neoplasia: One of the most difficult of all problems related to cytotoxic agents is the potential threat of neoplasia,[18a, 50a, 57a, 117a] perhaps first becoming apparent after years have passed since drug exposure. It took many years to recognize the increased risk of leukemia in patients who had received radiation therapy for ankylosing spondylitis.

The increased prevalence of neoplasia in the immunosuppressed patient after organ transplantation is an unequivocal fact. Admittedly this information cannot necessarily be extended to cover those patients with diseases who receive more modest doses of cytotoxic drugs.

The explanation for the development of malignant disease in patients treated with cytotoxic drugs is not clear. The most commonly expressed view is that, in their immunosuppressed state, immune surveillance is defective and that mutant or perhaps virus-transformed cells that would, in the normal person, be promptly destroyed, are instead permitted to survive and multiply.

Other Therapies

Heparin Therapy. Heparin therapy has been utilized only rarely in patients with AIHA, although, surprisingly, the early case reports indicated that it had been effective. The effects of heparin therapy have been reported in a total of 15 patients (including one with cold agglutinin syndrome), and the results are summarized in Table 11-5.

In 1949 Owren[108] treated a patient with severe hemolytic anemia for 7 days at a dose of 350 mg per day. No therapeutic effect was noted. When heparin was increased to 800 mg per day, hemolysis decreased. Hemorrhage necessitated a discontinuation of therapy and subsequently severe hemolysis recurred. Storti and associates[198] in 1956 described the results of heparin therapy in a patient with idiopathic acquired hemolytic anemia without demonstrable erythrocyte autoantibodies. Heparin, 250 mg intravenously daily, was given for 30 days. Hemolysis markedly decreased. Discontinuation of heparin therapy resulted in a return of the hemolytic process. Roth and Frumin[127] in the same year reported that a single 50 mg intravenous dose of heparin reduced the direct antiglobulin titer, serum bilirubin, and plasma hemoglobin in a patient with autoimmune hemolytic anemia. The effect was rapid and could be demonstrated six hours after heparin administration. The patient was concomitantly treated with ACTH.

McFarland and associates[96] observed therapeutic benefits from heparin in autoimmune hemolytic anemia associated with Hodgkin's disease. Corticosteroids and splenectomy had failed in this patient. Heparin, 150 mg daily subcutaneously, led to striking improvement of the hemolytic process. Positive direct and indirect antiglobulin tests reverted to negative. Temporary discontinuation of heparin was followed by a severe relapse. The patient was then maintained on 20 mg daily for 3 months but developed thrombocytopenia. When heparin was increased to 50 mg daily, severe thrombocytopenia was partially corrected. Discontinuation of heparin was followed by a return of severe thrombocytopenia and hemolysis and the patient died.

Hartman [60] reported a patient with autoimmune hemolytic anemia in whom heparin was substituted for maintenance prednisone on two occasions. Hematologic improvement was noted and antiglobulin tests were negative during therapy, but they reverted to positive two days after cessation of heparin administration on each occasion. The patient refused further injections and he was maintained on prednisone.

TenPas and Monto [153] reported a patient with a small cell lymphoma and autoimmune hemolytic anemia. The hemolytic process responded poorly to cyclophosphamide, corticosteroids, and splenectomy. Heparin, 100 mg administered subcutaneously 3 times daily, induced hematologic remission. The antiglobulin test became negative two days after the start of heparin therapy. Maintenance doses of heparin, 25 mg twice daily, and prednisone, 10 mg daily, were continued, and remission persisted for 8 months.

In marked contrast to the encouraging reports in the first 6 patients reported, heparin has produced no discernable benefit in 9 subsequently reported patients.[8,52] On the basis of the report by Bardana, Bayrakci, Pirofsky, et al.[8] of therapeutic failure in 6 patients with warm antibody AIHA and 1 patient with cold agglutinin syndrome, Pirofsky has concluded that its routine use does not appear indicated.[115]

A number of mechanisms have been offered to explain the apparently successful results of heparin in some patients. Reports of Roth,[125] Roth and Frumin,[127] McFarland and associates,[96] Hartman,[60] and TenPas and Monto [153] indicate that heparin can modify the antiglobulin test *in vitro* and *in vivo*. In addition, Johnson and Beneze[76] noted that heparin in excess of 1mg/ml would inhibit the LE cell and antinuclear factor tests.

Storti and Vaccari [148] suggested that the antihemolytic effect of heparin was due to its anticomplementary activity, and Rosenfield and associates [121] noted that heparin administration in rats prevented organ sequestration of transfused lysin-sensitized erythrocytes. Inhibition of lysis following a single dose of heparin lasted for less than 4 hours. Heparin did not appear to block antibody uptake by erythrocytes or increase antibody dissociation from lysin-erythrocyte complexes. Heparin's protective effect was thought to result from its anticomplementary action.

However, Roth in 1965, published a report on the relationship between therapeutic and anticomplementary effects of heparin in acquired hemolytic anemia and found an insignificant lowering of serum complement after parenteral administration of the drug.[126] He concluded that any beneficial effect of heparin was "definitely not due to inhibition of complement."

Table 11-5. SUMMARY OF LITERATURE REGARDING HEPARIN IN AUTOIMMUNE HEMOLYTIC ANEMIA

Author	Age, Sex, Diagnosis Other Than AIHA	Drugs Prior to Heparin	Heparin Dosage	Pertinent Physical and Laboratory Findings	Major Response in Laboratory Data	Comments
Owren,[56] 1949	74, male	None	a) 350 mg/day for 7 days b) 800 mg/day for 6 days	Splenomegaly; Hb 3.5 gm/dl; Retics 7.5%	a) No effect b) Decreased hemolysis	b) When heparin discontinued because of hemorrhage patient relapsed
Storti et al.,[148] 1956	32, male	None	250 mg/day intravenously in divided doses for 30 days	No autoantibodies demonstrated	Decreased bilirubin Increase in RBC count	When heparin discontinued patient relapsed
Roth et al.,[24] 1956	15, female	ACTH	50 mg intramuscularly for one dose	Hb 6.2 gm/dl, Retics 33%, Positive direct antiglobulin test	Decrease in direct and indirect titers Decrease Hb Decreased bilirubin	–
McFarland et al.,[96] 1960	19, male Hodgkin's Disease	Prednisone, Exchange Transfusion, ACTH, Splenectomy	a) 150 mg/day b) 20–50 mg/day	Hb 4 gm/dl Retics 60%	a) Reversal of direct and indirect antiglobulin tests to negative b) Increased Hb 5 gm/dl to 9 gm/dl; Decreased bilirubin	Cessation of heparin caused relapse on 2 occasions

Reference	Age, sex	Treatment	Dose	Pretreatment values	Response values	Comments
Hartman,[60] 1964	39, male	a) Prednisone discontinued during heparin therapy	50–300 mg/day for 17 days	Hb 8.9 gm/dl Retics 7%	Hb 11.5 gm/dl Retics 2.5%	Antiglobulin test neg. twice when on heparin, but most recent positive test not indicated; antiglobulin test positive a day after stopping heparin
Same patient 8 months later		b) Prednisone discontinued during heparin therapy	200 mg/day for 7 days, then 100mg/day for 7 days	Retics 14% RBC 2.5 million/μl; Bilirubin 3.0 Plasma Hb 30 mg/dl	Retics 2–4%; RBC 3.8 million/μl; Bilirubin 0.9; plasma Hb 5.2 mg/dl	Pretreatment antiglobulin test titer 128, became transiently negative 2 hours after starting heparin and was negative at 7 and 14 days Positive again 2 days after discontinuing heparin.
TenPas et al,[153] 1966	27, male Lymphosarcoma	Fluronethalone, Vinblastine sulfate, cyclophosphamide, corticosteroids, splenectomy	a) 100 mg, q8H subcutaneously b) 25 mg BID for 8 months	Hb 6 gm/dl; Retics 0.2% Bone marrow 60% infiltrated with lymphosarcoma cells	Reversal of direct and indirect antiglobulin test to negative in 2 days. Increased complement levels from 133 to 180 units/ml	Maintained on heparin 22mg BID for 8 mos; also concomitantly treated with prednisone
Frimmer et al,[52] 1969	33, male	Corticosteroids, Splenectomy	a) 50 mg q8H subcutaneously b) 300 mg/day for 3 days	Hb 8.3 gm/dl Retics 7%	a) Increased ^{51}Cr survival from 2.2 days to 8.8 days b) Increased ^{51}Cr survival from 8.9 days to 11.9 days	Responded to prednisone

Table 11-5. (CONTINUED)

Author	Age, Sex, Diagnosis Other Than AIHA	Drugs Prior to Heparin	Heparin Dosage	Pertinent Physical and Laboratory Findings	Major Response in Laboratory Data	Comments
Bardana et al.,[8] 1970	a) 80, female, Waldenström's Disease	$FeSO_4$	75 mg/day initially; increased to 300 mg/day for at least 3 days. Total duration of therapy = 5–8 days	PCV 25 Retics 6.1% ^{51}Cr T/2 = 16.5 days	None	Subsequently responded to prednisone
	b) 60, female chronic lymphocytic leukemia	Vit B$_{12}$ Prednisone	"	PCV 19 Retics 3.4% ^{51}Cr T/2 = 9 days	None	Failed to respond to azathioprine and splenectomy
	c) 57, female Systemic lupus erythematosus	Imferon	"	PCV 18 Retics 1.7% ^{51}Cr T/2 = 20 days	None	Failed to respond to prednisone, azathioprine and splenectomy; responded to antilymphocyte serum

Bardana et al.,[8] 1970	d) 67, male Cold agglutinin syndrome; dermatitis herpetiformis	None	75 mg/day initially; increased to 300 mg/day for at least 3 days. Total duration of therapy = 5–8 days	PCV 28 Retics 3.2% Cold agglutinin titer = 16,000	None	Responded to epsilon aminocaproic acid
	e) 72, male, Adenocarcinoma of lung	None	"	PCV 35 Retics 1.9% ^{51}Cr T/2 = 15 days	None	Antiglobulin test and anemia reverted with lobectomy
	f) 52, male, Acute myocardial infarction	Methyldopa	"	PCV 25 Retics 22%	None	Responded to prednisone and cessation of methyldopa
	g) 44, female	Prednisone	"	PCV 27 Retics 47% ^{51}Cr T/2 = 5 days	None	Responded to azathioprine

Garratty [53] in *in vitro* studies indicated that 10 units of heparin per ml caused measurably weaker reactions in the indirect antiglobulin test using a complement fixing Lewis antibody, and that when more than 50 units of heparin per ml were present, the anti-Le[a] was barely detectable. However, patients receiving heparin for anticoagulant therapy rarely, if ever, reach these levels.

More recently we [113] have studied serum complement levels in 10 normal volunteers (5 men and 5 women, aged 25 to 36) who received heparin on two separate occasions one week apart. One hundred units per kg of beef lung or pork gut heparin were given as an intravenous bolus. The effects of this dose of heparin on various coagulation tests are listed in Table 11-6, and these results indicate that therapeutically effective concentrations had been reached. Serum hemolytic complement assays, using a standard sensitized sheep cell assay and measured at 15, 45, and 120 minutes after heparin administration, revealed no significant changes in any subject compared with baseline measurements.

Thus, we have been unable to detect an effect of heparin on hemolytic complement activity *in vivo* even after therapeutic doses. Furthermore, most of the case reports suggesting a favorable effect of heparin in patients with AIHA have used heparin in less than anticoagulant dosage. [52]

In summary, heparin showed promise on the basis of early case reports indicating favorable effects on both clinical and serologic findings in patients with warm antibody AIHA. However, the speculation that its mechanism of action is related to its anticomplementary effects does not seem valid, and all 9 case reports after 1969 have indicated a lack of benefit. Perhaps further study is warranted, but at present heparin cannot be recommended with enthusiasm.

Thymectomy. The results of thymectomy in patients with AIHA are summarized in Table 11-7.

In 1963, Wilmers and Russell [163] reported a 2½ month old infant with autoimmune hemolytic anemia; the infant was unresponsive to splenectomy or corticosteroids. Thymectomy induced hematologic remission. The antiglobulin test was still positive 8 weeks after surgery, but it reverted to negative 3 weeks later. Cure of AIHA in an infant was also reported after thymectomy by Karaklis et al. [78] Subsequently, cases in which the operation produced benefit were reported by Hancock, [59] Dacie and Worlledge, [30] and Hirooka. [63] No benefit was recorded in patients described by Oski and Abelson [106] and Johnson and Abildgaard. [75]

Ross et al. [122] performed a thymectomy in a patient with a thymoma, erythroid aplasia, and AIHA. The surgery did not influence the hemolysis, positive antiglobulin tests, or erythrocytic aplasia. Pirofsky [114] also reported therapeutic failure of thymectomy in a similar patient. There are no reports of benefit of thymectomy in patients with AIHA associated with a thymoma.

It is difficult to derive firm conclusions on the basis of these meager and rather unimpressive results. Perhaps the operation should be considered after

Table 11-6. EFFECTS ON COAGULATION TESTS OF 100 UNITS OF HEPARIN PER KG GIVEN AS AN INTRAVENOUS BOLUS IN 10 NORMAL SUBJECTS

Test		Baseline	15 Minutes	45 Minutes	120 Minutes
Prothrombin time	A*	11.4 ± 0.4 sec	27.8 ± 6.5	19.2 ± 2.6	14.0 ± 1.0
	B*	11.1 ± 5.9	25.0 ± 5.9	17.7 ± 2.0	13.6 ± 0.8
Activated partial thromboplastin time	A	30.0 ± 3.4 sec	> 200	> 200	103.8 ± 52.9
	B	30.0 ± 3.6	> 200	> 200	112.6 ± 53.1
Thrombin time	A	13.7 ± 1.0 sec.	> 200	> 200	> 200
	B	13.8 ± 1.0	> 200	> 200	> 200
Template bleeding time	A	5.5 ± 1.4 min.	7.4 ± 1.4 min.	7.3 ± 3.1	6.3 ± 2.4
	B	5.5 ± 1.2	11.5 ± 5.6	11.2 ± 5.5	9.2 ± 4.9

* A = beef lung heparin; B* = port gut heparin

Table 11-7. THYMECTOMY IN AUTOIMMUNE HEMOLYTIC ANEMIA

Authors (year)	Age	Course	Reference Number
Wilmers and Russel (1963)	2½ months	Cured	163
Hancock (1963)	infant	Successful	59
Karaklis et al. (1964)	infant	Cured	78
Oski and Abelson (1965)	6 weeks	No benefit	106
Dacie and Worlledge (1969)	7 months	Cured	30
Hirooka (1970)	8 years	Marked clinical improvement	63
Johnson and Abildgaard (1976)	7 months	No benefit	75
Rose et al.* (1954)	44 years	No benefit	122
Pirofsky (1969) *	59 years	No benefit	114

* Associated with thymoma and erythrocytic aplasia.

more usual therapy has failed, especially in infants with severe hemolysis. Pirofsky comments that the surgery is technically easier than splenectomy.[114]

Antilymphocyte Globulin. The use of antilymphocyte globulin is an experimental form of therapy, and scanty data exist concerning its effectiveness in AIHA. Pirofsky has treated two patients with AIHA secondary to systemic lupus erythematosus and Hodgkin's disease, respectively. Both patients were said to respond surprisingly well after being unresponsive to all other therapies.[115]

Marmont et al.[93] describe the use of commercial antilymphocyte globulin of equine origin in 14 patients with a variety of autoimmune blood diseases and point out that after 15 to 21 days therapy was generally discontinued due to the onset of a "mild anaphylactic reaction." They treated one patient who had autoimmune hemolytic anemia associated with ulcerative colitis. The AIHA improved but the patient was also treated with corticosteroids and cyclophosphamide. These authors also cite favorable results in 10 further patients reported only in abstract form by Mauri et al.[94]

Splenic Irradiation. Splenic irradiation has been used on occasion in patients with AIHA, especially in those with secondary AIHA associated with malignant disease of the reticuloendothelial system. Although some success has been reported, remissions were generally incomplete and only transient in duration.[115]

Vinblastine-Laden Platelets. Ahn and associates have devised a new strategy to treat patients with refractory idiopathic thrombocytopenic purpura,[2] and they have also applied it to the treatment of AIHA.[1] The rationale for the method is based on the recognition of the key role of the macrophage in the pathogenesis of immune cytopenias. The macrophage participates in both the efferent and afferent arms of the immune response because of its role in antigen processing and its collaboration with B and T lymphocytes to activate or potentiate immune responses. Further, the macrophage plays an important role in extravascular cellular destruction as reviewed in Chapter 4. Their hypothesis is that vinca alkaloids can be concentrated by platelets that are then consumed by macrophages, thereby affecting direct delivery of these agents and resulting in modification of macrophage function. Vinblastine-laden platelets are prepared *in vitro*, and when administered to a patient with idiopathic thrombocytopenic purpura, the patient's antiplatelet antibodies (IgG) react with the platelets. The antibody-coated vinblastine-laden platelet reacts with IgG receptors of the macrophage. Favorable therapeutic responses were reported in idiopathic thrombocytopenic purpura.[2] The improvement noted was not ascribed to the known effects of vinca alkaloids in inducing thrombocytosis, since a larger amount of vinca alkaloid administered by intravenous injection had a lesser effect, both in degree and in duration of the increase in platelet count.

For patients with AIHA, the technique is modified by *in vitro* incubation of the vinblastine-laden platelet with plasma from a patient with idiopathic thrombocytopenic purpura to allow for IgG coating. Successful treatment in two patients with AIHA has been reported in an abstract.[1]

Most patients treated for thrombocytopenic purpura tolerated therapy well, but side effects were observed. Among 28 treatments, neutropenia (absolute granulocyte count less than 1,000 per μl) occurred on three occasions. Recovery was prompt within a few days. In one patient with severe chronic obstructive lung disease and a history of recurrent bronchial infections, pneumonia developed that resolved with antibiotics. Transient mild decreases in hemoglobin and white cell counts after the second and third treatments were followed by prompt recovery. In eight cases, febrile reactions reminiscent of buffy-coated reactions were observed when homologous platelets were employed, but they were not seen when the patient's own platelets were later harvested and returned. Three episodes of mild confusion were observed in three elderly patients. A definitive relation between treatment and the confusion was not clear in any case, but it was assumed to have been a contributing factor. Partial hair loss occurred in six patients; all had had two or more treatments. Three patients experienced jaw pain and one complained of a burning tongue.

No notable side effects were seen when the doses of vinblastine of 1 to 2 mg were employed with autogenous platelets in seven infusions. All side effects disappeared after discontinuance of therapy.

The authors are careful to emphasize that further refinements of the technique are needed for optimal use of platelet-vinblastine complex,[2] and the therapy should be considered experimental and reserved for patients who are refractory to more conventional therapies.

Plasma Exchange. Plasma exchange and plasmapheresis have been utilized in the therapy of a wide variety of disorders, particularly those associated with a well documented or suspected immunologic pathogenesis.[15, 70, 87] The two procedures differ in concept; plasma exchange involves the removal of plasma and the replacement of it with various fluids, whereas phasmapheresis involves only the removal of plasma.[18] It would seem worthwhile to maintain this distinction, although the two terms are often used synonymously in the medical literature. Blood cell separators, originally developed for the collection of granulocytes and platelets from normal donors, have facilitated large volume plasma exchange, and the list of conditions for which this technique has been utilized has been growing rapidly in recent years. As with many new approaches, enthusiasm and high hopes have often been more prominent than well documented evidence of benefit. Nevertheless, the procedure seems certain to have a role in the management of some disorders, and studies concerning the mechanism of benefit may lead to a better understanding of the pathogenesis of these disorders.[7, 54, 71, 88] Data concerning the effectiveness of plasma exchange in warm antibody AIHA are extremely limited. Branda et al.[15] reported a patient who developed warm antibody AIHA while convalescing from a viral illness. The patient was treated on one occasion only with 3,000 ml plasma exchange followed by transfusion of two units of whole blood. The hemoglobin that had been rapidly falling stabilized, and an auto-anti-e antibody, which had a titer of two before exchange, became negative. The patient recovered from the hemolytic anemia without further therapy.

Patten et al.[110] reported benefit from plasma exchange in a 45-year-old woman with Evans' syndrome. Prior to plasma exchange the patient's hematocrit level could not be raised over 10 percent despite 8 units of red cells administered over a four day period. Following plasma exchange, the hematocrit level rose to 29 percent, the platelet count rose from 14,500 per μl to 222,000 per μl, and the transfusion requirements declined to only 2 units of red cells over the next 37 days. However, the patient subsequently had a severe exacerbation of hemolysis which did not respond to plasma exchange and she expired.

Rosenfield and Jagathambal [120] commented that plasmapheresis has not been useful in their experience in patients with warm autoimmune disease.

We have used plasma exchange in two patients with warm antibody AIHA.

Patient J.P., referred by Dr. Marian A. Koerper, was a 13-year-old boy who first had an episode of autoimmune hemolytic anemia at age 3. This responded to a course of prednisone therapy. Between the ages of 3 and 6 his hemoglobin and reticulocyte counts were normal although his direct antiglobulin test was strongly positive with anti-IgG antiserum (titer 2048, score 30) and weakly positive with anti-C3 (titer 4, score 3). However, he had recurrent episodes of thrombocytopenia that responded to corticosteroid therapy and for which he underwent splenectomy at age 8. At age 10 parotid swelling was noted, and at age 12 a diagnosis of Sjögren's syndrome was made on the basis of a biopsy of labial accessary salivary glands. At age 13, he developed fever, cough, and malaise which persisted for 1 week, he was treated with ampicillin orally, and 5 days later was hospitalized because of the development of jaundice, fatigue, and tachycardia.

Laboratory data confirmed the presence of warm antibody AIHA. The hemoglobin level was 7.2 gm/dl, reticulocytes 5.8 percent, total bilirubin level 8.2 mg/dl, lactic dehydrogenase 405 U, serum C3 66 mg/dl and hemolytic complement less than 10 CH_{50} units. He also had a leukocytosis and thrombocytosis with 21,800 white cells and 800,000 to 1,000,000 platelets/μl. The direct antiglobulin test was positive with anti-IgG, -IgA, and -C3 antisera, and warm autoantibody was demonstrable in the serum by indirect antiglobulin test and by agglutination of enzyme-treated red cells.

He was treated with high doses of corticosteroids—beginning with 100 mg Solu-Cortef intravenously every 6 hours and later with 100 mg prednisone orally daily. Two units of red cells were transfused every 24 to 48 hours during the first 10 days of hospitalization but, nevertheless, his hematocrit repeatedly dropped below 25 percent. On the tenth day of hospitalization, plasma exchange was performed by Dr. C. H. Mielke, and this procedure was repeated six times during the subsequent 11 days. An average of 2,550 ml of plasma was removed during each procedure. The patient's need for transfusions continued unchanged until after the seventh plasma exchange at which time his transfusion requirement decreased; after one more week, no further transfusions were required. He was discharged and remained in remission after reduction of his prednisone dosage.

During the period of plasma exchanges, his direct antiglobulin test titration score decreased from 25 to 14 using anti-IgG antiserum and from 33 to 14 using anti-C3 antiserum. The serum antibody agglutination score using enzyme treated red cells decreased from 18 to 10.

Whether the patient's improvement is attributable at least in part to the plasma exchanges is conjectural because high doses of corticosteroids were given concomitantly.

Patient J.G., studied in association with Drs. Neal Birnbaum and C. H. Mielke, is a 24-year-old woman who has had warm antibody AIHA for seven years. Even after splenectomy she continued to have acute hemolytic episodes, which were controlled with difficulty. Her hemoglobin level frequently dropped to 5 to 6 gm/dl and reticulocytes frequently were 20 to 30 percent with counts occasionally as high as 80 to 95 percent. While receiving daily doses of 200 mg of azathioprine and 30 mg of prednisone episodes recurred and were controlled with intermittent courses of high doses of prednisone (100 mg daily) and intensive plasma exchange (about 3,000 ml every 2 to 3 days). Ultimately a program of regular plasma exchanges (about once weekly) was begun and a constant dose of prednisone (30 mg) and azathioprine (200 mg) was administered in the hope of preventing acute hemolytic episodes. On this regimen, no acute hemolytic episodes have occurred during the last 10 months.

The direct antiglobulin test titration scores with anti-IgG and anti-C3 have not changed significantly nor has the titer or score of her serum autoantibody. Thus, if plasma exchanges are contributing to her more stable course, the effect would seem more likely to be related to altered macrophage function.[88]

One modification of plasma exchange warrants further consideration in patients with AIHA. Since the red cell autoantibodies found in patients with

AIHA usually react readily with all normal red cells, specific *ex vivo* absorption of the autoantibody by red cell stroma should be feasible. This technique of extracorporeal absorption of antibody has already been utilized in other disorders.[7, 154] A theoretical advantage exists in that all blood components are returned to the patient except for the autoantibody. Thus an unlimited volume of plasma can be treated, and no deficiency of any plasma proteins will occur. We have performed preliminary experiments in one patient with warm antibody AIHA who has had splenectomy and still has life-threatening episodes of hemolysis while receiving high doses of corticosteroids and immunosuppressive drugs, as well as weekly three liter plasma exchanges. We have determined that incubation of the patient's plasma with an equal volume of papainized red cell stroma will absorb all autoantibody after just five minutes incubation at room temperature, even though the autoantibody titer is relatively high as tested by indirect antiglobulin test. Red cells that have been used for more than 21 days may be utilized for the *ex vivo* absorption, thus potentially putting to use red cells that would otherwise be wasted. Our experiments also indicate that the stroma become saturated after just one absorption so that very large volumes may be necessary to absorb all of the patient's autoantibody, including that which can be expected to return to intravascular spaces from the extravascular compartment after absorption of the autoantibody from the plasma. Further studies are necessary to test the validity of this approach.

COLD AGGLUTININ SYNDROME

Avoidance of Cold

Therapy for cold agglutinin syndrome is generally unsatisfactory. It is fortunate that the disorder is frequently not severe and, instead, results in a chronic mild hemolytic anemia with a hemoglobin level of 9 to 12 gm per dl. Such patients require no therapy other than avoidance of cold.[112] If patients go out in cold weather, they must clothe themselves well, including earmuffs, warm socks, and warm mittens. These measures will prevent the development of acute hemolytic crises,[28, 89] but even with strict avoidance of cold, some hemolysis usually persists.[112] Patients with significant degrees of anemia should usually be urged to learn to tolerate the symptoms rather than embark on therapeutic trials that have greater potential risk than probable benefit.

Corticosteroid Therapy

Corticosteroids are less effective in cold agglutinin syndrome than in warm antibody syndromes, and they probably should not be used in chronic cold antibody syndromes.[30] Lack of success of corticosteroid therapy in cold agglutinin syndrome has been reported by Pisciotta,[116] Firkin et al.,[49] Dausset and Colombani,[35] and Dacie.[28] Schubothe points out that there are only a few reports of allegedly successful treatment, and he questions whether the constant warm temperature of the hospital has not been the true cause of the limitation of hyperhemolysis.[137] Indeed, Dacie has shown that during simple bed rest the improvement of the hemoglobin values and of the patient's general condition is about the same as with treatment with corticosteroids.[27]

Recently, Schreiber et al. reported two patients that they classified as having cold agglutinin syndrome with atypical serologic reactions.[136] In each case the direct antiglobulin test was strongly positive with anti-C3 antiserum and negative with anti-IgG antiserum. The patients had only a modest elevation of the cold agglutinin titer at 4° C, but the antibodies reacted up to 37° C. Such serologic findings do, indeed, occur in a number of patients with cold agglutinin syndrome (page 214 and Tables 6-16 and 6-19). (However, the authors did not exclude the presence of warm hemolysins active against enzyme-treated red cells which are present in about 10 percent of the patients who have warm antibody AIHA and have C3 but not IgG on their red cells; see page 211.) The authors utilized the C1 fixation and transfer technique and determined that the amount of antibody fixed to homologous erythrocytes by the patient's plasma at 37°C seemed adequate to explain the *in vivo* hemolysis. They reasoned on the basis of prior experiments that the effects of corticosteroids on macrophage C3 receptors may be of clinical importance in these patients with relatively limited amounts of antibody. Prednisone administration at a dose of 100 mg per day on two occasions to the first patient produced a "remission" characterized by a rise in hemoglobin of more than 2 gm per dl, and, in case two, similar doses of prednisone caused a more impressive increase in the hemoglobin level. However, case one required "at least" 20 mg of prednisone and case two required 40 to 60 mg of prednisone to maintain a hemoglobin level of 10 gm per 100 ml. The authors suggested that patients with high titers of cold agglutinins with a high thermal amplitude would be expected to be resistant to even high concentrations of corticosteroids

The high maintenance doses of prednisone required to maintain a hemoglobin level of greater than 10 gm per dl even in these "responsive" patients illustrates a major problem. Pirofsky,[114] in a retrospective review of his own series of patients, has strongly emphasized that the maintenance of a partial remission in patients with AIHA by prolonged administration of prednisone at dose levels over 15 mg per day results in "disatrous side effects." The tendency to devleop such side effects is often underestimated by physicians. In cold agglutinin syndrome, educating the patient to tolerate a lower than normal hemoglobin level is likely to ultimately be preferable to chronic prednisone therapy. Patients with a hemoglobin level of 7 to 10 gm per dl are often capable of tolerating the symptoms of anemia, and they should be strongly urged to do so rather than to be treated with high doses of prednisone (see Case Report VW, Chapter 6). If patients are more anemic, have intolerable symptoms, and are refractory to cytotoxic drug therapy (described later), a program of chronic transfusions is probably the optimal means of management (see Chapter 10). In most instances, prednisone in acceptable doses (15 mg per day for maintenance therapy) will be of no significant benefit.

Immunosuppressive Drugs

Cytotoxic drugs have been employed in the treatment of the cold agglutinin syndrome by several investigators with favorable responses recorded in a minority of patients. Schubothe [137] described the use of cyclophosphamide in four patients. In two patients the cold agglutinin titer decreased, but no clinical details are given except that "neither patient showed the picture of chronic cold agglutinin syndrome." Dacie and Worlledge [30] reported that three of nine patients responded well to chlorambucil therapy with a sustained rise in hemoglobin level, alleviation of symptoms, reduction in cold agglutinin titer, and diminution in IgM concentrations. In one of these patients the rise in hemoglobin level and fall in reticulocyte count were sustained for at least 12 months after the chlorambucil was discontinued.

Hippe et al. [62] reported the use of chlorambucil in four patients with cold agglutinin syndrome. Some of the results are indicated in Table 11-8. All four patients presented with Raynaud's phenomenon and hemoglobinuria, and patient four also had gangrene of the fingertips. After therapy, none of the patients had Raynaud's phenomenon or hemoglobinuria, and two patients were able to work outdoors in winter (in Denmark). Dosage schedules varied, and the patients were treated intermittently or continuously. Effects were most pronounced during the first six months, but in two patients, essentially normal values of IgM were obtained only after treatment for periods of one year and three years, respectively.

Olesen [105] described one patient in whom therapy caused a reduction in plasma cold agglutinins from a titer of 128,000 to 32,000, and a decrease in their thermal amplitude by 3° C. There was also a subjective improvement in the intensity of the patient's Raynaud's phenomenon. However, her hemoglobin did not change during one course of therapy and, during a second course, dropped from 12.0 to 9.5 gm per dl.

Evans et al. described a patient with a chronic cold agglutinin syndrome of varying severity over a 20 year period. [45] Chlorambucil therapy (6 mg per day for 3 months) resulted in a decrease in cold agglutinin titer from 64,000 to 2,000, increase in hematocrit from 29 percent to normal levels, a decrease in reticulocytes from 15 percent to 2.5 percent, and an increase in serum complement levels toward normal. Cessation of chlorambucil was followed by relapse, and a second course again produced marked improvement. The patient was subsequently able to maintain an adequate hematocrit level without therapy.

In patients who do not respond satisfactorily to therapy, bone marrow depression and temporary worsening of anemia result. Therefore, it is wise to begin with daily doses of 2 or 4 mg per day. Bi-weekly blood counts including a reticulocyte count should be obtained, and the daily dose may be increased by 2 mg every 2 months until favorable effects or limiting adverse reactions result. The latter effects usually consist of marrow suppression, although anorexia and nausea may limit dosage as well. If a favorable response does result, maintenance therapy may be advisable, although an alternative approach is to use therapy intermittently as needed. [62, 164]

Table 11-8. LABORATORY DATA BEFORE AND AFTER TREATMENT OF COLD AGGLUTININ SYNDROME WITH CHLORAMBUCIL [62]

Patient (age)	Dates of Laboratory Tests	Serum IgM Concentration N = 0.11 – 1.23 gm/L	Cold Agglutinin Titer in Percent of Initial Titer	Decrease in Thermal Amplitude (°C)	Hemoglobin gm/dl
1 (78)	1962	7.2	100	–	11.5
	1968	1.0	17	3.3	13.5
2 (65)	1966	6.6	100	–	9.0
	1968	1.8	37	2.2	10.0
3 (62)	1967	8.2	100	–	11.0
	1968	1.3	14	2.6	12.5
4 (63)	1968	13.2	100	–	10.5
	1969	4.7	3	7.2	13.7

Plasma Exchange

There is some logic to the use of plasma exchange in those hemolytic anemias caused by IgM antibodies since IgM has a predominantly intravascular distribution, and experience has been favorable, with treatment of IgM-induced hyperviscosity syndrome and hemostatic defects in Waldenström's macroglobulinemia.[70, 160] However, the results in patients with cold agglutinin syndrome have been far from impressive.

Taft et al.[150] have reported the results of plasma exchange in two patients with the cold agglutinin syndrome. In this disorder, the technique is complicated by the rapid formation of red cell agglutinates when blood is withdrawn and maintained at room temperature. In treating their first patient, a 66-year-old man with histocytic lymphoma, they used a manual technique of withdrawing blood into bags that were kept in a 37° C water bath. Plasma was separated and red blood cells washed at 37° C in a walk-in incubator before readministration of the cells to the patient through a 37° C coil. This required two technicians full-time for the three days during which the procedure was done. Removal of 3,770 ml of plasma during a 1 week period was said to reduce the cold agglutinin titer from 8,000,000 (!) to 8,192 but the patient died 4 days later of widespread lymphoma and an acute myocardial infarction.

For their second patient, a 54-year-old woman with lymphocytic lymphosarcoma, they warmed the pheresis room to 37° C and used a mechanical cell separator modified with two fans to circulate air over the electronic components to prevent overheating. Water baths at 37° C were also used for anticoagulant lines and plasma return lines. Before plasma exchanges, the patient's hemoglobin level was 4 gm/dl and transfusion was attempted on several occasions using washed or unwashed red cells through a warming coil. The blood was not tolerated, and the patient became toxic after each attempted transfusion. Plasma exchange of 4,820 ml resulted in the reduction of cold agglutinin titer from 1,000,000 to 16,000 at 4° C and from 512 to 32 at 37° C. Three subsequent transfusions were said to be tolerated "fairly well," but the patient's post-transfusion hemoglobin level was only 5 gm/dl. The cold agglutinin titer rose to 64,000 and, 10 days after the first procedure, another exchange of 4,830 ml was performed. The cold agglutinin titer decreased to 4,000 and she was given 2 units of blood two days later. She was said to be "doing well," but expired five days after the second plasma exchange after developing abdominal distention and hypotension. Autopsy revealed widespread lymphoma and atherosclerosis of the left descending coronary artery.

Isbister et al.[70] describe results in three patients with cold agglutinin syndrome. In the first patient, a four liter plasma exchange and institution of corticosteroid therapy resulted in control of "severe autoimmune hemolytic anemia." No cold agglutinin titers are mentioned. The second patient, with immunoblastic lymphadenopathy, had an IgM agglutinin and hemolysin reactive up to body temperature. Corticosteroid therapy and plasma exchange were associated with a fall in agglutinin titer at 4° C from 128 to 8, disappearance of autoagglutination at 37° C, and sustained response to blood transfusion. A third patient with a wide thermal range IgM autoagglutinin failed to show any clinical response to plasma exchange "despite a fall in antibody titer." The authors comment that the value of the plasma exchange procedures in the first two cases is difficult to assess. This is particularly true since no serologic data are given in the first patient and the second patient, with a cold agglutinin titer of only 128, may have had an atypical warm antibody AIHA with a warm hemolysin (likely to respond to corticosteroid therapy) rather than cold agglutinin syndrome.

Logue, Rosse, and Gockerman [89] reported the results of large volume plasma exchange performed on two occasions in a patient with cold agglutinin syndrome. The procedure was performed in a room heated to 37° C. After exchange of 3,000 ml of plasma, there was a 70 percent fall in cold agglutinin level, as measured by the ability of the cold agglutinin and fresh serum to lyse red cells of a patient with paroxysmal nocturnal hemoglobinuria. However, within one week the antibody level returned to its original level. The rate of endogenous carbon monoxide production fell following the plasma exchange, indicating that the hemolytic rate decreased; [90] carbon monoxide production increased as the plasma antibody concentration subsequently rose.

Rosenfield and Jagathambal [120] comment that the level of cold agglutinins can be reduced by double unit plasmapheresis thrice weekly, but clinical improvement in patients with kappa chain IgM cold agglutinin syndrome has not been very great. Buskard [18] states that treatment by plasma exchange of cold hemagglutinin disease that is resistant to chemotherapy has been disappointing; the response is brief and the reduction in hemolysis is minimal. Neither Rosenfield and Jagathambal nor Buskard supply any further clinical details.

Thus, the procedure appears to offer a modest degree of temporary benefit in some patients with cold agglutinin syndrome.

Penicillamine

There have been several reports of benefit in cold agglutinin syndrome with the use of d-penicillamine. Edwards and Gengozian [42] described a patient with severe hemolytic anemia who did not respond to a 6 week course of 60 mg of prednisone daily or to 6-mercaptopurine given at a dose of 50 mg four times daily for 12 days. Serologic details are scanty, but cold (4° C) and warm (25° C) autoagglutinins (titers of 128 and 32, respectively) were completely inactivated *in vitro* by 2-mercaptoenthanol or d-penicillamine. The patient's hemogloblin level was 3.8 gm per dl, red cell count 910,000 per μl, and a ^{51}Cr red cell survival study indicated only one third of administered cells were circulating after two hours. Blood transfusion given simultaneously with hydrocortisone failed to increase the patient's hemoglobin and he became deeply icteric. He was treated with d-penicillamine 500 mg four times daily orally for 7 days. The autoagglutinin titer decreased by the eighth day and the antibody was not demonstrable by day 14 (although anti-A and anti-B titers did not change). The autoantibody did not recur during a 60 day follow-up period. This result permitted transfusion without evidence of excessive destruction of transfused red cells, and the patient's red blood cell count was greater than 2,000,000 per μl. He then expired, and autopsy revealed malignant lymphoma and carcinoma of the lung with metastases. The authors point out that the duration of effectiveness of the therapy indicate that the mechanism of action of d-penicillamine was not likely to be *in vivo* depolymerization and inactivation of the macroglobulin cold agglutinins. A similar conclusion was reached by Jaffe,[72] who reported that penicillamine treatment caused reductions in rheumatoid factor titers for four weeks to three months. Ritzmann and Levin [118] reported on clinical improvement and reduction of cold agglutinins and hemolysins in a patient whose original serum antibody titer was 500,000. The cold agglutinin titer returned to pretreatment levels within seven weeks after treatment.

Unfortunately, other authors have all reported that therapy with penicillamine or related compounds was of no benefit. Evans et al.[46] reported failure in one patient, Dacie [28] describes treatment as ineffective in two patients, and Schubothe records negative results in three patients followed personally and cites further failures in an unstated number of patients treated by Krug. Lind et al.,[86] in a detailed report of two patients, recorded no effect of the treatment with penicillamine on the clinical state or on the laboratory findings including the cold agglutinin titer, ultracentrifugal, and immunoelectrophoretic results. In *in vitro* experiments, on the other hand, the effect of penicillamine could be clearly shown by serologic and immunochemical tests.

Penicillamine seems to have little role in the management of patients with cold agglutinin syndrome.

Splenectomy

Splenectomy is generally considered ineffective in patients with cold agglutinin syndrome. McCurdy and Rath reported failure in one patient.[95] Bell et al.[9] described the outcome in three patients; two died of sepsis and one died of lymphoma. Pirofsky [114] described one patient who derived no clinical benefit. Dacie cites additional cases in which splenectomy has been unsuccessful.[28]

However, Dacie also described three patients with "atypical" cold agglutinin syndrome who demonstrated marked clinical improvement after splenectomy.[28] One patient had a complete and lasting remission (except for a persistently positive direct antiglobulin test). A second patient had a remission that lasted for two years and, when hemolysis recurred, she responded well to corticosteroids. The third patient had a chronic hemolytic anemia that was influenced favorably by ACTH and splenectomy. Remarkably, these patients had similar unusual serologic features in common. The serum antibodies of all patients failed to cause agglutination of normal red cells above 30° C, but nevertheless caused lysis of enzyme-treated red cells at 37° C. Furthermore, one of the sera caused lysis to a higher titer at 37° C than at 20° C (the other two sera were not tested at 20° C). The finding of lysis at 37° C but not at 20° C suggested that the lysis was being produced by a factor that was distinct from the cold agglutinin. That warm hemolysins (i.e., optimally active at 37° C) are unusual in cold agglutinin syndrome is further emphasized by the study of von dem Borne et al.[158] These authors described warm hemolysins in 69 patients; none of the patients had cold agglutinin syndrome. However, lysins reactive at 37° C against trypsinized cells but reactive to a higher titer at 20° C do occur in a minority of patients with cold agglutinin syndrome. Such findings were recorded in four of 16 patients described in detail by Dacie.[28]

Evans et al.[46] described a further patient with cold agglutinin syndrome who had marked improvement lasting for 18 months [46a] after splenectomy, and this patient's serum was also capable of causing lysis at 37° C, whereas agglutination was negative above 31° C. However, lysis was more pronounced at 20° C than at 37° C in contrast to Dacie's patients. The serologic findings in the patients described by Dacie and Evans are summarized in Table 11-9.

Since the total number of patients with cold agglutinin syndrome who have had a favorable response to splenectomy is small, it is impossible to draw firm conclusions regarding the significance of the unusual serologic features observed. Nevertheless, it is evident that splenectomy has been of benefit in only a small number of patients with cold agglutinin syndrome, and all these patients had hemolysins reactive at 37° C. It is conceivable that the serologic features described in these patients may be of some value in selecting patients for the operation.

PAROXYSMAL COLD HEMOGLOBINURIA

Acute post-infectious forms of paroxysmal cold hemoglobinuria usually terminate spontaneously, and the patient requires only temporary protection from cold exposure. Protection from cold is also of importance in preventing attacks in those rare patients who have the idiopathic chronic form of the disease. There are many reports in the earlier literature of clinical improvement caused by anti-syphilitic drugs in chronic paroxysmal cold hemoglobinuria associated with syphilis,[28] although not all patients respond.[6] Data concerning the use of corticosteroids are too scanty to allow for conclusions concerning their effectiveness.

We are aware of the results of splenectomy in only two patients. Both patients had chronic paroxysmal cold hemoglobinuria and, surprisingly, both benefited from the procedure. Banov[6] described a 51-year-old man who had frequent episodes of hemoglobinuria after cold exposure over a period of 10 years. He then sustained a splenic laceration as a result of an automobile accident, and splenectomy was therefore performed. He had no further episodes of hemoglobinuria despite continued exposure to cold. It was not until four years later during hospitalization for pneumonia that his intriguing history led to the performance of laboratory tests that documented the presence of a positive Donath-Landsteiner reaction as well as serologic evidence

Table 11-9. SEROLOGIC FINDINGS IN FOUR PATIENTS WITH COLD AGGLUTININ SYNDROME WHO RESPONDED TO SPLENECTOMY

| Reference | Age, Sex | Agglutination Normal Cells | | | Lysis | | | | |
| | | 2–4°C (Titer) | 20°C (Titer) | 31°C (Titer) | Normal Cells (pH 6.5–7.0) | | Enzyme-treated Cells | | |
					20°C	37°C	20°C (Titer)	37°C (Titer)	
Dacie,[28] pp. 487–488	73 F	512	32	0	0	0	NT*	32	
Dacie,[28] pp. 487–488	56 F	1,024	32	0	0	0	NT*	32	
Dacie,[28] pp. 487–488	32 F	256	32	0	0	0	0	64	
Evans et al.,[46, 46a]	57 M	500,000	NT*	0	2+	1+	NT*	NT*	

* NT = Not tested.

for syphilis. The authors speculated that reduction in total antibody formation was a possible explanation for the patient's improvement.

The other patient who responded well to splenectomy is our patient, L. Z., whose course is described on page 341.

SECONDARY AUTOIMMUNE HEMOLYTIC ANEMIAS

Mycoplasma Pneumoniae Infections and Infectious Mononucleosis

In some forms of secondary autoimmune hemolytic anemias, a spontaneous remission may be confidently predicted, e.g., hemolytic anemias associated with *Mycoplasma pneumoniae* infections and infectious mononucleosis. Cold antibodies with a high thermal maximum are always present with the former and often present with the latter, so that keeping the patient warm is a logical and uniformly recommended therapeutic maneuver. In patients with severe anemia, the hospital room should be warmed to as high a temperature as is tolerable, and mittens and warm slippers worn as well. These measures will prevent acute exacerbations that result from cold exposure, although more severely affected patients, whose disease is perhaps associated with antibodies of particularly high thermal amplitude, may have continued hemolysis and progressively more severe anemia even while being kept as warm as possible. Therefore, close observation and consideration of additional therapy is warranted.

Corticosteroid therapy is of dubious value in patients with cold agglutinin syndrome associated with *Mycoplasma pneumoniae* infection but, as Dacie and Worlledge comment,[30] it is difficult to resist the temptation to give corticosteroids since complications are minimal in a short term illness. Antibiotics have produced more impressive results than corticosteroids in those patients who still have evidence of unresolved pneumonia at the time of development of hemolytic anemia.[48] Erythromycin or tetracycline therapy should certainly be used in all patients with persisting evidence of pneumonia, but in many cases, the infection will have resolved before the onset of the hemolytic anemia.

In contrast to hemolytic anemia secondary to *Mycoplasma pneumoniae* infections, corticosteroids have been reported to be of distinct value in the management of patients with hemolytic anemia associated with infectious mononucleosis.[17, 57, 81, 98, 155] Tonkin [155] reported three patients with severe acute hemolytic anemia. In one patient steroids were not used and the hemolysis resolved spontaneoulsy over seven weeks. The two other patients were treated with corticosteroids and demonstrated marked improvement within a week. Keyloun and Grace [81] reported a patient who was started on therapy with corticosteroids after two weeks of illness; prompt improvement was noted, with defervescence of the patient's fever, relief of airway obstruction caused by lymphoid enlargement, a general feeling of well-being, and improvement in the hematocrit level. A less dramatic effect of corticosteroid therapy was noted by Bowman et al.;[17] in their patient, therapy with 60 mg of prednisone resulted in the stabilization of the hematocrit level at 22 percent but there was no improvement for the subsequent nine days.

Ovarian Tumors

Hemolytic anemia associated with ovarian tumors has been recognized since the report of West-Watson and Young in 1938.[161] Twenty-four cases were reviewed by Dawson et al.[36] The ages of patients ranged from 19 to 61 years. Evidences of autoimmunization are present in that the direct antiglobulin test is almost always positive, and serologic findings identical to those of idiopathic warm antibody AIHA have been reported.[29, 30, 36] Characteristically, the hemolytic anemia is refractory to corticosteroid therapy and to splenectomy, but remission is obtained after the removal of the tumor. Usually the remission is complete, but in a few cases only a partial remission has been recorded. In almost all cases the ovarian tumor has been a teratoma or dermoid, and the mechanism by which its presence leads to autoimmunization remains obscure. Although the association of AIHA with ovarian tumors is rare, its recognition is obviously important, and the possibility should be considered in all women who develop AIHA of unknown origin.

Ulcerative Colitis

The association of AIHA with ulcerative colitis was first reported by Lorber et al. in 1955.[91] Shashaty and co-workers reviewed the literature in 1977.[143] Although a positive direct antiglobulin test had been reported in association with ulcerative colitis in 34 individuals, only 14 patients, including 3 reported by the authors, had convincing evidence of hemolytic anemia. The patients ranged in age from 12 to 57 years, with a mean of 33 years. Ten were female and 4 were male. The diseases occurred simultaneously, or the diagnosis of AIHA followed the diagnosis of ulcerative colitis by six months to 16 years, with one exception in which AIHA antedated ulcerative colitis by three years. The direct antiglobulin test was positive in all patients and, in the five instances in which antiglobulin tests were performed utilizing monospecific antiglobulin reagents, red cell sensitization by IgG was demonstrated. Serologic testing has usually been incomplete, but autoantibodies in serum or eluate were reported in eight patients.

Based on results in the reported cases, the therapeutic approach should be similar to that for idiopathic AIHA. Corticosteroids produced a remission in about 50 percent of the cases, and for those patients who failed to respond to steroids, splenectomy was usually effective. If hemolysis is not responsive to either of these modalities, total proctocolectomy seems effective. Although only four patients have been reported in whom the indication for colectomy was persistence of hemolysis, hemolysis invariably abated after the surgery.[143]

Systemic Lupus Erythematosus

AIHA has been reported in 3 to 10 percent of the cases of systemic lupus erythematosus.[132] Often the management of these disorders is identical, in that steroid therapy may be effective in producing palliation of both entities. However, an adequate remission of the hemolytic state does not necessarily occur, even though the other manifestations of systemic lupus erythematosus may be under good control. Sarles and Levin [132] reported three patients with AIHA and systemic lupus erythematosus in whom hematologic improvement did not occur during treatment with steroids but did ensue following splenectomy. Other reports are also available in which hemolytic anemia was ameliorated by splenectomy without adversely affecting the course of the underlying systemic lupus erythematosus.[41, 61, 77, 117] Thus, if hemolysis does not respond to therapy utilized for systemic lupus erythematosus, the AIHA should be treated as a separate entity, as described for the management of patients with idiopathic AIHA.

Lymphoreticular Malignant Disease

Two different therapeutic relationships exist between AIHA and associated malignant diseases of the lymphoreticular system. In some instances, therapy directed toward the associated disease may lead to hematologic and serologic remission. In others, however, the AIHA appears to be clinically and therapeutically independent. Frequently therapy of the neoplastic disorder, even when successful, has little effect in correcting the hemolytic process. In such instances, the best approach is to treat the patient as if two unrelated disease processes were present.[114]

A SUMMARY OF THERAPEUTIC PRINCIPLES IN THE MANAGEMENT OF PATIENTS WITH AUTOIMMUNE HEMOLYTIC ANEMIA

Idiopathic Warm Antibody Autoimmune Hemolytic Anemia

1. Initial therapy should be prednisone at a dose of 1.0 to 1.5 mg per kg daily (or an equivalent dose of another corticosteroid drug).
2. If there is no response, higher doses of corticosteroids have greater potential harm than potential benefit.
3. If no response occurs in three weeks, the treatment should be considered to have failed.
4. For patients who respond to treatment, tapering of steroid dosage should begin after the hematocit level reaches 30 percent and should be carried out slowly over a period of months.
5. If more than 10 mg of prednisone per day (or, at most, 15 mg prednisone per day) is required to maintain an adequate remission (hematocrit

level greater than 30 percent), therapy with corticosteroids should be considered to have failed and splenectomy should be performed or immunosuppressive drug therapy should be initiated. This decision should be made in a matter of weeks or months after initiating therapy. The most common therapeutic error is the prolonged administration of prednisone (i.e., greater than four to six months) at a dose of over 15 mg per day to maintain a partial remission.

6. Splenectomy should not be performed because of the development of complications of corticosteroid therapy; it should have been done to prevent the development of such complications.

7. The decision to perform splenectomy should be made primarily on the basis of clinical findings rather than on the basis of a splenic sequestration study using radiolabelled red cells.

8. Immunosuppressive drugs have a definite role in management of patients with warm antibody AIHA, generally in those who have an inadequate response to corticosteroids even after splenectomy.

9. Blood transfusion should be performed reluctantly, but it is essential in some patients and should be performed even though the compatibility test may reveal gross incompatibility (see Chapter 10).

Idiopathic Cold Agglutinin Syndrome

1. Exposure to cold should be avoided; this may be the only therapy necessary even though a chronic hemolytic anemia may persist.

2. The patient should be encouraged to tolerate the presence of mild or moderate symptoms of anemia because of the high risk to benefit ratio of therapeutic maneuvers that have been used in this disorder.

3. Chlorambucil (or cyclophosphamide) produces benefit in a minority of patients and should be tried if significant symptoms of anemia are present.

4. Patients who have anemia with intolerable symptoms and who do not respond to chlorambucil are probably best managed by a chronic program of transfusion.

5. Corticosteroids are generally ineffective. In a few patients, high doses may cause some benefit, but the hazards of prolonged corticosteroid therapy usually greatly outweigh the benefits. The degree of improvement must justify the considerable long term risks.

6. Splenectomy is generally ineffective, although a few reports of success have been published, particularly in patients with atypical serologic findings including the presence of warm hemolysins.

7. Other therapies are of unproven value.

Paroxysmal Cold Hemoglobinuria

1. Most patients with this disorder have an acute and transient hemolytic anemia so that often only supportive care is necessary. Meticulous attention should be given to keeping the patient warm.

2. The severity of hemolysis may dictate the need for blood transfusion (see Chapter 10).

3. A short course of corticosteroid therapy is warranted empirically if hemolysis is severe.

4. Diagnostic tests for syphilis should be performed and antiluetic therapy given if definitive tests are positive.

5. In the extraordinarily rare patient with chronic paroxysmal cold hemoglobinuria, very limited data (two patients) suggest that splenectomy may be of benefit.

Secondary Autoimmune Hemolytic Anemias

1. Cold agglutinin syndrome associated with *Mycoplasma pneumoniae* infection should be treated by keeping the patient warm and administering antibiotics if signs of infection are still present. Corticosteroids are not likely to be of benefit. Transfusion may be necessary.

2. Hemolytic anemia associated with infectious mononucleosis should be treated with corticosteroids unless the anemia is mild. If cold reactive antibodies with high thermal maximum are demonstrated, the patient should be kept warm.

3. The possibility of an ovarian tumor should be considered in women with acquired hemolytic anemia. Surgical removal can be expected to ameliorate the hemolysis.

4. In patients with systemic lupus erythematosus, ulcerative colitis, or reticuloendothelial neoplasms, therapy for the underlying disorder may cause remission of hemolysis. If not, the hemolytic anemia should be treated as a separate entity.

REFERENCES

1. Ahn, Y. S., Byrnes, J. J., Brunskill, D. E., et al.: Selective injury to macrophages: A new treatment for idiopathic autoimmune hemolytic anemia. Clin. Res., *26:*340, 1978.
2. Ahn, Y. S., Byrnes, J. J., Harrington, W. J., Cayer, M. L., Smith, D. S., Brunskill, D. E., and Pall, L. M.: The treatment of idiopathic thrombocytopenia with vinblastine-loaded platelets. New Engl. J. Med., *298:*1101, 1978.
3. Ahuja, S., Lewis, S. M., and Szur, L.: Value of surface counting in predicting response to splenectomy in haemolytic anaemia. J. Clin. Path., *25:*467, 1972.
4. Allgood, J. W., and Chaplin, H.: Idiopathic acquired autoimmune hemolytic anemia: A review of forty-seven cases treated from 1955 through 1965. Am. J. Med., *43:*254, 1967.
5. Atkinson, J. P., Schreiber, A. D., and Frank, M. M.: Effects of corticosteroids and splenectomy on the immune clearance and destruction of erythrocytes. J. Clin. Invest., *52:*1509, 1973.
6. Banov, C. H.: Paroxysmal cold hemoglobinuria: Apparent remission after splenectomy. JAMA, *174:*1974, 1960.
7. Bansal, S. C., Bansal, B. R., Thomas, H. L., Siegel, P. D., Rhoads, J. E., Cooper, D. R., Terman, D. S., and Mark, R.: *Ex vivo* removal of serum IgG in a patient with colon carcinoma. Cancer, *42:*1, 1978.

8. Bardana, E. J., Bayrakci, C., Pirofsky, B., and Henjyoji, H.: The use of heparin in autoimmune hemolytic disease. Blood, *35:*377, 1970.
9. Bell, C. A., Zwicker, H., and Sacks, H. J.: Autoimmune hemolytic anemia. Amer. J. Clin. Path., *60:*903, 1973.
10. Ben-Bassat, I., Seligsohn, U., Leiba, H., Leef, F., Chaitchik, S., and Ramot, B.: Sequestration studies with chromium-51 labelled red cells as criteria for splenectomy. Israel. J. Med. Sci., *3:*832, 1967.
11. Bensinger, T. A., Logue, G. L., and Rundles, R. W.: Hemorrhagic thrombocythemia; control of postsplenectomy thrombocytosis with melphalan. Blood, *36:*61, 1970.
12. Bisno, A. L., and Freeman, J. C.: The syndrome of asplenia, pneumococcal sepsis, and disseminated intravascular coagulation. Ann. Intern. Med., *71:*389, 1970.
13. Bowdler, A. J.: The spleen and haemolytic disorders. Clinics Haematol., *4:*231, 1975.
14. Bowdler, A. J.: The role of the spleen and splenectomy in autoimmune hemolytic disease. Seminars Hematol., *13:*335, 1976.
15. Branda, R. F., Moldow, C. F., McCullough, J. J., and Jacob, H. S.: Plasma exchange in the treatment of immune disease. Transfusion, *15:*570, 1975.
16. Bossi, E., and Wagner, H. P.: Autoimmune hemolytic anemia and cytomegalovirus infection in a six-month old child, treated with azathioprine. Helv. Paediatr. Acta, *27:*155, 1972.
17. Bowman, H. S., Marsh, W. L., Schmacher, H. R., Oyen, R., and Reihart, J.: Auto anti-N immunohemolytic anemia in infectious mononucleosis. Amer. J. Clin. Path., *61:*465, 1974.
18. Buskard, N. A.: Plasma exchange and plasmapheresis. Canad. Med. Assoc. J., *119:*681, 1978.
18a. Casciato, D. A., and Scott, J. L.: Acute leukemia following prolonged cytotoxic agent therapy. Medicine, *58:*32, 1979.
19. Chaplin, H.: Clinical usefulness of specific antiglobulin reagents in autoimmune hemolytic anemias. Progr. Hematol., *8:*25, 1973.
20. Chaplin, H., and Avioli, L. V.: Autoimmune hemolytic anemia. Arch. Intern. Med., *137:*346, 1977.
21. Chertkow, G., and Dacie, J. V.: Results of splenectomy in auto-immune haemolytic anaemia. Br. J. Haematol., *2:*237, 1956.
22. Christensen, B. E.: The pattern of erythrocyte sequestration in immunohaemolysis: Effects of prednisone treatment and splenectomy. Scand. J. Haemat., *10:*120, 1973.
23. Coon, W. W., Penner, J., Clagett, G. P., and Eos, N.: Deep venous thrombosis and postsplenectomy thrombocytosis. Arch. Surg., *113:*429, 1978.
24. Coonrod, J. D., and Leach, R. P.: Antigenemia in fulminant pneumococcemia. Ann. Intern. Med., *84:*561, 1976.
25. Crosby, W. H.: Splenectomy in hematologic disorders. New Engl. J. Med., *286:*1252, 1972.
26. Crosby, W. H., and Rappaport, H.: Autoimmune hemolytic anemia. 1. Analysis of hematologic observations with particular reference to their prognostic value; a survey of 57 cases. Blood, *12:*42, 1957.
27. Dacie, J. V.: The cold haemagglutinin syndrome. Proc. Roy. Soc. Med., *50:*647, 1957.
28. Dacie, J. V.: The Haemolytic Anaemias: Part II, The Auto-Immune Haemolytic Anaemias. 2nd Ed. London, J. & A. Churchill, Ltd., 1962.
29. Dacie, J. V.: The Haemolytic Anaemias: Part III, Secondary or Symptomatic Hemolytic Anemias. 2nd Ed. London, J. & A. Churchill, Ltd., 1967.
30. Dacie, J. V., and Worlledge, S. M.: Auto-immune hemolytic anemias. Progr. Hematol., *6:*82, 1969.

31. Dameshek, W.: The management of acute hemolytic anemia and the hemolytic crisis. Clinics, 2:118, 1943.
32. Dameshek, W., and Komninos, Z. D.: The present status of treatment of autoimmune hemolytic anemia with ACTH and cortisone. Blood, 11:648, 1956.
33. Dameshek, W., and Schwartz, S. O.: Acute hemolytic anemia (acquired hemolytic icterus, acute type). Medicine, 19:231, 1940.
34. Dameshek, W., and Schwartz, R.: Treatment of certain "autoimmune" diseases with antimetabolites; a preliminary report. Trans. Ass'n. Amer. Physicians, 73:113, 1960.
35. Dausset, J., and Colombani, J.: The serology and the prognosis of 128 cases of autoimmune hemolytic anemia. Blood, 14:1280, 1959.
36. Dawson, M. A., Talbert, W., and Yarbro, J. W.: Hemolytic anemia associated with an ovarian tumor. Amer. J. Med., 50:552, 1971.
37. Devlin, H. B., Evans, D. S., and Birkhead, J. S.: Elective splenectomy for primary hematologic and splenic disease. Surg. Gynecol. Obstet., 131:273, 1970.
38. DeWeese, M. S., and Coller, F. A.: Splenectomy for hematologic disorders. West. J. Surg., 67:129, 1959.
39. Dickerman, J. D., Bolton, E., Coil, J. A., Chalmer, B. J., and Jakab, G. J.: Protective effect of prophylactic penicillin on splenectomized mice exposed to an aerosolized suspension of type III Streptococcus pneumoniae. Blood, 53:498, 1979.
40. Dreyfus, B., Dausset, J., and Vidal, G.: Étude clinque et hématologique de douze cas d'anémie hémolytique acquisé avec auto-anticorps. Rev. Hémat., 6:349, 1951.
41. Dubois, E. L.: Systemic lupus erythematosus. M. Clin. North Am., 36:1111, 1952.
42. Edwards, C. L., and Gengozian, N.: Auto-immune hemolytic anemia treated with d-Penicillamine: Report of a case. Ann. Intern. Med., 62:576, 1965.
43. Eichner, E. R.: Splenic function: Normal, too much and too little. Amer. J. Med., 66:311, 1979.
44. Evans, R. S.: Autoantibodies in hematologic disorders. Stanf. Med. Bull., 13:152, 1955.
45. Evans, R. S., Baxter, E., and Gilliland, B. C.: Chronic hemolytic anemia due to cold agglutinins: A 20-year history of benign gammopathy with response to chlorambucil. Blood, 42:463, 1973.
46. Evans, R. S., Bingham, M., and Turner, E.: Autoimmune hemolytic disease: Observations of serological reactions and disease activity. Ann. N.Y. Acad. Sci., 124:422, 1965.
46a. Evans, R. S., Turner, E., Bingham, M., and Woods, R.: Chronic hemolytic anemia due to cold agglutinins. II. The role of C' in red cell destruction. J. Clin. Inves., 47:691, 1968.
47. Eyster, M. E., and Jenkins, D. E.: Erythrocyte coating substances in patients with positive direct antiglobulin reactions. Am. J. Med., 46:360, 1969.
48. Fiala, M., Myhre, B. A., Chinh, L. T., Territo, M., Edgington, T. S., and Kattlove, H.: Pathogenesis of anemia associated with Mycoplasma pneumoniae. Acta Haematol., 51:297, 1974.
49. Firkin, B. G., Blackwell, J. B., and Johnston, G. A. W.: Essential cryo-globulinaemia and acquired haemolytic anaemia due to cold agglutinins. Australian Ann. Med., 8:151, 1959.
50. Floersheim, G. L.: A comparative study of the effects of anti-tumor and immunosuppressive drugs on antibody forming and erythropoietic cells. Clin. Exp. Immunol., 6:861, 1970.
50a. Foucar, K., McKenna, R. W., Bloomfield, C. D., Bowers, T. K., and Brunning, R. D.: Therapy-related leukemia. A Panmyelosis. Cancer., 43:1285, 1979.
51. Frank, M. M., Schreiber, A. D., and Atkinson, J. P.: Studies of the interaction of antibody, complement, and macrophages in the immune clearance of erythro-

cytes. In Phagocytic Cell in Host Resistance. Bellanti, J. A., and Dayton, D. H., Eds. New York, Raven Press, 1975.
52. Frimmer, D., and Creger, W. P.: Heparin and hemolytic anemia. Amer. J. Med. Sci., 259:412, 1970.
53. Garratty, G.: The effects of storage and heparin on the activity of serum complement, with particular reference to the detection of blood group antibodies. Amer. J. Clin. Path., 54:531, 1970.
54. Glassman, A. B.: Immune responses: The rationale for plasmapheresis. Plasma Therapy, 1:13, 1979.
55. Goldberg, A.: Radiochromium in the selection of patients with haemolytic anaemia for splenectomy. Lancet, 1:109, 1966.
56. Gopal, V., and Bisno, A. L.: Fulminant pneumococcal infections in 'normal' asplenic hosts. Arch. Intern. Med., 173:1526, 1977.
57. Green, N., and Goldenberg, H.: Acute hemolytic anemia and hemoglobinuria complicating infectious mononucleosis. Arch. Intern. Med., 105:108, 1960.
57a. Grünwald, H. W., and Rosner, F.: Acute leukemia and immunosuppressive drug use. A review of patients undergoing immunosuppressive therapy for non-neoplastic diseases. Arch. Intern. Med., 139:461, 1979.
58. Habibi, B., Homberg, J. C., Schaison, G., and Salmon, C.: Autoimmune hemolytic anemia in children: A review of 80 cases. Am. J. Med., 56:61, 1974.
59. Hancock, D. M.: Autoimmune haemolytic anaemia in an infant treated by thymectomy. Lancet, 2:1118, 1963.
60. Hartman, M. M.: Reversal of serologic reactions by heparin: Therapeutic implications. II. Idiopathic acquired hemolytic anemia (IAHA). Ann. Allerg., 22:313, 1964.
61. Haserick, J. R.: Modern concepts of systemic lupus erythematosus; a review of 126 cases. J. Chron. Dis., 1:317, 1955.
62. Hippe, E., Jensen, K. B., Olesen, H., Lind, K., and Thomsen, P. E. B.: Chlorambucil treatment of patients with cold agglutinin syndrome. Blood, 35:68, 1970.
63. Hirooka, V., Miki, K., Ono, T., et al.: Splenectomy and thymectomy for autoimmune hemolytic anemia in infants. Acta Paediatr. Jap., 74:513, 1970.
64. Hirsch, J., and Dacie, J. V.: Persistent post-splenectomy thrombocytosis and thrombo-embolism: A consequence of continuing anemia. Brit. J. Haematol., 12:44, 1966.
65. Hitzig, W. H., and Massimo, L.: Treatment of autoimmune hemolytic anemia in children with azathioprine (Imuran). Blood, 28:840, 1966.
66. Horster, J. A.: Die Korticosteroid-Behandlung Hematologische und Verwandter Erkrankungen. Stuttgart, Georg Theime Verlag, 1961.
67. Hughes-Jones, N. C., and Szur, L.: Determination of the sites of red-cell destruction using 51Cr-labelled cells. Brit. J. Haematol., 3:320, 1957.
68. Hyslop, N. E., Jr.: Fever and circulatory collapse in an asplenic man. Case records of the Massachusetts General Hospital. New Engl. J. Med., 293:547, 1975.
69. Ikkala, E., Kivilaakso, E., and Hästbacka, J.: Splenectomy in blood diseases: A report of 80 cases. Ann. Clin. Res., 6:290, 1974.
70. Isbister, J. P., Biggs, J. C., and Penny, R.: Experience with large volume plasmapheresis in malignant paraproteinaemia and immune disorders. Aust. N.Z.J. Med., 8:154, 1978.
71. Israel, L., Edelstein, R., Mannoni, P., Radot, E., and Greenspan, E. M.: Plasmapheresis in patients with disseminated cancer: Clinical results and correlation with changes in serum protein. Cancer, 40:3146, 1977.
72. Jaffe, I. A.: Comparison of the effect of plasmapheresis and penicillamine on the level of circulating rheumatoid factor. Ann. Rheum. Dis., 22:71, 1963.
73. Jandl, J. H., Greenberg, M. S., Yonemoto, R. H., and Castle, W. B.: Clinical determination of the sites of red cell sequestration in hemolytic anemias. J. Clin. Invest., 35:842, 1956.
74. Jandl, J. H., Jones, A. R., and Castle, W. B.: The destruction of red cells by

antibodies in man. I. Observations of the sequestration and lysis of red cells altered by immune mechanisms. J. Clin. Invest., *36:*1428, 1957.

75. Johnson, C. A., and Abildgaard, C. F.: Treatment of idiopathic autoimmune hemolytic anemia in children. Acta Paediatr. Scand., *65:*375, 1976.
76. Johnson, G. D., and Beneze, G.: The effect of heparin on nuclear immunofluorescence. Bibl. Haemat., *23:*40, 1965.
77. Johnson, H. M.: The effect of splenectomy in acute systemic lupus erythematosus. Arch. Dermatol. Syph., *68:*699, 1953.
78. Karaklis, A., Valaes, T., Pantelakis, S. N., and Doxiadis, S. A.: Thymectomy in an infant with autoimmune haemolytic anaemia. Lancet, *2:*778, 1964.
79. Karpatkin, S., Strick, N., and Siskind, G. W.: Detection of splenic anti-platelet antibody synthesis in idiopathic autoimmune thrombocytopenic purpura (ATP). Brit. J. Haematol., *23:*167, 1972.
80. Kay, N. E., and Douglas, S. D.: Monocyte-erythrocyte interaction in vitro in immune hemolytic anemias. Blood, *50:*889, 1977.
81. Keyloun, V. E., and Grace, W. J.: Acute hemolytic anemia complicating infectious mononucleosis. N.Y. State J. Med., *66:*273, 1966.
82. Kinlough, R. L., Bennett, R. C., and Lander, H.: The place of splenectomy in haematological disorders: The value of ^{51}Cr techniques. Med. J. Aust., *2:*1022, 1966.
83. Learmonth, J.: The surgery of the spleen. Br. Med., J., *2:*67, 1951.
84. Leddy, J. P., and Swisher, S. N.: Acquired immune hemolytic disorders (including drug-induced immune hemolytic anemia). In Immunological Diseases. 3rd Ed. Samter, M., Ed. Boston, Little Brown & Co., 1978, Vol. I, 1187.
85. Lewis, S. M., Szur, L., and Dacie, J. V.: The pattern of erythrocyte destruction in haemolytic anemia, as studied with radioactive chromium. Brit. J. Haematol., *6:*122, 1960.
86. Lind, K., Mansa, B., and Olesen, H.: Penicillamine treatment in the cold-haemagglutinin syndrome. Acta Med. Scand., *173:*647, 1963.
87. Lockwood, C. M.: Plasma-exchange: An overview. Plasma Therapy, *1:*1, 1979.
88. Lockwood, C. W., Worlledge, S., Nicholas, A., Cotton, C., and Peters, D. K.: Reversal of impaired splenic function in patients with nephritis or vasculitis (or both) by plasma exchange. New Engl. J. Med., *300:*524, 1979.
89. Logue, G. L., Rosse, W. F., and Gockerman, J. P.: Measurement of the third component of complement bound to red blood cells in patients with the cold agglutinin syndrome. J. Clin. Invest., *52:*493, 1973.
90. Logue, G. L., Rosse, W. F., Smith, W. T., Saltzman, H. A., and Gutterman, L. A.: Endogenous carbon monoxide production measured by gas-phase analysis: An estimation of heme catabolic rate. J. Lab. Clin. Med., *77:*867, 1971.
91. Lorber, M., Schwartz, L. I., and Wasserman, L. R.: Association of antibody-coated red blood cells with ulcerative colitis; report of four cases. Amer. J. Med., *19:*887, 1955.
92. Mappes, G., and Fischer, J.: Erfahrungen mit der splenektomie bei Blutkrankheiten. Dtsch. Med. Wochenschr., *94:*584, 1969.
93. Marmont, A., Giordano, D., Santini, G., Damasio, E., Carella, M., and Bacigalupo, A.: The treatment of autoimmune blood disease with antilymphocyte globulin. Postgrad. Med. J., *52* (Suppl 5): 139, 1976.
94. Mauri, C., Torelli, U., and Vaccari, G. L.: The treatment of autoimmune hemolytic anaemia with antilymphocytic globulin. Abstracts of XIIth International Congress of Haematology August 2–8, 1970.
95. McCurdy, P. R., and Rath, C. E.: Splenectomy in hemolytic anemia: results predicted by body scanning after injection of Cr^{51}-tagged red cells. N. Engl. J. Med., *259:*459, 1958.
96. McFarland, W., Galbraith, R. G., and Miale, A.: Heparin therapy in autoimmune hemolytic anemia. Blood, *15:*741, 1960.
97. McMillan, R., Longmire, R. L., Yelenosky, R., Donnell, R. L., and Armstrong, S.:

Quantitation of platelet-binding IgG produced in vitro by spleens from patients with idiopathic thrombocytopenic purpura. New Engl. J. Med., *291:*812, 1974.

98. Mengel, C. E., Wallace, A. G., and McDaniel, H. G.: Infectious mononucleosis, hemolysis, and megaloblastic arrest. Arch. Int. Med., *114:*333, 1964.

99. Miescher, P. A., Gerebtzoff, A., and Lambert, P. H.: Immunosuppressive therapy. In Textbook of Immunopathology. Miescher, P. A., and Mu, E. Eds. New York, Grune and Stratton, 1976, 343.

100. Mueller-Eckhardt, C. H., and Kretschmer, V.: Immunosuppressive therapy in blood diseases. In Immunosuppressive Therapy. Proceedings of the International Wiesbaden Symposium, 1972. New York, Schwabe, 1972, 85.

101. Murphy, S., and LoBuglio, A. F.: Drug therapy of autoimmune hemolytic anemia. Seminars Hematol., *13:*323, 1976.

102. Najean, Y., Cacchione, R., Dresch, C., and Rain, J. D.: Methods of evaluating the sequestration site of red cells labelled with ^{51}Cr: A review of 96 cases. Brit. J. Haematol., *29:*495, 1975.

103. Nightingale, D., Prankerd, T. A. J., Richards, J. D. M., and Thompson, D.: Splenectomy in anemia. Quart. J. Med., *41:*261, 1972.

104. Nordøy, A., and Neset, G.: Splenectomy in hematologic diseases. Acta Med. Scand., *183:*117, 1968.

105. Olesen, H.: Chlorambucil treatment in the cold agglutinin syndrome. Scand. J. Haematol., *1:*116, 1964.

106. Oski, F. A., and Abelson, N. M.: Autoimmune hemolytic anemia in an infant: Report of a case treated unsuccessfully with thymectomy. J. Pediatr., *67:*752, 1965.

107. Outeirino, J., Sanchez, J. F., Serrano, J., et al.: Risultati terapeutici di 45 casi di anemia emolitica asquisita, apparentemente extraglobulare. Minerva Med., *57:*3424, 1966.

108. Owren, P. A.: Acquired hemolytic jaundice. Scand. J. Clin. Lab. Invest., *1:*41, 1949.

109. Parker, A. C., MacPherson, A. I. S., and Richmond, J.: Value of radiochromium investigation in autoimmune haemolytic anemia. Brit. Med. J., *1:*208, 1977.

110. Patten, E., Reuter, F. P., Castle, R., and Mercer, C.: Evan's syndrome: Benefit from plasma exchange. Transfusion, *18:*383, 1978.

112. Petz, L. D.: Hemolytic anemias—immune. In Current Therapy. Conn, H. F., Ed., Philadelphia, W. B. Saunders, 1977, 256.

113. Petz, L. D., Rodvien, R., Yam, P., Jester, S., and Mielke, C. H.: Unpublished observations.

114. Pirofsky, B.: Autoimmunization and the Autoimmune Hemolytic Anemias. Baltimore, Williams & Wilkins Company, 1969.

115. Pirofsky, B.: Immune haemolytic disease: The autoimmune haemolytic anaemias. Clin. Haematol., *4:*167, 1975.

116. Pisciotta, A. V.: Cold hemagglutination in acute and chronic hemolytic syndromes. Blood, *10:*295, 1955.

117. Pisciotta, A. V., Giliberti, J. J., Greenwalt, T. J., and Engstrom, W. W.: Acute hemolytic anemia in disseminated lupus erythematosus. Amer. J. Clin. Path., *21:*1139, 1951.

117a. Plotz, P. H., Klippel, J. H., Decker, J. L., Grauman, D., Wolff, B., Brown, B. C., and Rutt, G.: Bladder complications in patients receiving cyclophosphamide for systemic lupus erythematosus or rheumatoid arthritis. Ann. Intern. Med., *91:*221, 1979.

118. Ritzmann, S. E., and Levin, W. C.: Effect of mercaptanes in cold agglutinin disease. J. Lab. Clin. Med., *57:*718, 1961.

119. Robson, H. N.: Medical aspects of splenectomy. Edinb. Med. J., *56:*381, 1949.

120. Rosenfield, R. E., and Jagathambal: Transfusion therapy for autoimmune hemolytic anemia. Seminars Hematol., *13:*311, 1976.

121. Rosenfield, R. E., Vitale, B., and Kochwa, S.: Immune mechanisms for destruction of erythrocytes in vivo. II. Heparinization for protection of lysin-sensitized erythrocytes. Transfusion, 7:261, 1967.
122. Ross, J. F., Finch, S. C. Street, R. B., Jr., and Strieder, J. W.: The simultaneous occurrence of benign thymoma and refractory anemia. Blood, 9:935, 1954.
123. Rosse, W. F.: Quantitative immunology of immune hemolytic anemia. II. The relationship of cell-bound antibody to hemolysis and the effect of treatment. J. Clin. Invest., 50:734, 1971.
124. Rosse, W. F., and Logue, G. L.: Immune hemolytic anemias. Modern Treatment, 8:379, 1971.
125. Roth, K. L.: Interaction of heparin with autoagglutinins in idiopathic acquired hemolytic anemia. Proc. Soc. Exp. Biol. Med., 86:352, 1954.
126. Roth, K. L.: Notes on the relationship between the therapeutic and anticomplementary effects of heparin in acquired hemolytic anemia. Ann. Allerg., 23:83, 1965.
127. Roth, K. L., and Frumin, A. M.: Effect of intramuscular heparin on antibodies in idiopathic acquired hemolytic anemia. Amer. J. Med., 20:968, 1956.
128. Rundles, R. W., Laszlo, J., Itoga, T., et al.: Clinical and hematologic study of 6-[(1-methyl-4-nitro-5-imidazolyl) thio] -purine (B.W. 57–322) and related compounds. Cancer Chemother. Rep., 14:99, 1961.
129. Rytel, M. W., Dee, T. H., Ferstenfeld, J. E., et al.: Possible pathogenetic role of capsular antigens in fulminant pneumococcal disease with disseminated intravascular coagulation (DIC). Amer. J. Med., 57:889, 1974.
130. Salmon, J., and Lambert, P. H.: Traitement immuno-suppressif au cours d'affections d' ordre immuno-pathologique. Acta Allergol., 22:220, 1967.
131. Sandusky, W. R., Leavell, B. S., and Benjamin, B. I.: Splenectomy: Indications and results in hematologic disorders. Ann. Surg., 159:695, 1964.
132. Sarles, H. E., and Levin, W. C.: The role of splenectomy in the management of acquired autoimmune hemolytic anemia complicating systemic lupus erythematosus. Amer. J. Med., 26:547, 1959.
133. Sedgwick, C. E., and Hume, A. H.: Elective splenectomy: An analysis of 220 operations. Ann. Surg., 151:163, 1960.
134. Schilling, R. F.: Hereditary spherocytosis: A study of splenectomized persons. Seminars Haematol., 13:169, 1976.
135. Schloesser, L. L., Korst, D. R., Clatanoff, D. V., and Schilling, R. F.: Radioactivity over the spleen and liver following transfusion of chromium ^{51}-labelled erythrocytes in hemolytic anemia. J. Clin. Invest., 36:1470, 1957.
136. Schreiber, A. D., Herskovitz, B. S., and Goldwein, M.: Low-titer cold-hemagglutinin disease. New Engl. J. Med., 296:1490, 1977.
137. Schubothe, H.: The cold hemagglutinin disease. Seminars Hematol., 3:27, 1966.
138. Schwartz, R., and Dameshek, W.: Drug-induced immunologic tolerance. Nature (London), 183:1682, 1959.
139. Schwartz, R., and Dameshek, W.: The treatment of autoimmune hemolytic anemia with 6-mercaptopurine and thioguanine. Blood, 19:483, 1962.
140. Schwartz, R., Eisner, A., and Dameshek, W.: The effect of 6-mercaptopurine on primary and secondary immune responses. J. Clin. Invest., 38:1394, 1959.
141. Schwartz, S. I., Adams, J. T., and Bauman, A. W.: Splenectomy for hematologic disorders. Current Prob. Surg. Chicago, Year Book Med Publishers, May, 1971.
142. Schwartz, S. I., Bernard, R. P., Adams, J. T., and Bauman, A. W.: Splenectomy for hematologic disorders. Arch. Surg., 101:338, 1970.
143. Shashaty, G. G., Rath, G. E., and Britt, E. J.: Autoimmune hemolytic anemia associated with ulcerative colitis. Amer. J. Hematol., 3:199, 1977.
144. Skinner, M. D., and Schwartz, R. S.: Immunosuppressive therapy. New Engl. J. Med., 287:221 and 281, 1972.
145. Steinberg, A. D., Plotz, P. H., Wolff, S. M., Wong, V. G., Agus, S. G., and Decker,

J. L.: Cytotoxic drugs in treatment of nonmalignant diseases. Ann. Intern. Med., *76:*619, 1972.

146. Stickney, J. M., and Heck, F. J.: Primary nonfamilial hemolytic anemia. Blood, *3:*431, 1948.

147. Sterzl, J., and Holub, M.: The influence of 6-mercaptopurine on antibody formation. Folia Biol. (Praha), *4:*59, 1958.

148. Storti, E., Vaccari, F., and Baldini, E.: Studies on the relationship between anticoagulants and hemolysis. Parts I and II. Acta Haematol. (Basel), *15:*12, 106, 1956.

149. Szur, L.: Surface counting in the assessment of sites of red cell destruction. Brit. J. Haematol., *18:*591, 1970.

150. Taft, E. G., Propp, R. P, and Sullivan, S. A.: Plasma exchange for cold agglutinin hemolytic anemia. Transfusion, *17:*173, 1977.

151. Tattersall, M. H. N.: Thrombocytopenic purpura in patients with autoimmune haemolytic anaemia, successfully treated with mercaptopurine. Br. Med. J., *3:*93, 1967.

152. Taylor, L.: Idiopathic autoimmune hemolytic anemia. Response of a patient to repeated courses of alkylating agents. Amer. J. Med., *35:*130, 1963.

153. TenPas, A., and Monto, R. W.: The treatment of autoimmune hemolytic anemia with heparin. Amer. J. Med. Sci., *251:*63, 1966.

154. Terman, D. S., Tavel, T., Petty, D., Racic, M. R., and Buffaloe, G.: Specific removal of antibody by extracorporeal circulation over antigen immobilized in collodion-charcoal: Clin. Exp. Immunol., *28:*180, 1977.

155. Tonkin, A. M., Mond, H. G., Alford, F. P., and Hurley, T. H.: Severe acute haemolytic anaemia complicating infectious mononucleosis. Med. J. Aust., *2:*1048, 1973.

156. Veeger, W., Woldring, M. G., VanRood, J. J., Eernisse, J. G., Leeksma, C. H., Verloop, M. C., and Nieweg, H. O.: The value of the determination of the site of red cell sequestration in hemolytic anemia as a prediction test for splenectomy. Acta Med. Scand., *171:*507, 1962.

157. Verma, I. C., Mittal, S. K., and Ghai, O. P.: Autoimmune hemolytic anemia in infancy and childhood. Indian J. Pediatr., *57:*326, 1970.

158. Von Dem Borne, A. E. G. Kr, Engelfriet, C. P., Beckers, D., Van Der Korthenkes, G., Van Der Giessen, M., and Van Loghem, J. J.: Autoimmune haemolytic anemias. II. Warm haemolysins—serological and immunochemical investigations and ^{51}Cr studies. Clin. Exper. Immunol., *4:*333, 1969.

159. Welch, C. S., and Dameshek, W.: Splenectomy in blood dyscrasias. N. Engl. J. Med., *242:*601, 1950.

160. Wells, J. V., and Fudenberg, H. H.: Paraproteinaemia. Disease-a-Month, *20:*2, 1974.

161. West-Watson, W. N., and Young, C. J.: Failed splenectomy in acholuric jaundice, and the relation of toxaemia to the haemolytic crisis. Brit. Med. J., *1:*1305, 1938.

162. Williams, E. D., Szur, L., Glass, H. I., Lewis, S. M., Pettit, J. E., and Ahuja, S.: Measurement of red cell destruction in the spleen. J. Lab. Clin. Med., *84:*134, 1974.

163. Wilmers, M. J., and Russell, P. A.: Autoimmune hemolytic anemia in an infant treated by thymectomy. Lancet, *2:*915, 1963.

164. Worlledge, S.: Immune haemolytic anemias. In Blood and Its Disorders. Hardisty, R. M., and Weatherall, D. J., Eds. Oxford, Blackwell, 1974, 714.

165. Worlledge, S. M., Brain, M. C., Cooper, A. C., et al.: Immunosuppressive drugs in the treatment of autoimmune haemolytic anaemia. Proc. R. Soc. Med., *61:*1312, 1968.

166. Young, L. E., Miller, G., and Swisher, S. N.: Treatment of hemolytic disorders. J. Chron. Dis., *6:*307, 1957.

Index

Page numbers followed by *t* represent tables. Page numbers followed by *f* represent figures. Throughout the index AIHA = autoimmune hemolytic anemia.

ABO blood grouping in AIHA, 159–160, 365–366

Absorption
  cold autoabsorption, 377–381*t*
  differential absorption, 371–372
  detection of alloantibodies in AIHA, 377–378*t*
  cell typing in AIHA, 161
  warm autoabsorption, 366, 368*t*, 369*f*, 370, 378–379*t*

N-Acetylneuraminic acid (NANA), 258

Acquired hemolytic anemia, definition of, 2

Acrocyanosis, 39, 41, 56, *See also* Raynaud's phenomenon

ACTH, 392, 408, 410*t*, 426

AIHA, *See* Autoimmune hemolytic anemia

Agglutination, *See also* Autoagglutination
  demonstration *in vivo*, 39
  grading and scores, 154*t*

Agglutinins, cold, *See* Cold agglutinin syndrome; Cold agglutinins; Autoagglutination

Albumin, role in antibody detection, 144–147

Aldomet, *See* Drug-induced immune hemolytic anemia, methyldopa

Alloantibodies,
  detection in warm-antibody AIHA, 366–372, *See also,* Transfusion in AIHA, selection of donor blood
  mimicking autoantibodies, 246–250
  subclasses of, 119*t*, 120. *See also* Immunoglobulins
  transfusion of, 335

Anaphylatoxin, *See* Complement, biologic activities

Anemia with a hemolytic component, definition, 2

Angioedema, hereditary (HAE), 82, 83*t*, 84, 193

Antibodies, *See* Alloantibodies; Autoantibodies; Immunoglobulins; Serologic investigation of AIHA; Complement, activation by; Specificity.

Antigens
  chemistry of Ii, 254–256
  chemistry of Pr, 258–259
  Chido blood group, 100
  development of I, 253*t*
  relative strength of i, I^F and I^D on red cells, 252*t*
  Rodgers blood group, 100

Antiglobulin test
  Anti-complement, *See* Antiglobulin test, complement
  Anti-IgA, 150, 155–156, 348–349
  Anti-IgG, 150, 153–155
  Anti-IgM, 150, 155–156
  complement-fixing antiglobulin consumption test, compared with, 307*t*
  complement, role of,
    anti-complement activity, standardization of, 156–158
    detection of red cell bound complement,
      direct antiglobulin test, 85, 87–90*f*, 91–92, 125, 150, 162–163*t*, 189–194, 195*t*, 196*f*, 197*f*, 198*f*, 199*f*, 200, 201–203*t*
      indirect antiglobulin test, 92–96
    detection on normal red cells, 100–101
    hereditary angioedema, 193
    in diagnosis of AIHA, *See* Differential diagnosis, antiglobulin test.
    potential detrimental effects, 96–99
  direct antiglobulin test (DAT), 13, 22,

Antiglobulin test (cont.)
148–153, 162–164, 188–206t, 344t
changes in reactivity during response to therapy, 204t, 395–396t
complement, role in, See Antiglobulin test, complement
differential diagnosis of AIHA, 188–206
false negative, causes of, 152–153
indirect (IAT) compared with,
in differentiation between delayed hemolytic transfusion reaction and AIHA, 329
in detection of alloantibodies in warm antibody AIHA, 366
infectious mononucleosis and hemolytic anemia, 44t
mechanisms of drug induced positive, 272–289
method, 162–164
methyldopa-induced hemolytic anemia, 190t, 191t, 204, 205t, 206t
monospecific antiglobulin reagents, 149–150, 163–164, 189–194, 195t
negative
in autoimmune hemolytic anemia, 305–321, See also AIHA with negative direct antiglobulin test
causes of false, 152–153
penicillin-induced immune hemolytic anemia, 190–191t, 273–282, 291–292t
polyspecific reagents, 150, 188–189
positive
anti-IgA antiserum only in warm-antibody AIHA, 192–193, 348–349
causes of, 151–152
drugs reported to cause, 271t
in normal persons, 22, 100–101
in patients without hemolytic anemia, 22, 151–152
significance of, 22, 151–152, 188–206
subclass specificity of IgG antibody,

determined by, 120t, 121
protein on red cells, determination of type and amount by, 163–164
See also Antiglobulin test, direct, monospecific antiglobulin reagents
scores, determination of, 154t
semi-quantitative, See Antiglobulin test, direct antiglobulin test, titrations and scores
sensitivity of, 306–307t
titrations and scores, 154t, 162, 163t, 164, 194–206
clinical interpretation, 196–206
comparison of commercial reagents with research reagents in, 194, 195t
during response to therapy, 204t, 395–396t
examples in three patients, 163t
method, 154t, 163–164
methyldopa-induced AIHA, 204, 205t, 206t
relationship to quantitative measurements of red cell sensitization, 194, 196f, 197f, 198f, 199f, 200f, 201–203t
indirect
complement, role in, 92–96
comparison with direct in AIHA, 366
comparison with direct in delayed hemolytic transfusion reaction, 329
principles, 148–150, 149f
quality control, 158
standardization of antiglobulin sera, 153–158
anti-complement, 156–158
anti-IgG, 153, 154t, 155
anti-IgA, 155–156
anti-IgM, 155–156
uses, 148t
Antilymphocyte globulin in management of warm-antibody AIHA, 416
Antithrombin III, 72
Autoabsorption technique
cold, 377, 379, 381t

warm, 366, 368–370

Autoagglutination, 34, 40, 186–187*f*

Autoanalyzer, use for studying AIHA, 178–181

Autoantibodies, *See also* Cold agglutinin syndrome; Immunoglobulins; Paroxysmal cold hemoglobinuria; Specificity of autoantibodies; Warm antibody AIHA

  anti-A, 242–243

  anti-B, 259

  anti-c, 232, 234, 237, 249, 250

  anti-C, 233, 234, 237, 249

  anti-CD, 236

  anti-Ce, 237, 249

  anti-D, 233, 234, 237, 249

  anti-e, 232, 233, 234, 236, 237, 238, 249, 250

  anti-E, 236, 237, 246, 247*t*, 248*t*, 249

  anti-En^a, 243, 244, 246

  anti-f, 237, 250

  anti-G, 237, 249

  anti-Gd, 259

  anti-HD, 257

  anti-HI, 260

  anti-Hr, 249

  anti-Hr$_0$, 249

  anti-hr^s, 248

  anti-hr^B, 248

  anti-H$_T$, 259

  anti-i, 43–46, 47, 251, 253, 257*t*

  anti-I, 43, 47, 247, 250, 251*t*, 252–254, 257*t*, 260

  anti-I^T, 241*t*, 242*t*

  anti-Jk^a, 233, 237, 243

  anti-Kell, 233, 237, 238–241, 246

  anti-LW, 234, 236, 238

  anti-M, 259

  anti-N, 242, 259

  anti-nl, -pdl, -dl, 233*t*, 234, 236, 237, 238, 244*t*, 245t, 246, 249

  "non-specific," 232, 236, 238, 250

  anti-O, 259

  anti-p, 260

  anti-P, 260

  anti-P$_1$, 259

  anti-PP$_1$P^k, 260

  anti-Pr, 48, 257*t*, 258

  anti-"Rh," 233, 234, 235, 236, 237, 238, 244*t*

  anti-Sd^x, 259

  anti-Sp$_1$, 257*t*

  anti-Tj^a, 260

  anti-U, 238, 244*t*

  anti-Wr^b, 237, 243, 244*t* 245*t*, 246

  anti-Xg^a, 237

  mimicking alloantibodies, 246–250

  Rh "relative specificity," 372, 373*t*, 374–375, 378–379*t*

  Rh specificity, 232, 233, 234, 236, 237, 244*t*, *See also* Rh

Autoimmune hemolytic anemia (AIHA), *See also* Cold agglutinin syndrome; Paroxysmal cold hemoglobinuria; Warm antibody AIHA; Drug-induced immune hemolytic anemia, autoimmune hemolytic anemia caused by drugs

  childhood, 349–351*t*

  clinical characteristics, 28–57

  development after immunization procedures, 129

  development after transfusion, 331–337

  diagnosis, *See* Differential diagnosis; Serologic investigation of AIHA

  drug induced, 190*t*, 191*t*, 192*t*, 204, 205*t*, 206*t*, 285–291*t*, 294–297

  in infancy and childhood, 349–351*t*

  in pregnancy, 321–327

  in patients whose direct antiglobulin test is positive only with anti-IgA antiserum, 348–349

  secondary, *See* Secondary AIHA

  with negative direct antiglobulin test, 305–321

    antibodies, measurement of red cell bound, 307–308

    antibody concentration, relationship to rate of hemolysis, 306

    case reports, 315–318, 324

    clinical and laboratory findings in 27 patients, 312–313*t*

    incidence, 306

    laboratory investigation of patients, 308–309

    measurement of small concentrations of red-cell bound IgG, 307–310, 311*t*, 312–313*t*, 314, 324–326*t*

Autoimmune hemolytic anemia with negative direct antiglobulin test
  sensitivity of direct antiglobulin test, 306–307
  serologic tests in diagnosis, 310
  therapy and course, 312–313*t*, 314–318
  with both IgG and IgM autoantibodies, 346, 347*t*, 348
Azathioprine, 404, 405, 407, 408

Bacteremia, fulminant, splenectomy and, 401–402
Bacterial endocarditis, 275–276
Bilirubin, 3, 4*f*, 5, 7–8, 20
Blood film in hemolytic anemias, 7, 13, 14*t*, 15–19*f*, 23, 40
Blood transfusion, *See* Transfusion
Bone marrow,
  erythroid hyperplasia, 9
  in cold agglutinin syndrome, 48
n-butanol in extraction of antigens, 255

Carbon monoxide, endogenous production, 9
Cephalosporin
  coated red cells, 293
  induced immunohematologic abnormalities, 283, 284*f*, 285*t*
  induced immune hemolytic anemia, 293
Chemistry of blood group antigens
  Ii Antigens, 254–256
  Pr Antigens, 258–259
Chemotaxis, 81
Chido blood group, 100
Childhood, AIHA in, 349–351
  clinical features, 351*t*
Chlorambucil, 404, 407
  cold agglutinin syndrome, 422, 423*t*
Chromium (⁵¹Cr), 9, 306, 382–384, 399–400
Cirrhosis of the liver, Laennec's, 86
Classification
  and clinical features of immune hemolytic anemias, 28*t*
  and differential diagnosis of AIHA, 177*t*
  hemolytic anemias, 10–11*t*, 12*t*

immune hemolytic anemias, 26, 27*t*, 28
Coagulation
  complement associations with, 81–83
  effect of heparin on complement and on coagulation tests, 409, 414, 415*t*
Cold
  association of AIHA with exposure to, 13, 55, 185–186
  avoidance of, in cold agglutinin syndrome, 420
Cold agglutinins, *See also* Cold agglutinin syndrome
  abnormal, 216*t*
    with warm-antibody AIHA, 344–346 347*t*, 348
  autoabsorption of, 377–378*t*, 381*t*
  clinically insignificant, with warm antibody AIHA, 345
  concentration, 48
  early descriptions of, 37–38
  immunochemistry, 47–48
  immune globulin class, 47–48
  in infectious mononucleosis, 42–46, 45*t*
  monoclonal, 26, 47, 48, 49, 50*t*
  polyclonal, 26, 47
  specificity
    determination of, 168–169, 174–175
    in cold agglutinin syndrome, 250, 251*t*, 252*t*, 253*t*, 254*t*, 255–259
  thermal range, 168–169, 174*t*, 214–216*t*, 217–218, 219–221*t*
  titer, 41, 168*t*, 174*t*, 219–221*t*, 223, 224*t*
Cold agglutinin syndrome, 37–50, *See also* Cold agglutinins
  acrocyanosis, 39, 41
  age, 38–39
  associated diseases, 41–47
  autoagglutination, 40, 186–187*f*
  autoantibody specificity, 250–259
    antibodies other than anti-I, i, or Pr, 259
    determination, 168–169, 174–175
    Ii blood group, 250–254
    Ii blood group antigens, chemistry of, 254–256

in 54 patients, 224*t*
other, 256–258
Pr blood group antigens, chemistry of, 258–259
bilirubinemia, 40
blood film, 18*f*, 19*f*, 40
blood transfusion in, 376–382, 387
See also Transfusion in AIHA
bone marrow, 48
case report, 218–222
complement metabolism in, 85
cryoglobulins, 40, 48
diagnosis of, 213–223
   characterization of antibodies in cold agglutinin syndrome 213–214
   compared with paroxysmal cold hemoglobinuria, 227–229
   direct antiglobulin test, 189–190*t*, 201–203*t*
   development of criteria to distinguish benign cold agglutinins from those associated with *in vivo* hemolysis, 214–216*t*
   essential diagnostic tests, 217–218
   further comments regarding serologic tests, 222–223
   serum screening tests in, 167*t*, 217*t*
   thermal range of autoantibody, *See* Cold agglutinins, thermal range titer of cold agglutinins, 213–223, *See also* Cold agglutinins
gangrene, 40
hemoglobinuria, 38, 39, 41
hemolysins, 214–215, 223
hemosiderinuria, 41
history, 37–38
immunochemistry of cold agglutinins, 47–48
incidence, 29*t*, 39
management of, 420–27
   avoidance of cold, 420
   corticosteroid therapy, 420–421
   immunosuppressive drugs, 422–423*t*
   laboratory data before and after treatment, 423*t*
   penicillamine, 425–426
   plasma exchange, 424–425

splenectomy, 426–427, 428*t*
   summary of therapeutic principles, 432
mononucleosis, infectious, 42*t*, 43, 44*t*, 45*t*, 46
Mycoplasma pneumoniae infections, 41–42, 43, 46–48, 141, 186, 227, 228
physical findings, 39–40
prognosis, 41, 49, 50*t*
Raynaud's phenomenon, 38, 39
red blood cell morphology, 18*f*, 19*f*, 40
reticuloendothelial neoplasia, 41
serologic findings in a patient with, 219–221*t*
serum screening tests, 167*t*, 217*t*
sex distribution, 39
symptoms, 39–40
transfusion in, *See* Transfusion in AIHA
Waldenstrom's macroglobulinuria compared with, 48–50*t*
warm-antibody AIHA, associated with, 345–346
Cold hemoglobinuria, paroxysmal. *See* Paroxysmal cold hemoglobinuria
Cold urticaria, 13, 56
Colitis, ulcerative, management of AIHA in, 430
Compatibility testing
   in AIHA, *See* Transfusion in AIHA
   in drug-induced immunohematologic abnormalities, 294–295
Compensated hemolytic disease, definition of, 1
Complement, 64–103
   abnormalities in human disease, 83*t*, 84
      acquired abnormalities, 84
      autoimmune hemolytic anemias, 337–338, 339*f*, 340*f*
      hereditary angioedema, 82–84, 193
      inborn abnormalities, 83–84
   activation, 64, 73–74, 87–89, 110–111, *See also* Complement, alternative pathway; Complement classical pathway.
      antibody class significance, 67, 75–76, 87–89

Complement (cont.)
  antibody subclass significance, 67, 74, 87, 111, 119, 142*t*
  activation unit, 68, 69
  activators, 68*t*, 76*t*
  alternative pathway of activation, 64, 73–79
    activators, 73–74, 76*t*
    biological functions which can result from, 80*t*
    reaction mechanisms, 75–79
  anaphylatoxins, *See* Complement, biologic activities
  antiglobulin test, role of, *See* Antiglobulin test, complement
  biological activities, 64, 79–83, 80*t*
    anaphylatoxins, 64, 69, 70, 71*f*, 79*f*, 80–81, 80*t*, 82
    associations with coagulation, 81–83
    chemotaxis, 81, 82
    immune adherence, 67, 81
    lysis, 64, 79, 87
    opsonization, 81
    phagocytosis, 67, 127
    virus neutralization, 81
  Chido blood group antigen, relationship to C4, 100
  classical pathway of activation, 64, 65–73
    activators, 68*t*
    effect of IgG subclass, 67, 74, 87, 111, 119, 142*t*
    physicochemical properties of proteins participating in, 65–67
    reaction mechanisms, 67–73
      activation unit, 69, 70*f*, 71*f*
      recognition unit, 68*f*, 69*f*
      membrane attack complex, 68, 71*f*, 72*f*, 73*f*, 78
  coagulation, associations with, 81–83
  cobra venom, 74, 76*t*
  components, *See* Complement proteins participating in reaction mechanisms
  definition of, 64
  destruction of red cells sensitized with, 122–128
    intravascular, 110–111
    extravascular, 111–113, 122–128, 129

"doughnut" hypothesis, 72
endotoxin, 74, 76*t*
-fixing antibody consumption test,
  autoimmune hemolytic anemia with a negative direct antiglobulin test, in, 310–311, 312–313*t*, 314
  comparison with antiglobulin test, 307*t*
  normal subjects, and patients with disorders other than idiopathic acquired hemolytic anemia, in, 311*t*
  patients with sickle cell anemia and other hemoglobinopathies, in, 318–321
  quantitation of red-cell bound IgG, use for, 308
  relapsing hemolytic anemia of pregnancy with a negative antiglobulin reaction, in, 324–326*t*
genetic deficiencies, 83*t*
guinea pig, C4 deficient, 74
heparin effect on, 102–103, 409, 414, 415*t*
inactivators, *See* Complement, proteins
inhibitors, *See* Complement, proteins
inulin, 76*t*
KAF (conglutinogen activating factor), *See* Complement, proteins, C3b inactivator
lysis, 64, 79
measurement, 84–87
  fractional catabolic rate, 85–87
  functional assays, 85
  hemolytic, 85
  immunodiffusion, 85
  immunohistochemical, 85
  metabolism in vivo, C3 and C4, 85–87
  red cell bound, *See also* Antiglobulin test, complement, 85, 125, 162–163*t*, 194, 196*f*, 197*f*, 198*f*, 199*f*, 200, 201–203*t*
  synthesis rate, C3, 85–87
membrane attack complex (MAC), 68, 71*f*, 72*f*, 73*f*, 78
metabolism, *See* measurement

proteins participating in reaction mechanisms, 64–79
  anti-thrombin III, 72, 73*f*
  BlH-globulin, 67, 75*t*, 76, 78*f*, 90*f*
  Cl, 64, 65, 68*f*, 69*f*, 70*f*
  Cl inhibitor, 64–65, 69*f*, 82
  Clq, 64, 65, 68*f*, 69*f*, 70*f*
  Clq inhibitor, 69*f*
  Clr, 64, 65, 68*f*, 69*f*
  Cls, 64, 65, 68*f*, 69*f*, 70*f*
  C2, 64, 65, 66, 68, 69, 70*f*, 71*f*
  C3, 66*f*, 67*f*, 69, 70, 75*t*, 76, 78, 90*f*
  C3a, 64, 66*f*, 69, 71*f*, 76, 77*f*, 79*f*, 81, 90*f*
  C3b, 64, 66*f*, 67, 69, 70, 71*f*, 75*t*, 76, 77*f*, 78, 79*f*, 90*f*
  C3c, 66*f*, 67, 75, 90*f*
  C3d, 66*f*, 67, 75, 78*f*, 80*t*, 90*f*
  C3b inactivator (C3bINA), 65, 66*f*, 67, 75*t*, 76, 78*f*,
  C3 convertase, 64, 66, 69, 70*f*, 71*f*, 76, 77*f*, 78, 79*f*
  C4, 64, 65, 66*f*, 67, 69, 70*f*
  C4a, 66*f*, 67, 69, 70*f*
  C4b, 66*f*, 67, 69, 70*f*, 81
  C5, 66*f*, 67, 70, 71*f*, 72*f*, 73*f*, 78, 79*f*
  C5a, 66*f*, 67, 70, 71*f*
  C5b, 66*f*, 67, 70, 71*f*, 72*f*, 73*f*, 79*f*
  C5 convertase, 66*f*, 67, 70, 71*f*, 78, 79*f*
  C6, 67, 71*f*, 72*f*, 73*f*, 79*f*
  C7, 67, 71*f*, 72*f*, 73*f*, 79*f*
  C8, 67, 72*f*, 79
  C9, 67, 72*f*, 79
  concentration in serum, 65*t*
  electrophoretic mobility, 65*t*
  factor B (proactivator), 64, 75*t*, 76, 77*f*, 78
  factor D (proactivator convertase), 64, 75*t*, 76, 77*f*, 79*f*
  fragments, 64, 66*f*, 70*f*, 71*f*, 72*f*, 73*f*, 77*f*, 78*f*, 79*f*, 90*f*, 91, 92
  lipoprotein, 72, 73*f*
  membrane attack complex, 68, 71*f*, 72*f*, 73*f*, 78
  membrane attack complex inhibitor, 72, 73*f*
  molecular weights, 65*t*
  participating in the alternative pathway, 75*t*
  participating in the classical pathway, 65*t*
  properdin (P), 64, 73, 74, 75*t*, 78, 79*f*
  S protein, 72
rabbit, C6 deficient, 81
reaction mechanisms, *See* Complement classical pathway; Complement alternative pathway.
reaction products of C3, 90*f*
receptors,
  Clq, 99
  C3, 122, 123, 124
  C3b, 64, 81, 99, 125–127, 130
  C3c, 113
  C3d, 99–100, 123, 126–127, 130
  C4, 81, 113, 130
  on lymphocytes, 81, 130
  on macrophages, 64, 81, 113, 122, 123
  on platelets, 82
recognition unit, 68*f*, 69*f*
red cell associated components, 100–101
red cell-bound, detection of, 85, 125, 162–163*t*, 194–200, 201–203*t*, *See also* Antiglobulin test, complement
red cell sensitization by non-immune mechanisms, 89, 275*t*, 283–285
Rodgers blood group antigen, relationship to C4, 100
stability in stored human serum, 101*f*–102
terminology, 64
zymosan, 73, 74, 76
Congenital hemolytic anemia, definition of, 2
Coombs test, *See* Antiglobulin test
Corticosteroid therapy,
  cold agglutinin syndrome, 420–421
  drug-induced immune hemolytic anemia, 296
  paroxysmal cold hemoglobinuria, 427
  warm-antibody AIHA, 392–397
Creatine, red cell, 9
Cryoglobulin, 40, 48
Cyclophosphamide, 403–405, 407
Cytotoxicity, 130–132

Differential diagnosis of AIHA, 185–229, See also Serologic investigation of AIHA
acute intravascular hemolysis in a child, 187
alloantibody induced immune hemolytic anemia, 188
antibodies in serum and red cell eluate, characterization of, 164–178, 206–229
antiglobulin test, direct in, 188–206
autoagglutination, 34, 40, 186–187f
classification, 10–11t, 12t, 27t, 177t
cold, association with exposure to, 13, 55, 185–186
cold agglutinin syndrome, See Cold agglutinin syndrome, diagnosis of
differentiation from delayed hemolytic transfusion reaction, See Transfusion reaction and AIHA, differentiation
distinctive clinical and routine laboratory features, 185–188
drug ingestion, 187–188
laboratory findings in, 188–229
paroxysmal cold hemoglobinuria, See Paroxysmal cold hemoglobinuria, diagnosis of
pneumonia, association with atypical, 186
summary of laboratory findings, 177t
warm-antibody AIHA, See Warm antibody AIHA, diagnosis of
Differential diagnosis of drug-induced immune hemolytic anemia, See Drug-induced immune hemolytic anemia, diagnosis
Differential diagnosis of hemolytic anemia, See Hemolytic anemia, diagnosis
Differential diagnosis of immune hemolytic anemia, See Hemolytic anemia, immune,
^{32}P-Diisopropyl fluorophosphate (DFP), 9
Dilution technique for alloantibody detection in warm-antibody AIHA, 370, 371t
Direct antiglobulin test, See Antiglobulin test, direct

Donath-Landsteiner antibody, See Paroxysmal cold hemoglobinuria
Donath-Landsteiner test, See Paroxysmal cold hemoglobinuria
Drug-induced immune hemolytic anemia, 267–297
antibodies, physicochemical characteristics of, 268–269
autoimmune hemolytic anemia caused by drugs, 26–27, 187–188, 274–275t, 285–291, 295–297, See also Drug-induced immune hemolytic anemia, methyldopa (Aldomet)-induced.
clinical features, 274–275t
AIHA caused by drugs, 285–289
compared with AIHA, 28t
hemolytic anemias caused by immune complex mechanism, 273
methyldopa-induced hemolytic anemia, 287–288
penicillin-induced hemolytic anemia, 273–283
compatibility testing, 294–295
AIHA caused by drugs, 294–295
hemolytic anemias caused by immune complex mechanisms or drug absorption mechanism, 294
diagnosis, methods of, 289–294
cephalosporin-coated red cells, preparation of, 293
cephalosporins, 285t, 293
history of drug ingestion, 13, 187–188, 289
L-dopa, 290–291
laboratory tests, 290–294
mefenamic acid, 290–291
methyldopa, 290–291t, See also Drug-induced immune hemolytic anemia, methyldopa (Aldomet)-induced.
other drugs, 293–294
penicillins, 291, 292t, 293, See also Drug-induced immune hemolytic anemia, penicillin-induced.
direct antiglobulin test results, 190t, 191t, 204–206, 271t, 272–294
drugs reported to cause a positive di-

rect antiglobulin test and hemolytic anemia, 271*t*
immunologic mechanisms, 267–289
  AIHA caused by drugs, 285–289
  correlation with clinical and labora-
    tory findings, 274–275*t*
  direct antiglobulin test (DAT)
    positivity, mechanisms of,
    272–289, 272*f*, 274–275*t*, 280*f*,
    284*f*
  drug adsorption mechanism, 273–
    283, 280*f*
  general concepts regarding cyto-
    penias, 267–272
  hapten mechanism, 268, 269–270
  immune complex mechanism, 268,
    269–270, 272*f*–273
  nonimmunologic protein absorp-
    tion, 283, 284*f*, 285*t*
incidence, 29*t*, 267
laboratory features, correlation with
    mechanisms of red cell sensiza-
    tion and clinical features, 274–
    275*t*
management and prognosis, 295–297
methyldopa (Aldomet)-induced,
  autoantibody specificity, 244, 286–
    287
  characteristic features, 275*t*, 285,
    287–288
  classification, 26–27
  compatibility testing in, 294–295
  direct antiglobulin test, 190*t*, 191*t*,
    204, 205*t*, 206*t*
  history of drug ingestion, 187–188,
    289
  incidence, 29*t*, 285
  indirect antiglobulin test results in,
    290, 291*t*, 294–295
  laboratory diagnosis of, 290–291
  management, 295–297
  mechanisms, proposed, 286–287
  prognosis, 295–297
  serum screening test results in 29
    patients, 291*t*
penicillin-induced, 273–283
  binding by red cells, 276–280*f*
  characteristic features, 282–283
  compatibility testing, 294
  complement activation in, 280–282
  course, 277*f*, 278*f*, 281*f*
  direct antiglobulin test, 190*t*, 191*t*,
    273–282, 291, 292*t*
  early reports, 273–276
  laboratory diagnosis of, 291, 292*t*,
    293
  management, 295–297
  mechanism of red cell sensitization,
    273–282
  penicillin-coated red cells, prepara-
    tion of, 292–293
  prognosis, 295–297

EDTA, collection of blood in, 159
Elliptocytosis, 15, 18*f*
Eluate, red cell
  characterization of antibodies in,
    206–213
  methods of preparation, 170–172
  showing anti-e "relative specificity,"
    173*t*, 373*t*
  specificity testing of, 172, 173*t*, 174
Endocarditis, bacterial, 275–276
Enzymes, proteolytic, role in antibody
    detection, 144–147
Epstein-Barr virus, 45, 99–100
Erythrocytes, *See* Red cells
Erythrophagocytosis, 56, *See also*
    Phagocytosis
Ether elution, method, 171
Evans' syndrome, 14, 19, 35
Extravascular hemolysis, definition of,
    3–4, *See also* Immune hemolysis

Factor XII (Hageman factor), 82
Fetal hazards of AIHA, 321–322

Gangrene, 40, 41
Genetic factors
  complement deficiencies, 83*t*
  development of AIHA, 335–337

Hageman factor (factor XII), 82
Hapten mechanism in drug-induced
    immune hemolytic anemia, 268–
    270, 279
Haptoglobin, 3*f*, 5, 8, 111
Heat elution, method, 170–171
Hemoglobin, 3–4, 8, 20, 359–361
  C, 15, 16*f*

Hemoglobin (cont.)
E, 15
plasma, 2, 3*f*, 20, 21, 111, 116
S, 17*f*
unstable, 14
Hemoglobinemia, *See* Hemoglobin,
plasma
Hemoglobinopathies, 10–11*t*, 12*t*, 15,
16*f*, 17*f*
complement-fixing antibody consumption test in, 318–321
Hemoglobinuria, 2–3*f*, 13, 20–22, 23,
33, 38, 39, 41, 55, 111, 116
causes, 20*t*
differentiation from hematuria, 21
paroxysmal cold, *See* Paroxysmal cold
hemoglobinuria
Hemolysins, *See also* Serologic investigation of AIHA
in warm antibody AIHA, 211–213
titration of, 169–170
Hemolysis
definition, 1
extravascular, definition of, 3–4*f*
factors affecting, 116*t*
intravascular, 3*f*, 13, 20–22, 110–111
acute, in a child, 187
definition, 2–3*f*
mechanisms of immune, *See* Immune
hemolysis, mechanisms of
red cell antibody concentration, relationship to rate of, 306
Hemolytic anemia, *See also* various
categories as, Autoimmune hemolytic anemia; Drug-induced; Warm
antibody; etc.
acquired, definition of, 2
characteristic features of AIHA and
drug-induced immune, 28*t*
classification, 10–11*t*, 12*t*
congenital, definition of, 2
definitions, 1–2, 3*f*, 4*f*
determination of hemolytic nature,
4–9
bilirubin, 7–8
blood count, 5–7
bone marrow hyperplasia, 9
red blood cell creatine, 9
red blood cell morphology, 7, 13,
14*t*, 15*f*, 16*f*, 17*f*, 18*f*, 19*f*

red blood cell survival studies, 5, 9
reticulocyte count, 5–7
serum haptoglobin, 8
serum lactic dehydrogenase, 8–9
diagnosis, 1–23
differential, 10–11*t*, 12*t*, 14*t*
establishing tentative, 9–22
specific confirmatory tests, 23
drug-induced immune, *See* Drug-
induced immune hemolytic
anemia
hereditary,
classification, 10–11*t*, 12*t*
definition of, 2
history and physical examination,
13–14
immune,
alloantibody induced, 188
characteristic features, 28*t*
classification, 26, 27*t*, 28, 177*t*
differential diagnosis, 185–229, *See
also* Differential diagnosis of
AIHA; Differential diagnosis
of drug-induced immune
hemolytic anemia.
incidence, 29*t*
mechanisms, *See* Immune hemolysis, mechanisms
intravascular hemolysis, 13, 20–22,
110–111, 187
mechanical, 2, 14*t*
peripheral blood film, 13, 14*t*, 15*f*,
16*f*, 17*f*, 18*f*, 19*f*
serum lactic dehydrogenase in, 8, 9*t*
Hemolytic transfusion reaction and
AIHA, differentiation, *See* Transfusion reaction and AIHA, differentiation
Hemosiderinuria, 3*f*, 21–22, 23, 55, 111
Heparin
complement, effect on, 102–103, 409,
414, 415*t*
therapy in warm-antibody AIHA,
408–414, 410–413*t*
Hepatomegaly, 34, 40, 49, 50*t*
Hereditary angioedema (HAE), 82, 83*t*,
84, 193
Hereditary hemolytic anemia, definition
of, 2
Herpes zoster infections, 406

History in diagnosis, medical
  cold agglutinin syndrome, 39–40
  drug-induced immune hemolytic
    anemia, 13, 289
  hemolytic anemia, 4, 13–14, 20
  warm antibody AIHA, 33
Hodgkin's disease, 41, 241, 407, 408

Idiopathic thrombocytopenic purpura,
  417
Ii blood group system, 250–254, *See also*
  Autoantibodies
  antigens, chemistry of, 254–256
  method of determining specificity,
    thermal range, and titer, 168–
    169, 174*t*
Immune adherence (IA), 67, 81
Immune complexes
  complement activation by, 89
  mechanism of drug-induced immune
    hemolytic anemia, 268–270,
    272–273, 294, 296
Immune hemolysis, mechanisms of,
    110–133, *See also* Drug-induced
    immune hemolytic anemia, im-
    munologic mechanisms; Immuno-
    globulins. .
  agglutination of red cells *in vivo*,
    132–133
  extravascular, 111–130
  factors effecting, 116*t*, 116–130
  intravascular, 110–111
  lymphocytes, possible role of, 130–
    131
  macrophage
    activity, variation in, 128–130
    development of, 112*t*
    /monocyte cytotoxicity, 131–132
    phagocytosis, 114*f*, 115*f*, 116,
      123–124
    receptors, 64, 81, 112–113*f*, 117,
      119–127
    rosettes, 113*f*, 123, 128–130
  quantitive factors, 118–121, 194–206,
    306
    complement sensitization of red
      cells, 125, 126, 127, 131–132,
      194, 199–200, 201–203*t*

IgG sensitization of red cells, 118–
    121, 131–132, 196–199
  methyldopa-induced   hemolytic
    anemia, 120–121, 204, 205*t*,
    206*t*
sensitization of red cells
  antibody subclass significance, 67,
    74, 87, 111, 119*t*, 120*t*, 142*t*,
    143
  complement components only,
    126–128
  IgA alone, 121, 348–349
  IgG and complement, 122–125
  IgG only, 117
  IgM alone, 121
  IgM and complement, 125–126
  protein type, 116–128
Immune hemolytic anemias, *See also* var-
    ious categories as Autoimmune
    hemolytic anemia; Drug-induced;
    Warm antibody AIHA; etc.
  characteristic features, 28*t*
  classification, 27*t*
  differential diagnosis, *See* Differential
    diagnosis
  incidence of various kinds, 29*t*
Immunoglobulins
  cold agglutinins, immunochemistry
    of, 47–48
  classes and subclasses of human,
    141–144, 142*t*, *See also* Comple-
    ment   activation;   Immune
    hemolysis, sensitization of red
    cells.
    differences between, 143–144
    IgA, 143
    IgD, 143–144
    IgE, 143–144
    IgG, 143
    IgM, 143
  destruction of sensitized red cells
    IgA alone, 121, 348–349
    IgG and complement, 122–125
    IgG only, 117
    IgM alone, 121
    IgM and complement, 125–126
  IgA autoantibodies, 48, 177*t*, 348–
    349
  IgG autoantibodies, 43–45, 48, 67,
    177*t*, 189, 204–206*t*, 211, 227*t*,

Immunoglobulins (cont.)
229, 234, 235t, 236, 241, 343, 346–348
IgM autoantibodies, 43–44, 47–49, 50t, 67, 177t, 211, 227t, 229, 346–348
monoclonal, 26, 47, 48, 49, 50t, 141
mixed IgG-IgM autoantibodies, 48
polyclonal, 26, 47
structure and function, 139, 140f, 141, 142t, 143–144
Immunologic mechanisms in drug-induced immune hemolytic anemia, 267–289
Immunization, development of AIHA following, 129
Immunosuppressive drugs
cold agglutinin syndrome, 422, 423t
warm-antibody AIHA, See Warm-antibody AIHA, management of, immunosuppressive drugs
Incidence
cold agglutinin syndrome, 29t, 38–39
drug-induced immune hemolytic anemia, 29t, 267
idiopathic and secondary warm antibody AIHA, 30–31t
paroxysmal cold hemoglobinuria, 29t, 54
warm antibody AIHA, 29t
Indirect antiglobulin test (IAT), See Antiglobulin test, indirect
Infancy, AIHA in, 349–351
Infection
as adverse effect of immunosuppressive drugs, 406
associated with hemolytic anemia, 13, 129
herpes zoster, 406
Mycoplasma pneumoniae, 41–43, 46–48, 141, 186, 227, 429–430
Pneumocystic carinii pneumonia, 406
Infectious mononucleosis, See Mononucleosis, infectious
Intravascular hemolysis, 20–22, 110–111
acute, in a child, 187
definition, 2–3
in cold agglutinin syndrome, 39
in paroxysmal cold hemoglobinuria, 39, 55–56, 187

in warm antibody AIHA, 33, 187
Irradiation, splenic, in warm-antibody AIHA, 416

Jaundice, 4, 14, 15, 33, 40

Kallikrein, 82
Kinins, 82

Laboratory diagnosis, See Serologic investigation; Differential diagnosis; Cold agglutinin syndrome; Warm antibody AIHA; etc.
Lactic dehydrogenase, serum, in hemolytic anemia, 5, 8, 9t
Landsteiner, Karl, 37, 267, See also Donath-Landsteiner
Leukocytosis, 34, 56
Leukopenia, 34, 56
Liver
hepatomegaly, 34, 40, 49, 50t
Laennec's cirrhosis, 86
Lupus erythematosus, systemic (SLE), 13, 14, 84, 191–192
management of AIHA in, 431
Lymphadenopathy, 34, 40, 49, 50t
Lymphocyte
cytotoxicity, 130–131
possible role in immune red cell destruction, 130–131
Lymphocytic leukemia, 13, 19, 27t, 32, 41
Lymphoma, 13, 27t, 41
Lymphoreticular malignant disease, 27t, 31, 34, 37, 41
management of AIHA in, 431, 433

Macroglobulinemia, Waldenström's, cold agglutinin syndrome compared with, 48–49, 50t
Macrophage, See Immune hemolysis, mechanisms
Management of AIHA, See also Cold agglutinin syndrome, management; Paroxysmal cold hemoglobinuria, management; Warm antibody AIHA, management
drug-induced autoimmune hemolytic anemia, 295–297

pregnancy, during, 327
secondary AIHA, 429–431, 433
  infectious mononucleosis, 46, 429–430
  lymphoreticular malignant disease, 431
  Mycoplasma pneumoniae infections, 42, 429
  Ovarian tumors, 430
  summary of therapeutic principles, 433
  systemic lupus erythematosus (SLE), 431
  ulcerative colitis, 430
  splenectomy, 344, 397–403, 426–427, 428*t*, 429
  summary of therapeutic principles, 431–433
  with negative direct antiglobulin test, 314–318
Marrow, bone, *See* Bone marrow
Maternal hazards of AIHA during pregnancy, 321
Matuhasi-Ogata phenomenon, 241, 246
Mechanisms of immune hemolysis, *See* Immune hemolysis, mechanisms; Drug-induced immune hemolytic anemia, immunologic mechanisms; Immunoglobulins
Membrane attack complex of complement, 68, 71*f*, 72*f*, 73*f*, 78
2-Mercaptoethanol, 216, 379
Methemalbumin, 3*f*, 20–21, 111
Methyldopa (Aldomet), *See* Drug-induced immune hemolytic anemia, methyldopa
Monocyte/macrophage, *See* Immune hemolysis, mechanisms of
Mononucleosis, infectious and hemolytic anemia, 13, 19, 42–46
  autoantibodies, 43–46
  clinical findings, 42*t*
  cold agglutinins, 45*t*
  course, 46
  direct antiglobulin test (DAT), 44*t*
  laboratory-findings, 43–46
  management, 46, 429–430
Mortality, *See* Prognosis
Mycoplasma pneumoniae infection
  cold agglutinin syndrome, 41–42, 43, 46–48, 141, 186, 227, 228
  management, 42, 429
  paroxysmal cold hemoglobinuria, 55, 186, 227

NANA (N-acetylneuraminic acid), 258
Neoplasia as adverse effect of immunosuppressive drugs, 408

Opsonization, 81, 123–124
Ovarian tumors, 31, 32*t*
  management of AIHA with, 430, 433
Oxyhemoglobin, 21

Pallor, 14, 40
Pancytopenia in warm antibody AIHA, 36
Paroxysmal cold hemoglobinuria (PCH), 2, 50–57
  associated diseases, 26, 55
  autoantibody, *See* Paroxysmal cold hemoglobinuria, Donath-Landsteiner antibody
  case reports, 225, 226*t*, 227, 341, 342*t*, 343*f*, 344*t*
  chronic idiopathic, 341–344
  comparison with cold agglutinin syndrome, 227–229
  diagnosis of, 223–229
    direct antiglobulin test, 189–190*t*
    distinctive clinical features, 185, 186, 187
    essential diagnosis tests, 223–224
    serum screening tests, 167*t*, 342*t*
  Donath-Landsteiner antibody, 50–57, 189–190
    compared with antibody in cold agglutinin syndrome, 227*t*, 228–229
    immunoglobulin class, 177*t*, 189–190
    specificity, 225*f*, 260
      determination of, 175–178
    thermal amplitude, 55, 341–342, 343*f*, 344*t*
  Donath-Landsteiner test
    method, 175–178
    original report, 51–53*f*
    value in diagnosis, 223–225*f*, 226
  hematologic findings, 56

Paroxysmal cold hemoglobinuria (cont.)
hemolysis, acute intravascular, 187
historical concepts, 50, 51–53f, 54
idiopathic and secondary types, 55
incidence, 54
management, 343–344, 427, 429, 432–433
Mycoplasma pneumoniae infection, 55, 186, 227
physical findings, 55
prognosis, 57
race, sex, and age, 55
serum screening tests, 167t
serologic findings in, 226t, 342t, 343f, 344t
summary of therapeutic principles, 432–433
symptoms, 55–56
transfusion in, 382, 387
warm blood use, 387
Paroxysmal nocturnal hemoglobinuria (PNH), 2, 79, 126
Penicillamine in cold agglutinin syndrome, 425–426
Penicillin, immune hemolytic anemia induced by, 273–283, See also Drug-induced immune hemolytic anemia, penicillin
Pentamidine isethionate, 406
Phagocytosis, 56, 113, 114f, 115f, 122–125, 126–130, 132
Physical examination in diagnosis
cold agglutinin syndrome, 39–40
hemolytic anemia, 4, 13–14
warm antibody AIHA, 33–34
Plasma exchange
cold agglutinin syndrome, 424–425
warm-antibody AIHA, 418–420
Plasmin, 82
Platelets, See also Thrombocytopenia; Thrombocytosis
in AIHA, 35–36
in hemolytic anemia, 19
thrombocytosis following splenectomy, 402–403
vinblastine-laden in management of warm-antibody AIHA, 416–417
Pneumococcus (Streptococcus pneumoniae), 401–402
Pneumocystis carinii pneumonia, 406

Pneumonia
association of AIHA with, 186, See also Mycoplasma pneumoniae
Pneumocystis carinii, 406
Pr blood groups, chemistry of, 258–259
Pregnancy, AIHA during, 321–327
case reports, 322–324
cause, 326–327
complement-fixing antiglobulin consumption test, 326t
fetal hazards, 321–322
management, 327
maternal hazards, 321
relapsing, 324–326
Prognosis
cold agglutinin syndrome, 41
drug-induced immune hemolytic anemia, 295–297
infectious mononucleosis with AIHA, 46
paroxysmal cold hemoglobinuria, 57
warm antibody AIHA, 37
Properdin (P), 64, 73, 74, 75t, 78, 79f
Purpura, in hemolytic anemias, 14, 17f, See also Platelets; Thrombocytopenic purpuria

Radiolabelled red cell studies, See Red cells, radiolabelled studies; Chromium (^{51}Cr)
Raynaud's phenomenon, 13, 38, 39, 56
Receptors, See also Complement, receptors
complement, 99–100
macrophage, 64, 81, 112–113f, 117, 119–127
Red cell(s)
creatine, 9
destruction of, See Hemolysis; Immune hemolysis, mechanisms of
enzyme deficiencies, 10–12t
fragmented, 14t, 15, 17f, 19, 56
irregularly contracted, 14t, 17f, 56
measurement of antibodies bound to, 307–308, See also Autoimmune hemolytic anemia with negative direct antiglobulin test
morphology in hemolytic anemias, 5, 7, 13, 14t, 15–19f

radiolabelled studies
  in diagnosis of hemolytic anemia, 9
  in selecting patients for splenec-
    tomy, 399–400
sensitization, *See* Immune hemolysis,
  mechanisms; Immunoglobulins;
  Complement
separating donor's and recipient's,
  330
spherocytes, 8, 14*t*, 15*f*, 16*f*, 19, 23,
  40, 43, 56
survival measurements, 5, 9, *See also*
  Carbon monoxide; Chromium;
  Red cells, radiolabelled studies
washed, use of, in AIHA, 388
Rosettes, 113*f*, 123, 128–130
Reticulocyte
  "corrected" count, 5
  count, 5–6
  production index, 6
  in cold agglutinin syndrome, 40
  in diagnosis of hemolytic anemia, 5,
    6
  in warm-antibody AIHA, 36–37
  reticulocytopenia, 6, 36–37, 40
  reticulocytosis, causes of, 6
Reticuloendothelial neoplasia, 41
Rh, *See also* Autoantibodies
  autoantibody specificity, 232–237,
    246–250, 286–287
    determination of, 172–174, 209
    significance in transfusion, 372–
      375, 377–378*t*
  typing in AIHA, 159–161, 365–366
Rodgers blood group, 100

Schistocytes, 14*t*
Scores, agglutination, 154*t*
Secondary AIHA,
  associated diseases, cold agglutinin
    syndrome, 41–47
  associated diseases, paroxysmal cold
    hemoglobinuria, 55
  associated diseases, warm antibody
    AIHA, 31, 32*t*
  classification, 27*t*
  definition, 26, 31–32
  incidence, warm antibody AIHA,
    30–31*t*

infectious mononucleosis, 42*t*, 43, 44*t*,
  45*t*, 46
lymphocytic leukemia, 13, 19, 27*t*, 32,
  41
lymphoma, 13, 27*t*, 41
Mycoplasma pneumoniae infections,
  41–42, *See also Mycoplasma
  pneumoniae*
reticuloendothelial neoplasia, 27*t*, 31,
  34, 37, 41
systemic lupus erythematosus, 13, 14,
  84, 191–192
  management, 429–431, 433, *See also*
    Management of AIHA
Waldenström's macroglobulinemia,
  48–50*t*
Serologic investigation of AIHA, 148–
  181, 188–229
See also Differential diagnosis; Cold
  agglutinin syndrome, diagnosis;
  Paroxysmal cold hemoglobinuria,
  diagnosis; Warm antibody AIHA,
  diagnosis.
antiglobulin test, *See* Antiglobulin test
characterization of antibodies in
  serum and eluate, 164–178,
  206–229
collection of blood, 159
eluate, methods of preparation,
  170–172
hemolysins,
  significance of, 211–213, 214–215,
    223
  titration of, 169–170
serum screening tests, 164–166
  cold agglutinin syndrome, 167*t*,
    217*t*
  methyldopa induced AIHA, 291*t*
  paroxysmal cold hemoglobinuria,
    167*t*
  warm antibody AIHA, 166*t*, 209*t*
specificity testing, 168, 170–178,
  179–180, *See also* Specificity of
  Autoantibodies
summary of findings, 177*t*
thermal range determination, 168–
  169, *See also* Cold agglutinins,
  thermal range; Paroxysmal cold
  hemoglobinuria, thermal amplitude

Serologic investigation of AIHA (cont.)
  typing of red cells
    antigens other than ABO and Rh,
      160–161*t*
    ABO typing, 159–160, 365–366
    Rh typing, 159–160, 161
Sickle cell anemia
  complement-fixing antibody con-
    sumption test, in, 318–321
  sickle cells, 15, 17*f*
Specificity of autoantibodies, 232–260,
    See also Autoantibodies
  antibodies other than anti-I, -i or -Pr
    associated with cold agglutinin
    syndrome, 259
  changes during AIHA, 250
  cold agglutinin syndrome, 174*t*, 175,
    250–259, 251*t*, 252*t*, 253*t*, 254*t*
  determination of, 170–178
  differentiation of AIHA and delayed
    hemolytic transfusion reaction,
    329–330
  early observations, 232, 233*t*, 234
  Ii blood group "system," 250–256
  method for determining Ii specificity,
    168–169
  mimicking alloantibodies, 246–247*t*,
    248*t*
  not associated with Rh, 237–246
  observations during last decade,
    234–237
  paroxysmal cold hemoglobinuria,
    175–176, 260
  Pr blood groups, 257–258
  relationship to complement sensitiza-
    tion, 234–235, 237
  warm antibody AIHA, 172, 173*t*, 174,
    232–250
Spherocytes, 8, 14*t*, 15*f*, 16*f*, 19, 23, 40,
    43, 56
Splenectomy, 344, 397–403, 426–427,
    428*t*, 429
  adverse effects, 400–403
  history of, 13
  cold agglutinin syndrome, 426–427,
    428*t*
  mortality in hematologic disorders,
    401*t*
  paroxysmal cold hemoglobinuria,
    344, 427, 429

warm-antibody AIHA. *See* Warm-
    antibody AIHA, management of,
    splenectomy
Splenic irradiation in warm-antibody
    AIHA, 416
Splenomegaly, 4–5, 14, 33, 40, 41, 49,
    55
Sterilization as adverse effect of im-
    munosuppressive drugs, 407
Steroids, *See* Corticosteroid therapy
Streptococcus pneumoniae (pneumo-
    coccus), 401–402
Symptoms, *See* History in diagnosis,
    medical
Syphilis, 26, 55, 344
Systemic lupus erythematosus (SLE), 13,
    14, 84, 191–192
  management of AIHA in, 431

T-cells in the development of AIHA,
    335–337
Teratogenic side reactions as adverse ef-
    fect of immunosuppressive drugs,
    407–408
Thalassemia, 10–11*t*, 12*t*, 15, 320
Therapy, *See* Management
Thermal range, *See* Serologic investiga-
    tion of AIHA, thermal range
Thrombocytes, *See* Platelets; Throm-
    bocytopenia; Thrombocytosis
Thrombocytopenia, 19, 35–36, 272
  mechanism of drug induced, 267–270
  quinidine and quinine, 269
Thrombocytopenic purpura
  idiopathic, 417
  thrombotic, 14*t*, 17*f*, 19
Thrombocytosis,
  splenectomy and, 402–403
  warm antibody AIHA, 35
Thymectomy in warm-antibody AIHA,
    414, 416, 416*t*
Transfusion, development of AIHA fol-
    lowing, 331–337
  autoantibodies developed following
    transfusion of foreign red cells,
    331–333
  autoantibodies produced by transfu-
    sion of alloantibodies, 335
  autoantibodies produced in recipient

by immune apparatus of donor,
333–335
genetic factors and T-cell responsiveness, 335–337
summary, 337
Transfusion in AIHA, 358–368
assessing need for, 362–364
acuteness of onset and rapidity of
progression, 362
appropriate use of blood, 362–364
chronic stable anemia, 363
fulminant hemolytic anemia, 363–
364
progressively severe anemia, 363
compatibility testing *in vivo*, 382–384
indications, general principles, 359–
362
optimal blood volume to be tranfused,
384–386
risks, 358, 364–365
selection of donor blood, 365–382
cold agglutinin syndrome, 376–382
cold autoabsorption, 377–379,
381*t*
compatibility test at 37°C in
saline, 376–377, 380*f*
other methods, 379–382
paroxysmal cold hemoglobinuria,
382
warm antibody AIHA, 365–376,
377–378*t*
ABO and Rh typing, 159–161*t*,
365–366
alloantibodies, detection of,
366–372
comparison of direct and indirect antiglobulin tests, 366
differential absorption technique, 371–372
dilution technique, 370, 371*t*
testing against red cell panel,
366, 367*t*
warm autoabsorption tech-
nique, 366, 368*t*, 369*f*, 370
autoantibody specificity,
autoantibodies without demonstrated specificity, 375
significance of Rh "relative
specificity," 372, 373*t*, 374–
375, 376, 377–378*t*

summary of methods, 378–379*t*
typing of red cells, 159–161*t*, 365–366
without serum autoantibody, 375–376
warm blood, use of, 387
washed red cells, use of, 388
Transfusion reaction and AIHA, differentiation, 327–331
additional approaches, 330–331
antibody specificity, 329–330
diagnostic aids, 328
direct and indirect antiglobulin test,
compared, 329
direct antiglobulin test (DAT), "mixed
field," 328–329
separating donor and recipient's red
cells, 330
Typing of red cells in AIHA, *See*
Serologic investigation of AIHA.

Ulcerative colitis, management of AIHA
in, 430
Urticaria, cold, 13, 56

Vinblastine-laden platelets in warm-
antibody AIHA, 416–417
Virus
cytomegalovirus, 45
Epstein, Barr (E-B), 45, 99–100
neutralization, complement, 81

Waldenström's macroglobulinemia, cold
agglutinin syndrome compared
with, 48–49, 50*t*
Warm-antibody AIHA, 29–37
age distribution, 30
associated diseases, 31–32*t*
autoagglutination, 186
autoantibody specificity, 232–250, *See
also* Autoantibody
alloantibodies mimicked by, 246–
250
changes, in 250
determination, 172–174
early observations, 232–234
observations during the last decade,
234–237
other than Rh, 237–246
significance in blood transfusion,
See Transfusion in AIHA

Warm-antibody AIHA (cont.)
blood picture, 16*f*, 34–36
blood transfusion, *See* Transfusion in AIHA
characterization of antibodies in serum and eluate, 164–166*t*, 169–174, 177*t*, 206–213
cold agglutinins, associated with abnormal, 344–346, 347*t*, 348
complement metabolism in, 85
diagnosis of, 208–213
essential diagnostic tests, 208–211
further important serologic tests, 211, 213
serum screening tests in, 166*t*, 209*t*
typical serologic findings, 212–213*t*
direct antiglobulin test (DAT) results, 190*t*, 193*t*, 205*t*, 206*t*
negative, 312–313*t*, *See also* AIHA with negative direct antiglobulin test
positive only with anti-IgA antisera, 348–349
disorders frequently associated with, 32*t*
hemolysins in, 211–213
incidence, 29*t*
incidence of idiopathic and secondary types, 30–31*t*
management of, 392–420
antilymphocyte globulin, 416
corticosteroid therapy, 392–397
antibody avidity, altered, 396
antibody-coated red cells, altered clearance of, 396–397
antibody synthesis, reduction of, 395–396
antiglobulin test titrations, 204*t*, 395–396*t*
initial management, 392–393
mechanisms of response, 394–397
remission maintenance, 393–394
response rate, 392–393*t*
heparin therapy, 408–414, 415*t*
effect on serum complement, 102–103, 409, 414, 415*t*
summary of literature, 410–413*t*
immunosuppressive drugs, 403–408

adverse effects, 405–408
effectiveness, 403–404
indications, 404–405
infection, 406
neoplasia, 408
regimens, 404–405
sterilization, 407
teratogenic side reactions, 407–408
plasma exchange, 418–420
secondary AIHA, 430–431, 433
splenectomy, 397–403, 397*t*
adverse effects, 400–403
bacteremia, fulminant, 401–402
clinical response, 397*t*, 398
mechanisms of response, 398–399
morbidity, 400
mortality, 400, 401*t*
radiolabelled red-cell studies in selection of patients, 399–400
surgical morbidity and mortality, 400–401
thrombocytosis, 402–403
splenic irradiation, 416
summary of therapeutic principles, 431–432
thymectomy, 414, 416*t*
vinblastine-laden platelets, 416–417
methyldopa-induced, serum screening tests, 291*t*
physical signs, 33–34
presenting symptoms, 33
prognosis and survival, 37
race distribution, 30
red blood cell morphology, 16*f*
reticulocytes, 36–37
secondary, 30, 31*t*, 32*t*, *See also* Secondary AIHA
serologic findings in a typical patient, 212–213*t*
serum screening tests, 166*t*, 209*t*
sex distribution, 30
transfusion in, *See* Transfusion in AIHA
Warm autoabsorption technique, 366, 368*t*, 369*f*, 370

Zeta potential theory, 144–145, 147